SECOND EDITION

FAMILY NURSE PRACTITIONER
Certification Review Guide

Editors

Susan M. DeNisco, DNP, APRN, FNP-BC, FAANP

Professor Emerita, Family Nurse Practitioner and Doctor of Nursing Practice Hybrid Program
Sacred Heart University
Fairfield, Connecticut
Family Nurse Practitioner, Southwest Community Health Center
Bridgeport, Connecticut

Nancy L. Dennert, MS, MSN, FNP-BC, CDCES, BC-ADM

Former Clinical Assistant Professor
Sacred Heart University
Fairfield, Connecticut

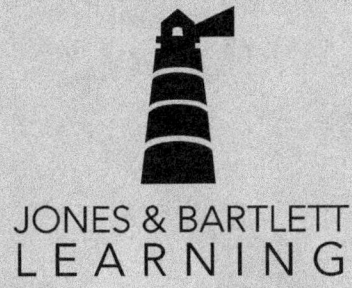

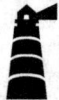

World Headquarters
Jones & Bartlett Learning
25 Mall Road
Burlington, MA 01803
978-443-5000
info@jblearning.com
www.jblearning.com

Jones & Bartlett Learning books and products are available through most bookstores and online booksellers. To contact Jones & Bartlett Learning directly, call 800-832-0034, fax 978-443-8000, or visit our website, www.jblearning.com.

Substantial discounts on bulk quantities of Jones & Bartlett Learning publications are available to corporations, professional associations, and other qualified organizations. For details and specific discount information, contact the special sales department at Jones & Bartlett Learning via the above contact information or send an email to specialsales@jblearning.com.

Copyright © 2027 by Jones & Bartlett Learning, LLC, an Ascend Learning Company

All rights reserved. Unauthorized use is prohibited. Materials protected by this copyright may not be reproduced adapted, transmitted, stored in a retrieval system, or utilized in whole or part, in any form or any means, electronic, mechanical, photocopied, recorded, or otherwise, without prior written permission from the copyright owner, except as permitted by U.S.A. copyright law.

The content, statements, views, and opinions herein are the sole expression of the respective authors and not that of Jones & Bartlett Learning, LLC. Reference herein to any specific commercial product, process, or service by trade name, trademark, manufacturer, or otherwise does not constitute or imply its endorsement or recommendation by Jones & Bartlett Learning, LLC and such reference shall not be used for advertising or product endorsement purposes. All trademarks displayed are the trademarks of the parties noted herein. *Family Nurse Practitioner Certification Review Guide, Second Edition* is an independent publication and has not been authorized, sponsored, or otherwise approved by the owners of the trademarks or service marks referenced in this product.

There may be images in this book that feature models; these models do not necessarily endorse, represent, or participate in the activities represented in the images. Any screenshots in this product are for educational and instructive purposes only. Any individuals and scenarios featured in the case studies throughout this product may be real or fictitious but are used for instructional purposes only.

The authors, editors, and publisher have made every effort to provide accurate information. However, they are not responsible for errors, omissions, or for any outcomes related to the use of the contents of this book and take no responsibility for the use of the products and procedures described. Treatments and side effects described in this book may not be applicable to all people; likewise, some people may require a dose or experience a side effect that is not described herein. Drugs and medical devices are discussed that may have limited availability controlled by the Food and Drug Administration (FDA) for use only in a research study or clinical trial. Research, clinical practice, and government regulations often change the accepted standard in this field. When consideration is being given to use of any drug in the clinical setting, the healthcare provider or reader is responsible for determining FDA status of the drug, reading the package insert, and reviewing prescribing information for the most up-to-date recommendations on dose, precautions, and contraindications, and determining the appropriate usage for the product. This is especially important in the case of drugs that are new or seldom used.

IT IS THE SOLE AND EXCLUSIVE RESPONSIBILITY OF THE HEALTHCARE PROVIDER OR READER TO ENSURE THAT ANY USE OF THIS INFORMATION AND RELATED CONTENT IS COMPLIANT WITH LAWS, REGULATIONS, POLICIES, AND APPLICABLE STANDARDS. THE AUTHORS, EDITORS, AND PUBLISHER DISCLAIM ANY OBLIGATION OR LIABILITY ARISING OUT OF THE HEALTHCARE PROVIDER OR READER'S FAILURE TO SO COMPLY.

The manufacturer's authorised representative in the EU for product safety is Mare Nostrum Group B.V., Mauritskade 21D, 1091 GC Amsterdam, The Netherlands.
Email: gpsr@mare-nostrum.co.uk

30582-1

Production Credits
Vice President, Innovative Learning and Assessment Solutions: Ada Woo
Senior Director, Content Production and Delivery: Christine Emerton
Director, Product: Melissa Kleeman Moy
Manager, Content Development: Bill Lawrensen
Product Manager: Sophie Fleck Teague
Senior Outsourcing Specialist: Carol Brewer Guerrero
Content Coordinator: Samantha Gillespie
Content Management: S4Carlisle Publishing Services
Manager, Intellectual Properties and Content Production: Kristen Rogers
Content Production Manager: Belinda Thresher
Content Production Manager, Navigate: Michael Lepera
Senior Intellectual Property Specialist: Angela Dooley
Senior Product Marketing Manager: Lindsay White
Director, Product Fulfillment: Aaron McKinzie
Purchasing Manager: Wendy Kilborn
Composition: S4Carlisle Publishing Services
Project Management: S4Carlisle Publishing Services
Text and Cover Design: S4Carlisle Publishing Services
Intellectual Property Specialist: Faith Brosnan
Intellectual Property Specialist: Lisa Passmore
Cover Image (Title Page, Part Opener, Chapter Opener):
    © s_maria/Shutterstock
Printing and Binding: Sheridan Michigan

Library of Congress Cataloging-in-Publication Data
Names: DeNisco, Susan M. editor | Dennert, Nancy L. editor
Title: Family nurse practitioner certification review guide / [edited by]
    Susan M. DeNisco, Nancy L. Dennert.
Other titles: Family nurse practitioner certification review (Stewart)
Description: Second edition. | Burlington, MA : Jones & Bartlett Learning,
    [2027] | Preceded by Family nurse practitioner certification review /
    edited by Julie G. Stewart and Nancy L. Dennert. First edition. [2017] |
    Includes bibliographical references and index.
Identifiers: LCCN 2025005815 | ISBN 9781284018950 paperback
Subjects: MESH: Family Nursing | Examination Questions | BISAC: MEDICAL /
    Nursing / Gerontology
Classification: LCC RT120.F34 F353 2027 | NLM WY 18.2 | DDC
    610.73076--dc23/eng/20250715
LC record available at https://lccn.loc.gov/2025005815

6048

Printed in the United States of America
29 28 27 26 25   10 9 8 7 6 5 4 3 2 1

Brief Contents

Introduction	xvii
Learning and Teaching Resources	xix
Contributors and Reviewers	xx

PART I Professional Issues and Achieving Success on Certification — 1

- **CHAPTER 1** Achieving Success on the National Certification Exam 3
- **CHAPTER 2** Test-Taking Strategies for Nurse Practitioner Students 9
- **CHAPTER 3** Professional and Legal-Ethical Issues 17

PART II Health Promotion and Pharmacology Review — 35

- **CHAPTER 4** Health Promotion and Disease Prevention 37
- **CHAPTER 5** Pharmacology 53

PART III Body Systems Review and Common Primary Care Issue — 79

- **CHAPTER 6** Head, Eyes, Ears, Nose, and Throat 81
- **CHAPTER 7** Respiratory System 117
- **CHAPTER 8** Cardiovascular Disorders in Primary Care 143
- **CHAPTER 9** Gastrointestinal System 165
- **CHAPTER 10** Musculoskeletal Review 191
- **CHAPTER 11** Nervous System 217

CHAPTER 12	**Endocrine System**	235
CHAPTER 13	**Hematology**	255
CHAPTER 14	**Renal and Genitourinary Urinary System**	273
CHAPTER 15	**Sexually Transmitted Infections**	287
CHAPTER 16	**Integumentary**	307

PART IV Reproductive Health, Pediatric and Adolescent Health, Gerontology, and Mental Health Review — 323

CHAPTER 17	**Women's Health and Female Reproductive System**	325
CHAPTER 18	**Men's Health**	365
CHAPTER 19	**Pediatrics**	381
CHAPTER 20	**Geriatrics**	403
CHAPTER 21	**Mental Health in Primary Care**	425

PART V Practice Exams — 461

Index 465

Contents

Introduction xvii
Learning and Teaching Resources.......... xix
Contributors and Reviewers................ xx

PART I Professional Issues and Achieving Success on Certification 1

CHAPTER 1 Achieving Success on the National Certification Exam 3
Susan M. DeNisco, DNP, APRN, FNP-BC, FAANP

Why Certification? 3
Which Examination? 3
Which Exam Should I Choose? 4
What Is the Difference Between the Two Exams?................................... 4
Making an Informed Decision 4
Family Nurse Practitioner Foci for Creating a Plan of Study.................... 4
Certification Exam Content Focuses on Common Diagnoses in Primary Care by Body System 4
Life Span Considerations for Exam Questions..................................... 5
Types of Exam Questions to Anticipate........ 6
    Lower-Level Thinking 6
    Higher-Level Thinking........................ 6
Exam Preparation and Taking the Exam 6
General Strategies............................ 7
Top Reasons for Failing the Exam 7
Retaking a Certification Exam................ 7
Recertification Requirements 7

CHAPTER 2 Test-Taking Strategies for Nurse Practitioner Students................. 9
Sherylyn M. Watson, PhD, MSN, RN, CNE

Where to Begin................................ 10
Best Practices for Test-Taking 11
    Know Your Test-Taking Type 11
Day Before the Examination 13
Day of the Exam 13
Day After the Exam 13

CHAPTER 3 Professional and Legal-Ethical Issues 17
Cynthia K. O'Sullivan, PhD, APRN, FNP-BC
Susan M. DeNisco, DNP, APRN, FNP-BC, FAANP

Nurse Practitioner Education 17
Nurse Practitioner Competencies 17
Licensure, Accreditation, Certification, and Education (LACE).................... 18
Scope of Practice............................. 18
Advanced Practice State Licensure 19
Drug Enforcement Agency Licensure........ 20
National Provider Identification 20
Reimbursement............................... 20
    Billing and Coding 20
Health Policy 21
    Affordable Care Act 21
    The Future of Nursing Report 21
Social Determinants of Health 22
Nurse Practitioner Policy-Related Competencies............................... 22
    American Association of Nurse Practitioners: Position on Terms such as Mid-Level Provider and Physician Extender 22

Responsibility to Patients/Care Priorities 23
    Ethical Terms. 23
    Minors. 24
The NP Role in End-of-Life Care 24
    Advanced Directives 24
Malpractice. 25
    Malpractice Insurance 25
    Malpractice Lawsuit Terminology 25
Nursing Research and Evidence-Based
    Practice. 25
    Nursing Research Terminology 25
Evidence-Based Practice 26
The PICOT Question. 26
Levels of Evidence. 26

PART II Health Promotion and Pharmacology Review 35

CHAPTER 4 Health Promotion and Disease Prevention............ 37

Susan M. DeNisco, DNP, APRN, FNP-BC, FAANP
Nancy L. Dennert, MS, MSN, FNP-BC, CDCES, BC-ADM

Disease Prevention 37
Health Promotion. 37
Health Promotion and Prevention
    Applied to Specific Diseases 38
    Levels of Prevention 38
Guide to Clinical Preventative Services:
    The USPSTF Recommendations 39
    Criteria for Screening. 39
    Characteristics of the Disease Targeted
        for Screening 39
    Characteristics of the Screening Test 39
Cancer Screening 40
Select United States Preventative Task Force
    Common Screening Recommendations
    for Adults in the Primary Care Setting 40
Immunizations Schedules and Exam Tips 42
Health Promotion and Disease Prevention
    Case Study. 42
    History of Present Illness. 42
    Pertinent Past Medical History. 42
    Pertinent Review of Systems 44
    Pertinent Physical Exam Findings 44
    Current Medications 44

    Treatment Recommendations 44
    Considerations for the NP Related to Health
        Promotion in This Case Study 44

CHAPTER 5 Pharmacology 53

Chrystyne Olivieri, DNP, FNP-BC, CDCES
Nancy L. Dennert, MS, MSN, FNP-BC, CDCES, BC-ADM

Introduction 53
Prescribing for Nurse Practitioners. 53
    Pharmacotherapeutics 54
    Pharmacokinetics 55
    Pharmacodynamics 56
Levels of Evidence 57
    Adverse Events 58
Commonly Used Medications in
    Primary Care. 62
    Hypertension. 62
    Anticoagulants. 65
    Hyperlipidemia 65
    Antimicrobials. 66

PART III Body Systems Review and Common Primary Care Issue........... 79

CHAPTER 6 Head, Eyes, Ears, Nose, and Throat 81

Marguerite Lawrence, DNP, FNP-BC, PHCNS-BC, MA
Susan M. DeNisco, DNP, APRN, FNP-BC, FAANP

General Approach to Ear, Nose, and Throat
    Health Problems. 81
Disorders of Balance. 81
    The Peripheral Vestibular System. 81
Defining Vertigo 82
Vertigo Pathophysiology 82
Benign Paroxysmal Positional Vertigo
    (BPPV) 82
    Definition 82
    Incidence/Prevalence. 83
    Etiology. 83
    Risk Factors. 83
    Historical Data. 83
    Physical Assessment 83
    Diagnostic Studies. 83
    Management 83
    Patient Education 84

Contents

- Indications for Referral 84
- Expected Course 84
- Other Peripheral Vertigo Etiologies 84
  - Vestibular Neuritis/Labyrinthitis 84
  - Ménière's Disease 84
- Hearing Loss 85
  - Conductive Hearing Loss 85
  - Historical Data 85
  - Physical Assessment 85
  - Differential Diagnosis 85
  - Diagnostic Studies 85
  - Complications 85
  - Management 85
  - Patient Education/Prevention 86
  - Indications for Referral 86
  - Expected Course 86
- Sensorineural Hearing Loss 86
  - Description 86
  - Etiology/Risk Factors 86
- Classification of Hearing Loss 86
  - Historical Data 86
  - Physical Assessment 87
  - Differential Diagnosis 87
  - Diagnostic Studies 87
  - Complications 87
  - Management 87
  - Patient Education/Prevention 87
  - Indications for Referral 87
  - Expected Course 87
- Acute Otitis Media/Otitis Media With Effusion 88
  - Definition 88
  - Incidence 88
  - Etiology 88
  - Risk Factors 88
  - Historical Data 89
  - Physical Assessment 89
  - Differential Diagnosis 89
  - Diagnostic Studies 90
  - Complications 90
  - Management 90
  - Acute Otitis Externa 90
- Epistaxis 92
  - Definition 92
  - Incidence 92
  - Etiology/Risk Factors 92
  - Physical Assessment 92
  - Differential Diagnosis 93
  - Diagnostic Studies 93
  - Complications 93
  - Management 93
- Patient Education 93
- Indications for Referral 93
- Follow-Up 93
- Acute Rhinosinusitis 93
  - Definition 93
  - Incidence 93
  - Etiology 93
  - Classifications of Rhinosinusitis 93
  - History of Present Illness 94
  - Clinical Presentation/Physical Assessment Findings 94
  - Differential Diagnosis 94
  - Diagnostic Studies 94
  - Complications 94
  - Management 94
  - Antibiotic Therapy 94
  - Patient Education 95
  - Indications for Referral 95
  - Follow-Up 95
- Allergic Rhinitis 95
  - Definition 95
  - Incidence 95
  - Risk Factors 95
  - Clinical Presentation 95
  - Physical Assessment Findings 95
  - Differential Diagnosis 96
  - Diagnostic Studies 96
  - Management 96
  - Indications for Referral 96
  - Follow-Up 96
- Aphthous Stomatitis (Canker Sores) 96
  - Etiology 96
  - Treatment 96
- Oral Candidiasis 96
  - Incidence/Etiology 96
  - Risk Factors 97
  - Clinical Presentation and Assessment Findings 97
  - Differential Diagnosis 97
  - Diagnostic Studies 97
  - Complications 97
  - Management 97
  - Prevention/Patient Education 97
  - Indications for Referral 98
  - Follow-Up 98
- Pharyngitis 98
  - Incidence 98
  - Etiology 98
  - Risk Factors 98
  - Bacterial Pharyngitis 98
  - Viral Pharyngitis 99
  - Differential Diagnosis 99

Diagnostic Studies............................ 99	Tuberculosis 130
Complications 99	Risk Factors for TB 130
Management 99	Tuberculosis Tests 131
Patient Education 100	Other Diagnostic Tests...................... 131
Indications for Referral 100	Treatment of Latent TB Infection and Active
Follow-Up................................. 100	TB Disease 132
Eyes... 100	Adverse Drug Considerations 132
Useful Tips and Terms When Performing	Cough 133
an Exam With an Ophthalmoscope 100	Management of Cough 133
Eye Exam 100	Acute Bronchitis 133
Common Eye Terminology 100	COVID-19 Infection 134
Common Eye Conditions 101	Respiratory Syncytial Virus 134
Age-Related Eye Diseases.................. 103	
Corneal Abrasion........................... 104	

CHAPTER 8 Cardiovascular Disorders in Primary Care 143

Heather Ferrillo, PhD, APRN, FNP-BC, CNE

Chalazion 104	
Differential Diagnosis 104	
Clinical Management....................... 104	Murmurs....................................... 143
Hordeolum (Stye) 105	Valvular Heart Disease 143
Dangerous Eye Conditions 105	Common Valvular Disorders.................... 144
	Aortic Stenosis............................. 144

CHAPTER 7 Respiratory System ...117

Susan M. DeNisco, DNP, APRN, FNP-BC, FAANP

	Mitral Regurgitation........................ 144
	Aortic Regurgitation 145
Review Basic Anatomy of the	Mitral Valve Prolapse....................... 145
Respiratory System......................... 117	Subacute Bacterial Endocarditis Prophylaxis 145
Gas Exchange 117	Heart Failure 145
Assessment of the Respiratory System 117	Treatment 146
History and Physical Examination........... 117	Follow-Up................................. 146
Diseases of the Respiratory System........ 117	Hypertension (2017 ACC/AHA Guidelines) ... 148
Asthma 117	Overview.................................. 148
Asthma Triggers............................ 119	Clinical Presentation 148
Asthma Physical Examination Findings........ 119	Goals for Treatment........................ 149
Diagnostic Testing.......................... 121	Treatment Recommendations 149
Asthma Treatment Goals 122	Follow-Up................................. 149
Treatment 122	Cholesterol Management 149
Assessment of Control...................... 124	Goals..................................... 149
Chronic Obstructive Pulmonary Disease 124	Assessment 149
Emphysema................................ 125	Treatment Guidelines (Stone et al., 2014) 150
Chronic Bronchitis 125	Follow-Up................................. 150
COPD Pharmacologic Treatment Plan 126	Evaluation of Chest Pain 152
COPD Education and Follow-Up 126	Pathogenesis 152
Pneumonia 126	Clinical Presentation 152
Pediatric Considerations 127	Coronary Artery Disease 153
Community-Acquired Pneumonia........... 127	Treatment 153
Diagnosing CAP 127	Atrial Fibrillation 154
CURB-65 Score for Pneumonia Severity	Etiology................................... 154
in Adult Patients 128	Clinical Presentation 154
Atypical Pneumoniae....................... 128	Diagnostics in New/Suspected AF 155
Viral Pneumonia and Pediatrics.............. 129	Treatment (Based on 2023 AHA/ACC/HRS
Prevention Guidelines 129	Guidelines for the Management of AF)...... 155
Lung Cancer 129	Prevention................................. 155
Screening Recommendations for Lung Cancer... 129	

Peripheral Vascular Disease—Atherosclerosis (PAD) 156
    Clinical Presentation 156
    Clinical Management...................... 156
Peripheral Vascular Disease—Venous Disorders............................ 156
    Varicose Veins 157

CHAPTER 9 Gastrointestinal System 165

Sylvie Rosenbloom, DNP, APRN, FNP-BC, CDCES

Nancy L. Dennert, MS, MSN, FNP-BC, CDCES, BC-ADM

Physical Examination.................... 165
Abdominal Content 165
Special Maneuvers..................... 166
Liver Enzymes 166
Cholecystitis.......................... 166
    Differential Diagnoses 167
    Treatment 167
    Patient Education 167
    Referral 167
Constipation......................... 167
    Differential Diagnosis 167
    Triggers............................. 167
    Management 167
    Complications......................... 167
    Treatment and Follow-Up 167
Gastroesophageal Reflux Disease 168
    Triggers............................. 168
    Clinical Manifestations 168
    Diagnostic Studies....................... 168
    Treatment 168
    Follow-Up and Education 169
    Complications......................... 169
Peptic Ulcer Disease, Gastric Ulcer, and Duodenal Ulcer Disease 169
    Clinical Manifestations 169
    Differential Diagnosis 169
    Diagnostic Studies....................... 169
    Treatment of *H. Pylori* 169
    Follow-Up and Education 170
Gastroenteritis........................ 170
    Etiology............................. 170
    Clinical Manifestations 170
    Differential Diagnosis 170
    Treatment and Follow-Up 170
Appendicitis 170
    Clinical Manifestations 171
    Diagnostic Testing....................... 171
    Differential Diagnosis 171
    Treatment and Follow-Up 171
Diverticulitis 171
    Clinical Manifestations 171
    Differential Diagnosis 171
    Outpatient Treatment and Follow-Up 171
    Guidelines for Outpatient Management........ 172
Colon Cancer 172
    Clinical Manifestations 172
    Differential Diagnosis 172
    Treatment and Follow-Up 172
Hepatitis 173
    History 173
    Clinical Manifestations 173
    Liver Function Tests 173
    Hepatitis A 173
    Hepatitis B........................... 173
    Hepatitis C 174
Nonalcoholic Steatohepatitis 174
    Risk Factors........................... 175
    Treatment and Follow-Up 175
Irritable Bowel Syndrome 175
    Clinical Manifestations 175
    Differential Diagnosis 175
    Management 175
    Patient Education 176
Acute Pancreatitis 176
    Clinical Manifestations 176
    Diagnostics 176
    Complications......................... 176
Clostridium Difficile Colitis 176
    Presenting Symptoms 176
    Clinical Presentation 176
    Diagnostics 176
    Treatment 176
Inflammatory Bowel Disease 177
    Risk Factors........................... 177
    Etiology............................. 177
    Clinical Manifestations 177
    Differential Diagnosis 177
    Diagnostic Testing....................... 177
    Treatment and Follow-Up 177
    Complications......................... 177
Crohn's Disease...................... 178
    Risk Factors........................... 178
    Etiology............................. 178
    Clinical Manifestations 178
    Differential Diagnosis 178
    Diagnostic Testing....................... 178

Contents

Treatment and Follow-Up 178
Complications. 178
Hemorrhoids 178
Clinical Manifestations 179
Differential Diagnosis 179
Diagnostic Testing. 179
Treatment 179
Patient Education 179
Anal Fissures 179
Clinical Manifestations 179
Differential Diagnosis 179
Treatment 179
Follow-Up. 180

CHAPTER 10 Musculoskeletal Review 191

Nancy L. Dennert, MS, MSN, FNP-BC, CDCES, BC-ADM

Foot and Ankle 191
Morton (Interdigital) Neuroma 191
Plantar Fasciitis. 192
Bilateral Heel Pain 192
Achilles Tendinopathy. 192
Charcot Neuropathic Osteoarthropathy
 (Charcot Foot) 192
Ankle Sprain Lateral/Medial 193
Compartment Syndrome. 193
Ottawa Ankle Rules. 193
Ottawa Foot/Ankle Rules. 194
Knee 194
Osgood Schlatter Disease. 194
Meniscus Tear 194
Patellar Fracture 194
Knee Osteoarthritis 195
Medial Tibial Stress Syndrome (MTSS)
 (Shin Splints). 195
Ottawa Knee Rules 195
Hip. 195
Legg-Calve-Perthes Disease 195
Intertrochanteric Fracture 196
Hip Dislocation. 196
Hip Impingement 196
Shoulder. 196
Labrum Tear 196
Acromioclavicular (AC) Joint Injury/
 Dislocation. 197
Rotator Cuff Injury 197
Adhesive Capsulitis (Frozen Shoulder) 197
Wrist and Hand 198
Distal Radius Fracture 198
Ligament Strain. 198
Carpal Tunnel Syndrome. 198
Deformities: Boutonniere Deformity, Mallet
 Finger, and Swan Neck Deformity 198
Trigger Finger (Stenosing Tenosynovitis) 199
Dupuytren's Contracture 199
Degenerative Joint Disease (DJD) 200
Osteomyelitis. 200
Ganglion Cyst 200
Raynaud's Phenomenon. 200
Pelvis and Sacrum. 201
Ankylosing Spondylitis 201
Lumbar Spine. 201
Degenerative Lumbar Disc Disease 201
Radiculopathy 201
Abdominal Aortic Aneurysm 202
Spinal Stenosis 202
Spondylolisthesis. 202
Cauda Equina Syndrome. 203
Clinical Lumbar Instability 203
Thoracic Spine 203
Rib Dysfunction: Costochondritis 203
Thoracic Disc Herniation. 203
Stress Fracture Ribs. 204
Shingles. 204
Scoliosis 204
Cervical Spine 205
Torticollis 205
Acute Cervical Disc Herniation/Radiculopathy . . . 205
Spinal Stenosis 205
Rheumatoid Arthritis. 206
Concussion. 206
Elbow 206
Lateral Epicondylalgia (Tennis Elbow). 206

CHAPTER 11 Nervous System 217

Nancy L. Dennert, MS, MSN, FNP-BC, CDCES, BC-ADM

Overview of Neurological Assessment. 217
Romberg Test. 217
Cranial Nerves 217
Brain Tumors 219
Stroke and Transient Ischemic
 Attack. 219
Sensitive Test for Stroke. 219
Transient Ischemic Attack 219
Stroke 219
Anticoagulants. 220
Concussion. 220
Clinical Management. 221

Meningitis... 221
   Etiology... 221
   Risk... 221
   Clinical Presentation... 221
   Prevention... 221
   Management... 221
   Treatment... 221
Progressive Degenerative Disorders... 222
   Dementia... 222
   Treatment of Moderate AD... 223
Acute Neurological Disorders... 223
   Delirium... 223
   Headache... 224
   Temporal Arteritis... 226
   Prompt Treatment... 226
Trigeminal Neuralgia... 226
   Treatment... 226
Bell's Palsy... 226
Motor Neuron Disorders... 226
   Multiple Sclerosis... 226
   Parkinson's Disease... 227
(Benign) Essential Tremor... 227
   Clinical Diagnosis... 227
   Treatment... 227

CHAPTER 12 Endocrine System ... 235
Nancy L. Dennert, MS, MSN, FNP-BC, CDCES, BC-ADM

Diabetes Mellitus... 235
   Etiology... 235
   Diabetes Facts... 235
   Diagnosis of Prediabetes... 235
   Clinical Presentation/Assessment Findings... 235
   Screening Recommendations for Both Prediabetes and Diabetes... 235
   Differential Diagnosis... 236
   Clinical Management (A, B, C)... 236
   Complication of Diabetes... 237
   Pharmacologic Agents for Type 2 Diabetes Mellitus... 238
   Hypoglycemia... 239
   Brief Case Study and Considerations for the Clinician... 240
Thyroid Disorders... 240
   Etiology... 240
   Clinical Presentation... 241
   Clinical Management... 241
   Hypothyroidism... 241
   Secondary Hypothyroidism... 242
   Hyperthyroidism... 242

Disorders of the Parathyroid Glands... 243
   Etiology... 243
   Clinical Presentation... 243
   Clinical Management... 243
Hypoparathyroidism... 244
   Etiology... 244
   Signs and Symptoms... 244
   Clinical Management... 244
   Pharmacologic Management... 244
   Nonpharmacologic Management... 244
Adrenal Disorders... 244
   Addison's Disease: Chronic Adrenal Insufficiency... 244
   Cushing Syndrome... 245

CHAPTER 13 Hematology... 255
Susan M. DeNisco, DNP, APRN, FNP-BC, FAANP

Laboratory Testing... 255
   Anemia... 255
   Laboratory Testing and Normal Ranges... 255
   Mean Corpuscular Volume Is Key!... 255
   Mean Corpuscular Hemoglobin Concentration... 256
   Peripheral Smear... 256
   Red Cell Distribution Width... 256
   Reticulocyte Count... 256
   Microcytic Anemia... 257
   Macrocytic Anemia... 258
   Normocytic Anemias... 259
Abnormalities of the White Blood Cells... 261
   Leukocytosis (Elevated WBC Count)... 261
   Leukopenia (Decreased WBC Count)... 262
   Neutrophils... 262
   Eosinophils... 262
   Basophils... 263
   Lymphocytes... 263
   Monocytes... 263
Abnormalities of Platelets... 263
   Thrombocytosis... 263
   Thrombocytopenia... 264

CHAPTER 14 Renal and Genitourinary Urinary System ... 273
Susan M. DeNisco, DNP, APRN, FNP-BC, FAANP

Review of Normal Kidneys Findings... 273
   Renal Function... 273
   Laboratory Findings... 273
Urinary Tract Infections... 273
   Acute Cystitis... 273
   Acute Pyelonephritis... 274

Risk Factors for Urinary Tract Infection....... 274
Diagnosis................................. 274
Differential Diagnosis 274
Treatment 274
Uncomplicated UTI........................ 274
Complicated UTI.......................... 275
Follow-Up................................ 275
Prevention............................... 275
Nephrolithiasis/Urolithiasis 275
Incidence and Risk Factors 275
Evaluation............................... 275
Differential Diagnosis 276
Treatment 276
Follow-Up and Prevention 276
Kidney Disease............................. 276
Classification........................... 276
Acute Kidney Injury 276
Chronic Kidney Disease................... 277
Urinary Incontinence 278
Epidemiology............................. 278
Risk Factors for UI 278
Evaluation............................... 279
Treatment 279
Follow-Up and Prevention 280

CHAPTER 15 Sexually Transmitted Infections 287

Shirley Kuan, MSN, APRN, AGNP-C

Chlamydial Infections 287
Etiology................................. 287
Clinical Presentation/Assessment Findings 287
Clinical Management...................... 287
Evaluation and Follow-Up................. 288
Gonococcal Infection 289
Etiology................................. 289
Clinical Presentation/Assessment Findings 289
Clinical Management...................... 289
Evaluation and Follow-Up................. 289
Trichomoniasis............................ 289
Etiology................................. 289
Clinical Presentation/Assessment Findings 290
Clinical Management...................... 290
Evaluation and Follow-Up................. 290
Herpes Simplex Virus (HSV-1 and HSV-2) ... 290
Etiology................................. 290
Clinical Presentation/Assessment Findings 290
Clinical Management...................... 291
Evaluation and Follow-Up................. 292
Human Papillomavirus 292
Etiology................................. 292

Clinical Presentation/Assessment Findings 292
Clinical Management...................... 292
Evaluation and Follow-Up................. 293
Syphilis................................... 293
Etiology................................. 293
Clinical Presentation/Assessment Findings 293
Clinical Management...................... 294
Evaluation and Follow-Up................. 295
Human Immunodeficiency Virus........... 295
Etiology................................. 295
Clinical Presentation/Assessment Findings 296
Clinical Management...................... 296
Evaluation and Follow-Up................. 297
Preexposure Prophylaxis 298
Postexposure Prophylaxis: Healthcare Workers... 298

CHAPTER 16 Integumentary 307

Nancy L. Dennert, MS, MSN, FNP-BC, CDCES, BC-ADM

History................................... 307
Terminology 307
Actinic Keratosis 308
Seborrheic Keratoses 308
Skin Cancers 308
Basal Cell............................... 308
Squamous Cell Carcinoma................. 309
Melanoma 309
Acne Vulgaris 309
Rosacea 310
Xerosis (Dry Skin)........................ 310
Cellulitis 310
Cysts 310
Folliculitis................................ 310
Dermatitis................................ 310
Atopic Dermatitis: Eczema................ 311
Seborrheic Dermatitis 311
Psoriasis 311
Pityriasis Rosea 312
Erythema Migrans 312
Characteristics of EM Rash 312
Warts: Verruca Vulgaris................... 313
Skin Tags................................ 313
Impetigo 313
Dermatophytosis 313
Tineas: Capitis, Corporis, Cruris, Pedis 313
Onychomycosis........................... 313
Tinea Versicolor......................... 313
Herpes Zoster (Shingles)................. 313

Vitiligo 314
　Three General Patterns of Depigmentation 314
Alopecia Areata 314
Urticaria (Hives) 314

PART IV Reproductive Health, Pediatric and Adolescent Health, Gerontology, and Mental Health Review 323

CHAPTER 17 Women's Health and Female Reproductive System 325
Sarah E. DeNisco, MSN, APRN, FNP-BC

Normal Findings 325
　Anatomy 325
Menstrual Cycle 326
　Phases 326
Routine Health Maintenance and Laboratory Procedures 327
　Mammogram 327
　Cervical Cytology ("Pap Test") 327
　Human Papillomavirus DNA Test 327
　The Bethesda System 327
　Colposcopy 328
Contraception 328
　Combined Hormonal Contraceptives 328
　Prescribing a Contraceptive 330
　Progesterone-Only Contraceptives 330
　Other Contraceptive Methods 331
Disease Review 332
　Fibrocystic Changes of the Breast 332
　Breast Cancer 333
　Galactorrhea 334
　Atrophic Vaginitis 334
　Lichen Sclerosus 335
　Vulvovaginal Candidiasis 336
　Bacterial Vaginosis 337
　Dysmenorrhea 338
　Amenorrhea 338
　Abnormal Uterine Bleeding 339
　Endometriosis 339
　Uterine Fibroids 340
　Polycystic Ovarian Syndrome 341
　Ovarian Cancer 341
　Menopause 342
　Osteoporosis 343

Pregnancy and Prenatal Care 344
　Obstetric History 344
　Signs of Pregnancy 344
　Prenatal Care 345
　Laboratory Testing/Expected Changes During Pregnancy 345
　Clinical Method for Dating Pregnancy ... 346
　Physiologic Changes During Pregnancy ... 346
　Drugs and Vaccines During Pregnancy ... 348
　Patient Education 348
Disease Review During Pregnancy 349
　Oligohydramnios vs. Polyhydramnios ... 349
　RH-Incompatibility 349
　Gestational Diabetes 350
　Preeclampsia (Pregnancy-Induced Hypertension) ... 351
　Urinary Tract Infection 352
　Uncomplicated Chlamydia Infection (Cervicitis, Urethritis) 352
　Abortion 353
Postpartum 354
　Uterine Involution 354
　Breastfeeding 354
　Postpartum Contraception 355
　Postpartum Depression 356

CHAPTER 18 Men's Health 365
Nancy L. Dennert, MS, MSN, FNP-BC, CDCES, BC-ADM

Anatomy of the Male Reproductive System .. 365
Urethritis 365
Dysuria 365
Prostate Disorders 365
　Prostatitis 366
　Benign Prostatic Hypertrophy 366
　Prostate Cancer 367
Disorders of the Scrotum/Testes 368
　Epididymitis 368
　Testicular Cancer 368
　Testicular Torsion 369
　Cryptorchidism 369
　Varicocele 369
　Hydrocele 369
　Spermatocele 370
Erectile Dysfunction 371
　Physiology of Erections 371
　Types of Erectile Dysfunction 371
　Medications for ED 371
Inguinal Hernias 372
　Diagnosis 372

CHAPTER 19 Pediatrics 381
Christopher Kennedy, DNP, FNP-BC, PMHNP-BC, CNE, APRN

Growth and Development 381
- Bright Futures/American Academy of Pediatrics Periodicity Schedule 381
- Physical Growth and Development 381
- Gross Motor Development 382
- Fine Motor Development 382
- Language Development 382
- Social and Emotional Development 382
- Social and Developmental Theorists 383
- Erikson's Stages of Development for Children ... 383
- Body Mass Index 383
- Immunizations 383
- Vital Signs 383
- Heart Rate 383
- Respiratory Rate 383
- Blood Pressure 383
- History 384
- Physical Exam 384
- Primitive/Primary Reflexes 385
- Important Terms 385
- Breastfeeding 385
- Anticipatory Guidance Topics 385

Congenital Heart Defects 385
- Acyanotic Defects—Left to Right Shunts 385
- Cyanotic Defects—Right to Left Shunts 386
- Obstructive Lesions 386
- Primary Care for Congenital Heart Defects 387
- Chest Pain in Children 387
- Pediatric Hypertension 388
- Treatment and Referral 388

Respiratory Conditions in the Pediatric Population 388
- Asthma 388
- Description of Asthma Levels 388
- Croup 389
- Bronchiolitis 389
- Respiratory Syncytial Virus 389
- Acute Bronchitis 390
- Pneumonia 390

Sports Physical/Preparticipation Physical Evaluation 391
- Sudden Death 391
- Causes 391
- History 391
- Physical 391

Pediatric Infectious Diseases Not Covered Elsewhere in Review Book 391
- Parvovirus B19 (Erythema Infectiosum, Fifth Disease) 391
- Measles (Rubeola) 392
- Impetigo 392
- Coxsackievirus (Hand, Foot, and Mouth Disease) 392

Child Maltreatment and Abuse 392
- Physical Abuse 393
- Emotional Abuse 393
- Sexual Abuse 393
- The Role of the Family Nurse Practitioner 393
- Differential Diagnoses 394

Additional Clinical Resources 394

CHAPTER 20 Geriatrics 403
Nancy L. Dennert, MS, MSN, FNP-BC, CDCES, BC-ADM

Considerations for the Older Patient 403

Geriatric Fast Facts: A Profile of Older Adults 403
- Oldest Old Is the Fastest Growing Segment of Older Adults 403
- Multiple Chronic Care Needs 403
- Marital Status 403
- Leading Causes of Death 403
- Income 403

Goals of Geriatric Care 405

Health Maintenance 406
- Communication Techniques 406
- Creating the Relationship 406
- Eliciting the Health History 406
- Geriatric Health Maintenance 406
- Welcome to Medicare Preventive Visit 406
- The Seven Components 406
- Medicare Annual Wellness Visit 407
- Role of FNP 407

Medicare Basics 407

Prescribing Practices in Older Adults 408
- Pharmacokinetics 408
- Pharmacodynamics 408

Adverse Drug Events in the Older Patient ... 409
- Commonly Prescribed Drug Categories for Older Adults Resulting in Potential Side Effects 409
- Associated Problems With Medication Use 410

Assessment Tools to Reduce Medication Risks in Older Adults 410
- STOPP/START Tool 410
- Psychiatric 410

Neurocognitive Disorders 411

Classify: Mild, Moderate, or Severe 411
Neurocognitive Domains 411
Treatment Interventions 411
Treatment Options 411
N-methyl-D-aspartate (NMDA)
  Antagonist 411
Combination Pill 411

Depression 412
Symptoms of Depression 412
Risk Factors for Depression 412
Criteria for Diagnosis of Depression
  in Long-Term Care 412
Workup for Depression in Long-Term Care 412
Pharmacological Treatment 413

Chronic Disease and Older Adults 413
Stats at a Glance 413
Hypertension 414
Diabetes 414
Osteoarthritis 414
Treatment Modalities Include Pharmacologic
  and Nonpharmacologic Therapies 414
Osteoporosis 415
FRAX WHO Fracture Risk Assessment Tool 415
Falls 415
Risk Factors 415

Atypical Presentation of Disease
  in Older Adults 415
Urinary Tract Infections 415
Acute Abdomen 416
Pneumonia 416
Other Atypical Presentations 416

End-of-Life Care/Advance Care Planning . . . 416

CHAPTER 21 Mental Health in Primary Care 425

Melissa Scollan-Koliopoulos, EdD, DNP, FNP, PMHNP, CDCES

Mood Disorders 425
Etiology 425

Major Depressive Disorder and Persistent
  Depressive Disorder Facts 425
Diagnosis of Depression 425
Clinical Presentation/Assessment Findings 425
History of Present Illness 426
Physical Assessment Findings 426
Screening Recommendations 426
Differential Diagnosis 426
Clinical Management Laboratory and Diagnostic
  Studies 426
Pharmacologic 427
Nonpharmacologic 427
Evaluation and Follow-Up 430
Prescribing SSRIs, SNRIs, and Norepinephrine-
  Dopamine Reuptake Inhibitors (NDRIs) 430

Serotonin Syndrome 430

Postpartum Depression 430
Clinical Presentation and Assessment
  Findings 430
History of Present Illness 430
Physical Assessment Findings 430
Differential Diagnosis 431
Clinical Management 431
Nonpharmacologic 431
Patient Education 431
Pharmacologic 431
Indication for Referral 431
Evaluation and Follow-Up 431

Bipolar Disorder 431

Cyclothymic Disorder 432

Disruptive Mood Dysregulation
  Disorder 432
Clinical Presentation/Assessment Findings . . . 432
Physical Assessment Findings 432
Clinical Management 432
Pharmacologic 433
Indication for Referral 433
Evaluation and Follow-Up 433

Attention-Deficit/Hyperactivity Disorder 434
Etiology 434
ADHD Facts 434
Diagnosis of ADHD 434
Clinical Presentation/Assessment Findings 434
Screening Recommendations for ADHD 434
Differential Diagnosis 435
Clinical Management 435
Evaluation and Follow-Up 435

Psychotic Disorders 435
Etiology 435
Diagnosis of Psychosis 436
Schizophrenia 436
Other Disorders With Psychotic Features 436
Differential Diagnosis 436
Clinical Management 436

Neuroleptic Malignant Syndrome 440
Treatment and Follow-Up 440

Anxiety Disorders 440
Etiology 440
Screening 440
Assessment 440
Type of Anxiety Disorders 441

Contents

    Differential Diagnosis 442
    Clinical Management. 442
Posttraumatic Stress Disorder 442
    Etiology. 442
    PTSD Facts 442
    Diagnosis of PTSD. 442
    Screening for PTSD 442
    Differential Diagnosis 443
    Clinical Management. 443
Pediatrics: Posttraumatic Stress Disorder
   in Children. 443
    Treatment and Follow-Up 443
Substance Abuse 443
    Etiology. 443
    Screening. 444
    Opioid Use Disorder 444
    Diagnosis. 444
    Clinical Management. 444
    Alcohol Misuse Therapy 445
    Evaluation and Follow-Up. 445
Suicide Risk and Prevention 445
    Etiology. 445
    Suicide Facts 445
    Warning Signs. 446
    Patient Education and Safety Measures 446
    Evaluation and Follow-Up. 446
Neurodevelopmental Disorders 446
    Etiology. 446
    Tourette Syndrome 446
    Tourette Syndrome Facts. 446
    Diagnosis of Tourette Syndrome 446
    Screening. 446
    Differential Diagnosis 446
    Clinical Management. 446
    Evaluation and Follow-Up. 446
    Autistic Spectrum Condition 447
    Autism Facts 447
    Diagnosis of Autism. 447
    Clinical Presentation/Assessment Findings 447
    Assessment 447
    Differential Diagnosis 447
    Clinical Management. 447
    Evaluation and Follow-Up. 447
Domestic Violence and Intimate
   Partner Violence 449
    Etiology. 449
Personality Disorders 449
    Etiology. 449
    Diagnosis. 449
    Clinical Management. 450
    Evaluation and Follow-Up. 450

PART V Practice Exams 461

Navigate TestPrep 461
    Practice Tests. 462
    AANPCB and ANCC Predictor Exams 463
    Complete Assessment Tests 463

Index **465**

Introduction

It is so exciting to offer the second edition of this certification review book to family nurse practitioner (FNP) students in preparation for their board examination and subsequent certification as an FNP. Since the first edition, there have been many changes in how we educate the future generation of nurse practitioners (NPs) to influence healthcare outcomes. This book has undergone significant revision to reflect current evidence-based practice guidelines, COVID-19 clinical guidelines, changes in pharmacologic agents, and insight into changes in the professional and legislative landscape. This new text is aligned with the blueprints for the newest American Academy of Nurse Practitioner Certification Board (AANPCB) and the American Nurses Credentialing Center (ANCC) certification exams.

Also, of importance, on April 6, 2021, the American Association of the Colleges of Nursing (AACN) endorsed *The Essentials: Core Competencies for Professional Nursing Education*, which delineates competency expectations for graduates of baccalaureate and graduate nursing programs. This historic and courageous move is transforming how nurses are educated for advanced roles. These "new" essentials are built on the strong foundation of nursing as a discipline, the foundation of a liberal education, and principles of competency-based education. The content areas of this revision align with the AACN competency-based essentials and the National Organization for Nurse Practitioner Faculties (NONPF) core competencies. **Table I-1** compares the Essentials of Professional Nursing Education, Domains, Advanced Practice Competencies, NONPF, ANCC/AANPCB Certification Domains, and book content.

We have incorporated questions with topics from the ANCC and AANPCB content outlines. Each chapter was written by a colleague who works and/or specializes in that specific area. Therefore, we can provide the most current evidence-based information for primary care practice. As FNP educators, we take pride in our students' scores on their certification exams consistently exceeding the national percentage pass rate year after year. We are confident you will pass your certification exam if you apply yourself by studying each chapter's course materials and answering the practice questions that follow. Additionally, you will find that Chapters 1 and 2 contain vital information regarding test-taking strategies.

We are grateful to all the contributing authors, as well as our family and colleagues, for their support in writing this book.

Table I-1 Comparison of Essentials of Professional Nursing Education, Domains, Advanced Practice Competencies, NONPF, ANCC/AANP Certification Domains and Book Content

Domains/Competencies AACN	NONPF	ANCC/AANP	Book Chapter(s)
Domain I: Knowledge for Nursing Practice	Scientific Foundation Competencies Independent Practice Competencies	Assessment (ANCC, AANP) Diagnosis (ANCC, AANP) Clinical Management (ANCC, AANP) Evaluation (AANP)	Chapters 3–21
Domain II: Person-Centered Care	Independent Practice Competencies	Assessment (ANCC, AANP) Diagnosis (ANCC, ANNP) Clinical Management (ANCC, AANP) Evaluation (AANP)	Chapters 4–21
Domain III: Population Health	Policy Competencies Health Delivery System Competencies	Assessment (ANCC, AANP) Diagnosis (ANCC, ANNP) Clinical Management (ANCC, AANP) Evaluation (AANP)	Chapters 3, 5–21
Domain IV: Scholarship for Nursing Practice	Scientific Foundation Competencies	Assessment (ANCC, AANP) Diagnosis (ANCC, ANNP) Clinical Management (ANCC, AANP) Evaluation (AANP)	Chapters 4–21
Domain V: Quality and Safety Descriptor	Quality Competencies Ethics Competencies	Evaluation (AANP)	Chapter 3
Domain VI: Interprofessional Partnerships	Quality Competencies Ethics Competencies	Clinical Management (ANCC, AANP) Evaluation (AANP)	Chapters 3–21
Domain VII: Systems-Based Practice	Practice Inquiry Competencies	Assessment (ANCC, AANP) Diagnosis (ANCC, ANNP) Clinical Management (ANCC, AANP) Evaluation (AANP)	Chapters 4–21
Domain VIII: Information and Healthcare Technologies	Technology and Information Literacy Competencies	Evaluation (AANP) Professional Role (ANCC)	Chapters 1, 2, and 3
Domain IX: Professionalism	Independent Practice Competencies	Professional Role (ANCC)	Chapters 1, 2, and 3
Domain X: Personal, Professional, and Leadership Development	Leadership Competencies Independent Practice Competencies	Professional Role (ANCC) Procedures (AANP) Evaluation (AANP)	Chapters 1, 2, and 3

Learning and Teaching Resources

Student Resources

Each new purchase of the print textbook includes Navigate curriculum access code with Navigate TestPrep and Navigate eBook. See Part V of this text for a detailed description of TestPrep.

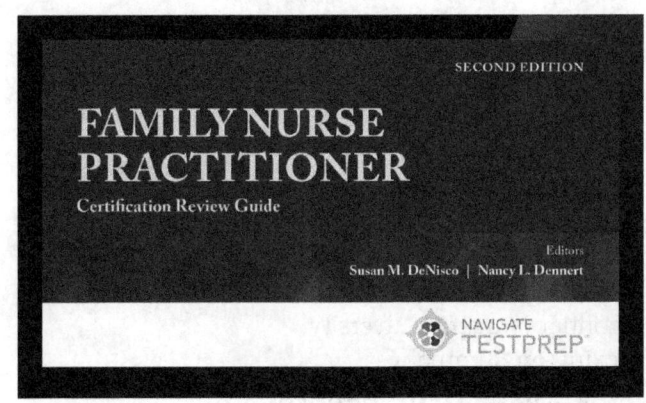

We Value Your Feedback

Do you love this text? Spot an error you'd like to report? Follow this QR code to give us your observations and suggestions for improvement.

Contributors and Reviewers

Contributors

Sarah E. DeNisco, MSN, APRN, FNP-BC
Family Nurse Practitioner
Southwest Community Health Center
Bridgeport, Connecticut

Heather Ferrillo, PhD, APRN, FNP-BC, CNE
Chair–Undergraduate Programs
Sacred Heart University
Fairfield, Connecticut

Christopher Kennedy, DNP, FNP-BC, PMHNP-BC, CNE, APRN
Family Nurse Practitioner
Psychiatric/Mental Health Nurse Practitioner
Frontier Nursing University
Lexington, Kentucky

Shirley Kuan, MSN, APRN, AGNP-C
Nurse Practitioner
South Central Family Health Center
Los Angeles, California

Marguerite Lawrence, DNP, FNP-BC, PHCNS-BC, MA
Clinical Associate Professor
The Susan L. Davis, RN, and Richard J. Henley College of Nursing
Sacred Heart University
Fairfield, Connecticut

Chrystyne Olivieri, DNP, FNP-BC, CDCES
FNP-DNP Hybrid Program
Sacred Heart University
Fairfield, Connecticut

Cynthia K. O'Sullivan, PhD, APRN, FNP-BC
Associate Dean of Academic Affairs & Global Nursing
The Susan L. Davis, RN, and Richard J. Henley College of Nursing
Sacred Heart University
Fairfield, Connecticut

Sylvie Rosenbloom, DNP, APRN, FNP-BC, CDCES
Associate Professor Nursing and Program Director
Family Nurse Practitioner Program
School of Nursing
Mercy University
Dobbs Ferry, New York

Melissa Scollan-Koliopoulos, EdD, DNP, FNP, PMHNP, CDCES
Associate Professor/Assistant Director
Sacred Heart University
Fairfield, Connecticut

Sherylyn M. Watson, PhD, MSN, RN, CNE
Director of Nursing
Associate Dean
NewYork-Presbyterian Iona School of Health Sciences
Associate Professor
Department of Nursing
Iona University
New Rochelle, New York

Reviewers

David Campbell-O'Dell, DNP, APRN, FNP-BC, FAANP
Professor
Keiser University
Fort Lauderdale, Florida

Kim Kuebler, DNP, APRN, ANP-BC, FAAN
Nell Hodgson Woodruff School of Nursing
Emory University
Atlanta, Georgia

Jennifer L. Mabry, PhD, MSN, FNP-BC
Associate Professor
Tennessee Tech University
Cookeville, Tennessee

Tanya Tanzillo, DNP, APRN-BC
Clinical Assistant Professor
Northern Illinois University
DeKalb, Illinois

Sheryl Winn, DNP, APRN, ANP-BC
Georgia College and State University
Milledgeville, Georgia

PART I

Professional Issues and Achieving Success on Certification

CHAPTER 1	Achieving Success on the National Certification Exam	3
CHAPTER 2	Test-Taking Strategies for Nurse Practitioner Students	9
CHAPTER 3	Professional and Legal-Ethical Issues	17

CHAPTER 1

Achieving Success on the National Certification Exam

Susan M. DeNisco, DNP, APRN, FNP-BC, FAANP

Congratulations on your success as you complete the rigors of your graduate degree and prepare to take one of the two national board certification examinations: American Nurses Credentialing Center Examination (ANCC) Family Nurse Practitioner (FNP) Board Certification Examination or the American Academy of Nurse Practitioner Certification Board (AANPCB) Family Nurse Practitioner Certification Examination. This chapter will focus on deciding which examination to take, the test blueprint and what to study, the examination process, and recertification requirements. Chapter 2 will focus on specific test-taking strategies.

Why Certification?

Certification is the process by which a nongovernmental agency recognizes an individual who has demonstrated the broad knowledge and application of the predetermined standards of care for entry-level nurse practitioner practice in a primary care setting. These examinations are competency based and population focused. If you purchased this review book, it is because you are preparing for the population foci "family." As a candidate, you are preparing to be tested on your ability to deliver primary care services across the lifespan, including prenatal and postpartum care, pediatric primary care, and care of the older adult. You are not preparing for specialties like acute care or emergency medicine.

The purpose of the examination is to test your broad knowledge, clinical reasoning, and decision-making in the following areas:

- assessment
- diagnosis
- planning
- implementation
- evaluation

See **Table 1-1** for distribution of questions per domain.

Which Examination?

You have two choices for becoming board certified as a family nurse practitioner.

The American Nurses Credentialing Center Examination (ANCC) Family Nurse Practitioner Board Certification Examination.

https://www.nursingworld.org/our-certifications/family-nurse-practitioner/

OR

The American Academy of Nurse Practitioner Certification Board (AANPCB) Family Nurse Practitioner Certification Examination

https://www.aanpcert.org/certs/fnp

Each organization has certified nurse practitioners since the 1990s and is widely respected. I encourage you to explore each website where you can read their

Table 1-1 AANP FNP and AANC FNP Exam Domains for 2024

Domain	ANCC	AANP
Assessment	19%	32%
Diagnosis	18%	26.5%
Planning	19%	26.5%
Implementation	29%	Not listed
Evaluation	15%	15%

Table 1-2 ANCC vs AANP Certification Examinations

American Nurses Credentialing Center (ANCC)	American Academy of Nurse Practitioners (AANP)
175 questions in 3.5 hours	150 questions in 3 hours
150 questions are scored	135 questions are scored
25 pretest questions (not scored)	15 pretest questions (not scored)
60 seconds allotted per question	60 seconds allotted per question
Computer tutorial prior to exam	Computer tutorial prior to exam
Free practice exam online	Complimentary test questions at end-of-test blueprint
Pass rate 2023 (85%)	Pass rate 2022 (74%)
Prometric test center	Prometric test center
Recertify every 5 years	Recertify every 5 years

certification requirements, test blueprints, costs, accommodations, retest requirements, and additional review materials.

Which Exam Should I Choose?

Both examinations are equally recognized as national specialty certifying bodies and acceptable to all government entities such as state boards of nursing, Medicare, Medicaid, the Veterans Administration, and private health insurance plans. If you are more clinically oriented, take the AANP exam; if you are considering a future career in research or academia, take the ANCC exam. However, both exams test the same clinical competencies.

There is no best test.

What Is the Difference Between the Two Exams?

The key difference between the examinations is that the ANCC exams tend to have more nonclinical questions, such as questions on ethics, regulatory guidelines, and scope of practice. Students also cited that the questions on the AANP examination seem shorter and ask only clinical questions. Each organization typically releases a new exam version every 3 years.

Making an Informed Decision

I encourage you to download the respective test blueprints, which include the content domains, body system focus, patient age, and applied FNP knowledge areas, to decide which examination is right for you.

Table 1-2 compares certification exam details.

Family Nurse Practitioner Foci for Creating a Plan of Study

Table 1-3 shows the broad areas that structure a primary care encounter: assessment, diagnosis, planning (implementation), and evaluation. Under these domains, you learned the competencies and skills associated with those terms related to common primary care diagnoses. When organizing your studying, consider reviewing the following per domain.

Certification Exam Content Focuses on Common Diagnoses in Primary Care by Body System

As you work through this review book, it is organized by body system representing the most common primary care diagnoses you may be tested on. **Table 1-4** represents some of the most commonly tested content areas in the systems chapters.

Table 1-3 Major Exam Domains With Study Tips

Assessment	Diagnosis	Planning and Implementation	Evaluation
History Taking: - PMH - HPI - ROS - OLD CARTS (symptom analysis) - Normal physical exam findings per age and ethnicity - Abnormal physical exam findings per common primary care diagnoses - Screening - Risk assessment - Lifestyle behaviors - Cognition and behavior	Differential Diagnosis: - Narrow down to most likely in the primary care setting given history and physical exam findings - Pathophysiology normal and abnormal - Diagnostic test selection and interpretation	Pharmacology: - Medication safety for most prescribed medication - Life span questions related to pharmacokinetics - Major adverse drug effects per drug class - Recognize both generic and brand names - Nonpharmacologic treatment modalities - Therapeutic communications - Culturally responsive care - Standards of care and evidence based guidelines - Scope of practice and regulatory guidelines - Referrals	- Assess patient response to treatment - Understand when to adjust treatment plan - Evaluation of lab results - Legal and ethical principles

Table 1-4 Body Systems

Cardiovascular - Hypertension - Hyperlipidemia - Coronary atherosclerosis - Hematopoietic anemia	Musculoskeletal - Back Pain - Osteoarthritis - Joint Pain - Fibromyalgia
Endocrine - Diabetes - Hypothyroidism - Obesity	Neurological - Headaches - Dementia - Tremors
Gastrointestinal - GERD Integumentary - Dermatitis - Eczema fungus	Psychiatric - Depression - Anxiety Reproductive - STIs - Contraception - Amenorrhea - Abnormal Vaginal Bleeding
Genitourinary and Renal - Urinary Tract Infection - BPH - Kidney Stones	
Head, Eyes, Ears, Nose, and Throat - Acute Pharyngitis - Acute Sinusitis - Allergic Rhinitis - Conjunctivitis - Visual Refractive Errors	

Table 1-5 AANP/ANCC FNP 2024

AANP Age Group	# of Questions	ANCC Age Group	# of Questions
Newborn	3	Infant	Not Specified
Infant	4	Preschool	Not Specified
Toddler	5	School Aged	Not Specified
Child	6	Adolescent	Not Specified
Adolescent	12	Young Adult	Not Specified
Young Adult	30	Adult	Not Specified
Middle Adult	35	Older Adult	Not Specified
Older Adult	40	Frail Elderly	Not Specified

Life Span Considerations for Exam Questions

New in 2024, AANP has changed the breakdown of questions by age group. Prenatal has been removed as an age category, and prenatal health knowledge will be assessed in questions about adolescent, young adult, and middle adult populations rather than as stand-alone test items. The new blueprint also introduced a toddler category and removed the elder adult category. **Table 1-5** represents the age groups you will be tested on and the anticipated percentage of exam questions.

The AANP question breakdown, shown above, is a reminder that success on the FNP exam requires pediatric knowledge: 20 percent of the exam covers newborns through adolescents. Pregnancy-related questions are now embedded into adolescent, young adult, and middle adult categories.

> **Exam Tip**
>
> Review your growth and development and life stages, and you will ace this category!

Types of Exam Questions to Anticipate

Test questions are typically arranged into two categories:

Lower-Level Thinking

- straight knowledge questions
- requires memorization and information recall
- one correct answer

Example:
Which tumor marker is specifically elevated in prostate cancer?

a. Prostate cancer tumor marker (PCTM)
b. Cancer antigen (CA) 125
c. Carcinoembryonic antigen (CEA)
d. Prostate-specific antigen (PSA)*

Which cognitive change is expected in healthy older adults age 65 and older?

a. Decrease in IQ
b. Slower information processing*
c. Low capacity for learning
d. Decreased attentional focus

Higher-Level Thinking

- Assesses clinical reasoning
- Problem-solving situations
- There may be two correct answers, but one best answer

Marvin, age 47, has just been given a diagnosis of diabetes. To increase his adherence to a healthy lifestyle, you:

a. initially have him come in weekly for a urinalysis and point of care glucose fingerstick to see how he is doing.
b. tell him to do an HgbA1C every 3 months to assess his blood glucose control.
c. instruct him on self-monitoring blood sugar.*
d. refer him to a nutritionist.

Your 75-year-old patient with osteoarthritis of the knee will be starting on a course of NSAIDs for pain management. What is the most important teaching point for your patient today?

a. Start with a high dose first and taper the dose down as needed.
b. Continue to take your Warfarin (Coumadin) as you have been.
c. Report any excessive stomach upset or if you notice bloody or dark stools.*
d. At this point, it will not be helpful to lose weight.

You may find the following four types of exam questions on both the AANP and ANCC Certification Exams. Traditional multiple choice is the predominant type, but the "select all" questions have been exceedingly popular. Depending on which exam you take, you may get a photograph of a rash to diagnosis or a chest X-ray or a basic electrocardiogram (EKG) rhythm to interpret.

- Multiple-choice questions: Select one option from many
- Multiple-answer questions: Select all the options that apply
- Hot-spot questions: Mark a certain area of an image
- Drag-and-drop questions

Exam Preparation and Taking the Exam

- Carefully review the chosen credentialing organization's website for test requirements, the scheduling process, and the FNP exam blueprint.
- While you have been studying throughout your education, start exam preparation 3 months before you intend to take the exam.
- Develop a study schedule of at least 2 hours daily.
- List each day's study topic and your goal for the session.
- Read and understand your topic and rewrite what you learned.
- Make a list of your areas of weakness and topics you need to focus on.
- Take advantage of a good certification review course and accompanying materials.
- Review all your resources (i.e., primary care textbook, clinical practice guidelines, advanced health assessment textbook, and diagnostic and lab interpretation references).

- Do not leave answers blank.
- Make an educated guess by process of elimination.
- Select the first answer that pops into your head (usually correct).
- Flag questions that you can go back to before exam completion.

General Strategies

- Review basic diagnostic imaging; the most common question may be for you to identify a chest film with Community Acquired Pneumonia (CAP), Tuberculosis (TB), or Chronic Obstructive Pulmonary Disease (COPD) (see chapter 7, Respiratory).
- Learn the basic significance of abnormal lab results and follow-up testing. (See pertinent review chapters.)
- Don't memorize drug dosages, but understand what first-line treatments are and what to use when a drug is contraindicated (i.e., Penicillin (PCN) allergic patient or patient with Angiotensin-converting enzyme (ACE) cough)
- Understand broad drug categories and reasons for starting or discontinuing treatment. (See chapter 5, Pharmacology review.)
- Review national treatment guidelines that are referenced in pertinent chapters.

Top Reasons for Failing the Exam

- Taking insufficient time to review all available resources
- Studying by only taking board review questions
- Memorizing but not understanding nor applying your knowledge to the clinical situation

Retaking a Certification Exam

- If you fail the certification exam, you should remediate the "weak" and "medium" areas of knowledge for which you scored on the respective exam.
- ANCC allows candidates to take the exam up to three times in any 12-month period; you must wait 60 days after failing an exam to retake it.
- AANP's policy limits a candidate to two (2) testing attempts per calendar year (January to December). There is no waiting period; however, you must submit 15 completed contact hours in the exam areas of weakness.

Recertification Requirements

- **Recertification comes fast!**
- Set up a Continuing Education Unit (CEU) folder on your computer and gather all CEUs, practice information, number of practice hours, lectures given, precepting hours, and so on.
- ANCC and AANP certification is valid for 5 years.
- All contact and clinical hours must be completed within the current 5-year certification period.
- ANCC and AANP require a minimum of 1,000 hours of clinical practice within your specialization within the 5 years of certification.
- ANCC requires 75 CEUs in the 5-year period, and 25 CEUs must be in pharmacology.
- ANCC also requires one or more of the following renewal categories to count toward recertification (i.e., academic credits, presentations, preceptor hours, publication, research, examination retake, etc.)
- AANP requires 100 CEUs in the 5-year period, and 25 CEUs must be in pharmacology.
- **Don't let your certification lapse!**

Resources

American Academy of Nurse Practitioners Certification Board (AANPCB). (2024). Annual reports. https://www.aanpcert.org/certs/pass

ANCC pass rates. American Nurses Credentialing Center. 2023 ANCC certification data. https://www.nursingworld.org/globalassets/docs/ancc/ancc-cert-data-website.pdf

APEA Staff. (2023, December). AANPCB introduces new FNP test blueprint. Advanced Practice Education Associates. https://www.apea.com/blog/FNP-test-blueprint-changes-in-2024-49/

Fitzgerald Health Education Associates. (2025). Pass your FNP exam the first time. https://www.fhea.com/pass-your-fnp-exam/#chapter5

Fitzgerald, M. A. (2020). *Nurse practitioner certification exam prep* (6th ed.). F.A. Davis.

Leik, M. C. (2025). *Adult-gerontology nurse practitioner certification intensive review* (5th ed.). Springer Publishing.

Springer Publishing Exam Prep. (2023). *FNP and AGNP certification: Practice Q&A*. Springer Publishing.

CHAPTER 2

Test-Taking Strategies for Nurse Practitioner Students

Sherylyn M. Watson, PhD, MSN, RN, CNE

As a nurse practitioner (NP) student, preparing for one of the national credentialing exams requires preparation and perseverance. Adequately preparing for the examination is similar to training for a marathon. With proper strategies, a systematic approach, and time, success is attainable!

Although all the coursework and clinical experience have prepared the student for this exam, NP students may find the national exam a new experience. Several best practices should help the NP student focus on the appropriate content and how to study. Several common questions arise when beginning this process:

1. What areas should I concentrate on when studying?
2. What should I review first?
3. What material, like textbooks, should I use in my review?
4. Should I review all class notes from the past 2 to 3 years?
5. How much time should I dedicate to studying?
6. Do I have to learn an entirely new way of studying for this exam?

This book was written to answer those questions and assist the NP student in preparing for the exam by offering a systematic approach to relevant content and outlining effective test-taking strategies. Use this book to review content you already learned, fill in content gaps, and take practice questions.

As you begin your marathon training, a few reminders will help you be successful:

1. **Quality Over Quantity**—Quality studying means minimizing distractions. No cell phones, no studying on the beach, no drinking your favorite drink or snacking, and no listening to music or watching television. The test-taker will not be allowed anything in their cubicles when taking the actual exam, so you should study under the same conditions. Second, study at your "best" time of the day.

    If you are a morning person, study during morning hours and plan to take your examination at the same time. If you are most alert during the afternoon, this is when you should study and plan your examination time. Studying after a long day of work or late in the evening is not ideal because you will have more reasons to be distracted.
2. **Practice Makes Perfect**—Do as many questions as possible. Questions, questions, questions!
3. **Believe in Yourself**—You know the content and have been successful throughout your NP program.

Where to Begin

- All information written in the question is critical to answering the question. If the question gives you the age, gender, or ethnicity of the patient or family, these items are relevant to the answer, or they would not be added.
- Ask yourself, "What is the question really asking?" Summarize this in your own words.
- Identify keywords. All the answer choices may be correct or reasonable; therefore, when reading the question stem the first time, look for keywords. Specific ones that are important are:
  - Immediate concern,
  - first,
  - best,
  - or additional instructions.
- Answer the question objectively.
- Do not add information to the scenario. These questions were designed for NP candidates nationwide; therefore, consider standard replies rather than the atypical patient you may have seen in clinical practice.
- Sometimes, you may not know the answer due to a true knowledge deficit. Answer the best you can and move to the next question.
- Have one *notebook* where you can write down content topics you need to review throughout your preparations.
- Formulate a realistic, achievable *study plan*!
- Start preparing for the NP certification exam 4 to 6 months ahead of time. You will still be taking classes; therefore, it is good to sit down and develop a plan. This plan can be flexible while finishing the program but set target goals to measure achievement. Starting early to prepare, reviewing content, and taking practice exams weekly are setting yourself up for success.
- Upon completion of your program's coursework, an effective approach is to create a plan for 4 to 6 weeks, culminating with the taking of the actual exam. Marathons are not won by training for one day! Quality studying is more important than quantity; therefore, you should study only 5 days a week. Take 1 to 2 days off to rest your mind; studying constantly is a mental workout, and the resulting fatigue may undermine your efforts. Throughout your day, take breaks to remain focused when studying.
- Approach your preparation systematically. Use different modes of preparation such as content review, practice questions, computer testing, videos, and note taking. The best practice is to divide your time between practicing questions and reviewing content. Also, decide if you are studying by body systems or health condition. No approach is wrong as long as you are consistent. Filling in gaps in your knowledge is necessary; however, minimize passive reading. Deep dive into specific, focused areas you need to review for content. When taking practice questions, it is most important to have time to review the rationales provided to learn why the answer is correct and why the others are not.
- There are many resources available. Using this review book is an excellent choice you made for yourself in preparing to be successful on your certification exam! Review the list of text resources that both credentialing bodies provide as references for you to look up information as needed. There is no need to reread any book!
- Answer questions ALL in one sitting to mimic the exam. Do not underestimate how difficult this will be. There are many competing demands; thus, sitting quietly for 2.5 to 3 hours without a break is challenging. Similar to training for a marathon, use your plan to increase the number of questions in one sitting over 4 weeks. Since each exam will be either 150 questions (American Association of Nurse Practitioners [AANP]) or 175 (American Nurses Credentialing Center [ANCC]), the best strategy is to prepare to sit without any distractions for that amount of questions. For example, in week 1, start taking 100 questions in one sitting. In week 2, plan for 125 questions; by week 4, plan to sit for 175 questions. By increasing increments and finishing as refreshed as you started, you will not answer questions incorrectly due to being distracted or tired.
- Review the exam content outline for your specific certification posted on its websites. The certification topics are outlined with percentages for each exam. When developing your study plan, consider the topics and percentages. For instance, on the AANP NP exam, there are three questions on newborns, or 2 percent of the exam; whereas, there are 35 questions on middle adults, or 26 percent of the exam; and 40 questions on older adults, or 30 percent of the exam. Because no one has an infinite amount of time and it is impossible to know everything, one way to approach this is to review newborn content but, more importantly, schedule more time to concentrate on middle and older adult content.

- Set target dates for each week. Review and revise as needed. This strategy is necessary, so build up to taking 175 questions in one sitting. You will likely feel tired initially, but practicing this for the actual certification exam gives you more opportunities to succeed.

A typical plan looks like the following:

Day 1	■ Answer 100 practice questions on a specific topic in one sitting. ■ Read the rationales. ■ Identify any knowledge deficit areas that need more review.
Day 2	■ Answer 100 practice questions on a specific topic in one sitting. ■ Read the rationales. ■ Identify any knowledge deficit areas that need more review.
Day 3	■ **"Content Day"**—Review content identified in your practice questions or in your coursework as "knowledge deficit."
Day 4	■ Depending on how much content is identified in gap analysis, continue to study information that needs to be reviewed. ■ (or) Take a 100-question comprehensive examination. ■ Review the rationales. ■ Identify knowledge deficit areas that need more review.
Day 5	■ Answer 100 practice questions on a specific topic in one sitting. ■ Read the rationales. ■ Identify knowledge deficit areas that need more review.

Best Practices for Test-Taking

Specific test-taking strategies assist the NP student in effectively preparing for the exam. Although there is always room for improvement, changing your approach to prepare for and take the exam is not recommended. You have been successful in reaching this point! Therefore, these strategies will support your current knowledge, offer a path to improve your approaches, and review the content.

- All information written in the question is critical to answering the question. If the question gives you the age, gender, ethnicity of the patient or family, diagnosis, comorbidity, and timeframe, these items are relevant to the answer, or they would not be added. The certification exams are not designed to trick you.
- Ask yourself, "What is the question really asking?" Summarize this in your own words.
- Identify keywords. All the answer choices may be correct or reasonable; therefore, when reading the question stem the first time, look for keywords. Specific ones that are important are: assess, evaluate, implement, immediate concern, first, or best.
- Answer the question objectively. Do not add information to the scenario. These questions were designed for NP candidates nationwide; therefore, consider evidence-based practice, not the atypical patient you may have seen in clinical practice.
- Sometimes, you may not know the answer due to a true knowledge deficit. Answer the best you can and move to the next question. Always answer all the questions.
- You should have one *notebook* or *document on your laptop* where you can write down content topics you need to review throughout your preparations.

Know Your Test-Taking Type

Once an individualized plan is established, determine which type of test-taker you are to minimize answering questions inaccurately other than knowledge deficits.

- The first step is to take a 100-question practice exam. When reviewing the answers, complete a spreadsheet noting which questions you answered incorrectly and the reason why. The three reasons to use are: K—Knowledge Deficit, C—Changed Answer, M—Misread the Question.
- The second step is to analyze why you answered incorrectly.
  - **Did you answer any questions wrong because of a "knowledge deficit"?** If reviewing the rationale was sufficient to understand the concept, move on. If the rationale left you realizing you need to look up this content, write the topic down for further studying on "content day." Always have a notebook ready to write down missed concepts so you can look them up later.
  - **Did you answer any questions wrong because of a "changed answer"?** A recommendation is to reread the question stem again, looking for new and compelling information that would make you change your initial

answer. Most people should not change their answer. Trust your instinct and, thus, your initial answer. Only after rereading the question stem and perhaps finding a keyword you initially missed should you change your answer. Trusting yourself and not changing answers takes practice; therefore, apply this strategy for 2 weeks before expecting marked improvement.

- **Did you answer any questions wrong because of a "misread"?** It is time to slow down. Perhaps you were distracted at that moment or rushing to finish. In either case, more than an occasional misread is a concern. A strategy to counteract this is to reread the stem of the question if you find yourself answering the question quickly. After picking the answer quickly, read the stem of the question to ensure that the answer fits. Typically, this issue can be resolved by taking questions for longer periods; this paces you and decreases distractions.
- Now complete a visual assessment of your answer key. This is a mock one of only 40 questions, but it will help you understand how important a visual assessment can be in recognizing how you approach examinations.

1.	11.	21.	31. x
2. x	12.	22. x	32.
3. x	13.	23. x	33.
4.	14.	24.	34. x
5.	15.	25.	35. x
6.	16.	26.	36.
7. x	17.	27.	37.
8. x	18.	28. x	38.
9.	19.	29.	39. x
10.	20.	30.	40.

- **Were most questions between 1 and 20 wrong?** Typically, this occurs because of test anxiety. A strategy to counteract this is to begin each exam the same, creating a routine that can be mimicked for the actual examination. A proven strategy is to take three deep breaths before reading the first question. Say positive statements to yourself before beginning, such as "I know this material!" "I am prepared!" "Trust my initial instinct!" The key is to use the same exercise each time to settle your nerves and put your mind in the same setting as all the other exams.
- **Were most questions wrong in the middle, between 40 and 60?** Your mind may be wandering. To address this issue, check back in during the exam when your mind drifts. Because you know you drift at a certain point, stop and close your eyes for 3 to 5 seconds. Stretching your neck and arms, closing your eyes, and counting to 10 are small ways to recharge and refocus on the exam. Do *not* get up and take a break. You cannot take a break on the day of the national exam; therefore, do not train yourself to stop whenever you feel distracted. Remember the "training for a marathon" analogy: runners do not stop on mile 4 when they begin to get fatigued; they push on and refocus.
- **Were most questions at the end between 80 and 100 wrong?** Test-takers know when the ending is near and sometimes lose focus to simply be done. The best approach is already what you agreed to do in your plan: extend the number of questions you take for each seating. If you start to get distracted and rush around question 85, remember that if you sit for 150 questions, #85 is still in the middle of the exam. Because we already know how long each exam will be, extend your exams to that many questions to practice sitting for that long and minimize rushing in the end. Also, when taking your practice questions, allow yourself enough time to finish. Using the formula of 1 minute for each question should guide you on how long you will need to take the examination.
- **Were most of your answers wrong in pairs or triples?** This indicates that although you answered a question and moved to the next, your mind remained on the preceding question. Allow yourself the full opportunity to answer the next question. Focus only on that: one question at a time. Here is an example of how you might stumble: Question #10 is difficult, and you know the answer may be wrong, but you choose an answer and move on to question #11. Because you are still thinking about question #10, you haphazardly read question #11 and choose an answer without using your test training to

find the correct answer. This happens subconsciously. The good news is that you can correct the problem. The goal is to clear your mind about the difficult preceding question so that you can refocus on the next one. The physical act of clearing your mind works best. When you note a difficult question, answer the question and write the # of the question down on a blank piece of paper. Using this same example, write down #10. This physical act will stop your mind, clear it, and allow you to refocus for the next question. This strategy usually takes some practice before seeing improvement.

The following are some helpful reminders as you begin reviewing the content in each of these chapters and taking practice questions:

- Do as many practice questions as possible.
- Read the rationales carefully. They will help you understand other concepts as well.
- Review the content at the beginning of each chapter. If you are still struggling to understand the information, read your textbook or review class notes about that specific topic.
- Sometimes, you must memorize certain information, such as lab values and medication classifications. Otherwise, the best practice is to learn how to apply the content to patients in different contexts.
- If you are a visual learner, draw out a patient with clinical features, diagnostic tests, and a treatment plan to help recall the information.
- Keep thinking positive thoughts.
- Proper preparation for the national examination will take some time; however, the successful outcome is worth the dedication and time investment!

Day Before the Examination

The goal is to be fresh for the next day. Therefore, it is important to relax your mind beforehand, so you are not drained of energy. You must conserve your strength and build up your endurance for the exam.

A few simple suggestions to consider when planning for this day include the following:

1. Limit your exposure to emotional situations with friends or family for the next 2 days that could distract you from focusing on yourself. Ask close relatives not to share any upsetting news with you this evening or tomorrow until the exam is over.
2. Avoid peers in the same situation because positive thinking is of the utmost importance. The day before the examination is not the time for you and a peer to compare how much prep time each of you dedicated to studying. Everyone takes examinations differently, and you have made your own concerted effort toward your preparation.
3. Double-check directions to the testing center, any IDs you must bring, and what time you must leave for the exam, considering traffic and road construction.
4. Eat well-balanced meals, stay hydrated, and go to bed early to get a good night's rest.

Day of the Exam

1. Eat a well-balanced breakfast and reduce caffeine. Caffeine can make you alert, but too much can make some people lose focus and need to go to the restroom during the examination.
2. Do not take phone calls from people who may cause you anxiety.
3. Be confident! Think positive thoughts. Tell yourself you can do this: "I know this material! I am prepared! I will pass!"
4. As you sit in front of the exam, close your eyes and think of a safe place. Begin the exam just as you have practiced it over the past months.

Day After the Exam

1. Plan a fun, relaxing, and energy-draining activity to keep your mind off the exam. You deserve this day!

Exam Success Tips

1. Know the certification's content topic plan.
2. Design a study plan 4–6 months in advance.
3. Apply best practices for preparing and taking questions.
4. Take up to 175 practice exams in one sitting to mimic the real exam.
5. Quality studying is more important than quantity.
6. Minimize distractions when studying.
7. Have confidence in yourself!

Review Questions

1. An 8-year-old with a known allergy history has been experiencing a nonproductive cough for 9 days. On day 9, the child's temperature rose to 103.5°F with an oxygen level of 92 percent on room air. Upon assessment, the child does not complain of ear or throat pain and wheezes. The family nurse practitioner (FNP) manages this patient by first:
   A. ordering an immediate chest X-ray.
   B. prescribing systemic antibiotics.
   C. administering a bronchodilator via nebulizer.
   D. referring the patient to a hospital for admission.

2. An older patient's family requests the nurse practitioner (NP) start her on a medication to help with agitation, behavior problems, and sleep issues. The NP counsels the family on the use of second-generation antipsychotics. Which statement is true regarding these medications?
   A. "While they help with sedation, they have an increased cardiovascular risk."
   B. "These medications will help her sleep but lower her blood glucose levels."
   C. "While this will help with one problem, they place her at high risk for weight loss."
   D. "These medications will help her sleep, but we must monitor for suicidal ideations."

3. A 27-year-old male client with Hodgkin's lymphoma in the abdominal and pelvic regions is about to start radiation therapy. Which information is the most important for the NP to address?
   A. Sperm production being permanently disrupted
   B. Constipation that will be continuous throughout therapy
   C. Baldness resulting from the radiation therapy will be permanent
   D. The treatment will increase the risk for prostate cancer later in life

4. What is the most common source for hepatitis A infection?
   A. Needle sharing
   B. Consuming raw shellfish
   C. Contaminated water supplies
   D. Intimate person-to-person contact

5. The NP is evaluating a pregnant person who was bitten by a deer tick and will receive treatment. Which medication would not be appropriate to prescribe for this patient?
   A. Amoxicillin
   B. Azithromycin
   C. Doxycycline
   D. Cefuroxime axetil

6. An 18-year-old Chinese exchange student presents to student health for a wellness visit to follow up on his immunization record and the reading of his purified protein derivative (PPD) result from 3 days ago. The PPD result is a 6-mm area of induration. What is the best initial intervention by the NP?
   A. Order an immediate chest radiograph
   B. Ask the student if he received the Bacillus Calmette-Guerin (BCG) vaccine before
   C. Prescribe isoniazid therapy immediately
   D. Request the student return in 1 month to repeat the PPD test

7. The FNP is reviewing results with a patient who has received a positive rapid human immune deficient virus (HIV) test. What would be the most appropriate response by the provider?
   A. "You will need a Western blot test to confirm a positive diagnosis of HIV."
   B. "You will need to have your CD4 count tested immediately."
   C. "You have acquired human immunodeficiency virus (HIV)."
   D. "Rapid tests have false positives."

8. What is the common presentation between uncontrolled diabetes mellitus and HIV?
   A. Pneumonia
   B. Vaginal candidiasis
   C. Retinopathy
   D. Gastric ulcer

9. Governing guidelines require that all patients seen in a primary care setting be routinely screened for domestic violence. During the screening, privacy and confidentiality are essential components. Which of the following statements by the FNP may help create a nonthreatening environment when asking the adult client?
   A. "I will ask you some questions that may make you uncomfortable, but you must answer them honestly."
   B. "I see that there is a strong history of drug and alcohol use in your personal history. This places you at risk for domestic violence. Do you want to discuss this further?"
   C. "I noticed that you were seen several times this past year by other providers in this office for complaints of abdominal pains and headaches. These can be indicators of domestic

violence. Should I review these records so that we can discuss this?"
D. "Since domestic violence is so prevalent, and it may be difficult for patients to bring up, I have started routinely screening all my patients."

10. The NP evaluates a new patient who is an African American with hypertension who has been taking lisinopril (Prinivil). His current BP is 160/90. Which medication does the NP prescribe to create a more effective treatment plan?
A. Angiotensin-converting enzyme inhibitor
B. Angiotensin II receptor blockers
C. Calcium-channel blocker
D. Beta blocker

Answers and Rationales

1. Answer C is correct. This is the **first** decision. The keyword in this question is *first* because the NP may take all these actions, but the immediate issue is improving breathing.

   Answer B is incorrect. Prescribing antibiotics without a source is not recommended.

   Answer A is incorrect. The differential diagnosis is pneumonia, thus requiring an order for a chest X-ray.

   Answer D is incorrect. A referral for a hospital admission is not necessary at this time, as the goal is to keep the child out of the hospital as long as possible. The other keyword is a child's age because the decision tree would be different if the patient were an 88-year-old.

2. Answer A is correct. The keyword is *true*. The learner needs to know about the medication before answering this question. This is an example of a question that if you do not know the answer, write it in your notebook to review the content. Also, make an educated guess. Older patients are at most risk for cardiovascular issues; therefore, this is a great concern for any older person.

   Answers B and C are incorrect. Do not read too much into the question and choose an answer based on the possibility that the patient has diabetes mellitus or is too thin. There is no indication that weight loss would be a bad issue for this patient. Be careful when adding your own subjectivity to the questions.

   Answer D is incorrect. There is no indication that the patient is depressed or has suicidal tendencies. Second generation antipsychotics have side effects that are cardiac in nature such as arrhythmias or cardiac arrest.

3. Answer A is correct. Although all these answers are true, addressing an immediate and life-changing issue is the most important keyword. The patient's age, which is noted in this question, clues you into the importance of this: having no future to produce a family once undergoing radiation treatment is extremely important. The NP should address this immediately and suggest banking sperm for later use if desired so that the patient has the option of a family.

   Answers B, C and D are all correct but the question asks what is the most important information that this patient needs prior to starting radiation therapy. Radiation therapy to the pelvic region could cause sterility. This would be of primary concern for a 27-year-old male.

4. Answer C is correct. Although raw shellfish is a source of contracting hepatitis A, and the other two answers are other ways to transmit hepatitis B and C, the keywords in this question are *most common*. This is an easy error to make when quickly answering the question after reading "raw shellfish" and not taking time to read the rest of the possible answers. After choosing the answer, the other strategy is to reread the question if you are deciding between B and C and pick up on the most common words. Another way to determine between B and C is to consider the entire world population and view this question in general terms because eating raw shellfish does not happen in all cultures.

5. Answer C is correct. Although all these antibiotics may be used in a treatment plan for Lyme disease, the keywords in this question are *pregnant person* and *not*. Including pregnancy is important and should always be used when making the critical decision. In reading carefully, the stem of the question should have had you identifying the word *not*. If you missed them the first time, reread the question to see what the keywords are because all these answers are associated with treatment of the disorder.

6. Answer B is correct. The keyword in this question is *Chinese*. The CDC recommends anyone with a positive PPD, regardless of receiving the BCG vaccine, be treated the same due to the false positives. Since this student is in a high-risk category, the FNP must know what is positive for

this group. The 6-mm induration would be read as negative. To account for the induration, the next step is asking about a history of receiving the BCG vaccine. An Interferon-Gamma Release Assay (IGRA) could be ordered to evaluate if the student has been infected with *M. tuberculosis*. The patient's Chinese ethnic background was important; otherwise, it would have been omitted from the question stem.

7. Answer A is correct. Requiring a Western blot test is important for a confirmed positive HIV diagnosis. The keywords are *most appropriate*.

   Answer B is incorrect. The patient does not need an immediate CD4 count; however, this will be part of the comprehensive workup later if the Western blot is positive for HIV. Therefore, the word *immediate* in answer B rules out this answer as correct.

   Answer C is incorrect. The patient should not be told they are positive for HIV without a confirming diagnosis.

   Answer D is incorrect. They should not be given false hope that the first test was false positive.

8. Answer B is correct. Vaginal candidiasis is a shared clinical presentation because of the high glucose levels with uncontrolled diabetes and being immunocompromised. When answering this question, ask yourself if each one of these disorders is common (not atypical).

   Answers A and C are incorrect. Retinopathy can occur with diabetes mellitus. Pneumonia can be associated with HIV/AIDS but not necessarily with diabetes.

   Answer D is incorrect. Gastric ulcers are not associated with either disease.

9. Answer D is correct. This is the most nonthreatening answer that creates a nonjudgmental atmosphere.

   Answer A is incorrect. The first answer would create an immediate defensive response because the NP calls the client a liar before the question.

   Answers B and C are incorrect. A judgment is made about certain behaviors, and blame is placed on the client. When answering questions about statements you should make to the client, repeat the answers out loud if you are unsure. Would anyone understand or accept that as a response? It is also helpful to think about a layperson who is not familiar with medical terminology and does not possess medical knowledge and repeat those questions. It is important not to think of yourself as the client because you already have a background in health care; therefore, *your* reactions would always be different from a regular person accessing health care.

10. Answer C is correct. Calcium-channel blockers work well with African Americans. In this situation, the keyword addresses the client's cultural aspect to determine the correct answer.

Resources

American Academy of Nurse Practitioners Certification Board. (2024). *FNP, AGNP & PMHNP certification handbook*. https://www.aanpcert.org/resource/documents/AGNP%20FNP%20PMHNP%20Candidate%20Handbook.pdf

American Nurses Credentialing Center. (2023a). *Certification: general testing and renewal handbook*. https://www.nursingworld.org/~4a9ce2/globalassets/certification/renewals/ancc-generaltestingrenewalrequirements.pdf

American Nurses Credentialing Center. (2023b). *How to prepare for your ANCC certification exam*. https://www.nursingworld.org/~498d51/globalassets/certification/ancc-1788_certification-seven-tips_fnl.pdf

Coppa, D., & Barcelos Winchester, S. (2020). Diagnostic readiness tests: Preparing nurse practitioner students for national certification examinations. *Journal of the American Association of Nurse Practitioners, 32*(1), 52–59. https://dx.doi.org/10.1097/JXX.0000000000000191

Thompson, D. L. (2016). Useful test-taking strategies when preparing for the WOCNCB continence examination. *Journal of Wound, Ostomy, & Continence Nursing, 43*(4), 425–426. https://dx.doi.org/10.1097/WON.0000000000000246

CHAPTER 3

Professional and Legal-Ethical Issues

Cynthia K. O'Sullivan, PhD., APRN, FNP-BC
Susan M. DeNisco, DNP, APRN, FNP-BC, FAANP

The American Nurses Credentialing Center (ANCC) Examination certification examination will have approximately 15 questions (10 percent) on professional issues, including ethics, regulatory guidelines, evidence-based practice (EBP), and scope of practice issues.

Nurse Practitioner Education

The goal of becoming a nurse practitioner (NP) can take several educational pathways. Most commonly, Bachelor of Science in Nursing (BSN) graduates complete either a Master of Science in Nursing (MSN) or Doctor of Nursing Practice (DNP) NP program. MSN or DNP-prepared nurses who are not NPs can also complete post-MSN certificates in an NP program, as can an NP who wishes to obtain an additional specialty. Additionally, direct entry into practice programs prepares students with nonnursing baccalaureate degrees to complete coursework and take the registered nurse (RN) state licensure board exam, which allows them to begin a graduate program for their NP education. The common denominator for all these programs is that they must meet standard criteria that prepare graduates to take national certification exams required for state licensure.

Nurse Practitioner Competencies

The National Organization for Nurse Practitioner Faculties (NONPF) and the American Association of Colleges of Nursing (AACN) define the competency statements for NPs at the basic level of practice. In addition, population-focused competencies for the various specialty areas articulate the requisite knowledge and skills for unique populations based on their age or clinical needs, which require that NP educational programs meet those competencies through their curriculum (for example, family nurse practitioner [FNP], pediatric nurse practitioner [PNP], psychiatric mental health nurse practitioner [PMHNP], etc.). Minimum practice hours for NP programs vary based on student needs, type of program, and curriculum requirements. While some programs at the MSN level require no more than 500 direct-care hours, the expectation is that this number will increase, primarily due to the National Task Force on Quality Nurse Practitioner Education (2022).

The National Task Force (NTF) comprises 19 professional nursing organizations, which are made up of experts in practice, certification, regulation, and education. Every 3 to 5 years, the organization reviews and sets NTF Standards and criteria to guide and facilitate NP educational programs to meet quality expectations and assist them with program assessment and planning.

Their work has been facilitated by the NONPF and the AACN since 1997. NONPF is a professional organization devoted to promoting the highest-quality NP education and leadership in NP education among its members. Since 1990, NONPF has identified Core Competencies for NPs entering practice, which represent knowledge and skills to be achieved during NP education to ensure safe entry into practice following graduation. The most recent version of the NONPF NP Role Core Competencies is aligned specifically with AACN's Advanced Level 2 Competencies. Details of the alignment may be found on the NONPF and AACN websites. Explicating essential requirements for NPs to be practice-ready, competencies in clinical knowledge and skill, as well as professional knowledge, skill, and professional behaviors, when used in practice, are expected to have positive impacts on the nation's health, as NPs' expanded roles allow them to practice at the full scope of their education and licensure. AACN's (2022) most recent standards are anticipated to be fully incorporated within 3 to 5 years of publication, but some requirements will require time to incorporate. One major change is the recommendation for a minimum of 750 direct-care hours required for all NP programs, while the previous criteria required a minimum of 500 direct-care practice hours. AACN practice requirements at the advanced Level 2 (MSN and DNP) require a minimum of 500 practicum hours beyond Level 1 for all graduate level nursing programs. The combined practicum requirements for AACN and the NTF standards contain overlapping clinical hour expectations, with some advanced Level 2 requirements for AACN including nondirect care.

As the NTF criteria become fully incorporated, educational programs must carefully review both NTF standards and the competencies outlined in the AACN Essentials, as aligned with the NONPF Nurse Practitioner Role Core Competencies, to ensure that they meet these requirements to remain accredited. Graduates of NP programs must have attended a program that is accredited by either the Commission on Collegiate Nursing Education (CCNE, an affiliate of AACN) or the Accreditation Commission for Education in Nursing (ACEN [formerly NLNAC | National League for Nursing Accrediting Commission]) to qualify to take one of the certification exams.

Licensure, Accreditation, Certification, and Education (LACE)

As advanced practice nursing evolved over the past several decades, professional nursing organizations recognized a need to define and standardize important aspects of advanced nursing roles. The current model requiring Licensure, Accreditation, Certification, and Education for regulating the advanced practice registered nurse (APRN) profession was developed by the Advanced Practice Nursing Consensus Work Group and the National Council of State Boards of Nursing (NCSBN, 2008) APRN Committee, with input from nearly 50 professional nursing organizations in 2008. The group formed what was known as the APRN Joint Dialogue Group or Licensure, Accreditation, Certification & Education (LACE). The group specified that requirements for licensure (granting authority to practice via state regulations), accreditation (achieved by nursing programs through the formal review and approval by a recognized agency, such as NLNAC or CCNE), certification (formal recognition of achievement of knowledge, skills, and experience to meet professional standards, by passing a certification examination), and education (required formal preparation in graduate degree-granting or postgraduate certificate programs). The goal was consistency in LACE in all states. While an APRN may specialize in an area such as diabetes or palliative care, they must be licensed in one of the four roles with a population focus. All advanced practice educational programs must be accredited and provide the core courses, including advanced pathophysiology, advanced pharmacology, and advanced physical assessment (the "3 Ps"). Certification must meet the standards given by the LACE guidelines, which would assure entry-level competency of the APRN role and population focus (DeNisco, 2023).

Scope of Practice

At this time, NPs have the authority to evaluate and diagnose, order and interpret diagnostic tests, initiate and manage a treatment plan consisting of nonpharmacological interventions, and prescribe medications without physician collaboration or oversight in 27 states, the District of Columbia, Guam, and the Northern Mariana Islands. In 11 states, NP practice is considered "Restricted" because at least one element of NP practice (assessment, diagnosis, or treatment) requires physician supervision, management, or delegated activities, despite the Institute of Medicine's (IOM) recommendations to allow nurses to practice to the full extent of their education and training. The other 11 "Reduced Practice" states require career-long collaboration or reduction in scope of one of the elements of NP practice. The scope of practice for NPs

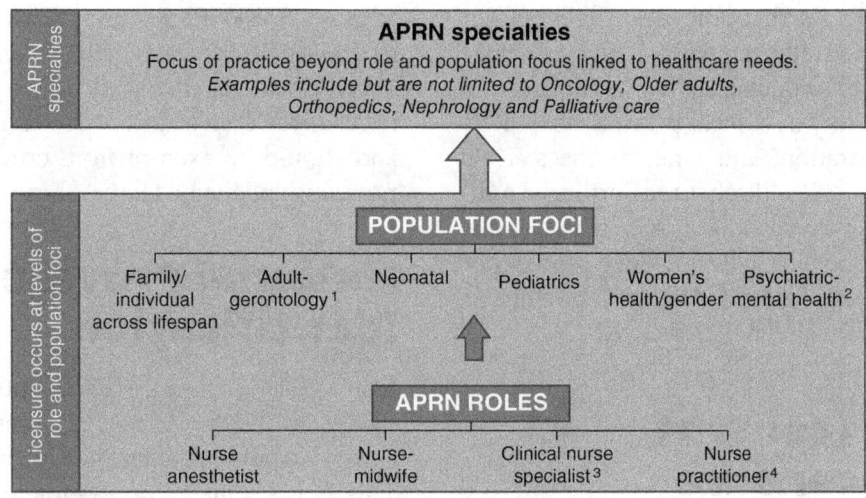

Figure 3-1 APRN Consensus Regulatory Practice Model.
Reproduced from American Nurses Association. (2008). *Consensus Model for APRN Regulation: Licensure, Accreditation, Certification & Education.* (July 7, 2008). p. 10.

can be found on the AANP website, although each state can define the scope of practice in their state statutes, which may be very specific or quite general. It is essential that NPs review the most current scope of practice legislated by the state where they practice. (DeNisco, 2024).

Not only did the work by the Consensus Model from the APRN Joint Dialogue Group Report (APRN Consensus Work Group & the NCSBN APRN Advisory Committee) determine the LACE criteria to set standards for entry into practice, but they also identified the professions that were considered APRNs (ANCC, 2008). The APRN title includes certified registered nurse anesthetists (CRNAs), certified nurse-midwives (CNMs), clinical nurse specialists (CNSs), and certified nurse practitioners (CNP/NPs). To date, each state has been able to define the legal scope of practice for each, recognize the roles and titles of each and define the criteria for practice entry, and authorize appropriate certification examinations (See **Figure 3-1**).

Advanced Practice State Licensure

The process for APRN licensure requires four steps. The educational program must be accredited to ensure that NP graduates have the requisite knowledge for practice. The NP must complete their graduate degree and then successfully pass the certification exam. For the final step, a graduate who successfully passes the certification exam sends the required documentation for APRN licensure to the state where they are applying to practice. Of note, in August 2020, the NCSBN adopted the APRN Compact for multistate licensure. Not every state is a Compact state, and there are specific requirements, such as having a minimum of 2,080 practice hours completed, for NPs who seek Compact licenses. States wishing to join the APRN Compact also need to enact the APRN Compact model legislation and implement a federal criminal background check for candidates seeking APRN licensure. NPs are advised to learn about their state's membership in the Compact as they pursue various professional opportunities in neighboring states.

For individual state licensure, most states require that the applicant hold an RN license; has successfully completed 30 hours of education in pharmacology for advanced nursing practice; and holds a minimum of an MSN or a related field recognized for certification as an NP, a clinical nurse specialist, or a nurse anesthetist by one of the above-recognized certifying bodies. Most states will want the application to be notarized and have photo identification. The American Association of Nurse Practitioners (AANP) is an excellent reference for all NPs. It provides an annual state-by-state national overview of NP legislation and healthcare issues, as well as the definition of the legal scope of practice for each individual state. It is important that the FNP understand the specific functions included in their state's definition of FNP scope of practice related to diagnosis, treatment, prescribing practices, hospital admission privileges, referrals, education, and ordering diagnostic tests. Each state's scope of practice also delineates what the legal role and requirements are of physician involvement in the NP practice. Language, such as "collaboration," "supervision," "independent practice," "delegation to the APRN," and "consultation," are examples of varying forms of physician involvement with the

NP (DeNisco, 2023). Furthermore, specific attention should be paid to the state's regulations on such practices as telehealth, therapeutic use of marijuana, the use of the title "Doctor" in clinical practice by APRNs with doctoral preparation, and whether the state is a Compact state for APRN licensure. Further, AANP provides a wealth of information on such topics and is instrumental in supporting NPs who may encounter fluctuations in various aspects of their roles as shifts in social, legal, and professional perspectives.

Drug Enforcement Agency Licensure

An NP must apply for the State Controlled Substances licensure and the Drug Enforcement Administration (DEA) licensure to practice. Through the Department of Justice (DOJ) and DEA, the NP must apply for a DEA number pursuant to Title 21, Code of Federal Regulations, Section 1300.01(b28), which states, "the term *mid-level practitioner* means an individual practitioner, other than a physician, dentist, veterinarian, or podiatrist, who is licensed, registered, or otherwise permitted by the United States or the jurisdiction in which he/she practices, to dispense a controlled substance in the course of professional practice" (DEA, 2024). Examples of "mid-level" practitioners include, but are not limited to, healthcare providers, such as NPs, CRNAs, CNMs, and physician assistants who are authorized to dispense controlled substances by the state in which they practice.

The scope and practice of an NP includes prescribing and some states limit NPs' ability to prescribe medications. The AANP advocates for NP prescriptive authority to be regulated only by state boards of nursing and confluent with the NP role, education, and certification. Any limitations on prescribing legal and controlled medications, devices, healthcare services, durable medical equipment, and other equipment and supplies curtails the ability of NPs to deliver essential services for timely, cost-effective, and high-quality health care.

Patients looking to manage their symptoms seek treatment from their healthcare providers for a variety of options. Evidence regarding the therapeutic use of marijuana and related compounds is limited. AANP supports efforts to review the efficacy and safety of marijuana and cannabinoids through systematic scientific review and evidence-based therapeutic recommendations. Further, nurses at all levels need continued education on marijuana and cannabinoids, and AANP endorses that this be included in nursing education. AANP supports policies that authorize NPs to discuss treatments and treatment alternatives in open and direct dialog with their patients. AANP believes these conversations are essential to patient care and should be exempt from criminal or professional prosecution, such as loss of licensure.

National Provider Identification

The Health Insurance Portability and Accountability Act of 1996 (HIPAA) mandated the adoption of a standard unique identifier for healthcare providers. This is particularly important for reimbursement of healthcare services that the NP provides. In 2004, the Center for Medicare/Medicaid (CMS) adopted the National Provider Identifier (NPI) as the standard unique identifier number for all healthcare providers to use when filing and processing healthcare claims (CMS, 2022). All NPs are required to apply for an NPI and be assigned only one number, which will follow the NP wherever they practice. NP students are permitted to apply for an NPI while in their NP educational programs because RNs are also eligible for NPIs. The number obtained as an RN will remain the same when the NP begins their practice. It is advisable to apply for the NPI relatively early in the process for licensure to avoid any potential error that could delay billing and reimbursement as an NP (DeNisco, 2023).

Reimbursement

Fiscal responsibility is vital for NPs to understand. Correct coding can increase revenue and decrease liability. The 1997 Balanced Budget Act (BBA) liberalized Medicare coverage of NP services. Effective January 1, 1998, NPs and CNSs became authorized to bill directly for their professional services and be reimbursed at 85 percent of the physician rate for services provided to a patient (Department of Health & Human Services, 2007).

Billing and Coding

Understanding proper medical record documentation and billing procedures for an office visit can maximize reimbursement for services, affecting both the practice's and the NP's bottom line.

"Incident-to billing" allows NPs to provide follow-up services under the direction of a supervising physician and bill under the doctor's NPI, resulting in a greater Medicare reimbursement rate at 100 percent instead of 85 percent if billed under the NP's NPI.

Medical Billing and Coding Terminology

- International Classification of Diseases (ICD-10) Codes
  - The foundation of medical billing and coding, ICD-10 codes indicate the patient's diagnosis.
- Current Procedural Terminology (CPT) Codes
  - Essential to the billing process and tell insurance companies which procedures a healthcare provider wants reimbursement (e.g., EKG, injections, suturing, etc.).
    - If a bill is missing the ICD-10 or CPT code, the bill will be rejected by the insurance company and will have to be resubmitted with the correct information.
    - Services rendered must show the medical necessity of the visit and the appropriateness of the diagnostic and/or therapeutic services rendered at the time of the visit.

Evaluation and Management (E&M) Service Codes

- CPT codes from 99202 to 99499 represent services provided by the healthcare provider. These medical codes apply elements such as complexity of the visit; new versus established visit; and total time of visit, including face-to-face time, time spent reviewing the medical record, prescribing medication, doing referrals, and so on.

Clinical Pearl

The International Classification of Diseases, 11th Revision (ICD-11) became available globally on January 1, 2022. While there is an expectation that countries will start planning for the transition, currently, there is no mandatory implementation date in the United States.

Health Policy

Affordable Care Act

In March 2010, the Affordable Care Act (ACA) became law. The ACA and the Health Care and Education Reconciliation Act (HCERA) have had the greatest impact on the United States healthcare system since Medicaid and Medicare were enacted in the 1960s. The ACA intended to allow more Americans access to quality health insurance, reduce the number of uninsured people, and lower the cost of health insurance. In addition, the ACA instituted efficiencies that were targeted to encourage hospitals and primary care practices to improve technology and clinical outcomes; ultimately, all improvements were intended to increase access to care, lower costs, increase patient satisfaction with their health care, and ultimately, improve health outcomes. Currently, 40 of the 50 states have expanded Medicaid to offer health insurance to those who would not otherwise be eligible. While this practice has been found to improve outcomes, states cannot be forced to expand Medicaid and will not lose Medicaid funding if they choose not to. Since 2010, the number of uninsured has dropped from 45.2 million in 2013 to 26.4 million in 2022, a reduction from nearly 16 percent of the population to less than 8 percent. Gains were seen throughout racial and ethnic groups and among people, with estimates indicating that there are over 19 million fewer people who are uninsured.

The Future of Nursing Report

The legendary report from the IOM (2011), *The Future of Nursing: Leading Change, Advancing Health*, was released in 2010, which recommended that nurses should

- practice to the full extent of their education and training.
- achieve higher levels of education and training through an improved education system that promotes seamless academic progression.
- be full partners with physicians and other healthcare professionals in redesigning health care in the United States.
- understand effective workforce planning and policymaking that require better data collection and information infrastructure.

A second report released in 2016 reviewed progress from the 2011 report and further emphasized the need to broaden awareness by gaining support from organizations that could disseminate information supporting nurses' value in advancing positive health outcomes. Allowing NPs to practice to their full potential in clinical practice, education, professional collaboration, and leadership scenarios and reviewing progress in strengthening the quality and availability of data to inform improvements, the report strengthens the body of knowledge on NP value. The report also underscores the need to prioritize promoting a diverse nursing workforce.

The recommendations detailed in the IOM report have been further expanded in the next report, *The Future of Nursing 2020–2030: Charting a Path to*

Achieve Health Equity (National Academies of Sciences, Engineering, and Medicine et al., 2021). This report outlines the essential role of nurses, including APRNs in improving health equity, access, and quality through efforts to address social determinants of health (SDOH). It continues to support the four key messages outlined in the original report.

Social Determinants of Health

As numbers of NPs grow and their value is recognized, it is important to note that primary care NPs are often the only source of care for low-income or uninsured patients, people receiving Medicaid, and other groups in both urban areas and throughout rural settings where they have been historically underserved. However, NPs have reported that they would benefit from learning more about SDOH—sometimes called social drivers of health. With proper intervention, negative effects of certain societal factors may be lessened rather than "determined." NPs are encouraged to seek out professional conferences on topics related to SDOH to be better equipped to address the needs of underserved patients. Similarly, content on mental health has been cited by FNPs and other specialties outside of behavioral health as an area where more education is needed (Kueakomoldej et al., 2022). The AACN and NONPF NP Role Core Competencies advocate for these areas to receive closer attention in NP education. Both organizations expect NPs to regularly identify areas of need and obtain education and support to address any deficits in knowledge and practical skills.

Nurse Practitioner Policy-Related Competencies

While the previous NONPF Core Competencies include "policy" as a discrete competency area, the new NONPF NP Role Core Competencies integrate policy matters throughout the 10 Domains. The side-by-side presentation of NONPF NP Role Core Competencies and AACN's Advanced Level 2 Competencies can be viewed on the NONPF website. Several descriptions of required NP policy knowledge, behaviors, and skills as integrated into the AACN Domains and NONPF NP Role Competencies are presented below:

- **Domain 2, Patient-Centered Care**: NPs coordinate care, incorporating evidence-based guidelines while also considering the influence of system and policy factors on transitions of care.
- **Domain 3, Population Health**: NPs ascertain how ethical, legal, and socioeconomic factors affect care delivery, develop interventions to improve population health, and contribute to health policy development to achieve health equity.
- **Domain 4: Scholarship for the Nursing Discipline/ Practice Scholarship and Translational Science**: NPs use the most current scholarly evidence to develop or update current health policies to improve healthcare delivery and patient outcomes.
- **Domain 5, Quality and Safety**: NPs use knowledge of quality, safety, and outcome metrics to inform policy recommendations, including how access to health care, population factors, cost, quality, and safety affect health outcomes.
- **Domain 6, Interprofessional Partnerships/ Interprofessional Collaboration in Practice**: NPs collaborate with multiple stakeholders, including policymakers, to positively impact the healthcare system for all, including diverse populations.
- **Domain 7, Health Systems/Systems-Based Practice**: NPs evaluate health policies using an ethical framework that considers cost-effectiveness, health equity, and care outcomes; they implement strategies to change practices and systems that perpetuate structural racism and other forms of discrimination in health care.
- **Domain 9 Professionalism/Professional Acumen**: NPs need to abide by applicable laws, policies, and regulations; they are expected to advocate for policies which would allow all NPs to practice to the full extent of their education; they are responsible for evaluating policies within the professional practice environment related to how NP practice impacts health outcomes.

American Association of Nurse Practitioners: Position on Terms such as Mid-Level Provider and Physician Extender

As seen in several notable examples, such as the DEA's Title 21, Code of Federal Regulations on prescribing practices, the term "mid-level provider" is often used in regulatory language and other documents regarding NP practice. The AANP strongly endorses eliminating terms such as "mid-level provider" and "physician extender" in reference to NPs individually or to an aggregate inclusive of NPs. AANP calls on employers, policymakers, healthcare professionals, and other parties to use "nurse practitioner" when referring to our profession because other terms are inaccurate and misleading (AANP, 2022). When the IOM developed a blueprint for the future of nursing, a key recommendation of this report was that NPs should be full partners with physicians and other healthcare professionals. Achieving this recommendation requires using clear and accurate nomenclature for the nursing profession. AANP stands with the IOM, the NCSBN, and other nursing associations that recognize nursing's role in the healthcare system and only endorses the term "nurse practitioner." AANP further endorses the title of "Doctor" being used for nonphysicians practicing in a clinical setting, including NPs who are prepared at the doctoral level.

As licensed, independent practitioners, NPs practice throughout the entirety of health care—from health promotion and disease prevention to diagnoses that prevent and limit disability. These inaccurate terms originated decades ago in bureaucracies and/or organized medicine; they are not interchangeable with the use of the NP title and fail to recognize the established national scope of practice for the NP role and authority of NPs to practice according to the full extent of their education. Further, these terms confuse healthcare consumers and the public due to their vague nature and are not a true reflection of the role of the NP.

The term "mid-level provider" implies an inaccurate hierarchy within clinical practice. NPs practice at the highest level of professional nursing practice. It is well established that patient outcomes for NPs are comparable or better than those of physicians. NPs provide high-quality and cost-effective care.

The term "physician extender" originated in the physician community and was related to the extension of physician services by other providers. The NP role, however, evolved in response to identified healthcare needs across populations. NPs continue to meet the current and evolving future needs within a complex healthcare system. NPs are independently licensed, and their scope of practice is not designed to be dependent on or an extension of care rendered by a physician.

In addition to the terms cited above, other terms that should be avoided in reference to NPs include "limited-license providers," "nonphysician providers," and "allied health providers." As it would be inappropriate to call physicians "nonnurse providers," it is similarly inappropriate to call all providers by something that they are not. Similarly, the term "allied health provider" has no clear definition or purpose in today's environment.

When it is necessary to group providers for policymaking or other purposes, more appropriate terms may instead include "primary care providers," "healthcare providers," "healthcare professionals," "advanced practice providers," "clinicians," and/or "prescribers." Best practices call for clearly informing patients and referring to each healthcare provider by their individual title to recognize their unique but overlapping roles. Now is the time to eliminate outdated terms to ensure clarity and public understanding of the title of NP.

Responsibility to Patients/Care Priorities

The FNP has a variety of responsibilities, roles, and priorities for care. As a primary care provider, educator, mentor, researcher, administrator, and advocate for the NP profession, their role incorporates both direct and indirect care activities. AANP's priorities for the NP practice model incorporate patient and family education, which includes assisting their participation in care and promoting optimal health. NPs also need to provide culturally competent care, help patients access health care, and promote a safe environment. As expressed by AANP, NP accountability is to patients, the nursing profession, and their state board of nursing. The scope of practice for NPs requires that they practice according to their national certification, evidence-based principles, and current practice standards. Further, NPs must practice according to an ethical code of conduct. Specific ethical principles important to NPs are defined in the following section.

Ethical Terms

Autonomy—the patient has the right to self-determine choices and actions.

Beneficence—doing good/helping others.

Confidentiality—keeping patient information private unless sharing is required by legal need to share and/or to protect children and older people from domestic violence, psychiatric violence, and so on.

Fidelity—developing and maintaining trust in the patient–provider relationship based on truthfulness.

Justice—a complex term that simply means that equals should be treated equally.

Nonmaleficence—the obligation to avoid harm; protecting a patient from harm. The benefit(s) outweigh the risk(s).

Paternalism—in the case of the healthcare provider, it means the provider knows better than the patient and therefore would make decisions for the patient. This directly contradicts the concept of autonomy.

Utilitarianism—the obligation to act in a way that is useful to or benefits the majority (e.g., the Supplemental Nutrition Assistance Program [SNAP] and Supplemental Nutrition Program for Women, Infants, and Children [WIC]).

Veracity—the obligation to present information honestly and truthfully so that patients can make an informed and rational decision about their health care.

For a complete review of nursing ethics please refer to Grace and Uveges (2023) in the reference list.

Test Tip

Review the Health Insurance Portability and Accountability Act Privacy Rule
Understand scenarios where the Health Insurance Portability and Accountability Act (HIPPA) is applied to your work as an NP. It is a HIPPA violation to access a patient's medical record when you are not the patient's healthcare provider (U.S. Department of Health and Human Services, 2024).

Minors

A minor is a person under the age of 18. Federal and state laws outline the provision of health care to a minor without parental/guardian consent. Any person who is going to receive health care must provide informed consent; this means that the patient needs to understand their condition and the options being offered for treatment, as well as the risks for declining treatment. Many states allow adolescents to obtain care without parental consent. The American Academy of Pediatrics has valuable information regarding confidential healthcare services for minors. It is vital for FNPs to be aware of the laws pertaining to minors and health care in the state in which they practice.

The NP Role in End-of-Life Care

FNPs focus on the care of patients throughout their lifespan. Their relationship with patients in various settings, especially in primary care, can allow for fully engaged discussions with patients and their families about their end-of-life wishes, an important component of high-quality care. The Physician Orders for Life-Sustaining Treatment (POLST) Paradigm Program is a system that communicates patients' wishes about treatment preferences through portable medical orders, with the intention of allowing patients with advanced progressive frailty and chronic illnesses to identify treatment preferences in advance of the time when their illness may make such conversations difficult or impossible.

POLST orders are only intended for patients with serious, life-limiting illness, not for the general population. Alternatively, advanced directives and living wills can be completed by any individual capable of making their own decisions, but they are a different form of documentation; they state a person's wishes for end-of-life care, but they are not medical orders for treatment. POLST orders are actionable medical orders that travel wherever the patient receives their care and are written at a time when details about a patient's specific health conditions at the end of their life are more clearly understood.

Do Not Resuscitate Orders are designated for a specific healthcare facility and are not portable. National POLST outlines specific statements to help provide clarity for NPs and other healthcare providers, patients, and their families on this important topic. These statements on the National POLST website include the term "physician" rather than any other professional group. NPs are encouraged to review their own state's regulations about the role of NPs in initiating and signing POLST orders, which are summarized on the POLST website (National POLST, 2022).

Clinical Pearl

A Medical Order for Life-Sustaining Treatment (MOLST) is synonymous with a POLST order depending on the state you practice in.

Advanced Directives

Advance directives are legal documents that provide instructions for medical care and only go into effect when an individual cannot communicate their own wishes.

The two most common advanced directives for health care are the living will and the durable power of attorney for health care.

- A living will is a legal document that tells healthcare providers how a patient wants to be treated

if they can no longer make their own decisions about emergency treatment. A living will outlines medical treatment or care the patient would want rendered and what to avoid given certain conditions (e.g., do not resuscitate, do not intubate, do not hospitalize, etc.)
- A durable power of attorney for health care is a legal document that names a patient's healthcare proxy, a person who can make healthcare decisions for the patient if they cannot communicate their wishes. The proxy is also known as a representative, surrogate, or agent and should be familiar with the patient's values and wishes. A proxy can be chosen in addition to or instead of a living will.

Malpractice

The NP needs to become familiar with malpractice insurance, lawsuits, and elements of a case.

Malpractice Insurance

- The two major types of medical malpractice coverage are a claims-based policy or an occurrence-based policy.
- An occurrence-based policy will pay a claim on acts of medical malpractice based on the period during which you had the insurance regardless of if you are still currently with the policy.
- A claims-based policy will only cover a payout if a claim is brought against you during the term of the policy.
- Tail coverage added to a claims-based policy will cover the NP for malpractice claims that can be filed against them in the future.

Malpractice Lawsuit Terminology

- Failure to meet the standard of care. For example,
  - misdiagnosis or failure to diagnose.
  - failure to order appropriate tests or to act on results.
  - not following up with the patient.
  - prescribing the wrong dosage or the wrong medication.
- The plaintiff is the person who complains; this can be the patient or a legally designated person who acts on the patient's behalf.
- The defendant is the healthcare provider who is being sued for injury or damage (physical and/or emotional)

NPs should review elements of a case, such as phases of medical malpractice trial and expert witnesses who practice in the same specialty. A great resource for a deeper understanding of legal and ethical issues is Carolyn Buppert's (2023) textbook *Nurse Practitioner's Business Practice and Legal Guide*, Eighth Edition.

Nursing Research and Evidence-Based Practice

- Nursing research is the process of systematic study or investigation to discover new knowledge or expand on existing knowledge
- The evidence-based-practice (EBP) approach helps NPs and other clinicians provide the highest-quality and most cost-efficient patient care possible.

Nursing Research Terminology

- **Primary sources** are research from where the original data originated (**PREFERRED**).
- **Secondary sources** are created when the original data is interpreted by another researcher.
- The **Institutional Review Board** (IRB) is an administrative body established to protect the rights and welfare of human research subjects recruited to participate in research activities conducted under the auspices of the institution with which it is affiliated.
- **Population vs. Sample**: A population includes all members of interest, whereas the sample includes only a portion (subset) of the population.
- **Sampling** is the process of selecting a subset of participants from the pool of all potential participants.
- A **variable** is an attribute or characteristic that can be measured and takes on different values (changes) among and between participants.
- An **independent variable** is an attribute or characteristic that the researcher manipulates or changes and which the researcher expects affects the dependent variable(s).
- A **dependent variable** is an attribute or characteristic that changes as a result of another variable (typically the independent variable).
- A **hypothesis** is an informed and educated prediction or explanation about a relationship or phenomena.
- **Qualitative** methods refer to a research approach that emphasizes nonnumerical data.
- **Quantitative** methods refer to a research approach that emphasizes numerical data.

- **Validity** is the degree to which we observe or measure what we think we are (precision).
- **Reliability** is the degree to which we will obtain the same results with repeated observations or measures (accuracy).
- **Bias** happens during a study that is not part of the research protocol and alters the results.
- **Generalizability** is the degree to which research results or patterns found in a sample population will also be found in the wider population that the sample represents.
- **Statistical significance** measures the probability of the null hypothesis being true compared to the acceptable level of uncertainty regarding the true answer. Usually represent as "P" value < .05 (5 percent probability that the results are due to chance) or < .01 (1 percent probability that the results are due to chance). For more information on nursing research, please refer to the work of Melnyk and Fineout-Overholt (2023) in the reference list.

Evidence-Based Practice

EBP is a process founded on the collecting, interpreting, appraising, and integrating of valid, clinically significant, and applicable research.

The seven steps of EBP process are

1. encouraging and supporting a spirit of inquiry.
2. asking questions.
3. searching for evidence.
4. appraising the evidence.
5. integrating evidence into practice.
6. evaluating outcomes.
7. sharing results.

The PICOT Question

The foundation of EBP is developing a PICOT question, which identifies the terms to be used to search for the best evidence to answer a clinical question.

P is for Patient, Population, or Problem (i.e., a disease or condition)
I is for Intervention (e.g., therapy, procedure, drug, exposure, test, strategy)
C is for Comparison (i.e., compared to an alternative intervention or an experimental control)
O is for Outcome (i.e., the consequence, effect, or improvement of interest and the measurement thereof)
T is for Time frame of treatment and/or measurable outcome (optional)

Levels of Evidence

Studies are assigned evidence levels (sometimes called a hierarchy of evidence) based on their research design, quality, and applicability to patient care. Higher levels of evidence have less risk of bias (Melnyk & Fineout-Overholt, 2023).

- Level I: Evidence from systematic reviews or meta-analysis of randomized control trials
- Level II: Evidence from well-designed randomized control trials
- Level III: Evidence from well-designed control trials that are not randomized
- Level IV: Evidence from case-control or cohort studies
- Level V: Evidence from systematic reviews of descriptive or qualitative studies
- Level VI: Evidence from a single descriptive or qualitative study
- Level VII: Evidence from expert opinions

> **Exam Tip**
>
> Other EBP models are the Iowa Model, the Advancing Research and Clinical Practice through Close Collaboration (ARCC) Model, the Star Model of Knowledge Transformation, and the John Hopkins Nursing Evidence-Based Practice (JHNEBP) Model.

Review Questions

1. The term "LACE" stands for which of the following?
   A. Licensure, accommodation, consensus, and education
   B. Licensure, accreditation, certification, and education
   C. Liberation, accommodation, consensus, and education
   D. Liberation, accreditation, certification, and education

2. A family nurse practitioner (FNP) sees a patient, Mr. A, who is HIV+. After the patient is gone, the next patient to be seen mentions she knows Mr. A and is aware he is HIV+ and is in an intimate relationship with someone who is unaware of the patient's status. Of the available choices below, choose the best response for the FNP.
   A. Mr. A is not HIV+, and I am not sure where you got that information.
   B. Please report your concerns to the local public health department, which can follow up on Mr. A's inappropriate behavior.
   C. Patient confidentiality and privacy are the basis for our clinical practice. Therefore, I do not discuss your or any other patient's information unless it is necessary for your health care.
   D. Thank you for the information. I will follow up on this.

3. Ms. J is being seen for various vague complaints, including malaise and mild body aches that have not gone away for several weeks. The initial workup included a complete blood count (CBC), comprehensive metabolic panel, mono-spot, and Lyme antibody. All tests were negative and/or within normal limits. Ms. J. wants a full-body magnetic resonance imaging test ordered and a prescription for an antibiotic "just in case." While formulating an appropriate response, the FNP is aware that balancing the basis for her response will depend on which of the following ethical concepts?
   A. Nonmaleficence and beneficence
   B. Virtue and action
   C. Justice and altruism
   D. Ecocentrism and procedural justice

4. A 15-year-old female patient is seen in the office. She discloses she has been having unprotected sexual intercourse with a 15-year-old male she has known for many years. She would like to discuss contraceptive options, but she is afraid to tell her mother. The best next step for the FNP is to:
   A. let the minor know the FNP cannot discuss contraception with her unless one parent or guardian is present.
   B. make an appointment for the patient to go to an STD clinic.
   C. assure the patient that the discussion will be confidential and review contraceptive options as well as possible STD testing.
   D. make a separate appointment in 2 weeks for the patient to return and have a full gynecological examination and discussion of options at that time.

5. Ms. K is a 28-year-old female patient who is very shy and can be indecisive. She has a small, nontender lump on her right breast. When the FNP recommends an ultrasound and possible mammogram, Ms. K is tearful and says she needs time to decide. After a few days of being unable to decide, the FNP calls her and says she made the appointments for her, so she has to go for testing. This concept is best described as which of the following?
   A. Aggressive medicine
   B. Nonmaleficence
   C. Paternalism
   D. Distributive justice

6. The Health Insurance Portability and Accountability Act of 1996 (HIPAA) mandated the use of which of the following to improve the efficiency and effectiveness of electronic records transmissions?
   A. National Provider Identification
   B. Medicare Provider Unique Number
   C. Healthcare Privacy Identifier
   D. Unique Insurance and Portability Number

7. An FNP is moving from Maine to Ohio. In addition to applying for a license in the new state, he is aware of the need to know which of the following?
   A. The Consensus Model enforces each state to provide the same licensing and scope of practice for all APRNs.
   B. Although many states have incorporated portions of the Consensus Model, there are varying requirements and practice acts among states.
   C. His license from Maine will be honored in most other states.
   D. All states have some form of physician supervision in the practice act.

8. A local medical center is advertising an advanced practice registered nurse (APRN) position. The FNP requests further information before applying for a position. The need to ask about the role for this position is important because:
   A. APRNs are not just nurse practitioners (NPs) but also certified nurse midwives (CNMs), certified registered nurse anesthetists (CRNAs), and clinical nurse specialists (CNSs).
   B. APRNs include NPs and clinical nurse leaders (CNLs).
   C. APRNs are specifically identified in each state and have the same scope of practice across the United States.
   D. All APRNs are nurses with master's degrees.

9. As an NP, you consistently strive for the best outcome in patient care. This highest standard of care is accomplished by:
   A. clinical expertise, skill, and good judgment.
   B. interprofessional collaboration, research, and patient history.
   C. research, clinical skill, and patient adherence.
   D. patient values, clinical expertise, and research knowledge.

10. A 45-year-old male and a 52-year-old male are seeking treatment options for increased prostate-specific antigen (PSA) levels. One of these men has no health insurance, and the other has very comprehensive coverage. The FNP knows they must offer both men the same options/recommendations based on which ethical principle?
    A. Maternalism
    B. Nonmaleficence
    C. Deontology
    D. Justice

11. A newly graduated, certified, and licensed FNP has taken a position in a large medical practice. The physicians repeatedly refer to him as a "mid-level provider" when introducing him to patients and the office staff. What is an appropriate next step to help inform the physicians and staff about using the term "mid-level"?
    A. Make copies of the position paper about using the term "mid-level" from AANP and leave it on the physicians' desks.
    B. Ask for a meeting with the lead physician of the practice to discuss some positive feedback about the role and the negative use of the term "mid-level." Offer other terms that would reflect a more positive image to patients and staff, such as "primary care or healthcare provider" and/or "clinician."
    C. Plan to discuss this at the next full staff meeting to let everyone know how insulting this has been and threaten to quit if it continues.
    D. Because this is the FNP's first job, it would be better to let them continue calling him a "mid-level" and address this in a year or so when they realize how competent he is.

12. Select two of the following examples of the FNP role as it relates to health policy and practice:
    A. Joining the local community center's board of directors
    B. Serving as a leader in the local Girl Scout troop
    C. Volunteering to work on increasing access to care for the local shelter for the unhoused
    D. Advocating for concussion evaluations and best-fit helmets for the local youth football league

13. The newly licensed FNP is seeing a patient with acute pain related to a severe ankle strain. The collaborating physician recommends that she write the patient a prescription for Tylenol #3 (acetaminophen with codeine). The FNP is aware of her state's law that requires which of the following to prescribe this medication?
    A. A state controlled-substances license and a Drug Enforcement Agency (DEA) registration certificate for Schedule III drugs
    B. A state APRN license and NPI registration number
    C. A federal license to practice and a state APRN license allowing her to prescribe Schedule I and II drugs.
    D. A state controlled-substances license and a state APRN registration license for Schedule II to IV drugs.

14. What must you do as an NP before billing visits?
    A. Establish a collaborative agreement with the physician
    B. Obtain a provider number and familiarize yourself with the rules and policies of the third-party payer
    C. Provide evidence of continuing medical education
    D. Have a DEA number.

15. An FNP is completing paperwork for a new position in a large hospital-based outpatient center. Forms to be signed include strict guidelines about physician supervision of the FNP and patient care. Which of the following statements is true?
    A. The institution can dictate whatever restrictions on physician oversight they prefer, even if FNPs are allowed to practice without supervision in that state.
    B. The institution cannot dictate that the FNP must be supervised when providing care in an outpatient setting if that state allows completely unsupervised practice.
    C. The FNP must report to the supervising physician on each patient seen before the end of the patient's medical visit.
    D. The FNP can sign the forms and then make an agreement with the chief medical officer about which patients can be seen without supervision.

16. The primary purpose of professional licensure is to:
    A. protect the public by ensuring a minimum standard for competency.
    B. ensure high nursing care standards.
    C. standardize nursing programs.
    D. grant prescriptive privileges.

17. Which of the following are ways one may risk breaching patient confidentiality?
    A. Leaving a patient's record within view
    B. Discussing the patient with the consulting surgeon
    C. Shredding duplicate records
    D. Confirming the patient's diagnosis over the telephone with the pharmacist

18. The levels of evaluation and management (E/M) services are based on which types of histories?
    A. Medical surgical
    B. Psychosocial
    C. Expanded problem focused
    D. Preoperative

19. In the primary care setting, the most common reason for a malpractice lawsuit is failure to:
    A. refer properly.
    B. diagnose correctly and in a timely manner.
    C. obtain informed consent.
    D. manage fractures and traumas correctly.

20. Advanced directives, such as a healthcare proxy and durable power of attorney, are important for all clients to consider. Unmarried persons may preserve their healthcare wishes by:
    A. executing a durable power of attorney for health care.
    B. drafting a letter stating that their next of kin is not this authorized decision maker.
    C. signing an institutional document stating that the healthcare provider can make all healthcare decisions for the client.
    D. having one partner declared legally incompetent.

21. The research function of the NP may be operationalized as both a consumer of research findings and a researcher. Being a consumer of research findings involves several activities, including:
    A. reading the literature, analyzing its clinical applicability, and using new interventions.
    B. organizing and conducting a research study.
    C. collecting data.
    D. ensuring protection of human subjects.

22. What conditions must be met for the nurse practitioner (NP) to bill "incident-to" in order to receive 100 percent reimbursement for Medicare?
    A. The NP must initiate the plan of care for the patient.
    B. The physician must be on-site and engaged in the patient care.
    C. The NP must be employed as an independent contractor.
    D. The NP must be the main healthcare provider who sees the patient.

23. The term "collaboration" is best defined as:
    A. intra-professional teamwork.
    B. a signed protocol agreement with a physician.
    C. case management approach to care.
    D. a cooperative relationship with another provider to achieve mutual goals and provide the best patient care.

24. Social determinants of health (SDOH) are influenced by the following factors (select all that apply):
    A. Adequate housing
    B. Access to affordable, healthy food
    C. Access to comprehensive health care
    D. Treatment of infectious disease

25. What is the difference between an advanced directive and a physician order for life-sustaining treatment (POLST)?
    A. There is no difference; they are both documents that help ensure patients receive the care they want and avoid the care they don't want.
    B. The patient completes the advanced directive at any stage of life, while the family signs a POLST form when the patient is near death.
    C. A POLST form is a medical order focusing on end-of-life decisions that require immediate medical attention.
    D. A POLST form is required for hospice care, and advanced directives are not required.

Answers and Rationales

1. Answer B is correct. "LACE" stands for licensure, accreditation, certification, and education.

   Answers A, C, and D are incorrect.

2. Answer C is correct. Of the available choices, the FNP should respond, "Patient confidentiality and privacy are the basis for our clinical practice. Therefore, I do not discuss your or any other patient's information unless it is necessary for your health care."

   Answers A, B, and D are incorrect.

3. Answer A is correct. The FNP is balancing the ethical concepts of nonmaleficence (do no harm

by ordering unnecessary procedures and medications) and beneficence (NP's obligation to act for the benefit of their patient).

Answer B is incorrect. Virtue and action concern a person's entire life, not just a point in time and specific action. A virtuous person would act the same way in the same situation.

Answer C is incorrect. Justice involves fairness, equality, and equitable treatment, and altruism concerns the welfare and well-being of others.

Answer D is incorrect. Ecocentrism emphasizes the importance of environmental factors in health, and procedural justice concerns fairness in the processes of resource allocation.

4. Answer C is correct. The FNP should assure the female patient that the discussion will be confidential and then review contraceptive options, as well as possible STD testing.

Answer A is incorrect. The NP must review the applicable state law of medical treatment for minors. NPs have an ethical duty to promote minors' developing autonomy by involving them in decisions about their health care to the degree that's appropriate for their abilities. They also have a responsibility to protect the confidentiality of their minor patients.

Answer B is incorrect. Referring the patient to an STD clinic may cause the patient to lose trust in the NP.

Answer D is incorrect. While it may be appropriate to have the patient return in 2 weeks for an examination and discussion of treatment options, the NP didn't address the patient's concerns during the visit, and she may get pregnant before the follow-up visit.

5. Answer C is correct. The concept is best described as paternalism when the NP makes decisions for a patient without their explicit consent, based on the belief that the decisions are in the patient's best interest.

Answer A is incorrect. "Aggressive medicine" is typically reserved for treatments that are more severe or intense than normal and could potentially cause harm (e.g., feeding tubes, resuscitation, emergency surgery).

Answer B is incorrect. Nonmaleficence requires the NP to consider the benefits of procedures and weigh them against the potential risks and burdens on the patient.

Answer D is incorrect. Distributive justice is the fair distribution of resources, goods, and opportunities within a society, accounting for factors such as wealth, income, and social status, and does not fit in this case.

6. Answer A is correct. HIPAA mandated using National Provider Identification to improve the efficiency and effectiveness of electronic records' transmissions.

Answers B, C, and D are incorrect.

7. Answer B is correct. Although many states have incorporated portions of the Consensus Model, there are varying requirements and practice acts among states.

Answers A, C, and D are incorrect.

8. Answer A is correct. APRNs are not just NPs but also CNMs, CRNAs, and CNSs.

Answer B is incorrect. CNLs have master's degrees with some overlap in curricula but do not have prescribing privileges and are not considered APRNs.

Answer C is incorrect. APRNs' roles vary according to individual state statutes, rules, and regulations.

Answer D is incorrect. APRNs may hold both master's degrees and doctoral degrees.

9. Answer D is correct. Evidence-based practice aims for the best outcome. Combining clinical expertise, research findings, and the patient's preferences will lead to individualized care and, thus, high-quality results.

Answers A, B, and C are incorrect. While skill, good judgment, and interprofessional collaboration are important elements of patient care, they are not key elements for meeting standards of care.

10. Answer D is correct. Justice involves fairness, equality, and equitable treatment.

Answer A is incorrect. Maternalism is the public expression of domestic values associated with motherhood.

Answer B is incorrect. Nonmaleficence is an ethical principle that means to avoid or minimize harm.

Answer C is incorrect. Deontology is the philosophy that judges an act as moral or good based on the intentions of the individual committing the act and the duties the person is obligated to uphold.

11. Answer B is correct. The FNP should ask for a meeting with the practice's lead physician to discuss positive feedback about the role, discuss the negative use of the term "mid-level," and offer other terms that would reflect a more positive image to patients and staff, such as "primary care or healthcare provider" and/or "clinician."

    Answer A is incorrect. Leaving copies of a position paper on the physicians' desk is passive and may not get read.

    Answer C is incorrect. Bringing the issue to a full staff meeting and threatening to quit is unprofessional.

    Answer D is incorrect. Saying nothing because you are a new graduate is passive and will reinforce using the term in the office.

12. Answers C and D are correct. Two examples of the FNP role as it relates to health policy and practice are volunteering to work on increasing access to care for the local shelter for the unhoused and advocating for concussion evaluations and best-fit helmets for the local youth football league.

    Answers A and B are incorrect. While joining the local community center's board of directors and serving as a leader in the local Girl Scout troop are examples of community service, they have a local impact on the community but not at the health policy level.

13. Answer A is correct. A state controlled-substance license and a DEA registration certificate for schedule III drugs would be needed.

    Answer B is incorrect. While a state APRN license and NPI registration number are needed to practice, a DEA registration certificate is mandatory to prescribe a controlled substance.

    Answer C is incorrect. NPs hold a state APRN license and not a federal license, and it is mandatory to have a DEA registration certificate to prescribe a controlled substance.

    Answer D is incorrect. Most states require a state controlled-substances license in addition to a federal DEA number to prescribe Schedule II–V drugs.

14. Answer B is correct. To bill clients for services, the NP must obtain a provider or panel membership as needed and familiarize themselves with each payer's rules and policies.

    Answers A, C, and D are incorrect. Some, but not all, states require a collaborative agreement with the physician for you to practice. In some states, you can provide controlled substances, which requires a DEA number. Other states do not allow you to prescribe controlled substances. Currently, you are not required to have a specific number of continuing medical education credits to bill for services provided.

15. Answer A is correct. The institution can dictate whatever restrictions on physician oversight they prefer, even if FNPs can practice without supervision in that state. Answers B, C, and D are incorrect.

16. Answer A is correct. The primary purpose of professional licensure is to protect the public from unsafe practitioners by ensuring a minimum standard for competency. Licensure is the legal status granted by a regulating authority.

    Answer B is incorrect. Licensure does not ensure high nursing standards; passage of a national certification exam is designed to assess minimum competency for safe practice.

    Answer C is incorrect. Nursing programs retain autonomy over their curricula.

    Answer D is incorrect. Although the licensing statutes may spell out prescriptive privileges for nurse practitioners, they do not necessarily do that, nor is that the primary purpose of professional licensure.

17. Answer A is correct. Leaving a patient's record within view, talking about a patient within close proximity to others, discussing the patient's medical condition with a family member, and leaving a detailed message on an answering machine are examples of breaching patient confidentiality.

    Answer B is incorrect. Discussing the patient with the consulting surgeon is necessary to provide proper care.

    Answer C is incorrect. Shredding duplicate records is a way of protecting patient confidentiality.

    Answer D is incorrect. To provide proper patient care, the client must confirm the pharmacist's diagnosis over the telephone.

18. Answer C is correct. The levels of evaluation and management (E/M) services are based on four types of histories: (1) problem focused, (2) expanded problem focused, (3) detailed, and (4) comprehensive.

    Answers A, B, and D are incorrect.

19. Answer B is correct. Failure to diagnose in the primary care setting is the most common reason for a malpractice lawsuit. Approximately one-third of malpractice cases brought against nurse practitioners involve cases of failure to diagnose in a timely manner. These cases typically involve breast and lung cancer.

    Answers A, C, and D are incorrect. Failure to refer, failure to manage fractures, and lack of informed consent may also be reasons for malpractice but are not as common as failure to diagnose.

20. Answer A is correct. The durable power of attorney authorizes another person or agent to make medical decisions on behalf of an individual if the client becomes unable or unwilling to make those decisions.

    Answers B, C, and D are incorrect.

21. Answer A is correct. Reading the literature, analyzing its clinical applicability, and using new interventions are consistent with evidence-based practice and being a good consumer of that process.

    Answers B, C, and D are incorrect. These are all steps in the nursing research process.

22. Answer B is correct. The term "incident-to" implies that your services as an NP are performed in connection with a physician. The physician must be on-site when the care is provided.

    Answer A is incorrect. The physician, not the NP, must have initiated the patient's care plan.

    Answer C is incorrect. If the NP is employed as an independent contractor, they can only be reimbursed at 85 percent from Medicare.

    Answer D is incorrect. The physician must have input and ongoing patient involvement.

23. Answer D is correct. The term "collaboration" is best defined as cooperation with another to achieve mutual patient goals without the individual's personal agenda getting in the way.

    Answer A is incorrect. While collaboration is the foundation of interprofessional teamwork, it is not the definition of "collaboration."

    Answer B is incorrect. A signed protocol agreement with a physician implies a hierarchical relationship.

    Answer C is incorrect. The case management approach to care is the coordination of services for a patient.

24. Answers A, B, and C are correct. These are key factors that can support the health of the community at large. Adequate housing; access to affordable, healthy food; and access to health care, safe community, economic stability, and education are all essential components of SDOH.

    Answer D is incorrect. Activities to prevent infectious disease would be an example of an SDOH, not treatment.

25. Answer C is correct. A POLST form is a medical order that focuses on end-of-life decisions that require immediate medical attention. POLSTs are intended for people who are seriously ill, frail, or near the end of their lives.

    Answer A is incorrect. While they both ensure the patient's wishes for treatment are followed, advanced directives are patient initiated or initiated by an appointed legal healthcare agent who can make medical decisions if the patient can't communicate. A medical order signed by a healthcare professional, usually a doctor or NP, outlines a patient's wishes for medical treatment in a medical emergency.

    Answer B is incorrect. The patient can complete the advanced directive at any stage of life; however, the medical professional signs a POLST form when the patient is near death.

    Answer D is incorrect. A POLST form is not required for hospice or palliative care. While advance directives are not required for hospice care, they can help ensure the patient's wishes are respected and the best care is rendered.

Resources

American Association of Nurse Practitioners (AANP). (2025). Practice Information by States: What you need to know about NP practice in your state. https://www.aanp.org/practice/practice-information-by-state

American Association of Colleges of Nursing (AACN). (2023). *2022–2023 enrollment and graduations in baccalaureate and graduate programs in nursing.* AACN.

American Association of Nurse Practitioners. (2022). *Use of terms such as mid-level provider and physician extender.* https://www.aanp.org/advocacy/advocacy-resource/position-statements/use-of-terms-such-as-mid-level-provider-and-physician-extender

American Association of Colleges of Nursing (AACN). (2008). Consensus Model for APRN Regulation: Licensure, Accreditation, Certification & Education. https://www.aacnnursing.org/Portals/0/PDFs/Teaching-Resources/APRNReport.pdf

Buppert, C. (2023). *Nurse practitioner's business practice and legal guide* (8th ed.). Jones & Bartlett Learning.

Center for Medicare and Medicaid Services (CMS, 2022). *NPI: what you need to know.* https://www.cms.gov/outreach-and

-education/medicare-learning-network-mln/mlnproducts/downloads/npi-what-you-need-to-know.pdf

DeNisco, S. (2024) *Advanced practice nursing: Evolving roles for the transformation of the profession* (5th ed.). Jones & Bartlett Learning.

DeNisco, S. (2023). *Role development of the nurse practitioner* (3rd ed.). Jones & Bartlett Learning.

Department of Health and Human Services. (2007). Direct Billing and Payment for Non-Physician Practitioner Services Furnished to Hospital Inpatients and Outpatients. https://www.hhs.gov/guidance/document/direct-billing-and-payment-non-physician-practitioner-services-furnished-hospital

Drug Enforcement. (2024). *Mid-level practitioners authorization by state.* Office of Diversion Control. https://www.deadiversion.usdoj.gov/drugreg/practioners/practioners.html#:~:text=Examples%20of%20mid%2Dlevel%20practitioners,state%20in%20which%20they%20practice

Grace, P., & Uveges, M. K. (2023). *Nursing ethics and professional responsibility in advanced practice* (4th ed.). Jones & Bartlett Learning.

Institute of Medicine. (2011). *The future of nursing: Leading change, advancing health.* National Academies Press.

Kueakomoldej, S., Turi, E., McMenamin, A., Xue, Y., & Poghosyan, L. (2022). Recruitment and retention of primary care nurse practitioners in underserved areas: A scoping review. *Nursing Outlook, 70*(3), 401–416. https://doi.org/10.1016/j.outlook.2021.12.008

Melnyk, B., & Fineout-Overholt, E. (2023). *Evidence-based practice in nursing & healthcare: A guide to best practice* (5th ed.). Wolters Kluwer.

National Academies of Sciences, Engineering, and Medicine; National Academy of Medicine; Committee on the Future of Nursing 2020–2030; Flaubert, J. L.; Le Menestrel, S.; Williams, D. R.; & Wakefield, M. K. (Eds.). (2021). *The future of nursing 2020-2030: Charting a path to achieve health equity.* National Academies Press.

National Council of State Boards of Nursing. (2008). *The consensus model for APRN regulation: A guide for advanced practice registered nurses (APRNs).* https://www.ncsbn.org/nursing-regulation/practice/aprn.page

National Task Force. (2022). *Standards for quality nurse practitioner education. A report of the National Task Force on Quality Nurse Practitioner Education* (6th ed.). https://cdn.ymaws.com/www.nonpf.org/resource/resmgr/ntfstandards/ntfs_final.pdf

National Organization of Nurse Practitioner Faculties. (2024). *Competency implementation guide for nurse practitioner faculty.* https://cdn.ymaws.com/www.nonpf.org/resource/resmgr/np_competencies_&_ntf_standards/NP_Competency_Implementation.pdf

National Organization of Nurse Practitioner Faculties. (2025). *NP Competencies & DNP Resources.* https://www.nonpf.org/page/DNP_NPCompetencies

National POLST. (2022). *Directory of POLST programs.* https://polst.org/state-polst-programs/

National Task Force on Quality Nurse Practitioner Education. (2022). *Standards for quality nurse practitioner education* (6th ed.). American Association of Colleges of Nursing. https://cdn.ymaws.com/www.nonpf.org/resource/resmgr/ntfstandards/ntfs_final.pdf

U.S. Department of Health and Human Services. (2024, September 27). *The HIPAA Privacy Rule.* https://www.hhs.gov/hipaa/for-professionals/privacy/index.html#:~:text=The%20HIPAA%20Privacy%20Rule%20establishes,care%20providers%20that%20conduct%20certain

PART II

Health Promotion and Pharmacology Review

CHAPTER 4	Health Promotion and Disease Prevention	37
CHAPTER 5	Pharmacology	53

CHAPTER 4

Health Promotion and Disease Prevention

Susan M. DeNisco, DNP, APRN, FNP-BC, FAANP
Nancy L. Dennert, MS, MSN, FNP-BC, CDCES, BC-ADM

Since the role's inception, health promotion and disease prevention have been the cornerstone of nurse practitioner (NP) practice. Health promotion requires a thorough understanding of an individual's past and present medical history and an assessment of their physical, mental, psychosocial, and educational needs. The focus of health promotion is to help the individual make informed decisions about their health and well-being and empower them to make better health choices and lifestyle changes to help prevent chronic disease.

Much of the information that the family nurse practitioner (FNP) can obtain regarding health promotion and disease prevention may be found by using established and recognized guidelines.

- The National Center for Chronic Disease Prevention and Health Promotion of the Centers for Disease Control and Prevention (CDC) provides recommendations for individuals throughout their lifespan (NCCDPHP, 2025).
- The USPSTF (United States Preventative Services Task Force) is an organization that makes evidence-based recommendations for primary and secondary prevention strategies. (USPSTF, 2025a).
- Through the CDC, the Advisory Committee on Immunizations Practices (ACIP) makes recommendations for vaccinations (CDC, 2025).
- The Women's Preventive Services Initiative (WPSI) makes appropriate recommendations for females (WPSI, 2024).
- The American College of Obstetrics and Gynecology (ACOG, 2025).
- The American Cancer Society (ACS, 2023).
- American Academy of Pediatrics (AAP) *Bright Futures: Guidelines for Health Supervision of Infants, Children and Adolescents*, Fourth Edition (Hagan et al., 2017).

Disease Prevention

Disease prevention, understood as specific, population-based, and individual-based interventions for primary and secondary (early detection) prevention, aims to minimize the burden of diseases and associated risk factors.

Health Promotion

Health promotion empowers people to increase control over their health and its determinants through health literacy efforts and multisectoral action to increase healthy behaviors. This process includes activities for the community or populations at increased risk of negative health outcomes.

Health promotion activities are targeted at the following behavioral risk factors:

- tobacco use
- obesity, diet, and physical inactivity
- mental health, injury prevention, drug use control, alcohol control
- health behavior related to HIV and sexual health

Health Promotion and Prevention Applied to Specific Diseases

- Coronary artery disease
- Stroke
- Alcohol and substance misuse
- Cancers
- Osteoporosis
- Sexually transmitted diseases
- Infectious diseases
- Chronic obstructive pulmonary disease
- Accidents
- Diabetes
- Glaucoma

See **Table 4-1** for the leading causes of death in the United States (CDC, 2022).

Levels of Prevention

Primordial Prevention

- Policy efforts that target the underlying social conditions that promote disease onset
- Improving access to safe sidewalks and playgrounds in urban neighborhoods to promote physical activity in children and prevent childhood obesity and type 2 diabetes, and so on.
- Education aimed to prevent children and adolescents from adopting unhealthy behaviors (e.g., tobacco and illicit drug use)

Primary Prevention

Primary prevention aims to prevent a disease or injury before it occurs. This can be done by changing risky or unhealthy behaviors and increasing disease resistance to infectious diseases. Some examples of primary prevention are

- using seat belts and helmets and banning hazardous products;
- providing education about healthy habits, such as quitting smoking, eating healthy meals, and exercising regularly;
- immunizing against infectious diseases; and
- promoting micronutrient supplementation programs for pregnant and lactating women, young children, and nonpregnant women, especially adolescent girls.

Secondary Prevention

Secondary prevention aims to reduce the impact of the disease or the injury that has already occurred. This is done by treating the disease as soon as possible to slow or halt the progression, encouraging strategies to prevent recurrence, and implementing programs to return people to their original health. Some examples of secondary prevention are

- screening tests to detect disease in the early stages, such as mammograms, colonoscopies, or Papanicolaou (Pap) smears;
- blood pressure screening;
- bone density screening;
- lipid screening;
- a daily low dose of aspirin in appropriate populations to prevent MIs or strokes; and
- modifications in the workplace so that an injured worker may continue safely doing their job.

Tertiary Prevention

The goal of tertiary prevention is to decrease the impact of an ongoing illness or injury. This is done by helping the patient manage their chronic disease or permanent impairment to let them function as much as possible and improve their quality of life and life expectancy. Examples include

- chronic disease management programs, such as diabetic programs, arthritis, or depression;
- occupational and physical therapy in burn patients;
- Cardiac rehab in postmyocardial infarction patients;
- diabetic foot care; and
- vocational rehabilitation programs to assist workers in new jobs once they have recovered as much as possible.

Table 4-1 Leading Causes of Death in the United States Age Adjusted (Center for Disease Control, 2022)

- Heart disease
- Cancer
- Accidents (unintentional injuries, suicide)
- COVID-19
- Stroke (cerebrovascular diseases)
- Chronic lower respiratory diseases (COPD, influenza, pneumonia)
- Alzheimer's disease
- Diabetes
- Nephritis, nephrotic syndrome, and nephrosis
- Chronic liver disease and cirrhosis

Center for Disease Control (CDC). (2022). *National Center for Health Statistics: Leading Causes of Death.* https://www.cdc.gov/nchs/fastats/leading-causes-of-death.htm

Quaternary Prevention

Quaternary prevention is the set of health activities that mitigate or avoid the consequences of unnecessary or excessive intervention of the health system. Examples include

- the appropriate use of antibiotics in upper respiratory tract infections,
- protection against unnecessary interventions, and
- avoidance of screening without evidence, such as in prostate cancer.

Guide to Clinical Preventative Services: The USPSTF Recommendations

1. Recommendations are based on a review of current best evidence.
2. Suggest criteria for screening.
3. Provide classification codes regarding the strength of recommendation and the quality of the evidence (**Table 4-2**).

Criteria for Screening

- Screening is to be distinguished from diagnostic evaluation.
- Screening presumes that the patient has no symptoms.
- Screening should be based on the patient's risk factor profile.

Characteristics of the Disease Targeted for Screening

- The targeted disease should be serious and sufficiently prevalent in the screened group to justify the costs and risks of screening.
- The patient's risk of future morbidity and mortality must be reduced due to early detection of the condition.
- The screening maneuver itself must be acceptable to the patient.

Characteristics of the Screening Test

Sensitivity

- A sensitive test will identify people with the disease or the percent of positive test results.

Table 4-2 USPTF Strength of Recommendations

- Grade A = Good Evidence: The USPSTF recommends the service. There is high certainty that the net benefit is substantial.
- Grade B = Fair Evidence: The USPSTF recommends the service. There is high certainty that the net benefit is moderate, or there is moderate certainty that the net benefit is moderate to substantial.
- Grade C = No recommendation: The USPSTF recommends against routinely providing the service. There may be considerations that support providing the service in an individual patient. There is at least moderate certainty that the net benefit is small.
- Grade D = Recommends against in asymptomatic: The USPSTF recommends against the service. There is moderate or high certainty that the service has no net benefit or that the harms outweigh the benefits.
- Grade I = Insufficient Evidence: The USPSTF concludes that the current evidence is insufficient to assess the balance of benefits and harms of the service. Evidence is lacking, of poor quality, or is conflicting, and the balance of benefits and harms cannot be determined.

Modified from U.S. Preventive Services Task Force. (2018). Grade Definitions. https://www.uspreventiveservicestaskforce.org/uspstf/about-uspstf/methods-and-processes/grade-definitions

- Sensitive tests show a positive result when an asymptomatic condition is truly present.
- A test with 95 percent sensitivity will generate a positive result for 95 percent of people with the disease but will return a negative result (a false negative) for 5 percent of people with the disease.
- Urine HCG is 99 percent sensitive for detection of early pregnancy if done correctly.
- The sensitivity of digital mammography is about 87 percent (i.e., mammography correctly identifies about 87 percent of women who have breast cancer).

Specificity

- A specific screening test will reveal a negative result when the disease is absent.
- A specific test can eliminate people who do not have the disease.
- Nonspecific tests will yield many false positives.
- Rapid strep tests have very high specificity—in the 98 to 99 percent range—so there are very few false positives.
- Breast biopsy is the most specific test for breast cancer.

Cancer Screening

- The top cancer deaths for all ages and sexes are lung, colorectal, pancreatic, and breast cancer.
- Cancer is more common in older adults; 80 percent of all cancer diagnoses in the United States are in people 55 years and older.
- Around one-third of deaths from cancer are due to tobacco use, high body mass index, alcohol consumption, low fruit and vegetable intake, and lack of physical activity.
- **Table 4-3** (USPTF, 2025b) provides select USPTF recommendations for cancer screening.
- Review other screening guidelines mentioned on the first page of this chapter.

Select United States Preventative Task Force Common Screening Recommendations for Adults in the Primary Care Setting

Recommendation for Aspirin ASA in Adults to Prevent Cardiovascular Disease

- For adults aged 40 to 59 years with an estimated 10 percent or greater 10-year cardiovascular disease (CVD) risk: The decision to initiate low-dose

Table 4-3 United States Preventative Task Force Cancer A and B Cancer Screening Recommendations

Topic	Description	Grade	Release Date of Current Recommendation
Colorectal Cancer: Screening: adults aged 45–49 years	The USPSTF recommends screening for colorectal cancer in adults aged 45–49 years.	B	May 2021*
Breast Cancer: Screening: women aged 40–74 years	The USPSTF recommends biennial screening mammography for women aged 40–74 years.	B	April 2024*
Cervical Cancer: Screening: women aged 21–65 years	The USPSTF recommends screening for cervical cancer every 3 years with cervical cytology alone in women aged 21–29 years. For women aged 30–65 years, the USPSTF recommends screening every 3 years with cervical cytology alone, every 5 years with high-risk human papillomavirus (hrHPV) testing alone, or every 5 years with hrHPV testing in combination with cytology (cotesting). See the Clinical Considerations section for the relative benefits and harms of alternative screening strategies for women 21 years or older.	A	August 2018*
Lung Cancer: Screening: adults aged 50–80 years who have a 20 pack-year smoking history and currently smoke or have quit within the past 15 years	The USPSTF recommends annual screening for lung cancer with low-dose computed tomography (LDCT) in adults aged 50–80 years who have a 20 pack-year smoking history and currently smoke or have quit within the past 15 years. Screening should be discontinued once a person has not smoked for 15 years or develops a health problem that substantially limits life expectancy or the ability or willingness to have curative lung surgery.	B	March 2021*
Skin Cancer Prevention: Behavioral Counseling: young adults, adolescents, children, and parents of young children	The USPSTF recommends counseling young adults, adolescents, children, and parents of young children about minimizing exposure to ultraviolet (UV) radiation for persons aged 6 months to 24 years with fair skin types to reduce their risk of skin cancer.	B	March 2018*

Data from U.S. Preventive Services Task Force. (2018). Final recommendation statement: Unhealthy alcohol use in adolescents and adults: Screening and behavioral counseling interventions. Retrieved from https://www.uspreventiveservicestaskforce.org/uspstf/recommendation/unhealthy-alcohol-use-in-adolescents-and-adults-screening-and-behavioral-counseling-interventions

aspirin use for the primary prevention of CVD in this group should be an individual one. (Grade C)
- For adults 60 years or older: Do not initiate aspirin for the primary prevention of CVD. (Grade D)

Recommendation for Screening for Abdominal Aortic Aneurysm in Adult Men

- Screen males aged 65 to 75 years once with abdominal ultrasound if any history of smoking. (Grade B)
- Selectively offer screening for abdominal aortic aneurysm (AAA) for men aged 65 to 75 years who have never smoked rather than routinely screening all men in this group. (Grade C)

Recommendation for Screening for Prostate Cancer

- For men aged 55 to 69 years, the decision to undergo periodic prostate-specific antigen (PSA)-based screening for prostate cancer should be an individual one. Before deciding whether to be screened, men should have an opportunity to discuss the potential benefits and harms of screening with their clinician and incorporate their values and preferences in the decision. (Grade C)
- The USPSTF recommends against PSA-based screening for prostate cancer in men 70 years and older. (Grade D)

Recommendation for Screening for Ovarian Cancer

- For asymptomatic women without a known high-risk hereditary cancer syndrome, do not screen for ovarian cancer. (Grade D)

Recommendations for Fall Prevention in Community Dwelling Adults

- The USPSTF recommends exercise interventions to prevent falls in community-dwelling adults 65 years or older who are at increased risk for falls. (Grade B)

Recommendations for Osteoporosis Screening to Prevent Fractures in Women

- For women 65 years and older, the USPSTF recommends screening for osteoporosis with bone measurement testing to prevent osteoporotic fractures. (Grade B)

Recommendations for Screening for Prediabetes and Type 2 Diabetes: Screening

- For adults aged 35 to 70 years who are overweight or obese, screen for prediabetes and type 2 diabetes and offer or refer patients with prediabetes to effective preventive interventions. (Grade B)

Recommendations for Screening for Human Immunodeficiency Virus (HIV) Infection

- Screen for HIV infection in all pregnant persons, including those who present in labor or at delivery whose HIV status is unknown. (Grade A)
- Screen for HIV infection in adolescents and adults aged 15 to 65 years. (Grade A)
- Younger adolescents and older adults at increased risk of infection should also be screened. (Grade A)

Recommendations for Depression and Suicide Risk Screening in Adults

- Screen for major depressive disorder (MDD) in adults, including pregnant and postpartum persons and older adults (65 years or older). (Grade B)

Recommendations for Screening and Behavioral Counseling and Interventions: Unhealthy Alcohol Use in Adolescents and Adults

- Screen for unhealthy alcohol use in primary care settings in adults 18 years or older, including pregnant women, and provide persons engaged in risky drinking with brief behavioral counseling interventions to reduce unhealthy alcohol use. (Grade B)
- The current evidence is insufficient to assess the balance of benefits and harms of screening and brief behavioral counseling interventions for alcohol use in primary care settings in adolescents aged 12 to 17 years. (Grade I)
- Audit C-screening tool that detects unhealthy alcohol use in adults.
- CAGE questionnaire for alcohol use.

See Chapter 7 for Screening and Treatment of Tuberculosis.

See Chapter 15 for Sexually Transmitted Disease Guidelines.

Interventions for Tobacco Users Based on Patient's Willingness to Quit

- Ask
- Advise
- Assess
- Arrange

Immunizations Schedules and Exam Tips

The review of immunizations will focus on ACIP through the CDC recommendations for vaccinations (CDC, 2025).

See **Table 4-4** for the recommended adult immunization schedule for people aged 19 or older (CDC, 2025).

This review is not inclusive, and you should refer to the CDC for complete information.

General Principles of Immunizations

- Defer vaccine for any person with a history of anaphylactic reaction to a vaccine.
- When in doubt of patient's vaccine history, re-immunize.
- Do not defer a vaccine if patient has a minor illness.
- Only defer a vaccine if patient has a moderate to severe illness with or without fever.
- Anaphylaxis following a vaccine may include hives, angioedema, respiratory compromise, sudden decreased blood pressure, and gastrointestinal (GI) symptoms.
- Administer vaccines in settings where there is personnel and equipment for rapid recognition and treatment of anaphylactic reactions.

Influenza Vaccine Fast Facts

- Do not give to infants ≤ 6 months old
- Do not give to people with severe life-threatening allergies to components of the influenza vaccine (i.e., gelatin, gentamycin preservative)
- Patients allergic to egg who only experience hives may receive the influenza vaccine.
- People with egg allergies no longer need to be observed for 30 minutes after the vaccine.
- Recombinant (RIV-4) or cell-cultured vaccines are an option for patients who refuse an egg-based vaccine.
- Avoid vaccine if patient has a history of Guillain-Barré syndrome (GBS) within 6 weeks of receiving a prior influenza vaccine.
- Antibodies take 2 weeks to develop following a flu vaccine.
- Administer from October to March (fall–winter season). Peak flu season is January but can last until May.
- Avoid getting vaccinated too early (July, August) because protection will decrease later in the season.

Active Versus Passive Immunity

Active Immunity	Passive Immunity
<ul><li>results when exposure to a disease organism triggers the immune system to produce antibodies to that disease.</li><li>can be acquired through natural immunity or vaccine-induced immunity.</li><li>takes time (usually several weeks) to develop.</li></ul>Examples:<ul><li>Resistance developed due to acquiring the common cold</li><li>Developing chicken pox</li><li>Varicella vaccine</li></ul>	<ul><li>acquired when a person is given antibodies to a disease rather than producing them through their own immune system.</li><li>gives immediate protection from a specific disease.</li><li>only lasts a few months.</li></ul>Examples:<ul><li>Newborn baby acquires passive immunity from its mother through the placenta.</li><li>Monoclonal antibodies to treat cancer.</li><li>Antibody-containing blood products such as immune globulin.</li></ul>

Health Promotion and Disease Prevention Case Study

History of Present Illness

A 65-year-old female has a history of 20 pack-years of cigarette smoking and quit smoking 10 years ago. She has an established diagnosis of emphysema. She is seen in her primary care provider's office for complaints of increased fatigue, worsening cough, and a low-grade fever. The patient recently was on vacation and traveled by airplane. She returned home 7 days ago. The patient states that before traveling, she took a COVID-19 home test for screening purposes, and it was negative.

Pertinent Past Medical History

As noted above, the patient has an established diagnosis of emphysema. She had a lung cancer screening performed 15 months ago using low-dose computed tomography (LDCT). She is up to date with vaccinations, including PCV15 and PPSV 23. She received the current annual flu vaccination and four COVID-19 vaccinations, with the most recent vaccine being a booster 6 months ago.

Table 4-4 Adult Immunization Schedule by Age: Recommendations for Ages 19 Years or Older (CDC, 2025)

Immunization	Immunization Schedule and Information
COVID-19	Recommends 2024–2025 COVID-19 vaccines as authorized or approved by FDA in persons ≥ 6 months of age. Persons ≥ 65 years of age should receive an additional dose of 2023–2024 formula COVID-19 vaccine.
Influenza inactivated (IIV4) or Influenza recombinant (RIV4) Or Influenza live attenuated (LAIV4)	Administer from October to March (fall–winter season). Peak flu season is January. Routine annual influenza vaccination recommended for all persons ≥ 6 months who do not have contraindications. Contraindicated in patients with allergy to eggs (if allergy is only hives can administer). Fluzone high dose may be more effective in patients > 65 years old.
Respiratory Syncytial Virus (RSV)	A single dose of RSV vaccine recommended for adults ≥ 75 years old. A single dose of RSV vaccine recommended for adults 60–74 years old who are at an increased risk of severe RSV disease.
Tetanus, diphtheria, pertussis (Tdap or Td)	Every 10 years 1 dose Tdap each pregnancy 1 dose Td/Tdap for wound management
Measles, mumps, rubella (MMR)	No evidence of immunity to measles, mumps, or rubella: 1 dose
Varicella (VAR)	2 doses if born in or after 1980
Zoster recombinant (RZV) Shingrix	Age ≥ 50 years: 2-dose series RZV (Shingrix) 2–6 months apart (minimum interval: 4 weeks; repeat dose if administered too soon) regardless of previous case of herpes zoster or history of zoster vaccine live (Zostavax)
Human papillomavirus (HPV)	2 or 3 doses depending on age at initial vaccination or condition (9–26 years old) or (27–45 years old)
Pneumococcal (PCV15, PCV20, PPSV23)	Age ≥ 65 years: Give pneumovax (PPSV23) Previously received a dose of PCV13, PCV15, or PCV20 or whose previous vaccination history is unknown: 1 dose PCV15 OR 1 dose PCV20. Do not give PPSV23 if patient is immunocompromised, has a cochlear implant, or cerebrospinal fluid (CSF) leak
Hepatitis A (HepA)	2, 3, or 4 doses depending on vaccine
Hepatitis B (HepB)	2, 3, or 4 doses depending on vaccine or condition Check immunity status for booster vaccine
Meningococcal A, C, W, Y (MenACWY)	1 or 2 doses depending on indication
Meningococcal B (MenB)	Ages 16–23 years old; 2 or 3 doses depending on vaccine and indication
Haemophilus influenzae type b (Hib)	1 or 3 doses depending on indication
Mpox	Any person at risk for Mpox infection: 2-dose series, 28 days apart Risk factors for Mpox infection include persons who are gay, bisexual, men who had sex with men (MSM), transgender or nonbinary people who in the past 6 months have had high-risk sexual activity and/or an STD.

Data from Center for Disease Control and Prevention. (2024). Adult Immunization Schedule by Age (Addendum updated June 27, 2024) Recommendations for Ages 19 Years or Older, United States, 2024. https://www.cdc.gov/vaccines/hcp/imz-schedules/adult-age.html?CDC_AAref_Val=https://www.cdc.gov/vaccines/schedules/hcp/imz/adult.html

Pertinent Review of Systems

The patient reports an increase in cough and sputum production × 3 days. She reports increased fatigue, which she attributes to interrupted sleep due to coughing. She denies any increase in shortness of breath, chest pain, or dyspnea on exertion. She is sleeping on two pillows, which she states is normal for her.

Pertinent Physical Exam Findings

The patient appears moderately ill. She is wearing an N95 mask and coughing intermittently. Respiratory rate is 22, temperature = 100.8°F, pulse ox = 94%, blood pressure (BP) = 130/86, pulse = 100 and regular.

A COVID-19 test is performed in the office and is positive.

Current Medications

Trelegy Ellipta 100 mcg/62.5 mcg/25 mcg. One inhalation daily.

Treatment Recommendations

Pharmacologic

Paxlovid 300 mg/100 mg 1 tablet po BID × 5 days.
Acetaminophen 500 mg 2 tablets po Q 6 hours.
Over-the-counter (OTC) antitussive medication, if needed.

Nonpharmacologic

Rest and increase activity as tolerated.
Encourage fluids and avoid dehydration.
Continue wearing N95 while at home and around other individuals. Isolate from others and remain home for 5 days. Wear an N95 or high-filtration mask for a total of 10 days. Continue to wear an N95 mask for 5 days after a negative COVID-19 test.
Contact EMS if symptoms worsen.

Considerations for the NP Related to Health Promotion in This Case Study

- The patient used **primary prevention** strategies by obtaining vaccinations to prevent pneumonia, COVID-19, and influenza.
- COVID-19 vaccine that was received less than 6 months ago and has likely lost its efficacy.
- **Secondary Prevention:** LDCT lung scan should be performed annually for high-risk individuals (i.e., smokers with 20 pack-year history and who quit smoking less than 15 years ago).
- **Tertiary Prevention:** Treatment with Paxlovid to minimize the effects of the illness and with antipyretic or antitussive to reduce symptomology.
- **Primary Prevention of Others Within the Community:** Masking and isolating from others who are not sick with COVID-19 decreases the risk of transmission to others.
- Health promotion considerations are related to age, gender, and social factors. There should be variations in the approach to health promotion based on these factors.
- See Chapter 7 for respiratory guidelines and recommendations.

Review Questions

1. The probability that the test says a person has the disease, when in fact they do have the disease, is known as:
   A. specificity.
   B. sensitivity.
   C. diagnostic.
   D. probability.

2. The probability that the test says a person does not have the disease, when in fact they are disease-free, is known as:
   A. specificity.
   B. sensitivity.
   C. diagnostic.
   D. probability.

3. A patient with type 2 diabetes enrolls in a diabetes program that includes information on nutrition, exercise, and general wellness strategies. What type of prevention is this considered to be?
   A. Primary prevention
   B. Secondary prevention
   C. Tertiary prevention
   D. Type 2 diabetes prevention

4. Bone density studies to screen for osteoporosis should be performed on which of the following clients?
   A. Perimenopausal women who used to smoke but no longer do
   B. Only on women after menopause
   C. All women who have had hysterectomies
   D. Women who consume more than 3 ounces of alcohol a day

5. Immunizations are what type of prevention?
   A. Primary
   B. Secondary
   C. Tertiary
   D. Quaternary

6. A 67-year-old female visits the wellness clinic for an annual gynecological exam and Pap smear. She has no history of abnormal Pap smears or any STIs. She states that she feels fine and has no concerns. She is in a monogamous relationship with her male partner. It is appropriate for the primary care provider to inform the patient that:
   A. she should get a Pap smear and HPV screening now and then again in 5 years.
   B. she should continue to get annual Pap smears, but she no longer needs HPV screening.
   C. she no longer needs gynecological exams since she has no history of gynecological problems.
   D. she no longer needs to have a Pap smear.

7. According to the U.S. Preventative Services Task Force (USPSTF) guidelines, which of the following is the appropriate screening test for lung cancer for a 65-year-old male patient with a 25-pack-year history of cigarette smoking?
   A. Chest X-ray
   B. MRI of the lungs with and without contrast
   C. Low-dose CT scan of the lungs
   D. Bronchoscopy

8. A 58-year-old hypertensive female patient has been placed on ASA 81 mg by her PCP. This is:
   A. primary prevention.
   B. secondary prevention.
   C. tertiary prevention.
   D. active intervention.

9. A 67-year-old woman visits your office for a routine annual examination. She denies any allergies, tobacco use, alcohol use, or drug use. She takes Tylenol once or twice a week for "aches and pains," which are in her lower back and knees. She denies any acute problems. She reports she had the Shingrix vaccine series 2 years ago. Immunizations for this patient should include:
   A. yearly Td or tetanus, diphtheria, Tdap, and pneumococcal every 2 years.
   B. pneumococcal yearly, influenza once only.
   C. Td or tetanus, diphtheria, Tdap every 10 years, influenza once only, pneumococcal yearly.
   D. Td or tetanus, diphtheria, Tdap every 10 years, influenza yearly, pneumococcal (PCV13) once, followed a year later by the PPSV23.

10. A 48-year-old male presents to the clinic after having his cholesterol checked at a health fair. He states that they told him it was > 300 and that he needed to see his PCP for further testing. Appropriate interventions for the nurse practitioner include:
    A. prescribing a cholesterol-lowering agent.
    B. ordering an electrocardiogram and an exercise stress test.
    C. starting the client on an exercise program.
    D. performing a thorough history and physical and ordering a fasting lipid profile.

11. According to the USPSTF, blood pressure screenings should begin at:
    A. 16 years.
    B. 18 years.
    C. 21 years.
    D. 25 years.

12. The nurse practitioner is teaching the parents of a pediatric patient about vaccine recommendations. Which sexually transmitted disease can be prevented by this vaccine?
    A. Human papillomavirus (HPV)
    B. Meningococcal B
    C. Pertussis
    D. Hepatitis A

13. Which diagnostic test should be performed annually after age 45 to screen for colon cancer?
    A. Complete blood count (CBC)
    B. Abdominal X-ray
    C. Colonoscopy
    D. Fecal immunochemical test (FIT) blood testing

14. Which hepatitis immunization will the nurse practitioner administer to a patient who will be visiting Africa?
    A. Hepatitis C
    B. Hepatitis A
    C. Hepatitis D
    D. Hepatitis E

15. A 46-year-old Black male with no family history of prostate cancer presents to the clinic for an annual Wellness visit. Which prostate cancer screening tool is recommended for this patient?
    A. Prostate-specific antigen test (PSA)
    B. Transurethral ultrasound
    C. Digital rectal exam (DRE)
    D. No screening indicated

16. The nurse practitioner is preparing to create a plan of care to vaccinate a 16-year-old patient who has never had a human papillomavirus (HPV) vaccine. Which vaccination plan will the nurse practitioner recommend to the patient?
    A. Administer 2 doses over 12 months
    B. Administered 2 doses over 3 months
    C. Administer 3 doses over 6 months
    D. Administer 3 doses over 3 months

17. Swim therapy (aqua therapy) for a 13-year-old patient with cerebral palsy is an example of which type of prevention?
    A. Primary
    B. Secondary
    C. Tertiary
    D. Quaternary

18. A 67-year-old patient who is in excellent health is concerned about staying healthy in their retirement years. They are unsure of their vaccine history. Which vaccines will the nurse practitioner recommend? (Select all that apply.)
    A. Shingles/Zoster vaccine
    B. Annual influenza vaccine
    C. Pneumococcal vaccine
    D. Measles, mumps, rubella (MMR)

19. A 22-year-old pregnant patient has been diagnosed with gonorrhea. The nurse practitioner should test the patient for:
    A. Herpes simplex virus one (HSV-1)
    B. Genital warts
    C. Syphilis
    D. Chlamydia

20. Which of the following is a true contraindication to immunizations?
    A. Mild to moderate local reaction to a previous immunization
    B. Mild acute illness without a low-grade fever
    C. Moderate or severe illness with or without a fever
    D. Recent exposure to an infectious disease

21. Which is the leading cause of cancer deaths?
    A. Lung cancer
    B. Prostate cancer
    C. Colon cancer
    D. Breast cancer

22. A 25-year-old nurse states that she does not want to get the hepatitis B virus vaccine because of its adverse side effects. You tell her that the most common side effect is:
    A. fatigue.
    B. headache.
    C. pain at the injection site.
    D. elevated temperature.

23. For primary prevention of skin cancer, the NP would recommend a sunscreen with how much ultraviolet (UVA and UVB) wave protection?
    A. 15
    B. 25
    C. 30
    D. 45

24. A 90-year-old independent woman is moving into her daughter's home. Her daughter comes to see you seeking information to help keep her mother from falling. Which of the following interventions would help to prevent falls?
    A. Install an intercom system or have the mother use a pendant connected to EMS
    B. Limit the time the mother is home alone
    C. Higher an aide to assist the mother with her activities of daily living (ADLs) 24 hours a day.
    D. Remove all loose rugs from the floors and install hand grips in bathtubs and near toilets.

25. For which individuals does the USPSTF recommend the screening depression question?
    A. Adults who are experiencing gender issues
    B. Adults who have already tried unsuccessfully to commit suicide
    C. All adults
    D. If the NP suspects depression, the individual should be referred to a specialist rather than screening in the primary care office.

Answers and Rationales

1. Answer B is correct. By definition, the probability that the test says a person has the disease when they do have the disease is known as the sensitivity. (positive-positive)

    Answer A is incorrect. Specificity is the probability that the person does not have the disease when they do not. (negative-negative)

    Answer C is incorrect. Diagnostic is the clinician's process of identifying a disease, condition, or injury. It is not based on probability.

    Answer D is incorrect. Probability is defined as the likelihood of something happening.

2. Answer A is correct. The probability that the test says a person does not have the disease when they are disease-free is defined as specificity. (negative-positive)

    Answer B is incorrect. Sensitivity is defined as the probability that the person has the disease and they do have the disease. (positive-positive)

    Answer C is incorrect. Diagnostics are used to identify a disease or condition.

    Answer D is incorrect. Probability is a mathematical term used to identify the likelihood that something will happen.

3. Answer C is correct. The patient with type 2 diabetes has a chronic disease and, therefore, would benefit from strategies that help manage the disease and improve their quality of life. This is known as tertiary prevention.

    Answer A is incorrect. Primary prevention concerns actions used to prevent disease or injury before it can occur. Examples of primary prevention are immunizations and educational and preventative services.

    Answer B is incorrect. Secondary prevention aims to prevent disease from occurring before symptoms appear to reduce the long-term severity of the disease. Examples of secondary prevention services are mammograms, colonoscopies, and Pap smears.

    Answer D is incorrect. The patient is already diagnosed with type 2 diabetes. A diabetes program will provide education to prevent further disease progression and assist the patient in participating in the management of their disease.

4. Answer A is correct. The USPSTF recommends screening for osteoporosis in women aged 65 years and older. For women younger than 65, the evidence supports screening only for perimenopausal women with risk factors that include Caucasian or Asian race, history of bilateral oophorectomy before menopause, a slender build, smoking or having a smoking history, low calcium intake, sedentary lifestyle, and a positive family history of the condition. Women who had a hysterectomy but not an oophorectomy are not considered a particular risk. Alcohol negatively impacts bone health by interfering with the absorption and use of calcium and vitamin D. Because there are several negatives about drinking and bone density, it would be wise for persons with problems with bone loss to decrease or eliminate alcohol.

    Answer B is incorrect. Postmenopausal women are at higher risk for developing osteoporosis, but there are many other factors as outlined above.

    Answer C is incorrect. A hysterectomy alone is not a risk factor. It is important to ascertain whether the patient has had a bilateral oophorectomy since the presence of estrogen is known to protect against bone loss.

    Answer D is incorrect. Alcohol negatively affects bone density, but if the patient is not perimenopausal or menopausal, it is only one risk factor. Alcohol alone should not cause osteoporosis in a premenopausal woman without other risk factors.

5. Answer A is correct. Immunizations are a primary prevention strategy that aims to prevent a disease or injury before it occurs.

    Answer B is incorrect. Secondary prevention is used to identify a disease before the patient experiences symptoms. Colonoscopies, mammograms, and Pap smears are good examples of secondary prevention.

    Answer C is incorrect. Tertiary prevention is used for patients who are symptomatic with a disease, and it aims to reduce the severity of the symptoms of the illness. Attending rehabilitation classes is a good example of tertiary prevention.

    Answer D is incorrect. Quaternary prevention is an action taken to protect individuals from medical interventions that are likely to cause more harm than good. An example of this would be performing routine screening with a PSA test for men who do not have any symptoms of prostate cancer.

6. Answer D is correct. According to the USPSTF guidelines, the patient no longer needs a Pap smear since she has no previous history of abnormal gynecological findings. (Grade D)

   Answer A is incorrect. Per the guidelines, the patient is unlikely to develop cervical cancer and has no previous history of HPV; therefore, per the USPSTF guidelines, the patient no longer needs annual Pap smears.

   Answer B is incorrect. Per the guidelines, she does not need further screening for cervical cancer.

   Answer C is incorrect. A Pap smear is no longer recommended; however, if the patient has an intact uterus and ovaries, she should continue to have gynecologic exams.

7. Answer C is correct. A low-dose CT (LDCT) scan of the lungs is the preferred test to screen for lung cancer. The USPSTF recommends annual screening for lung cancer with LDCT in adults aged 50 to 80 years who have a 20-pack-year smoking history and currently smoke or who have quit smoking within the last 15 years.

   Answer A is incorrect. A chest X-ray will not show very small nodules and cannot distinguish between cancer and other benign conditions such as a lung abscess.

   Answer B is incorrect. An MRI may be helpful after the patient has undergone LDCT scanning and there is a high index of suspicion for lung cancer. It is not used routinely in early lung cancer diagnosis, staging, treatment, or surveillance.

   Answer D is incorrect. A bronchoscopy may be part of a workup for a patient who has undergone a screening LDCT scan and there is a high index of suspicion for lung cancer. A bronchoscopy will allow the doctor to obtain a biopsy and view the airway passages and lungs.

8. Answer A is correct. Primary prevention is designed to prevent the occurrence of a disease or illness. The patient is at a higher risk of stroke due to her age and hypertensive condition. ASA 81 mg is an appropriate recommendation to prevent the occurrence of a stroke. (Grade B)

   Answer B is incorrect. Secondary prevention is an intervention that will reduce the impact of a disease that is not yet symptomatic.

   Answer C is incorrect. Tertiary prevention is an intervention used to alleviate the impact of the disease or illness.

   Answer D is incorrect. An active intervention does not define the type of prevention being used and is not necessarily based on scientific evidence.

9. Answer D is correct. Per the guidelines, a 67-year-old woman should have a Tdap every 10 years, an annual influenza vaccine, and, for those getting the pneumococcal vaccine for the first time after age 65, the PCV13 followed a year later with PPSV23.

   Answer A is incorrect. It is not appropriate to get annual Tdap or Td vaccines. It is also not appropriate to get a pneumococcal vaccine every 2 years.

   Answer B is incorrect. An annual influenza vaccine is always necessary. This is needed due to the different prevalent strains each year and because influenza vaccines only provide effective protection for approximately 6 months.

   Answer C is incorrect. The influenza vaccine is needed annually, and it is not recommended to get the pneumococcal vaccine yearly.

10. Answer D is correct. The PCP should first perform a thorough history and physical and ensure that a lipid profile is repeated with fasting levels.

    Answer A is incorrect. Before prescribing a cholesterol-lowering agent, the cholesterol profile needs to be repeated with a 12-hour fast. Additionally, the patient should be advised on dietary changes or consider referral to a nutritionist.

    Answer B is incorrect. The patient is not experiencing cardiac symptoms, so an ECG or stress test is not appropriate at this time.

    Answer C is incorrect. While an exercise program is almost always beneficial, the PCP would first need further information regarding this patient's CV status and overall health condition.

11. Answer B is correct. According to the USPSTF, blood pressure screenings should start at age 18. The USPSTF recommends screening individuals 18 years and older for high blood pressure.

    Answer A is incorrect unless there is a reason to screen a patient under 18. For example, the CDC and the American Academy of Pediatrics (AAP) advocate that screenings begin as young as 3 years of age in response to the obesity and diabetes epidemics in the United States. Youth with obesity have the highest prevalence of hypertension.

    Answer C is incorrect because the recommendation is to begin screenings at age 18.

Answer D is incorrect. Waiting until the patient reaches 25 might delay preventative strategies that could have been implemented earlier.

12. Answer A is correct. Human papillomavirus (HPV) protects against nine HPV types, including those associated with cancer and genital warts.

    Answer B is incorrect. Meningococcal illness is acquired through contact with respiratory and throat secretions such as sharing utensils, cups, or kissing.

    Answer C is incorrect. Pertussis is transmitted via droplets that are released when sneezing or coughing.

    Answer D is incorrect. Hepatitis A is transmitted via the oral-fecal route, not sexually.

13. Answer D is correct. The current United States preventative task force guidelines for colorectal cancer screening recommend an annual FIT beginning at 45. Surface blood vessels of polyps and cancer are fragile and often bleed with the passage of stools.

    Answer A is incorrect. A CBC does not screen for colon cancer. Anemia may indicate the need for further testing to assess the etiology of the anemia.

    Answer B is incorrect. An annual abdominal X-ray is an inappropriate test for colon cancer. An abdominal X-ray can help establish tumor size and metastases after detection of colon cancer.

    Answer C is incorrect. A colonoscopy is recommended beginning at age 45 and is recommended to be repeated every 10 years unless polyps are identified or the patient has a high-risk family or personal history.

14. Answer B is correct. Patients planning to visit Africa, Mexico, or other endemic areas with hepatitis A should receive the hepatitis A (Havrix) vaccine. Hepatitis A and E are transmitted via contaminated water or the oral-fecal route. There is no FDA-approved vaccine for hepatitis C, D, or E.

    Answer A is incorrect. Hepatitis C is caused by parenteral contact with infected body fluids. Hepatitis C is transmitted via needles, sexual intercourse, and unsterile tattooing.

    Answer C is incorrect. Hepatitis B, C, and D are all transmitted through parenteral contact with infected body fluids.

15. Answer D is correct. No screening indicated. Risk factors for prostate cancer include being a Black male older than 50 years old, obesity, and positive family history.

    Answer A is incorrect. The USPSTF no longer recommends routine prostate cancer screening with PSA.

    Answer B is incorrect. Black men with no other risk factors would not warrant referral for more advanced screening such as a transurethral ultrasound. A prostate biopsy guided by a transurethral ultrasound is performed to confirm a suspected diagnosis of prostate cancer.

    Answer C is incorrect. The USPSTF states a patient with no symptoms of prostate cancer or enlargement would need an annual DRE.

16. Answer C is correct. Patients older than 15 years who have never received the HPV vaccine will receive 3 doses over 6 months. The second dose should be given 1 to 2 months after the first dose, and the third should be given 6 months after the first dose

    Answer A is incorrect. Patients aged 9 to 14 should receive a 2-dose series 6 to 12 months apart.

    Answer B is incorrect. The 2-dose vaccination is only appropriate for those aged 9 to 14, and the second dose must be given at least 6 months after the first dose.

    Answer D is incorrect. Administering 3 doses over 3 months is not an appropriate schedule for the HPV vaccine. The 3-dose schedule is done with an initial dose followed by a second dose 2 months later, and a third dose 6 months after the first dose.

17. Answer C is correct. Aqua therapy is a tertiary prevention rehabilitation program designed to prevent further complications of CP.

    Answer A is incorrect. Primary prevention consists of interventions to prevent disease or illness (i.e., vaccines).

    Answer B is incorrect. Secondary prevention is designed to provide early intervention through early screening, such as mammography or colonoscopy.

    Answer D is incorrect. Quaternary prevention prevents unnecessary medical interventions that may cause more harm than good.

18. Answers A, B, and C are correct. The vaccinations recommended by the CDC for individuals 65 or older are the Shingles/Zoster vaccine and annual influenza vaccine. Pneumococcal vaccine is also recommended for those whose previous vaccine histories are unknown.

Answer D is incorrect. Most adults over the age of 65 do not need the measles vaccine. The CDC considers those born before 1957 to have natural immunity and do not need vaccination.

19. Answer D is correct. If a pregnant patient is diagnosed with gonorrhea, they should also be evaluated for chlamydia due to the high rate of co-infection.

    Answer A is incorrect. HSV-1 is usually an oral infection and should be treated with antiviral medications.

    Answer B is incorrect. There is no need to treat genital warts unless they are present in the vagina, anus, or external glands.

    Answer C is incorrect. An individual who is infected with HIV should also be tested for syphilis.

20. Answer C is correct. According to the American Academy of Pediatrics, the only true contraindications to immunizations are a moderate or severe illness with or without a fever or an anaphylactic reaction to a vaccine.

    Answer A is incorrect. A mild to moderate reaction to a previous immunization is not a contraindication to receiving further vaccinations.

    Answer B is incorrect. Illnesses themselves are not contraindications to vaccines. Early symptoms may be a prodrome of something else; however, risks of the diseases are usually greater than the complications of the vaccine.

    Answer D is incorrect. Exposure to an infectious disease does not mean the vaccine should not be administered.

21. Answer A is correct. Lung cancer is the leading cause of cancer death, and cigarette smoking causes almost all cases. Compared to nonsmokers, men who smoke are about 23 times more likely to develop lung cancer. Women who smoke are about 13 times more likely. Smoking causes about 90 percent of lung cancer deaths in men and almost 80 percent in women.

    Answer B is incorrect. Prostate cancer is the most common cancer in men (1 in 8 men will develop prostate cancer in their lifetime). However, statistically, only 1 in 44 men will die of prostate cancer, and for some, it may be 100 percent curable with early detection and treatment.

    Answer C is incorrect. Colon and rectal cancer account for roughly 916,000 deaths per year and are the second most common cause of cancer deaths.

    Answer D is incorrect. While breast cancer is the most common cancer for women (1 in every 8 women will be diagnosed with breast cancer), it is responsible for roughly 685,000 deaths per year, significantly less than deaths from lung cancer.

22. Answer C is correct. The most common adverse reaction to the hepatitis B virus vaccine is pain at the injection site (13 to 20 percent in adults).

    Answer A is incorrect. Although postvaccination fatigue has been reported, it is typically a mild transient systemic side effect.

    Answer B is incorrect. Approximately 11 to 17 percent of adults report fatigue and headache after receiving the hepatitis B vaccine.

    Answer D is incorrect. Temperature elevation is reported in approximately 1 to 6 percent of adults posthepatitis B vaccination.

23. Answer C is correct. For primary prevention of skin cancer, a sunscreen with an ultraviolet wave protection factor of 30 or higher blocks 97 percent of the sun's UVB rays.

    Answer A is incorrect. Daily use of SPF 15 is effective; however, it must be applied every 2 hours to all exposed areas daily. This will decrease the risk of skin cancer by 40 to 50 percent and effectively blocks approximately 93 percent of the sun's UVB rays.

    Answer B is incorrect. The difference between SPF 25 and SPF 30 is minimal. However, most dermatologists will recommend SPF 30.

    Answer D is incorrect. Sunscreen with an SPF higher than 30 provides little additional protection. No sunscreen will block 100 percent of the sun's UV rays.

24. Answer D is correct. The correct answer is to allow the elderly mother her independence but provide a safe environment by removing loose rugs that she could easily trip over and installing handrails by the toilet and in the bathtub. The rails will support her as she goes from sitting to standing.

    Answer A is incorrect. An intercom or access to EMS will not decrease the risk of falling. However, if a fall occurs, this will allow for a more immediate response for assistance.

    Answer B is incorrect. Limiting the time the mother is home alone is not a preventative strategy to prevent falls.

    Answer C is incorrect. Hiring an aide 24 hours a day would decrease the mother's independence.

25. Answer C is correct. The USPSTF recommends screening all adults for depression in practices that have systems in place to assure accurate diagnosis, effective treatment, and adequate follow up. Evidence shows that screening improves the accurate identification of depressed patients in primary care settings and that treating depressed adults identified in primary care settings reduces clinical morbidity.

Answer A is incorrect. The adult experiencing gender issues should certainly be screened for depression, but screening all adults is the preferred answer because it is more inclusive.

Answer B is incorrect. Although this person would need to be screened regularly and receive psychiatric treatment, the answer is not inclusive enough.

Answer D is incorrect. Per the USPSTF guidelines, all adults should be screened for depression during an exam. Primary care practices should have systems in place to ensure accurate diagnosis, effective treatment, and adequate follow-up.

Resources

American Cancer Society. (2023, November 1). *American Cancer Society guidelines for the early detection of cancer*. https://www.cancer.org/cancer/screening/american-cancer-society-guidelines-for-the-early-detection-of-cancer.html

American College of Obstetricians and Gynecology (ACOG). (2025). *Screening & prevention*. https://www.acog.org/womens-health/healthy-living/screening-and-prevention

Center for Disease Control (CDC). (2022). *National Center for Health Statistics: Leading Causes of Death*. https://www.cdc.gov/nchs/fastats/leading-causes-of-death.htm

Center for Disease Control (CDC). (2025). *Adult immunization schedule by age*. https://www.cdc.gov/vaccines/hcp/imz-schedules/adult-age.html?CDC_AAref_Val=https://www.cdc.gov/vaccines/schedules/hcp/imz/adult.html

Center for Disease Control. (2025). *Advisory Committee on Immunization Practices (ACIP)*. https://www.cdc.gov/acip/?CDC_AAref_Val=https://www.cdc.gov/vaccines/acip/index.html

Hagan, J. F. Jr., Shaw, J. S., & Duncan, P. M. (Eds.) (2017). *Bright futures: Guidelines for health supervision of infants, children and adolescents* (4th ed.). American Academy of Pediatrics. https://www.aap.org/Bright-Futures-Guidelines-for-Health-Supervision-of-Infants-Children-and-Adolescents-4th-Edition

Kisling, L. A., & Das, J. M. (2024). *Prevention strategies*. StatPearls Publishing. https://www.ncbi.nlm.nih.gov/books/NBK537222/

Kochanek, K. D., Murphy, S. L, Xu, J. Q., & Arias, E. (2023). Mortality in the United States, 2022. National Center for Health Statistics. https://dx.doi.org/10.15620/cdc:135850

National Center for Chronic Disease Prevention and Health Promotion (NCCDPHP). (2025). Center for Disease Control. https://www.cdc.gov/nccdphp/index.html

U.S. Preventative Services Task Force (USPSTF). (2025a). https://www.uspreventiveservicestaskforce.org/uspstf/

U. S. Preventive Services Task Force (USPSTF). (2025b). *A & B recommendations*. https://www.uspreventiveservicestaskforce.org/uspstf/recommendation-topics/uspstf-a-and-b-recommendations

U.S. Preventive Services Task Force. (2018). *Final recommendation statement: Unhealthy alcohol use in adolescents and adults: Screening and behavioral counseling interventions*. https://www.uspreventiveservicestaskforce.org/uspstf/recommendation/unhealthy-alcohol-use-in-adolescents-and-adults-screening-and-behavioral-counseling-interventions

Women's Preventative Services Initiative (WPSI). (2024). *Homepage*. ACOG Foundation. https://www.womenspreventivehealth.org/

CHAPTER 5

Pharmacology

Chrystyne Olivieri, DNP, FNP-BC, CDCES
Nancy L. Dennert, MS, MSN, FNP-BC, CDCES, BC-ADM

Introduction

This chapter is designed to provide the nurse practitioner (NP) with a review of the concepts of prescribing pharmaceuticals and other drugs. It is not meant to be a review course of pharmacology, although specific drugs and disease processes may be discussed. In the medical world, "drug" and "medicine" are often used interchangeably. It must be understood that a drug is a *chemical substance that produces a biologic effect when given to an organism*, and a medication is a *chemical substance used to treat, cure, prevent a disease or to promote well-being* (Merriam-Webster.com). Therefore, for the purposes of education, this chapter will use the universal term "drug" since that is what the pharmaceutical industry manufactures.

The Food & Drug Administration (FDA) is the main regulating body that reviews and approves drug applications before approval and market distribution. It has nothing to do with specific prescribing rules as they are governed by the Drug Enforcement Administration (DEA). The FDA has put consumer protection laws in place to protect the public, and they regulate what is included on the pharmaceutical/drug package insert for all prescribed and nonprescribed drugs. They are also the organization that sets the standards for controlled substance prescribing.

Prescription drugs must go through a rigorous sequence of events to achieve approval from the FDA to ensure they are not harmful to the public. This process can take up to 10 years or so. Even once a drug is approved and enters the market, it is not guaranteed to stay on the market. Many drugs have been removed within a few years after approval due to adverse events in the larger population (FDA.gov). Over-the-counter (OTC) drugs are available without a prescription and are NOT formally approved or monitored by the FDA. However, they regulate if those products are generally recognized as safe (GRAS) (FDA.gov). This includes common household items such as aspirin, nonsteroidal anti-inflammatory (NSAID) agents, antacids, cold and cough treatments, herbs, and supplements. There is *no* strict government oversight on the efficacy of these drugs. Although they may have adverse effects, the FDA only determines that they are generally safe. Any NP needs to know about commonly used items and if they may harm their patients. Knowing drug–drug interactions, drug–food interactions, and major side effects are an important part of prescribing for NPs.

Many drugs prescribed by healthcare providers have more than one therapeutic use. This is the basis of the concept of "off-label use" (Greiwe et al., 2022). Prescribers often use a drug for another well-known issue that differs from what the drug was originally approved to treat. When NPs prescribe drugs, the patient is considered on many levels. The risk–benefit ratio considers the possible risks of using a drug and the benefit that may be gained. The risks include adverse events, interactions, and intolerances. Overall, the NP must prioritize patient safety first when prescribing.

Prescribing for Nurse Practitioners

As of January 1990, the first six states in the USA and the District of Columbia granted NPs statutory authority to independently prescribe medication. As of December 2022, NPs who meet state-specific requirements can prescribe pharmaceuticals, including Schedule II to V drugs in all states except Georgia and Oklahoma, where NPs can only prescribe Schedule III to V controlled substances (*Nurse Journal*, 2023). Each year, more and more states have been granting full practice authority to NPs and full prescriptive authority. Each NP should check with their State Board of Nursing for specific practice laws.

Controlled substance law includes the five prescription schedules. The drugs in Schedule II to V are generally prescribed under the DEA license of healthcare providers. Schedule I drugs are *not* prescribed. Marijuana for medicinal purposes remains a Schedule I drug under federal law, but it is now prescribed in many states either fully legal or partially restricted. NPs must review their specific state laws (Wadsworth et al., 2022). Despite each state law for marijuana use as of January 2024, it remains a Schedule I drug under federal law and is illegal. NPs must complete an "Office of Cannabis Management" approved educational course before prescribing (Celeste & Thompson-Dudiak, 2020). Emerging research is now being conducted on this Schedule I drug, expanding the knowledge base about prescribing. **Table 5-1** lists the classification of scheduled drugs as well as some examples.

NP prescriptive privileges come with rules that include using an official DEA prescription pad. They should be imprinted with the prescriber's name, license number, National Provider Identifier (NPI), and practice address; however, it is *never* recommended to preprint the prescriber's DEA number. This can be written in when prescribing controlled substances only. Prescription pads should always be locked up when not in use to avoid unauthorized use. This has never been more evident than during the opioid crisis, with rampant illegal prescriptions filled across the United States, which has led to the Controlled Substances Act of 2019 (Lampe & Attorney, 2021). There are legitimate reasons for patients needing strong pain drugs, but that choice is to be made between the NP and the patient alone. Because pain is subjective, there are many ways to ensure that opioid pain drugs are used properly. An NP may consider using a *pain contract* with their patients. This is a written agreement signed by both an NP and the patient that clearly outlines the responsibilities of each party so opioid pain drugs are properly and safely used.

Pharmacotherapeutics

Pharmacological therapy utilizes drugs to improve ongoing symptoms, treat an underlying condition,

Table 5-1 DEA Drug Scheduling

Schedules 1-5	Examples
Schedule 1 drugs have no acceptable medical use and a high potential for abuse and physical dependence.	LSD, heroin, ecstasy. Special note: marijuana remains a schedule 1 drug according to the DEA; however, many states have independently recognized and accepted medical uses for marijuana.
Schedule 2 drugs have a high potential for abuse and psychological and physical dependence.	Narcotics, such as hydromorphone (Dilaudid), meperidine (Demerol), hydrocodone, morphine, oxycodone, fentanyl. Amphetamines, such as methamphetamine, Adderall, Ritalin, Dexedrine, Cocaine.
Schedule 3 drugs are those with a low to moderate potential for abuse and a low to moderate risk of physical or psychological dependence.	Testosterone, anabolic steroids, codeine products containing < 90 mg of codeine.
Schedule 4 drugs have a low risk of abuse and a low risk for physical dependence.	Benzodiazepines, such as alprazolam (Xanax), diazepam (Valium), clonazepam (Klonopin), lorazepam (Ativan). Sedative-hypnotic medications, such as zolpidem (Ambien).
Schedule 5 drugs have the lowest risk of abuse potential and are typically drugs that are combination medications that are used for the treatment of diarrhea, coughs, and neuropathic pain.	Antidiarrhea agents: lomotil motofen, parepectolin. Antitussive agents: Robitussin AC (contains low-dose codeine). Nonnarcotic analgesic: pregabalin (Lyrica) used to treat neuropathic pain.

or prevent other diseases. This is governed by two concepts: pharmacokinetics (what the body does to a drug) and pharmacodynamics (what the drug does to the body). Drugs are created as targeted chemicals that produce a desired effect while minimizing undesired effects. These chemicals change how a protein, enzyme, or receptor site works in the human body. The therapeutic range is the minimum effective dose balanced with the minimum toxic concentration. Drugs may be agonists (increase an effect), partial agonists, or antagonists (reduce an effect).

Pharmacokinetics refers to how the body affects the drug and includes absorption, distribution, metabolism, and excretion of drugs (**Table 5-2**). The closer to the targeted site, the higher the drug concentrations (think about topical creams or inhaled drugs vs. oral drugs). Remember, prescribers want to give the least amount of drug to achieve the desired therapeutic result.

Pharmacokinetics

One phenomenon of metabolism that must be considered for all prescribers is to be aware that there is a lot of variability among individuals (absorption, distribution, metabolism, and excretion) and among routes of drug dosing. The natural variations from person to person may

Table 5-2 Lehne's Pharmacotherapeutics

	Considerations	Factors That Affect
Absorption	Movement of a drug from site of administration to the blood Rate of absorption will determine how fast and intense the effects will be	Rate of dissolution Surface area Blood flow Lipid solubility pH partitioning
Distribution	Movement of an absorbed drug in body fluids throughout the body to target tissues Drug moves from areas of high blood flow to low blood flow Based on protein binding, so low protein may affect distribution Based on tissue distribution: lipids, adipose tissue, and bone as some drugs have affinity for bone Blood-brain barrier Placental barrier	Requires a good blood flow Water and lipid solubility Size of the molecule Acid/base environment Transporters Volume of distribution
Metabolism	Enzymatic alterations of a drug Most take place in the liver Cytochrome P450 (CYP450)—Also 1A2, 2C9, 2C19, 2D6, 3A4 Half life Metabolism often involves a **prodrug:** Administered as inactive but becomes a prodrug (active drug) during metabolism	Age Genetic differences Pregnancy Liver disease status Time of day Environment Diet Alcohol Drug-drug interactions
Excretion	Removal of the drug from the body May be eliminated by kidneys, lungs, GI tract, sweat/saliva, breast milk Renal: Must know renal function prior to prescribing	*Renal*: drug must be unbound from protein to be filtered by kidneys. Age, hydration, and cardiac output affect kidney elimination *GI*: Biliary excretion—drug may be reabsorbed in the intestine *Lung*: Excreted as gases—rate is based on respiratory rate and pulmonary blood flow *Sweat/Saliva*: Not many drugs eliminated by this route but may cause rashes and "taste" in mouth *Breast Milk*: Many drugs are excreted in breast milk, lipid soluble

make a drug a great choice for one person and a poor choice for another. The bioavailability of a drug is based on many factors, which includes things like route (IV drugs are 100 percent bioavailable, but not so with oral, inhaled, and topical drugs), concomitant food intake, GI transit time, age, and renal/liver status. Since pharmaceutical companies only run studies on sample populations, the true test of a drug isn't known until it formally enters the market and large numbers of people use the drug.

Many oral drugs are sometimes quickly metabolized, requiring their doses to be much larger than intravenous dosages (which are usually the smallest). The "first-pass effect" is an example of the variability of drug metabolism. The first-pass effect is when a drug gets metabolized at a specific location in the body, which results in a reduced concentration of the active drug upon reaching its site of action or entering the systemic circulation. The liver is the main site of drug metabolism; however, the first-pass effect can occur in the lungs, vasculature, gastrointestinal tract, and other metabolically active tissues. Metabolism by the liver following oral drug intake can determine if a drug can be given orally. This system depends on liver enzymes called *cytochrome P450 (CYP450)* enzymes, which metabolize drugs. It is critical to understand which drugs experience the first-pass effect to allow for safe and effective drug dosing.

Pharmacodynamics

This term refers to the *therapeutic effects* of a drug and how it can help a patient. A prescriber needs to choose a drug that will be as specific as possible, target the problem, and have the greatest therapeutic effects with the least adverse effects. Evidence-based guidelines can help a prescriber to make the best choices for drugs. Some drugs require close monitoring or follow-up lab work as they may become toxic in some individuals (e.g., Digoxin, Ergocalciferol, Dilantin, Warfarin). Others have a wider therapeutic range and are generally safe for most people.

Prescribers must know special populations that need additional consideration. These populations include pediatrics, the elderly, and during pregnancy.

Pediatric Considerations

Gastrointestinal absorption does not reach adult levels until 20 to 30 months of age. This will affect the bioavailability of many drugs. Infants have increased intestinal motility and decreased plasma proteins for binding. Also, the blood-brain barrier is incomplete in young children and is very permeable. Due to higher lean-body mass and lower fat mass, distribution may be affected in some children. Metabolism using the CYP450 and CYP3A4 system is not as well known in children. Concurrent disease processes may affect the metabolism of drugs, and food often interacts with drug metabolism. Excretion is also affected until age 6 to 12 months, so dose adjustments may be necessary. It is good to keep in mind that many drugs are excreted in breast milk, so nursing is best done *before* dosing for the mother. **Table 5-3** identifies the pregnancy category of drugs according to their risks to the fetus or infant.

Pregnancy Considerations

Considering prescribing during pregnancy requires a knowledge of the disease and the drug to be prescribed. Most pharmaceutical drug trials exclude pregnant persons from their study populations, so there is little information available for many drugs and their use during pregnancy. Some drugs have been found to have teratogenic effects. One example is isotretinoin, an oral drug to treat severe cystic acne. This drug was found to be *highly* teratogenic, but only after almost 1,000 babies were born with a congenital condition. This data was discovered after it was released to the population. The bad outcomes changed the drug labels and warnings (Altıntaş Aykan & Ergün, 2020).

Some of the pregnancy dangers occur during specific stages of the pregnancy only. We know that drug absorption increases during pregnancy and that most drugs can cross the placenta. Insulin does not cross the placenta due to its large molecular weight. We also know that animal testing is not always transferable to humans. Therefore, many drug package inserts list pregnancy categories of fetal risk as "unknown."

Table 5-3 Pregnancy Category of Drugs

Medscape	www.medscape.com
A	Controlled studies show no risk.
B	No evidence of risk in humans; the chance of fetal harm is remote.
C	Risk not excluded. Adequate studies lacking. Chance of fetal harm, but benefits outweigh risks.
D	Positive evidence of risk. Studies in humans show fetal risk. Potential benefit in pregnant women may outweigh risk.
X	Contraindicated

Data from Cardiosource © 2007 by the American College of Cardiology Foundation

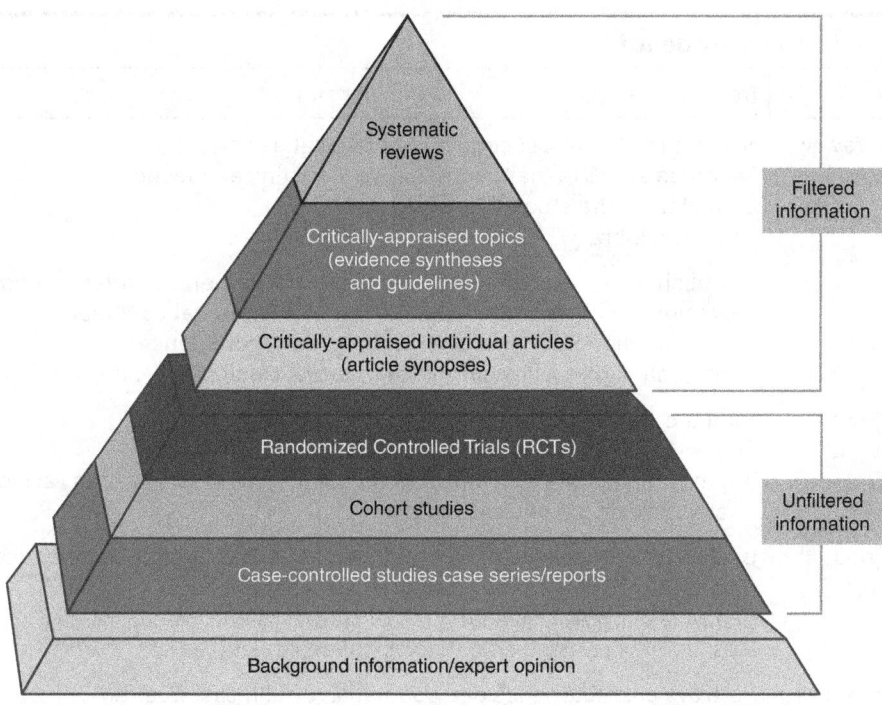

Modified from EBM Pyramid and EBM Page Generator, 2006 Trustees of Dartmouth College and Yale University. All Rights Reserved. Produced by Jan Glover, David Izzo, Karen Odato, and Lei Wang.

Elderly Considerations

Polypharmacy is a common problem for older people. When reviewing a drug list for an older patient, always look for drugs that may no longer provide therapeutic results for your patient and consider *deprescribing* whenever possible (Omuya et al., 2023). Since aging is too often associated with mental and sensory changes, reviewing drugs with your older patients is a good habit. Absorption is not known to be very different for aging patients; however, note the GI motility for each individual as this can affect bioavailability. Drug distribution can change due to increased fat stores and decreased muscle mass. Also, hydration and serum albumin (often low in the elderly) may affect drug distribution. Metabolism affects older people due to changes in cardiac output and decreased liver and/or kidney function. This may drastically alter the CYP450 system. Excretion is also affected by reduced renal function, so monitoring the glomerular filtration rate (GFR) is important.

Sometimes, older patients may not take their medications as prescribed. This may be due to intentional (e.g., cost or concern for unpleasant side effects) or unintentional (e.g., forgetfulness or dementia) reasons. It is good practice to refer to the *Beer's Criteria*, which is published by the American Geriatrics Society (2023). This is a list of drugs to avoid, adjust dosage, or use cautiously for your older patients. This list is updated periodically based on new evidence.

Levels of Evidence

The basis of pharmacology is scientific research, which provides clinical evidence for our practice. NPs are taught to refer to the many *guidelines*. The most comprehensive databases are the Agency for Healthcare Research and Quality (AHRQ, n.d.) and the National Guidelines Clearinghouse. In addition, individual organizations also weigh in on providing guidelines for practice. The American Heart Association, the American Diabetes Association, the American Cancer Society, and the U.S. Preventative Services Task Force (USPSTF) are only a few of the private and governmental organizations that provide guidelines for practice (USPSTF.org).

Evidence is graded on seven levels based on the quality, reliability, and validity of the research results. The highest level of evidence is Level 1, which is the most reliable and dependable for large populations (**Table 5-4**). Sometimes, evidence is presented as level A through D, with A being the highest quality and D being less reliable and generalizable. The USPSTF uses this rating system (**Table 5-5**). Clinical evidence A and B is widely accepted as strongly based, robust, and highly reliable. C and D level is considered weaker or simply opinion. The risk–benefit ratio of C and D level evidence may not show enough benefit compared with risk to justify a general recommendation; however, some providers may find it works in some situations and benefits some of their patients. All

Table 5-4 Clinical Levels of Evidence

Level of Evidence	Description
Level 1: Systematic review or meta-analysis of RCT	Highest level of evidence to base a clinical decision Searches all RCTs that address a similar clinical question Compiles all the studies Cochrane Library
Level 2: Single, well-designed RCT	Establishes cause of a disease, efficacy of treatment, or intervention Maintains a high degree of control with experimental conditions Random assignment allows a high degree of confidence Double-blinding further strengthens support for cause-and-effect relationship
Level 3: Well-designed controlled trials without randomization	Evaluate effectiveness of intervention or treatment Subjects are not randomly assigned Attempt to improve internal validity with control of extraneous variables and standardization of treatment
Level 4: Well-designed case control or cohort studies	Useful for answering clinical questions related to prognosis or causation Compares those with the "disease" to those without Risks introducing bias with no case control in study Most commonly used epidemiological design currently in literature
Level 5: Systematic reviews of descriptive or qualitative studies	Portrays characteristics of a population or clinical situation Quantitative (measurable characteristics) or qualitative (increasing understanding of the phenomena of a clinical question)
Level 6: Single descriptive or qualitative study	Case study Likelihood of decreased objectivity Used to alert an adverse event, a rare disease, or to add to the providers' knowledge base No inferences can be made to general population
Level 7: Opinion of authorities and/or expert committees	Follows the traditional approach May or may not be based on strong evidence Should NOT be the sole determination of changing practice May be the only evidence in rare situations

RCT: Randomly Controlled Trials

evidence is good. It's just that some have a higher level of validity and reliability (Schmidt & Brown, 2024).

Adverse Events

Drug-to-Drug Interactions, Food-to-Drug Interactions

An adverse drug reaction (ADR) is any undesirable or unintended effect occurring after using a pharmaceutical or OTC drug. There are two types of ADRs: pharmacological (about 90 percent of all ADRs) and idiosyncratic or unpredictable events (Uetrecht, 2013). The language used when discussing ADRs is important and includes side effects, toxicity, idiosyncratic, paradoxical, physical dependence, and teratogenic effects. When prescribing, it is important to know if there may be drug-to-drug interactions. Sometimes, changing one drug in the combination is all that is needed to avoid the interaction. One example is prescribing clopidogrel with omeprazole, which may decrease the effectiveness of the clopidogrel. Changing the omeprazole to pantoprazole eliminates the interaction (**Table 5-6**).

Also, prescribers must be very aware of liver and renal function before prescribing. Many drugs have *renal dosing*, which may indicate an undesired increase in the bioavailability of a drug due to altered metabolism or excretion. One example is rivaroxaban, which requires a lower dose for patients with liver or renal impairment. Another example is the many drugs used for type 2 diabetes. Metformin and other oral drugs require a lower dose for patients with GFR less than 45 and should not be used for patients with GFR less than 30.

Warfarin is one drug that has *many* drug-to-drug and drug-to-food interactions; however, it has only one side effect: bleeding. It is highly affected by many drugs, including some common antibiotics, NSAIDs, and prescription pain relievers. There are also *many* drug-to-food interactions: dark green leafy vegetables and other foods high in vitamin K, as well as alcohol.

Table 5-5 United States Preventative Services Task Force

The USPSTF has updated its definitions of the grades it assigns to recommendations and now includes "suggestions for practice" associated with each grade. The USPSTF has also defined levels of certainty regarding net benefit. These definitions apply to USPSTF recommendations released after May 2007.

Grade	Definition	Suggestions for Practice
A	The USPSTF recommends the service. There is high certainty that the net benefit is substantial.	Offer or provide this service.
B	The USPSTF recommends the service. There is high certainty that the net benefit is moderate or there is moderate certainty that the net benefit is moderate to substantial.	Offer or provide this service.
C	The USPSTF recommends against routinely providing the service. There may be considerations that support providing the service in an individual patient. There is at least moderate certainty that the net benefit is small.	Offer or provide this service only if other considerations support offering or providing the service in an individual patient.
D	The USPSTF recommends against the service. There is moderate or high certainty that the service has no net benefit or that the harms outweigh the benefits.	Discourage the use of this service.
I	The USPSTF concludes that the current evidence is insufficient to assess the balance of benefits and harms of the service. Evidence is lacking, poor quality, or conflicting and the balance of benefits and harms cannot be determined.	Read the clinical considerations section of USPSTF Recommendation Statement. If the service is offered, patients should understand the uncertainty about the balance of benefits and harms.

Reproduced from U.S. Preventive Services Task Force. October 2018. Grade Definitions. https://www.uspreventiveservicestaskforce.org/uspstf/about-uspstf/methods-and-processes/grade-definitions

Table 5-6 Common Drug–Drug Interactions

Drug 1	Drug 2	Potential Outcome
ACEIs	NSAID	Hyperkalemia, decline in renal function
Ciprofloxacin	Olanzapine	Cipro inhibits CYP1A2, which may result in increase in olanzapine plasma concentration
Digoxin	Furosemide	Hypokalemia may increase risk for digitalis intoxication
Nitroglycerin	Sildenafil	Increased risk of severe hypotension
Spironolactone	Potassium chloride	Hyperkalemia
Verapamil	Atenolol	Bradycardia and hypotension
Warfarin	Aspirin	Increased risk of bleeding

This can lead to very bad outcomes of either bleeding (warfarin levels too high) or blood clots (warfarin levels too low) when left unaddressed (Wang et al., 2021).

When discussing ADRs, it's also important to understand hypersensitivity reactions (Khalil & Huang, 2020). There are many levels of this "allergic" reaction type of adverse event (**Table 5-7**). This chart identifies the components of the immune system and the four major types of hypersensitivity reactions.

A type I reaction is anaphylactic and requires an immediate response. It is seen in a previously sensitized person and can be fatal if not treated immediately. A type II reaction is a cytotoxic reaction sometimes called an "autoimmune response." It can present as hemolytic anemia, thrombocytopenia, or drug-induced lupus. Improvement is seen when the drug is removed. A type III reaction is an "Arthus," or an acute, localized reaction. It is sometimes referred to as "serum sickness." It can cause angioedema, arthralgias, fever, swollen lymph nodes, and splenomegaly. This can occur 1 to 3 weeks after drug exposure, making identification of the offending agent quite challenging. A type IV reaction is a cell-mediated or delayed

Table 5-7 Hypersensitivity Types and Their Mechanisms

	Type I	Type II	Type III	Type IV
Immune reactant	IgE	IgE or IgM	IgE and IgM	T cells
Antigen form	Soluble antigen	Cell-bound antigen	Soluble antigen	Soluble or cell-bound antigen
Mechanism of activation	Allergen-specific IgE antibodies bind to mast cells via their Fc receptor. When the specific allergen binds to the IgE, cross-linking of IgE induces degranulation of mast cells.	IgG or IgM antibody binds to cellular antigen, leading to complement activation and cell lysis. IgG can also mediate ADCC with cytotoxic T cells, natural killer cells, macrophages, and neutrophils.	Antigen-antibody complexes are deposited in tissues. Complement activation provides inflammatory mediators and recruits neutrophils. Enzymes released from neutrophils damage tissue.	T_H1 cells secrete cytokines, which activate macrophages and cytotoxic T cells.
Examples of hypersensitivity reactions	Local and systemic anaphlaxis, seasonal hay fever, foot allergies, and drug allergies	Red blood cell destruction after transfusion with mismatched blood types or during hemolytic disease of the newborn	Poststreptococcal glomerulonephritis, rheumatoid arthritis, and systemic lupus erythematosus	Contact dermatitis, type I diabetes mellitus, and multiple sclerosis

IgE: Immunoglobulin E; IgM: Immunoglobulin E.
Reproduced from Open Stax. (n.d.). Allied Health Microbiology (1st ed.). Oregon State University. https://creativecommons.org/licenses/by/4.0/deed.en

hypersensitivity. This may present as a common skin reaction that occurs 1 to 2 days after drug exposure.

Nephrotoxicity is a consideration for patients with chronic renal insufficiency. Many drugs are considered "nephrotoxic" drugs (Kwiatkowska et al., 2021). These are known to cause some level of kidney injury. The more common nephrotoxic drugs are in **Table 5-8**.

Hepatotoxicity is another consideration. There are many drugs considered "hepatotoxic" drugs. It is one of the major causes of liver failure in the United States (Shah et al., 2024). There are over 50 pharmaceutical drugs that are in this category. During the metabolism phase of pharmacokinetics, there are toxic byproducts that can injure liver cells. It is important to understand that patients need to be warned about concurrent use of alcohol and/or OTC drugs while using some hepatotoxic prescriptions (Di Federico et al., 2023). Some patients need to monitor AST (aspartate aminotransferase) and ALT (alanine aminotransferase). It is also important to monitor for signs of liver injury. Educate patients about jaundice, dark urine, light-colored stool, nausea, vomiting, malaise, abdominal discomfort, and loss of appetite as these symptoms may indicate acute liver injury, and the drug should be stopped immediately.

Some pharmaceutical drugs may lead to arrhythmias. Prescribers need to know that most antiarrhythmic drugs can also *induce* arrhythmias. One of the more common side effects may be long QT syndrome. There are more than 100 drugs known to be associated with long QT intervals. They may change a normal sinus rhythm into an abnormal rhythm due to its effects (**Table 5-9**). If a drug is known to have this side effect, the mechanism of action may affect the depolarization of the QRS complex and change how the ventricles receive and express their electrical impulses. If the QT interval becomes too long, the T wave may occur so late in the cardiac cycle that the next QRS complex lands on top, resulting in a deadly arrhythmia such as Torsades de Pointes (TdP). Many of the drugs in this category have black box warnings due to their potential effects that can lead to fatal ventricular arrhythmias. It is essential to warn patients not to concurrently take other drugs (especially OTC drugs) that can trigger this side effect. Patients at higher risk for this include women; older adults; and patients with bradycardia, heart failure (HF), congenital QT prolongation or Wolf Parkinson's White Syndrome (WPW); low potassium; and low magnesium.

Adverse Drug Reaction Reporting

ADR reporting is the responsibility of all involved when prescribing and using drugs. That includes prescribers, nurses, pharmacists, and patients. The FDA

Table 5-8 Common Nephrotoxic Drugs

Drug	Effects	Patient Considerations
NSAIDs	Reduce renal blood flow	Elderly, heart failure, liver disease, pain management, avoid in renal impairment
Diuretics	Reduce blood volume	Elderly, polypharmacy, avoid in renal impairment
ACEIs	Reduces blood pressure. Cleared by kidneys	Avoid dehydration, watch renal function
Iodinated Radiocontrast	Used in some Radiology procedures. Can cause kidney injury 1–2 days after infusion	Renal impairment, increase hydration to facilitate elimination
Vancomycin	Injury can occur 4–17 days after treatment	Used to treat MRSA
Aminoglycosides (Gentamycin)		Avoid giving longer than 10 days at a time
HIV Medications (Truvada)		Avoid in renal impairment
Antivirals	Crystal formation may block renal filtration	
Reclast (Zoledronic Acid) and Zometa		Avoid in renal impairment

Table 5-9 Drugs Associated With QT Prolongation and TdP

Antiarrhythmics	Antimicrobials	Antidepressants	Antipsychotics	Others
Amiodarone	Levofloxacin	Amitriptyline	Haloperidol	Cisapride
Sotalol	Ciprofloxacin	Desipramine	Droperidol	Sumatriptan
Quinidine	Gatifloxacin	Imipramine	Quetiapine	Zolmitriptan
Procainamide	Moxifloxacin	Doxepin	Thioridazine	Arsenic
Dofetilide	Clarithromycin	Fluoxetine	Ziprasidone	Dolasetron
Ibutilide	Erythromycin	Sertraline		Methadone
	Ketoconazole	Venlafaxine		
	Itraconazole			

has an Adverse Event Reporting System (FAERS) and Medwatch (FDA, 2023). This is all based on post-market surveillance because it is only after a drug enters the market that all the adverse events can be known.

If a patient is having or is suspected to be having an ADR, regardless of the type or severity, it is best to discontinue the drug. If the drug is considered to be lifesaving and there are no other choices to change it to another, the risk–benefit ratio must always be discussed with the patient. It is also good practice to consult with experts in the field for the best outcomes.

One drug that has been suspected for years to cause allergy is penicillin (PCN). This is worth mentioning because there has been a lot of recent controversy on this topic. Many people continue to believe they have or have been told they have an allergy to PCN but do not. About 10 percent of the population historically claim they are allergic to PCN, but research reveals that less than 1 percent of the U.S. population had a true IgE reaction. And even after an allergy to PCN has been identified, the Centers for Disease Control (CDC) estimates that 80 percent of individuals with a true IgE reaction to PCN lose their sensitivity after around 10 years. Continuing to believe that a PCN allergy exists in an individual is a problem because other antibiotics will need to be used for a bacterial infection, which may be inferior to PCN. It has been studied that this may delay treatment, risk sepsis, prolong hospital length of stay, and lead to more opportunistic infections like *C. difficile* and methicillin-resistant Staphylococcus aureus (MRSA). Referral to an allergist for workup is the best way to assess if a true PCN allergy exists (Allergy Asthma Network, 2024).

Commonly Used Medications in Primary Care

Hypertension

Hypertension (HTN) is one of the most common reasons to use drugs in the United States today (Goodrx, n.d.). Several organizations weigh in with recommendations and guidelines regarding HTN (**Table 5-10**). Since there are many risk factors associated with HTN, it is best to provide treatment as soon as possible. The risk versus benefit must be discussed, including lifestyle modifications. Lifestyle changes in eating, sleeping, and physical activity rarely cause adverse reactions. This has been studied to be the most beneficial toward the initial treatment of HTN (Tam et al., 2020). Eating a whole food diet, daily physical activity, avoiding too much alcohol and processed/ultra-processed foods, sleeping well at night, managing stress, and maintaining a healthy weight should all be discussed before using pharmacological drugs (Di Federico et al., 2023). Left untreated (or poorly treated), HTN can lead to complications such as HF, left ventricular hypertrophy, chronic kidney disease, stroke, and myocardial infarction.

When considering the diagnosis of HTN for special populations, it's important to practice safe prescribing. **Table 5-11** identifies some important considerations for different populations when prescribing antihypertensive drugs. Also, to keep in mind, many Americans concurrently take other drugs that are known to *increase* blood pressure. They include contraceptives, nicotine, steroids, weight loss drugs,

Table 5-10 Guidelines for Hypertension Treatment

Organization	Target Population	Target Blood Pressure
American Academy of Family Physicians (AAFP)	Adults with hypertension with or without cardiovascular disease	< 140/90
International Society of Hypertension	Adults Adults < 65 years of age	< 140/90 < 130/80
American Heart Association (AHA)	Adults with established cardiovascular disease	< 130/80
American Diabetes Association	People with diabetes	< 130/80
U.S. Preventative Services Task Force (USPSTF)	No treatment guidelines Only guidelines based on screening	

Table 5-11 Special Populations and Hypertension Treatment

Population	Special Considerations
Pediatrics	Look for undiagnosed metabolic syndrome X, diabetes, or renal insufficiency Recommend electrocardiogram (EKG) (may be left ventricular hypertrophy), then echocardiogram Encourage whole food diet and increase exercise time Ask about sleep patterns Not all drugs have pediatric approval; do not give adult dosing Referral to pediatric specialist is recommended
Women	Look for undiagnosed metabolic syndrome X and/or diabetes Ask about diet and exercise time Ask about sleep patterns **NO angiotensin converting enzyme inhibitor or angiotensin receptor blocker (ACEi or ARBs) if childbearing age** Watch for concurrent smoking or contraception use
Elderly	Look for undiagnosed metabolic syndrome X and/or diabetes Look for renal and hepatic insufficiency Watch for slowing metabolism, fatigue, and polypharmacy
Pregnancy	Look for undiagnosed metabolic syndrome X and/or gestational diabetes Methyldopa and labetolol safest Atenolol and metoprolol safe after 20 weeks' pregnancy

ACEi: Angiotensin Converting Enzyme Inhibitor; ARBs: Angiotensin Receptor Blockers; EKG: Electrocardiogram.

tricyclic antidepressants, cyclosporine, nasal decongestants, and NSAIDs (Mayo Clinic, 2023).

First-line treatments for HTN in primary care include diuretics, angiotensin-converting enzyme inhibitors (ACEIs), angiotensin receptor blockers (ARBs), and calcium channel blockers (**Table 5-12**). Beta blockers are rarely first-line treatments due to their antiarrhythmic properties. However, they are good choices for patients with concomitant ischemic heart disease or HF.

Table 5-12 Antihypertensive Drugs Commonly Used in Primary Care

Drug	Category	Mechanism of Action	Common Side Effects	Special Consideration
ACE-I: • lisinopril • enalapril • captopril • ramipril • quinapril • benzepril • fosinopril	Angiotensin-converting enzyme inhibitors	Inhibits conversion of angiotensin I to angiotensin II, a potent vasoconstrictor	• Hypokalemia • Angioedema is a true allergic reaction	• Watch for chronic, dry cough • Monitor renal function • NOT ok in pregnancy/lactation • NSAIDs diminish control of HTN/HF • Antacids decrease bioavailability
ARBs: • losartan • valsartan • candesartan • irbesartan • olmesartan • telmisartan	Angiotensin II receptor blockers	Dilates arteries and veins and promotes renal excretion of sodium and water	Hypokalemia	• Watch for chronic, dry cough • Monitor renal function • NOT ok in pregnancy/lactation • NSAIDs diminish control of HTN/HF
Renin Inhibitor: aliskiren		Dilates arteries and veins	• Monitor potassium • Diarrhea	• Avoid with ACEI or ARB • Diuretic properties • Dry cough
Diuretics:	**Thiazide Diuretics:** • HCTZ • chlorthalidone • Potassium-sparing diuretics • spironolactone • eplerenone • triamterene **Loop Diuretics:** • furosemide • torsemide • bumetanide	Inhibit sodium-chloride transport in distal tubules Increase sodium and water loss	• Hypokalemia • Dehydration • Hyponatremia • Increased LDL and TG • Hyperglycemia • May exacerbate gout • Loop diuretics may cause ototoxicity	• Watch with digoxin • NSAIDs can reduce diuretic effects • Beta blockers can increase lipids/BG • Steroids can enhance potential hypokalemia
CCBs—Dihydropyridines: • amlodipine • felodipine • nifedipine • nisoldipine • nicardipine • isradipine	**Calcium Channel Blockers** Nondihyrdropyrides: Anti-arrhythmics	Binds to calcium channels in cardiac tissue and sinoatrial node (SA node) Decreases myocardium contractility and heart rate Causes vasodilation Good inhibitor of coronary artery spasms	• Constipation • Dizziness • Fatigue • Lower extremity edema	• Watch with Digoxin • NOT ok in pregnancy/lactation • Use caution with beta blockers

(continues)

Table 5-12 Antihypertensive Drugs Commonly Used in Primary Care *(continued)*

Drug	Category	Mechanism of Action	Common Side Effects	Special Consideration
BBs (cardio selective): - atenolol - metoprolol - nebivolol - bisoprolol - nadolol - propranolol **BBs (non-cardio selective):** - carvedilol - labetalol - sotalol - timolol	Beta Blockers	Decreases heart rate, myocardial contractility and relaxation rate Reduces smooth muscle contraction	- Bradycardia, AV node block - Reduces exercise capacity	- Monitor EKG - Watch BG, lipids, renal, and liver function - May be used in children - Watch for sedation and sleep issues in elderly - Use with caution in pregnancy/lactation

CCBs–Calcium channel blockers; BBs–Beta blockers; ACEIs–Angiotensin-converting enzyme inhibitor; ARB–Angiotensin receptor blocker; NSAIDs–Nonsteroidal anti-inflammatory drugs; HTN–Hypertension; HF–Heart failure; HCTZ–Hydrochlorothiazide; LDL–Low-density lipoprotein; TG–triglycerides; AV–Atrioventricular; BG–Blood glucose; EKG–Electrocardiogram

Beta blockers have two main categories: cardioselective and noncardioselective. Cardioselective beta blockers only affect Beta 1 receptors, which are mainly located in the heart. This means that these drugs may be better for patients with chronic obstructive pulmonary disease (COPD), asthma, peripheral vascular disease (PVD), and diabetes. Noncardioselective beta blockers affect both Beta 1 and Beta 2 receptors, which are located in the heart and lungs, vascular smooth muscle, kidneys, GI tract, and other systems. Although they are less likely to cause fatigue, they may NOT be appropriate for patients with lung issues, vascular disease, and diabetes.

Calcium channel blockers also have two main categories: dihydropyridines and nondihydropyridines. Dihydropyridines are commonly used for HTN and are often first-line therapy for patients of African American descent. The two main drugs in the nondihydropyridine category are Verapamil and Diltiazem. These drugs are used for arrhythmia control, specifically ventricular rate control, in patients with atrial fibrillation. They are typically not used for HTN.

Heart Failure

HF is becoming more common in primary care (Morris & Butler, 2022). HF is seen in two main categories: systolic HF and diastolic HF. Systolic HF results from cardiac damage, such as a myocardial infarction and uncontrolled/poorly controlled HTN, and is seen with a reduced ejection fraction (EF). It is also known as HFrEF. It is diagnosed due to increasing symptoms of dyspnea occurring even at rest. EFs below 40 require a cardiac workup, and when the EF drops below 30, the patient is at risk for sudden cardiac death from ventricular fibrillation. These patients may need an implantable cardiac defibrillator (ICD).

The second category of HF is diastolic HF, which has a preserved EF. It is highly associated with hyperglycemia, type 2 diabetes, and insulin resistance. Initially, it does *not* present with a reduced EF and is known as HFpEF (Redfield & Borlaug, 2023). It is also diagnosed due to increasing dyspnea symptoms. The same criteria for needing an ICD apply.

Digoxin, a cardiac glycoside, is among the oldest drugs used for HF since the late 18th century. Today, it is a drug that interacts with others that are commonly used in HF. Drugs like amiodarone, verapamil, and diltiazem used concurrently with digoxin can increase serum levels and risk digoxin toxicity. Digoxin use requires periodic blood testing of levels to avoid potential toxicity. If it is used for HF, it is used for patients with severe systolic dysfunction with EFs less than 40 percent and patients with symptoms unrelieved by ACE inhibitors and diuretics. In electrophysiology, digoxin has largely been replaced by beta blockers, which exert similar physiological goals to decrease preload and/or afterload, improve contractility, and decrease heart rate.

Control of underlying causes of HF is key to mitigating symptoms and preserving patient independence. Control of HTN (using drugs and lifestyle modifications), weight loss, blood glucose control, and any other factor that may be contributing to HF symptoms must be employed (Pandey et al., 2020)

Sacubitril/Valsartan, also known as Entresto, is a combination drug for HF that has a lot of success in keeping patients out of the hospital. It *cannot* be used in conjunction with an ACEI or ARB and is *not* recommended in pregnancy/breastfeeding. Due to its ARB component, the same side effects and warnings apply. Digoxin is also still used for patients with HF; however, it MUST be monitored periodically as the therapeutic range is narrow, and it also has renal dosing. Hydralazine and minoxidil are also used for HF due to their peripheral vascular effects. Thiazide diuretics are *not* used for HF; however, loop diuretics like furosemide reduce preload and overall volume but can only be used for patients with GFR greater than 30, so check renal function frequently.

Anticoagulants

Warfarin is one of the most effective, inexpensive, and widely prescribed anticoagulant drugs. It acts by inhibiting the enzyme vitamin K epoxide reductase, which prevents the formation of functional vitamin K. This inhibits the activation of clotting factors in the liver, causing prolonged PT/PTT clotting time. Prolonged bleeding time is the only side effect of warfarin, but it has many interactions with drugs and foods. It needs to be monitored regularly with its own blood test. The International Normalization Ratio (INR) monitors bleeding times and maintains a "therapeutic range." If the INR is too high, the patient may bleed excessively, and if it is too low, the patient may clot. The therapeutic range for most patients requiring warfarin is 2 to 3. The main diagnoses that require anticoagulation are atrial fibrillation, atrial flutter, deep vein thrombosis (DVT), pulmonary embolism (PE), and coagulopathies. Patients with mechanical heart valves must use warfarin as an anticoagulant, as the other oral anticoagulants have not yet been approved for this population. The INR therapeutic range for patients with mechanical heart valves is 2.5 to 3.5 (Syed et al., 2024).

In addition to the anticoagulant warfarin, the direct oral anticoagulants (commonly called the DOACs) are also used to prevent thrombus development. They are commonly used to prevent stroke in people with nonvalvular atrial fibrillation and to prevent and treat venous thromboembolism. They have fewer drug and food interactions than warfarin and do not require INR monitoring. They are also shorter acting than warfarin. They are more expensive than warfarin. **Table 5-13** lists the commonly used anticoagulants and any necessary monitoring, interactions, and precautions.

Patients are also often prescribed antiplatelet drugs. These act differently than anticoagulants and are used for different reasons. Sometimes, they are used together, significantly increasing the bleeding risk. It is important to note that the American Heart Association no longer recommends daily baby aspirin 81 mg for cardiovascular risk reduction in patients *without* established heart disease. The most common use for this class of drugs is for ischemic heart disease patients with cardiac stents, coronary artery bypass graft history, and peripheral vascular disease. These drugs include Aspirin 81 mg or 325 mg daily; clopidogrel (Plavix) 75 mg daily; ticagrelor (Brilinta) 60 mg or 90 mg daily; prasugrel (Effient) 5 mg or 10 mg daily; and cilostazol (Pletal) 50 mg or 100 mg BID.

Hyperlipidemia

Drugs to lower cholesterol and triglycerides are among the most commonly prescribed drugs in the United States (GoodRx, n.d.). Cardiology and primary care prescribe statins most frequently, and many are prescribed for people using them for the "primary prevention" of cardiovascular disease. This means there is no established disease yet. The USPSTF only gives a B to C grade for using statins as primary prevention (USPSTF, 2022). The American College of Cardiology and the AHA have developed a 10-year risk calculator to see if a patient meets the criteria for using a statin (AHA, n.d.).

The decision to provide a statin to a patient is often for a lifetime, so all efforts should be placed on helping the patient do lifestyle modifications, such as a diet low in carbohydrates and sugars, daily exercise, reducing alcohol, encouraging healthy sleep, and stress reduction techniques, before prescribing if possible. If a statin is needed, it is important to run a full set of bloodwork as elevated blood glucose, hypo or hyperthyroidism, and liver disease may be found to cause the elevated lipids. These issues need to be addressed prior to prescribing statins.

Adults who smoke cigarettes and those with existing ischemic heart disease and type 2 diabetes are considered the highest risk groups and may benefit the most from using a cholesterol-lowering drug (CDC, 2024). Because nonalcoholic fatty liver disease is a growing concern in the United States, always check liver function before starting one of these drugs (**Table 5-14**).

Many drugs can raise serum lipids, so doing a full set of blood work and getting a thorough history is important. Drugs known to raise serum lipids include beta blockers, steroids, oral contraceptives, estrogen

Table 5-13 Commonly Used Anticoagulants

Anticoagulant	Monitoring/Reversal?	Interactions	Precautions
Warfarin (Coumadin)	Regular INR testing Reversal: Vitamin K or FFP	Foods high in vitamin K OTC pain relievers Narcotic pain relievers Concurrent aspirin Some antimicrobials* Alcohol	No renal dosing
Dabigatran (Pradaxa) DIRECT thrombin inhibitor	No monitoring Reversal: idarucizumab (Praxabind)	Some antimicrobials* Concurrent aspirin Erythromycin Nondihydropyridine calcium channel blockers Phenobarbital and dilantin	Renal dosing Caution with bariatric patients
Rivaroxaban (Xarelto) Inhibitor of Factor Xa	No monitoring Reversal: adnexanet (Adnexxa)	Some antimicrobials* Concurrent aspirin Erythromycin Nondihydropyridine calcium channel blockers Phenobarbital and dilantin	Renal dosing Caution with bariatric patients
Apixaban (Eliquis) Inhibitor of Factor Xa	No monitoring Reversal: adnexanet (Adnexxa)	Some antimicrobials* Concurrent aspirin Erythromycin Nondihydropyridine calcium channel blockers Phenobarbital and dilantin	Renal dosing Caution with bariatric patients
Edoxaban (Savaysa) Inhibitor of Factor Xa	No monitoring No approved reversal agent	Some antimicrobials* Concurrent aspirin Erythromycin Nondihydropyridine calcium channel blockers Phenobarbital and dilantin	Renal dosing Caution with bariatric patients
Enoxaparin (Lovenox) Injection	No monitoring Dose based on weight	Pregnancy Category B	Renal dosing

High-risk antimicrobials: Bactrim, ciprofloxacin, levofloxacin, metronidazole, fluconazole, azithromycin, clarithromycin.
Low-risk antimicrobials: Clindamycin, cephalexin
FFP: Fresh frozen plasma

therapy, some antipsychotics, and thiazide diuretics (Herink & Ito, 2018). Lifestyle behaviors, which are known to raise serum lipids, include smoking cigarettes, obesity, type 2 diabetes (also prediabetes and insulin resistance), stress, internal inflammation (from poor diet and other/undiagnosed disease processes), and sedentary lifestyle (Franklin et al., 2020).

There is a lot of new research showing how eating the "Standard American Diet," which is estimated to be > 60 percent processed and ultra-processed food, is a large contributor to the problem of hyperlipidemia in the United States (Martinez Steele et al., 2017). Drinking alcohol frequently, even at the AHA's recommendations of one drink a day for a woman and two drinks a day for a man, is contributing to this problem. The newest data from the AHA now states that even one drink a day can increase risk, so no amount of alcohol may be considered safe (Di Federico et al., 2023).

Antimicrobials

Antibiotics, antivirals, and antifungal agents are a big part of primary care. Over the last several decades, antimicrobial resistance has become a growing problem, which now threatens the future use and success of these drugs. When using any antimicrobial agent, using the narrowest spectrum with the lowest potential

Table 5-14 Drugs for Hyperlipidemia

Drug	Mechanism of Action	Common Side Effect	Special Considerations
Statins: - atorvastatin - rosuvastatin - simvastatin - pravastatin - lovastatin - fluvastatin - pitavastatin	Inhibits 3-hydroxy-3-methylglutaryl-coenzyme A reductase, inhibiting cholesterol synthesis in the liver	- Myalgias, tendon - Rupture, pancreatitis - Type 2 diabetes - CK elevation - Cognitive impairment - Behavioral changes - AST/ALT elevation	- NOT ok in pregnancy/lactation - Do not use in liver disease
Ezetimibe:	Selectively inhibits absorption of dietary cholesterol in the intestine	- Diarrhea - Sore throat - Joint and leg pains	- Best used with a statin in patients with familial heterozygous hyperlipidemia - NOT ok in pregnancy
PCSK-9 Inhibitors: - alirocumab - evolocumab - inclisiran	Blocks the PCSK9 protein, which makes LDL receptors susceptible to degradation	- Angioedema - Muscle pains - Nasopharyngitis - Hyperglycemia - Diarrhea	- Best used in patients with familial heterozygous hyperlipidemia - Only injected
Fibrates: - *gemfibrozil - *fenofibrate	Inhibits cholesterol and triglyceride synthesis	- Myalgias - Pancreatitis - Nausea - Diarrhea - Cholelithiasis	Used for TG > 500 and familial heterozygous hyperlipidemia
Bile Acid Sequestrants: - cholesevelam - cholestyramine - colestipol	Convert cholesterol into bile acid and promotes bile acid excretion in feces	- Dyspepsia - Constipation - Bloating and abdominal pain	OK in liver disease
Omega-3 Fatty Acids: - icosapent ethyl - omega-3 acid - ethyl esters	Reduce serum triglycerides	- Diarrhea - Nausea - Heartburn - Upset stomach - Bloating - Constipation	Watch for arrhythmias and bleeding

for adverse effects is good practice. Narrow spectrum agents are effective against a limited number of organisms and are unlikely to disrupt normal flora. In contrast, broad-spectrum agents are effective against multiple organisms from more than a single class (Church & McKillip, 2021).

Antibiotics

Antibiotics are generally either bacteriostatic (inhibit the growth and replication of bacteria) or bactericidal (kill the bacteria independent of the immune system). These agents are used against Gram-positive (aerobic) and Gram-negative (anaerobic) bacteria. Common Gram-positive bacteria include *Staphylococcus aureus*, *Streptococcus pneumoniae*, listeria, and *Staphylococcus agalactiae*. Common Gram-negative bacteria include *Neisseria meningitidis*, *Haemophilus influenza*, *Klebsiella pneumonia*, and *Escherichia coli*. Specific antibiotics are best used against either Gram-positive or Gram-negative bacteria (**Table 5-15**).

Antifungals

These drugs inhibit fungal growth and use the CYP450 and CYP34A enzymes. The oral forms have multiple and frequent drug–drug interactions and therefore require close liver monitoring. Alcohol is not recommended when using these oral drugs, and they should always be taken with food. Griseofluvin V,

Table 5-15 Commonly Used Oral Antibiotics

Class	Common Use	Considerations
Penicillins (PCNs): amoxicillin amoxicillin/clavulanate piperacillin PCN G PCN VK dicloxacillin oxacillin	GABHS* (Strep Throat) Many upper respiratory infections, including CAP	Watch for *C. difficile* super infection Resistance is common
Cephalosporins: First generation: cephalexin cefadroxil Second generation: cefaclor cefprozil cefuroxime axetil Third generation: cefdinir cefixime Fourth and fifth generation: Only injectables	First generation: Use for skin and soft tissue infections, upper respiratory infections, impetigo, pharyngitis, and tonsillitis Second generation: Use for pneumonia, skin infections, and otitis media Third generation: Use for bronchitis, gonorrhea, skin/soft tissue, syphilis, meningitis	Beta-lactam: related to PCNs Monitor CBC and kidney function First generation: Does not penetrate cerebrospinal fluid Third generation: Can cross the blood/brain barrier. Not reliable against anaerobes
Fluoroquinolones: ciprofloxacin levofloxacin moxifloxacin ofloxacin	Use for CAP, chlamydia, epididymitis, traveler's diarrhea, joint infections, typhoid fever, and meningococcus	Beware: Tendon rupture (Achilles), tendonitis, muscle weakness/aches Beware: Long Q-T syndrome, may need renal dosing NOT recommended in children/pregnancy
Clindamycin	Reserved for severe infections First-line treatment of MRSA Often used as SBE prophylaxis, skin/soft tissue infections in patients with PCN allergy	NOT recommended in pregnancy
Macrolides/Azolides: erythromycin azithromycin clarithromycin	Used for *H. pylori* infections, often used for patients with PCN allergy, CAP	Erythromycin and azithromycin safe in pregnancy Clarithromycin NOT safe in pregnancy Watch liver and arrhythmias and other interactions
Tetracyclines: doxycycline minocycline tetracycline	Often used for skin infections	Avoid in children < 8 years old (can harm teeth) Photosensitivity May be hard to tolerate Watch for interactions
Sulfonamides, *Trimethoprim,* *Nitrofurantoin*	These are structurally related Used for upper respiratory infections Nitrofurantoin: First line for UTIs (watch for resistance)	May not be appropriate in pregnancy

GABHS–Group A-beta Hemolytic Streptococcus; CAP–Community-acquired Pneumonia; CBC–Complete blood count; MRSA–Methicillin-resistant Staphylococcus aureus; SBE–Subacute bacterial endocarditis prophylaxis; UTIs–Urinary tract infections fluconazole, itraconazole, clotrimazole, and ketoconazole are all are considered "broad spectrum." Fluconazole (Diflucan) is often prescribed for a vaginal yeast super infection following using an antibiotic. A locally applied antifungal drug may be a better choice as we now see antifungal-resistant fungi. *Candida aureus* was first identified in 2016 and is particularly deadly.

The topical forms of these drugs are not as convenient and may be messy, but they do the job well without the high risk of resistance. Topically applied creams and powders are available for most skin, mouth, and vaginal yeast infections.

Antivirals: NOT HIV

Oral and topically applied drugs are used for common viral infections such as herpes simplex I and II, herpes zoster (Varicella/Shingles), human papillomavirus (HPV), viral Hepatitis B & C, influenza, and COVID-19.

Common Oral Antivirals
- Acyclovir (Zovirax): Used for herpes simplex I and II and herpes zoster
- Famciclovir (Famvir): Used for herpes simplex I and II and varicella
- Valacyclovir (Valtrex): Used for herpes simplex I and II, herpes zoster, and varicella
  - Use caution in the elderly, hepatic/liver impairment, and immunocompromised

Common Topical Antivirals
- Penciclovir (Danavir): 1% Cream
- Docosanol (Abreva): Cream

Influenza Antivirals
- Oseltamivir (Tamiflu) 75 mg BID × 5 days
  - May use in pregnancy/breastfeeding
  - OK in children with pediatric dosing
  - Reduces flu symptoms × 20 to 24 hours and must be given within 1 to 2 days of symptom onset to be effective. It can be given prophylactically, but side effects include nausea, vomiting, diarrhea, and headache.
- Baloxavir (Xofluza) 40 to 80 mg × 1 (based on weight)
  - *not* in pregnancy/breastfeeding
  - OK in children with pediatric dosing
  - Nausea and diarrhea

Review Questions

1. The regulation of practice authority and prescriptive authority for the advanced practice registered nurse (APRN) is made by:
   A. the Federal Drug Enforcement Agency (DEA).
   B. the Food and Drug Administration (FDA).
   C. the American Medical Association (AMA).
   D. the state board of nursing.

2. The DEA license held by a nurse practitioner (NP) allows the NP to:
   A. prescribe marijuana (depending on state laws).
   B. prescribe drugs that are in Schedules II to V. (Some states do not allow NPs to prescribe Schedule II drugs.)
   C. prescribe drugs that are in Schedules I to V.
   D. only prescribe drugs that are not scheduled drugs.

3. Some drugs are agonist drugs. This means they bind with specific receptor cells in the body to produce an active response. Endorphins are the body's natural agonist for specific receptor cells. What is a synthetic agonist for these receptor cells?
   A. Naltrexone
   B. Selective Serotonin Reuptake Inhibitors (SSRIs)
   C. Nicotine
   D. Demerol

4. Some drugs have an antagonist effect. They block the receptor sites so that a chemical or drug is prevented from occupying the specific receptor. An example of a synthetic antagonist for endorphins is:
   A. naloxone.
   B. buprenorphine.
   C. methadone.
   D. nicotine.

5. An NP may decide to prescribe an opioid pain reliever for a patient with significant pain. The NP should make every effort to prevent abuse of opioid pain relievers. One proven technique that the NP can use is to:
   A. discuss with the patient that any abuse of the pain-relieving opioid drug will lead to being discharged from the practice.
   B. limit the amount of opioid pain reliever to a 1-month supply.
   C. have a written pain contract in place that outlines the responsibility of both the prescriber and the patient.
   D. discuss with the patient that nonnarcotic pain medication will be prescribed. If the patient does not get relief, they will need to see a pain specialist.

6. The term "pharmacokinetics" refers to:
   A. what the drug does to the body.
   B. what the body does to the drug.
   C. the goal of achieving therapeutic range.
   D. the first-pass effective.

7. Which area of the body is the main site of drug metabolism?
   A. Gastrointestinal tract
   B. Integumentary system
   C. Liver
   D. Kidneys

8. Which of the following statements is correct concerning the first-pass effect?
   A. The amount of drug entering the systemic circulation after undergoing the first-pass effect is increased.
   B. The amount of drug entering the systemic circulation after undergoing the first-pass effect is decreased.
   C. A patient with hepatic dysfunction will have fewer drugs entering the circulation.
   D. A patient with renal insufficiency may not effectively excrete a drug.

9. The NP prescribing medication for a pregnant person must consider many things. Pregnancy categories range from category A (no risk) to category X (contraindicated). Which category of drugs shows positive evidence of fetal risk and should only be used in pregnancy if the benefits clearly outweigh the risks?
   A. Category B
   B. Category C
   C. Category D
   D. The NP should not prescribe any medication to a pregnant person without first consulting with the patient's obstetrician.

10. Polypharmacy is a common issue with older persons. The NP should perform medication review and reconciliation at every visit. The American Geriatrics Society publishes a list of medications that should be used cautiously in older people. This list is known as:
    A. the Adverse Event Reporting System list.
    B. the Drug Enforcement Agency list.
    C. the Beers Criteria.
    D. the American Pharmacists Association (AphA) Criteria.

11. The NP is very responsible when prescribing medications. One aspect of this responsibility is reviewing the patient's most recent laboratory results. Which body system must be assessed before prescribing medications?
    A. Gastrointestinal
    B. Cardiovascular
    C. Renal
    D. Endocrine

12. Many drugs are hepatotoxic. Patients must be informed about this potential toxicity. What is the most appropriate response to a patient if they ask the NP what medications they can take for their cold symptoms?
    A. "Do not take ibuprofen within 8 hours of taking acetaminophen."
    B. "You can take acetaminophen as directed, but be aware that many cold-relieving preparations also contain acetaminophen. You should never exceed 4,000 mg of acetaminophen in a 24-hour period."
    C. "It is preferable not to take any oral medications for your cold symptoms. Your body will fight off the virus typically within 3 to 7 days."
    D. "You only need to take an antipyretic medication, such as ibuprofen or acetaminophen, if you develop a fever."

13. Some drugs are associated with QT prolongation, which can lead to dangerous arrhythmias and need to be used cautiously. One class of medications that is associated with QT prolongation is:
    A. fluoroquinolones.
    B. statins.
    C. loop diuretics.
    D. PDE5 inhibitors.

14. The NP evaluates a 35-year-old female patient with established hypertension (HTN). The patient takes three medications to reduce her blood pressure. In the office, her BP is 140/90. The patient

states that she doesn't want to add more medications since she already takes "too many pills." The NP reviews the medication list for this patient. The patient takes amlodipine, lasix, lisinopril, an oral contraceptive pill (OCP), phentermine for weight loss, and daily ibuprofen for "aches and pains." What is the most appropriate recommendation by the NP for this patient that addresses her concern?
   A. "We need to add one more antihypertensive medication because you have a disorder known as 'resistant HTN.'"
   B. "You will need to be evaluated by a cardiologist because the antihypertensives you take are not working well enough."
   C. "OCPs, phentermine, and ibuprofen are all medications that increase your BP, and we need to consider alternatives."
   D. " If you lose weight, your BP will come down, so let's focus on your weight loss for now."

15. A 33-year-old female patient with type 2 diabetes is being evaluated today by her PCP. She reports that she and her spouse have decided to start a family and are actively trying to get pregnant. A review of the patient's medications reveals that she is currently taking:
   Metformin 500 mg BID, lisinopril 5 mg daily, and Lantus 10 units at bedtime.
   The NP informs the patient that she should immediately:
   A. discontinue the Lantus at bedtime.
   B. discontinue the metformin 500 mg PO BID.
   C. continue the current medications and begin a prenatal vitamin.
   D. discontinue the lisinopril and discuss alternatives.

16. A 50-year-old male patient with HTN was recently prescribed lisinopril by his PCP. Two weeks later, he returned for a follow-up blood pressure check. His blood pressure in the office today is 118/76. The patient is now requesting to be evaluated for gastroesophageal reflux disease (GERD) and sleep apnea because he is not sleeping well and has developed a cough that is interfering with his sleep and daytime activities. With this information, what intervention should the NP now recommend?
   A. "I would like to order a PPI for you to take first thing in the morning. This should prevent GERD symptoms and alleviate the coughing symptoms."
   B. "I will order a sleep study to help tell us if you have sleep apnea or GERD."
   C. "I will stop the lisinopril and order a different antihypertensive medication to see if this alleviates the coughing symptoms."
   D. "Let's continue the lisinopril for now because it works well. We can follow up in 3 months to see if your cough has resolved."

17. The CYP450 pathway in the liver uses enzymes to metabolize drugs. Many drugs are considered to be CYP450 inhibitors, and this can lead to several negative effects. If a CYP450 inhibitor is taken along with a drug using the same enzyme pathway such as warfarin, the following may result:
   A. The anticoagulant effect of the warfarin will be reduced, and the patient will require higher dosing.
   B. The drugs will compete for the receptor sites, and the more potent drug will have a stronger effect.
   C. The anticoagulant effect of warfarin will be increased.
   D. If the patient doesn't take the drug at the same time as the other medication, there should not be any negative effects.

18. There are two main categories of beta blockers. The cardioselective beta blocker only blocks beta 1 receptors that are primarily located in the heart. If a patient would benefit from beta-blocker therapy, the cardioselective beta blockers would be the preferred choice for patients who have:
   A. hyperthyroidism.
   B. resistant HTN.
   C. diabetes.
   D. anxiety and/or panic attacks.

19. A 30-year-old female patient is being evaluated and treated for an uncomplicated UTI. The NP prescribes Bactrim DS 160 mg PO BID × 7 days. The NP discusses treatment and follow-up with the patient. Which of the following statements made by the patient is most critical?
   A. "I know I should get the urinalysis (U/A) and culture and sensitivity (C&S) first before starting the medication."
   B. "I understand that I should complete the entire course of antibiotic therapy even if I feel better."
   C. "I think I was told a long time ago that I might have a sulfa allergy."
   D. "I know that I should have repeat testing done after I finish this course of therapy."

20. Warfarin is a common anticoagulant. It is widely prescribed because it is inexpensive and effective. Patients on warfarin need to have frequent

International Normalization Ratio (INR) monitoring and understand bleeding precautions. A patient taking warfarin needs to understand that:
A. the therapeutic range for the INR is 3.0 to 4.0.
B. many foods contain vitamin K and may interfere with the effectiveness of warfarin.
C. there is no antidote for warfarin.
D. they should no longer engage in outdoor activities.

21. Drugs used to lower cholesterol are among the most common types of drugs prescribed in primary care. The most common category of antihyperlipidemic drugs are statin drugs. Before prescribing a statin drug, the prescriber should first obtain laboratory tests to assess for (select all that apply):
A. pregnancy.
B. renal diseases.
C. anemia.
D. liver disease.

22. Antifungal medications use the CYP450 and CYP34A enzymes. The oral forms of the antifungal medication have frequent drug–drug interactions that can hurt the liver. Which of the following statements, when made by the patient, indicates a good understanding of taking antifungal medication?
A. "I know I should take this medication on an empty stomach."
B. "I should limit my alcohol intake to no more than one ounce daily while I'm taking this medication."
C. "I should complete the course of therapy prescribed even if my symptoms have resolved."
D. "If I develop a headache or nausea, I know to discontinue the medication."

23. A 25-year-old female patient comes to the clinic complaining of fever, anorexia, body aches, and cold symptoms for the past 4 days. The patient gets a nasal swab and is positive for influenza-type A. The patient is asking for a prescription medication to treat her symptoms. What is the most appropriate treatment recommendation?
A. Prescribe Oseltamivir (Tamiflu) 75 mg BID × 5 days.
B. Prescribe Acyclovir 400 mg PO TID × 7 days.
C. Recommend supportive care such as rest, fluids, and acetaminophen or NSAIDs as directed for fever and body aches.
D. Prescribe azithromycin (Z-pack) 500 mg PO on day 1 and then 250 mg PO daily for the next 4 days.

24. A new patient is providing her medical history. She reports being allergic to codeine. The NP asks her what type of reaction she had when she took codeine, and the patient states that it made her very nauseated. The NP documents that the patient states she is allergic to codeine and recognizes that the reaction most likely:
A. is a common side effect of the medication.
B. is an allergic reaction that will become increasingly severe with repeated exposure to the medication.
C. could cause an anaphylactic reaction if she were to receive it again.
D. is due to a drug–drug interaction.

25. A patient who is also a nurse presents to the office complaining of severe back pain after lifting a heavy patient at work the day before. The patient is requesting a narcotic pain medication to help alleviate her pain. Before ordering the narcotic medication, the APRN should:
A. have the patient undergo a urinalysis test for toxic substances.
B. review the patient's history of controlled substance prescriptions through the PDMP (Prescription Drug Monitoring Program).
C. educate the patient that NSAIDs are far more effective than narcotics for relief of back pain.
D. refer the patient to a neurologist for possible treatment with a steroid injection.

Answers and Rationales

1. Answer D is correct. The individual states and the state board of nursing regulate prescriptive authority for the APRN.

   Answer A is incorrect. The DEA requires a practitioner to have a DEA registration number to dispense controlled substances.

   Answer B is incorrect. The FDA regulates medical products; prescriptions; and nonprescription drugs, food, and biologics. The FDA is responsible for protecting public health. It does not determine practice authority.

Answer C is incorrect. The American Medical Association opposes the expansion of the scope of practice (such as independent practice and prescriptive authority) by nonphysicians, arguing that this threatens patient safety. The association does not regulate APRN practice.

2. Answer B is correct. NPs with a DEA license may prescribe Schedule II to V drugs.

    Answer A is incorrect. Federal law continues to schedule marijuana as a Schedule I drug. Individual states that have legalized medical marijuana conflict with federal law. Most states that have legalized medical marijuana allow the APRN to certify a patient for a medical marijuana program. It is not prescribed; rather, the patient is enrolled in the program.

    Answer C is incorrect. Schedule I drugs include heroin, LSD, and other hallucinogens. Drugs listed as Schedule I are considered to have no safe accepted medical use in the United States.

    Answer D is incorrect. The NP is allowed to write prescriptions for medications in all 50 states. However, the state board of nursing decides whether the NP can prescribe scheduled drugs.

3. Answer D is correct. Demerol is a synthetic endorphin agonist and binds to those specific receptor cells.

    Answer A is incorrect. Naltrexone is an antagonist that blocks the chemicals from occupying the receptor sites.

    Answer B is incorrect. SSRIs work by increasing serotonin levels. They are not endorphins.

    Answer C is incorrect. Nicotine is a highly addictive stimulant drug found in tobacco products that speeds up the messaging traveling through the brain and body.

4. Answer A is correct. Naloxone is an antagonist for endorphin receptor sites and blocks endorphins or similar drugs, such as morphine, fentanyl, and so on, from the receptor cells.

    Answer B is incorrect. Buprenorphine is an opioid agonist and binds to those same opioid receptors.

    Answer C is incorrect. Methadone is an opioid agonist.

    Answer D is incorrect. Nicotine is an addictive stimulant drug and does not have an affinity for opioid receptor sites.

5. Answer C is correct. Before prescribing an opioid pain reliever, the NP should have a written pain contract that outlines the responsibility for both the patient and the NP. This should be in accordance with the NP's clinical practice organization.

    Answer A is incorrect. Threatening the patient that they will be discharged from the practice is inappropriate and does not promote a therapeutic relationship.

    Answer B is incorrect. The APRN needs to know what the state regulations are regarding the amount of opioid medication that the NP can prescribe. This varies from state to state.

    Answer D is incorrect. If the patient has "significant pain," it is appropriate for the NP to try to help the patient get effective pain control. Nonnarcotic pain medication may or may not be effective and may be tried initially. A pain specialist is needed if the patient's pain cannot be controlled with the medications that the NP is permitted to prescribe and has determined that the medication is not effective.

6. Answer B is correct. Pharmacokinetics describes what the body does to the drug and is related to many patient factors, such as renal function, sex, age, and genetic makeup.

    Answer A is incorrect. Pharmacodynamics is what the drug does to the body.

    Answer C is incorrect. Pharmacokinetics is a term used to describe what the body does to a drug. It is not a goal.

    Answer D is incorrect. The first-pass effect refers to the metabolism a medication undergoes in the body that decreases the amount of drug reaching circulation.

7. Answer C is correct. The liver is the primary site where drug metabolism occurs.

    Answer A is incorrect. While some drugs may be metabolized in the GI tract, this is not the main site of metabolism for most drugs.

    Answer B is incorrect. The integumentary system is the largest organ in the body, but transdermal medication passes through the deeper dermal layer to be absorbed in the circulation.

    Answer D is incorrect. The renal system is primarily responsible for the excretion of most medications.

8. Answer B is correct. The first-pass effect will reduce the amount of the drug entering the circulation by first metabolizing the drug. Most often, this metabolism occurs in the liver, but it can occur in other organs as well.

    Answer A is incorrect. The amount of drug that enters the circulation after the first-pass effect is decreased. The individual also influences this. Many factors, including sex and age, influence the first-pass effect.

    Answer C is incorrect. A patient with hepatic dysfunction will have *more* drugs entering the circulation because the liver is unable to function appropriately and metabolize the drug effectively.

    Answer D is incorrect. The ability of the body to excrete the drug is not a factor in the first-pass effect.

9. Answer C is correct. There is evidence of risk to the fetus, which has been demonstrated in studies on pregnant women who have received the drug. The potential benefit of the drug should outweigh the risks to the fetus.

    Answer A is incorrect. Category B states that there have been no risks to the fetus in animal studies. There is not enough information in human studies.

    Answer B is incorrect. Category C states that there have been risks to the fetus seen in animal studies. There are no satisfactory studies on pregnant people.

    Answer D is incorrect. The NP can prescribe medication to a pregnant person without consulting the obstetrician. Certain states in the United States may require physician oversight of prescriptive authority, but it is not necessarily the patient's obstetrician.

10. Answer C is correct. The American Geriatrics Society publishes a list of medications that should be used cautiously in older people. The list is called the "Beers criteria."

    Answer A is incorrect. Clinicians and the public can use the Adverse Event Reporting list to report an adverse reaction to medications.

    Answer B is incorrect. The DEA does not compile a list of drugs that should be used cautiously in elderly persons.

    Answer D is incorrect. The AphA works to ensure that patients have access to pharmacists' care and to upgrade the standards of pharmacy services.

11. Answer C is correct. While any body systems may affect the metabolism and effectiveness of drugs, most drugs are excreted via the renal system, and, therefore, the NP must review a patient's renal function before prescribing any medication.

    Answer A is incorrect. The gastrointestinal system may be involved in a medication's metabolism and excretion, but it is not the most essential body system. Additionally, assessing the GI function through reviewing laboratory values would be difficult.

    Answer B is incorrect. CV function is not the most essential body system for excretion of medications. CV function should be considered when prescribing any medication. However, it is difficult to assess through laboratory values and is not considered when reviewing the drug's information on medication dosing.

    Answer D is incorrect. Endocrine function should be considered when the drug directly affects the endocrine system. In hypothyroidism, increased medication circulating due to slowed metabolism may occur. However, renal function is the most important body system that needs to be assessed because this is the most common way that drugs are excreted from the body.

12. Answer B is correct. Many cold preparations contain acetaminophen; patients must be aware of this to prevent hepatic injury.

    Answer A is incorrect. Ibuprofen and acetaminophen are often taken alternately. The most common recommendation is to separate them by 3 to 4 hours.

    Answer C is incorrect. Patients need symptomatic relief from cold symptoms. Depending on the virus, their bodies will fight it off over time. This is independent of taking symptom relief medications.

    Answer D is incorrect. Patients with colds often need relief from congestion, cough, or body aches. Many OTC preparations, such as decongestants, antitussive medications, and pain relievers (e.g., ibuprofen or acetaminophen), are appropriate for them to take for symptom relief.

13. Answer A is correct. Many drugs in the fluoroquinolone class can prolong QT and should be used cautiously in patients with bradyarrhythmia or known long QT intervals.

    Answer B is incorrect. Statin drugs are not implicated in QT prolongation.

Answer C is incorrect. Loop diuretics are not associated with QT prolongation. However, patients on loop diuretics are at risk for hypokalemia, which can lead to arrhythmias.

Answer D is incorrect. PDE5 inhibitors cause vasodilation and must be used cautiously in patients who take any form of nitrates or have hypotension. PDE5 inhibitors are not associated with QT prolongation.

14. Answer C is correct. OCPs, phentermine, and ibuprofen are all implicated in causing HTN. To address the patient's concerns, alternative medications could be recommended, or options such as using barrier methods for birth control should be offered.

    Answer A is incorrect. Although the patient is considered to have resistant HTN, adding more antihypertensive medications does not address this patient's concerns of "taking too many pills."

    Answer B is incorrect. The patient may need to be evaluated by a cardiologist to help reduce her blood pressure; however, some of the medications implicated in raising it should be removed first.

    Answer D is incorrect. For this patient, focusing on weight loss is not the priority. She has expressed concern that she takes too many medications, and her BP currently remains elevated. Removing some of the medications known to elevate BP is the most appropriate response to address her concerns.

15. Answer D is correct. ACE inhibitors are a category D for a pregnant person. This is particularly true in the second and third trimesters.

    Answer A is incorrect. Lantus is safe to use during pregnancy and does not cross the placental barrier.

    Answer B is incorrect. Metformin is a category B for pregnant women and is considered a safe and successful treatment for patients with type 2 diabetes or gestational diabetes.

    Answer C is incorrect. The patient should start prenatal vitamins if she is actively trying to achieve pregnancy. However, she should be prescribed an alternative medication other than an ACE inhibitor.

16. Answer C is correct. The most common side effect of ACE inhibitors is a dry hacking cough. The patient should be prescribed a different class of medications for his BP.

    Answer A is incorrect. Although GERD may cause the patient's cough, it is preferable to first try a different hypertensive medication because ACE inhibitors commonly cause coughs as a side effect.

    Answer B is incorrect. The question does not provide any information (such as snoring or gasping when waking up) that would cause the NP to think his cough is associated with sleep apnea.

    Answer D is incorrect. Continuing the lisinopril (which is likely the cause of his cough) for an additional 3 months will interfere with his quality of life and may cause an unnecessary delay in intervening and eradicating the cause.

17. Answer C is correct. The anticoagulant effect of warfarin will be increased. This is because the CYP450 inhibitor will inhibit the metabolism of warfarin and subsequently increase the amount available to the body.

    Answer A is incorrect. The anticoagulant effect of the warfarin will be increased, not reduced, and the patient's INR will need to be carefully monitored.

    Answer B is incorrect. While the drugs may compete for the same enzyme receptor sites, deciding which drug is more potent does not affect the outcome. It depends on whether the drug is a CYP450 inhibitor.

    Answer D is incorrect. Warfarin has a long half-life of 20 to 60 hours. Taking a CYP450 inhibitor with warfarin will have a negative effect on the anticoagulant effect of warfarin even if they are taken 12 hours apart.

18. Answer C is correct. Patients with diabetes may experience hypoglycemia unawareness due to the blocking effects on their adrenaline response if they use a non-cardioselective beta-blocker.

    Answer A is incorrect. Patients who have symptomatic hyperthyroidism benefit from non-selective beta-1 and beta-2 adrenergic blockers.

    Answer B is incorrect. Although beta blockers are not the first-line choice for patients with HTN, if used, they would benefit from both beta-1 and beta-2 adrenergic blocking.

    Answer D is incorrect. The benefit of beta blockers, when used for stage fright, anxiety, or panic attacks, is the effect of both beta-1 and beta-2 adrenergic blocking.

19. Answer C is correct. The patient's most critical information is that they may have a sulfa allergy. Prescribing Bactrim (Sulfamethoxazole) could cause an anaphylactic reaction and should be avoided.

    Answer A is incorrect. While some clinicians prefer to get a urine C&S before the patient starts antibiotic therapy, this is not the most critical information that the patient needs to understand.

Answer B is incorrect. All patients should be educated to complete a prescribed course of antibiotic therapy even if symptoms resolve to prevent the development of resistant bacteria. This is important information that the patient should understand and agree to do.

Answer D is incorrect. Patients with an uncomplicated UTI who complete the course of therapy and have symptom resolution do not need to have repeat urine testing performed.

20. Answer B is correct. Vitamin K is the antidote for warfarin. If a patient consumes a large amount of foods in their diet that contain vitamin K, the effectiveness of the warfarin will decrease.

Answer A is incorrect. The therapeutic range for an INR is usually 2.0 to 3.0, depending on the reason for use. An INR of 4.0 is too high.

Answer C is incorrect. The antidote for warfarin is vitamin K. It can be administered orally or via a parental route.

Answer D is incorrect. While it is important to understand bleeding precautions, patients should not be restricted from outdoor activities, such as walking, gardening, or other low-impact outdoor activities.

21. Answers A, B, and D are all correct. Statin drugs are a category X in pregnancy. Renal function should be assessed with lower statin dosages used for those with a creatinine clearance less than 30. Statin drugs are metabolized by the liver where cholesterol is made; therefore, LFTs should be evaluated. Statins are contraindicated in acute liver failure or decompensated cirrhosis.

Answer C is incorrect. A CBC is not needed before initiating statin therapy, and anemia is not a contraindication.

22. Answer C is correct. Patients should always be aware that they must complete the therapy course to eradicate the fungus.

Answer A is incorrect. Many antifungals cause negative GI effects, which can be diminished by taking the medication with food.

Answer B is incorrect. A patient taking a medication that is metabolized in the liver, such as antifungal medication, should avoid alcohol altogether while taking the medication.

Answer D is incorrect. The patient should know that headaches and nausea are common side effects of antifungal medications. They should continue the medication as prescribed unless the side effects are severe enough to warrant discontinuation. If so, they should first contact the prescriber to discuss it.

23. Answer C is correct. The patient should be instructed on supportive care since they have had the virus for 4 days.

Answer A is incorrect. Oseltamivir (Tamiflu) is effective in shortening the duration of the flu symptoms if taken within the first 48 hours of illness. The patient has been sick for 4 days.

Answer B is incorrect. Acyclovir is an antifungal medication, not an antiviral medication.

Answer D is incorrect. Azithromycin is an antibiotic, so it will not benefit a patient who is sick with a virus.

24. Answer A is correct. Many patients feel nauseated when taking codeine and call it an "allergy." However, if the patient states that they are allergic to codeine, it is best to write it in the chart and avoid use. The NP could also indicate that the reaction is "nausea."

Answer B is incorrect. It is unlikely that this is a true allergic reaction rather than a side effect of the medication, as nausea is a common side effect of codeine.

Answer C is incorrect. An anaphylactic reaction occurs after sensitization and can occur at any time with any medication after the patient has received it once. It is preferable to avoid using codeine for this patient because they state that they have an allergy to it, but it is unlikely to be a true allergic reaction.

Answer D is incorrect. There is no information given in the question that states the patient is taking any other medication, so a drug–drug interaction is not a consideration.

25. Answer B is correct. All prescribers are required to first review the patient's controlled substance history using the PDMP before prescribing a scheduled drug.

Answer A is incorrect. This is unnecessary, and it is insulting to the patient.

Answer C is incorrect. While NSAIDs can be effective for alleviating some pain due to both their analgesic and anti-inflammatory properties, they are not considered to be more effective for pain control than narcotics.

Answer D is incorrect. While the patient may benefit from a referral to a neurologist for back pain later, this is not helpful to the patient currently complaining of "severe" pain.

Resources

American Geriatrics Society Beers Criteria® Update Expert Panel. (2023). AGS Beers Criteria® for potentially inappropriate medication use in older adults. *Journal of the American Geriatrics Society*, 77(7), 2052–2081.

Agency for Healthcare Research and Quality. (n.d.). *Home page*. U.S. Department of Health and Human Services. https://www.ahrq.gov/

Allergy Asthma Network. (2024, November 23). *The truth about penicillin allergy—and why it's important to get tested*. https://allergyasthmanetwork.org/news/the-truth-about-penicillin-allergy-and-why-its-important-to-get-tested/

Altmtaş Aykan, D., & Ergun, Y. (2020). Isotretinoin: Still the cause of anxiety for teratogenicity. *Dermatologic Therapy*, 33(1), e13192.

American Heart Association. *Prevent online calculator for 10-year CVD risk*. https://professional.heart.org/en/guidelines-and-statements/prevent-calculator

Celeste, M. A., & Thompson-Dudiak, M. (2020). Has the marijuana classification under the Controlled Substances Act outlived its definition? *Conn. Pub. Int. LJ*, 20, 18.

Centers for Disease Control & Prevention (CDC). (2024, October 24). *Heart disease facts*. https://www.cdc.gov/heart-disease/data-research/facts-stats/index.html

Centers for Disease Control & Prevention (CDC). *Antimicrobial-resistant fungal disease*. https://www.cdc.gov/fungal/antimicrobial-resistant-fungi/index.html

Church, N. A., & McKillip, J. L. (2021). Antibiotic resistance crisis: challenges and imperatives. *Biologia*, 76(5), 1535–1550.

Di Federico, S., Filippini, T., Whelton, P. K., Cecchini, M., Iamandii, I., Boriani, G., & Vinceti, M. (2023). Alcohol intake and blood pressure levels: a dose-response meta-analysis of nonexperimental cohort studies. *Hypertension*, 50(10), 1961–1969. https://doi.org/10.1161/HYPERTENSIONAHA.123.21224

Food & Drug Administration (FDA). (2022). *Development & approval process/drugs*. https://www.fda.gov/drugs/development-approval-process-drugs

Food & Drug Administration (FDA2). (2016). *How the FDA strives to ensure the safety of OTC products*. https://www.fda.gov/drugs/special-features/how-fda-strives-ensure-safety-otc-products

Food & Drug Administration. (2023, December 7). *FAERS—adverse event reporting system public dashboard*. https://www.fda.gov/drugs/questions-and-answers-fdas-adverse-event-reporting-system-faers/fda-adverse-event-reporting-system-faers-public-dashboard

Franklin, B. A., Myers, J., & Kokkinos, P. (2020). Importance of lifestyle modification on cardiovascular risk reduction: Counseling strategies to maximize patient outcomes. *Journal of Cardiopulmonary Rehabilitation and Prevention*, 40(3), 138–143.

GoodRx. (n.d.). *Top 20 most common medications*. https://www.goodrx.com/drug-guide?label_override=undefined

Greiwe, J., Honsinger, R., Hvisdas, C., Chu, D. K., Lang, D. M., Nicklas, R., & Apter, A. J. (2022). Boxed warnings and off-label use of allergy medications: Risks, benefits, and shared decision making. *The Journal of Allergy and Clinical Immunology: in Practice*, 10(12), 3057–3063. https://doi.org/10.1016/j.jaip.2022.08.033

Herink, M., & Ito, M. K. (2018). Medication induced changes in lipid and lipoproteins. In K. R. Feingold, B. Anawalt, M. R. Blackman, et al. (Eds.). *Endotext* [Internet]. https://www.ncbi.nlm.nih.gov/books/NBK326739/

Khalil, H., & Huang, C. (2020). Adverse drug reactions in primary care: A scoping review. *BMC Health Services Research*, 20, 1–13.

Kwiatkowska, E., Domanski, L., Dziedziejko, V., Kajdy, A., Stefanska, K., & Kwiatkowski, S. (2021). The mechanism of drug nephrotoxicity and the methods for preventing kidney damage. *International Journal of Molecular Sciences*, 22(11), 6109.

Lampe, J. R., & Attorney, L. (2021). *The Controlled Substances Act (CSA): a legal overview for the 117th Congress*. Congressional Research Service.

Martinez Steele, E., Popkin, B. M., Swinburn, B., & Monteiro, C. A. (2017). The share of ultra-processed foods and the overall nutritional quality of diets in the US: Evidence from a nationally representative cross-sectional study. *Population Health Metrics*, 15, 1–11.

Mayo Clinic. (2023, April 13). *Medications and supplements that can raise your blood pressure*. https://www.mayoclinic.org/diseases-conditions/high-blood-pressure/in-depth/blood-pressure/art-20045245

Merriam-Webster Dictionary. *Definition of drugs*. https://www.merriam-webster.com/dictionary/drug

Morris, A. A., & Butler, J. (2022). Updated heart failure guidelines: time for a refresh. *Circulation*, 145(18), 1371–1373.

National Institute on Alcohol Abuse and Alcoholism. *Alcohol-medication interactions: Potentially dangerous mixes*. https://www.niaaa.nih.gov/health-professionals-communities/core-resource-on-alcohol/alcohol-medication-interactions-potentially-dangerous-mixes#pub-toc2

Syed, R., Zaidi, H., & Rout, P. (2024, June 8). *Interpretation of blood clotting studies and values (PT, PTT, aPTT, INR, Anti-Factor Xa, D-Dimer)*. https://www.ncbi.nlm.nih.gov/books/NBK604215/

Nurse Journal. (2023). *Nurse practitioner prescriptive authority by state*. https://nursejournal.org/articles/nurse-practitioner-prescriptive-authority-by-state/

Omuya, H., Nickel, C., Wilson, P., & Chewning, B. (2023). A systematic review of randomised-controlled trials on deprescribing outcomes in older adults with polypharmacy. *International Journal of Pharmacy Practice*, 31(4), 349–368.

Pandey, A., Patel, K. V., Bahnson, J. L., Gaussoin, S. A., Martin, C. K., Balasubramanyam, A., Johnson, K. C., McGuire, D. K., Bertoni, A. G., & Kitzman, D. (2020). Association of intensive lifestyle intervention, fitness, and body mass index with risk of heart failure in overweight or obese adults with type 2 diabetes mellitus: An analysis from the Look AHEAD trial. *Circulation*, 141(16), 1295–1306.

Redfield, M. M., & Borlaug, B. A. (2023). Heart failure with preserved ejection fraction: A review. *Jama, 329*(10), 827–838.

Rosenthal, L. D., Burchum, J. R. (2020, March 12). *Lehne's pharmacotherapeutics for advanced practice nurses and physician assistants* (2nd ed.). Elsevier.

Schmidt, N. A., & Brown, J. M. (2024). *Evidence-based practice for nurses: appraisal and application of research.* Jones & Bartlett Learning.

Shah, N. J., Royer, A., & John, S. (2023, April 7). Acute liver failure. In *StatPearls* [Internet]. https://www.ncbi.nlm.nih.gov/books/NBK482374/

Tam, H. L., Wong, E. M. L., & Cheung, K. (2020). Effectiveness of educational interventions on adherence to lifestyle modifications among hypertensive patients: An integrative review. *International Journal of Environmental Research and Public Health, 17*(7), 2513.

Uetrecht, J., & Naisbitt, D. J. (2013). Idiosyncratic adverse drug reactions: Current concepts. *Pharmacological Reviews, 65*(2), 779–808. https://doi.org/10.1124/pr.113.007450

USPSTF. *Screening recommendations.* U.S. Preventative Services Task Force. https://www.uspreventiveservicestaskforce.org/uspstf/

USPSTF. (2022, August 23). *Statin use for the primary prevention of cardiovascular disease in adults: Preventative medicine.* U.S. Preventative Services Task Force. https://www.uspreventiveservicestaskforce.org/uspstf/recommendation/statin-use-in-adults-preventive-medication

Wadsworth, E., Hines, L. A., & Hammond, D. (2022). Legal status of recreational cannabis and self-reported substitution of cannabis for opioids or prescription pain medication in Canada and the United States. *Substance Abuse, 43*(1), 943–948. https://doi.org/10.1080/08897077.2022.2060431

Wang, M., Zeraatkar, D., Obeda, M., Lee, M., Garcia, C., Nguyen, L., Agarwal, A., Al-Shalabi, F., Benipal, H., & Ahmad, A. (2021). Drug-drug interactions with warfarin: A systematic review and meta-analysis. *British Journal of Clinical Pharmacology, 87*(11), 4051–4100.

PART III

Body Systems Review and Common Primary Care Issue

CHAPTER 6	Head, Eyes, Ears, Nose, and Throat	81
CHAPTER 7	Respiratory System	117
CHAPTER 8	Cardiovascular Disorders in Primary Care	143
CHAPTER 9	Gastrointestinal System	165
CHAPTER 10	Musculoskeletal Review	191
CHAPTER 11	Nervous System	217
CHAPTER 12	Endocrine System	235
CHAPTER 13	Hematology	255
CHAPTER 14	Renal and Genitourinary Urinary System	273
CHAPTER 15	Sexually Transmitted Infections	287
CHAPTER 16	Integumentary	307

CHAPTER 6

Head, Eyes, Ears, Nose, and Throat

Marguerite Lawrence, DNP, FNP-BC, PHCNS-BC, MA
Susan M. DeNisco, DNP, APRN, FNP-BC, FAANP

General Approach to Ear, Nose, and Throat Health Problems

- Always use proper equipment, including:
  - a pneumatic otoscope, and
  - an anterior rhinoscope.
- Treat acute presentations with antibiotics **only** after the appropriate history, physical examination, and testing are completed.
- Listen to the patient's story for important diagnostic clues.
- Do not rely on clinical data alone. Know your anatomical landmarks.
- Ear, nose, and throat (ENT) emergencies must be referred immediately. These include:
  - Epiglottitis—Inflammation of the epiglottis most often due to infection. It can rapidly result in airway obstruction. Attempting to examine the oral cavity or inserting a tongue blade to examine the pharynx may result in acute airway obstruction.
  - Angioedema—Abrupt onset of nonpitting, nonpruritic edema with lesions on lips, periorbital area, extremities, abdominal viscera, and genitalia. There may be associated urticaria. Either mast-cell or nonmast-cell–mediated mechanisms cause this and may lead to laryngeal edema.
  - Malignant otitis externa (OE)—Potentially life-threatening infection involving the external auditory canal, temporal bone, and surrounding structures. It has an aggressive course and can result in a high mortality rate.
  - Ludwig's angina—Rapidly progressive gangrenous cellulitis of the soft tissues of the neck and the floor of the mouth. It may result in airway obstruction.
  - Tympanic membrane perforation—**Never** try to remove cerumen if there is a suspicion or history of perforation.
  - Peritonsillar abscess.
  - Rhinosinusitis complications:
    - External facial edema
    - Erythema or cellulitis over a suspected sinus
    - Diplopia or difficulty with EOMs
    - Proptosis
- Abnormal neurological signs: facial drooping, drooling

Disorders of Balance

The Peripheral Vestibular System

The human ear has two divisions:

- Hearing portion (cochlea)
- Balance portion (peripheral meaning outside the central nervous system).

- This contains a network of tubes (semicircular canals) and sacs (the vestibule).
- These structures are filled with a fluid (endolymph).
- The inner ear is called the labyrinth due to its anatomic complexity.
- As the head position changes, endolymph moves within the inner ear and bends tiny hairs of sensory cells inside the canals.
- This initiates nerve impulses that pass along the vestibule-cochlear nerve to the brain.
- The brain then sends commands to initiate ocular movement. This enables clear vision and commands travel to muscles, allowing balance **as motion occurs**.

Defining Vertigo

The initial question must establish the person's perception of the word "dizzy." Once a subjective statement is precise, this early clue will lead to appropriate assessment strategies.

Knowledge of the four most common types of complaints will guide this evaluation:

- Type 1: **Vertigo** is a definite **rotational** sensation in which the person feels as if they or the environment are rotating. This may begin spontaneously, become episodic, and, when severe, may be accompanied by nausea, vomiting, and ataxia. These symptoms are almost always due to a problem in the peripheral labyrinth.
- Type 2: **Presyncope** is a sensation of an impending loss of consciousness, often beginning with vision loss and a roaring tinnitus. This usually implies inadequate blood perfusion to the brain rather than a focal event. It is usually gradual in onset and often is indicative of a metabolic disorder such as hypoglycemia or a rapid change in blood pressure (e.g., with postural hypotension).
- Type 3: **Disequilibrium** is a sense of impaired balance and gait, frequently due to impaired motor function control.
- Type 4: **Lightheadedness** is an ill-defined term often referred to as a sensation of "wooziness" or "feeling drunk" and is usually a diagnosis of exclusion. It occurs with psychiatric problems, hyperventilation, various encephalopathies, and as part of a geriatric syndrome that often reveals associations between vertigo and cardiovascular, neurological, psychological, and sensory disorders.

Vertigo Pathophysiology

Spatial orientation is automatic but complex. The five sensory modalities constantly sample position and motion: vision, vestibular sensation, proprioception, touch and pressure, and hearing. When the orienting image is unreliable, proprioception becomes impaired, resulting in a sensation of vertigo.

This could be central (brain) vertigo or, more commonly, peripheral (inner ear, eighth cranial nerve).

- **Central vertigo—least common type, usually caused by:**
  - ischemia—common after a cerebrovascular accident (CVA).
  - demyelination disorder—multiple sclerosis, Parkinson's disease.
  - neoplasms—rare cause. Even an acoustic neuroma (see Sensorineural Hearing Loss [SNHL]) causes vertigo in only about 20 percent of cases.
  - head trauma with concussion—acute problem and observable.
  - autoimmune diseases—Vertigo is part of the complex symptoms of Lyme disease, syphilis, and systemic lupus erythematosus when the disease affects the central nervous system.
- **Peripheral vertigo:**
  - Benign paroxysmal positional vertigo
  - Vestibular migraine
  - Ménière's disease
  - Head trauma, especially under 50 years of age
  - Otitis media, acute sinusitis, whiplash injury to the cervical spine, and degenerative changes associated with aging
  - High doses or long-term use of ototoxic antibiotics
  - Labyrinthitis, usually from a viral infection

Benign Paroxysmal Positional Vertigo (BPPV)

Definition

- A disorder of the inner ear that produces vertigo with certain head movements due to debris collected within the cochlea.
- This debris is thought to be small crystals of calcium carbonate derived from structures called "otoliths" that have been damaged by head trauma, infection, or aging-related inner ear degeneration.

Incidence/Prevalence

BPPV is common, with an estimated incidence of 64/100,000 cases/year and a lifetime prevalence of 2.4 percent. It is usually not a pediatric problem but can affect adults of any age, especially the older population. Most cases are idiopathic, with many people describing the room spinning sensation.

Etiology

- Idiopathic in more than 50 percent of cases
- Viruses affecting the ear—vestibular neuritis, TIAs, Ménière's disease
- Head trauma
- Degeneration of the vestibular system in the older patient

Risk Factors

- Aging
- Head injury
- Recent viral illness
- Occasionally following a surgical procedure—combination of trauma to the inner ear during surgery and a prolonged period of supine positioning
- Irrigating the ear with water can cause transient vertigo with presyncopal/syncopal sequelae

Historical Data

- Sudden onset
- Abrupt awakening with a spinning sensation while turning over in bed
- Nystagmus—rapid oscillation of the eyeballs
- Transient—episodic and lasting seconds to minutes
- Aggravated by head movements, changes in position, riding in a fast car or on an amusement park ride
- May be unilateral or bilateral
- May be associated with nausea and vomiting
- Hearing loss, tinnitus, and aural fullness may be present
- Asymptomatic between episodes

Physical Assessment

- Orthostatic blood pressure readings
- Otoscopic examination of the middle ear
- Weber and Rinne testing—see acute otitis media (AOM)/otitis media with effusion (OME)
- Nasal and sinus evaluation to rule out sinus disease
- Cranial nerve assessment
- Cervical spine assessment to rule out degenerative disease and trauma
- Romberg, tandem walk, and march-in-place testing
- Hyperventilation testing if psychiatric disorder is suspected
- Assessment of the eyes:
  - Pupils—especially following trauma
  - Extraocular movements testing for nystagmus
  - Vestibular testing; in primary care, the most common test is the Dix–Hallpike maneuver

Diagnostic Studies

- Dix–Hallpike maneuver is the gold standard test to identify BPPV:
  - A rapid change in head position from sitting to supine (with the head hanging over the edge of the examination table) will produce active rotary nystagmus when the head is turned so that the affected ear is facing the floor.
  - This may be accompanied by nausea.
  - A positive response is diagnostic for BPPV.
- Audiometric testing, if available.
- Weber and Rinne testing will be normal in BPPV.

Management

- Nonpharmacologic:
  - Epley maneuver or Semont maneuver:
    - Particle (canalith) repositioning maneuver may be performed.
    - The patient is placed in the supine position, with the head hanging as earlier, and the affected ear facing the floor.
    - At 30-second intervals, specific head rotations permit the misplaced otolithic material to transmit through the semicircular canal and be returned to the utricle, removing the cause of the problem.
    - The Epley maneuver eliminates vertigo in about 80 percent of patients after one treatment.
- Pharmacologic:
  - Meclizine 12.5 to 25 mg (antiemetic, antihistamine) PO in divided doses prn (*pro re nata*) for vertigo
  - Prochlorperazine by mouth, intramuscular, or rectal suppository for nausea and vomiting

Patient Education

- This is an anxiety-producing problem, and the patient will need a complete explanation of the etiology and natural course of the disease.
- Emphasize no driving for self-protection and to avoid posing a danger to others.
- Discuss the self-limited nature of BPPV.
- Discuss fall risk, especially with the older patient.

Indications for Referral

- Refractory vertigo lasting more than 2 weeks, becoming more intense, or occurring with greater frequency.
- If a central etiology is suspected, immediately refer to the appropriate healthcare provider.
- Physical therapy for vestibular therapy if peripheral vertigo becomes prolonged.

Expected Course

- Usually self-limited, with some less intense recurrence.
- Follow-up in 7 to 10 days for reevaluation.

Other Peripheral Vertigo Etiologies

Vestibular Neuritis/Labyrinthitis

Definition

- Inflammation of the vestibular portion of the eighth cranial nerve caused by viral or bacterial infection.
  - Neuritis affects the balance portion, resulting in vertigo but no change in hearing.
  - Labyrinthitis occurs when an infection affects both branches, resulting in hearing changes and vertigo. Etiologies include:
    - bacterial infections, usually associated with untreated otitis media. It usually manifests in mild symptoms.
    - viral infections, which are more common and may result from a systemic viral illness (infectious mononucleosis, rubeola), herpes (varicella, zoster), influenza, hepatitis, Epstein–Barr.

Symptoms

- Sudden onset of severe vertigo with nausea and vomiting and gait impairment
  - Unilateral hearing loss in labyrinthitis
  - Episodes can last from hours to days

Diagnostic Studies

- The Head Impulse-Nystagmus-Test of Skew (HINTS) exam is a bedside test that carefully assesses eye movements.
  - A benign HINTS exam is an abnormal HIT + direction-fixed horizontal nystagmus + absent skew.
- A normal Head Impulse test (HIT) strongly indicates a central cause for acute vestibular syndrome (AVS).
  - MRI may be warranted to rule out a vascular or central cause

Treatment

- Steroid taper
- Vestibular suppressants and antiemetics PRN for symptom management in the first 24 to 48 hours
- Broad spectrum antibiotic if suspicious for bacterial infection
- Antibiotics if there is AOM
- Refer to ENT specialist if unsure of etiology

Ménière's Disease

Definition

- A chronic peripheral vestibular disorder attributed to excess endolymphatic fluid pressure causing episodic inner ear dysfunction.
- Etiology is unknown.
- Theories include circulatory disease, allergies, autoimmune disorders, migraine headaches, and genetic predisposition.
- Episodes can be triggered by stress, overwork, fatigue, emotional distress, systemic illness, pressure changes, certain foods, and a large sodium intake.

Symptoms

- Vertigo
- Tinnitus
- Progressive hearing loss

During an attack:

- May have nausea and vomiting.
- No associated focal neurologic symptoms

Treatment

- Initial treatment includes lifestyle changes
  - Salt restriction (2 to 3 g/daily)
  - Avoid triggers (e.g., nicotine and MSG)
  - Minimize caffeine and alcohol intake (one serving a day)

- Vestibular suppressant and antiemetic medications as needed
- Vestibular rehabilitation
- Referral to otolaryngology may be necessary if attacks are persistent.

Hearing Loss

Conductive Hearing Loss

Description
This occurs when sound waves are not conducting properly anywhere along the channel from the ear canal through the tympanic membrane into the middle ear space. It may occur alone or with sensorineural hearing loss (mixed loss). It is usually temporary, fluctuating, and mild.

Incidence
Otosclerosis is the most common cause of progressive hearing loss in young adults. All ages are affected, and prevalence is equal among genders.

Etiology
- Malformation of the outer ear, ear canal, or middle ear structures (ossicles)
- Fluid in the middle ear from episodes of AOM
- Nasal allergies
- Eustachian tube dysfunction (ETD)
- Perforated tympanic membrane
- Benign tumors of the middle ear with ossicular erosion (cholesteatoma)
- Cerumen impaction
- Acute otitis externa (AOE)
- Foreign body in ear canal
- Otosclerosis

Historical Data
- Patient usually complains of unilateral hearing loss.
- Young children often have speech problems or language delay.
- Parents complain that children are not doing well in school.
- Patient often has a long history of AOM or OME.
- Often asymptomatic.

Physical Assessment
- *Always use a pneumatic otoscope to assess tympanic mobility.*
- Cerumen impaction or foreign body in ear canal.
- Tympanic membrane may be perforated because of AOM.
- Tympanic membrane may be dull and retracted or immobile due to the presence of fluid.
- Tympanometry (if available) will show negative pressure or the presence of fluid.
- Audiology (if available) shows the presence of an "air-bone gap," where hearing is superior when sound is transmitted so that it bypasses the ossicles in the middle ear.
- Nasal exam will often show the presence of congestion and clear drainage.

Differential Diagnosis
- Sensorineural hearing loss
- Mixed hearing loss
- Congenital hearing loss
- Superior canal dehiscence—very rare—surgery required

Diagnostic Studies
- Assess hearing acuity to a whispered or spoken voice.
- **Weber test**
  - Place the tuning fork midline on the forehead.
  - Normal finding: no lateralization. Lateralization (hearing the sound only in one ear or hearing the sound louder in one ear) is an abnormal finding.
- **Rinne Test**
  - Place the tuning fork first on the mastoid process and then at the front of the ear. Time each area.
  - Normal finding: Air conduction (AC) lasts longer than bone conduction (BC).

Complications
- Delayed speech
- Social problems
- Isolation from loss of communication, especially in older people
- Safety in the elderly
- Middle ear problems may progress to chronic problems—chronic otitis media
- Otosclerosis may worsen during pregnancy
- Untreated cholesteatoma can cause balance problems, facial nerve paralysis, meningitis, and brain abscesses.

Management
- Nonpharmacologic/pharmacologic:
  - Keep ear canals free of cerumen—Over-the-counter (OTC) drops are available; discuss dangers of self-irrigation.

- In cases of AOM and OME, see the AOM/OME section.
- In cases of a perforated tympanic membrane, invoke strict water precautions. See the AOE section.
- Surgical:
  - Head trauma
  - Cholesteatoma
  - Otosclerosis
  - Myringotomy tubes for protracted cases of OME
  - Hearing aids

Patient Education/Prevention

1. Avoid Q-tip, fingertip, and hair pin use in the external auditory canal.
2. Prompt treatment of all episodes of AOM.
3. Use protective measures when flying to prevent ETD.

Indications for Referral

- Any conductive hearing loss that does not respond after initial treatment
- Sensorineural hearing loss
- Sudden hearing loss
- Audiologist for hearing aid evaluation/hearing aid management
- Speech therapist if speech delay or impediment
- Neurology if an intracranial lesion suspected or surgery in middle ear is needed

Expected Course

- Temporary hearing problems are reversible when related to common health issues (i.e., ETD, AOM, cerumen impaction, foreign body in external auditory canal).

Sensorineural Hearing Loss

Description

- The dysfunction is in the inner ear (cochlea), the eighth cranial nerve, or both.
- Presbycusis or age-related hearing loss can be defined as a progressive bilateral SNHL of mid- to late-adult onset.
- The diagnosis of presbycusis is one of exclusion, and primary causes, such as otosclerosis, Meniere's disease, and cytotoxicity, among many others, must first be excluded.
- Noise-induced hearing loss is due to excessive noise exposure, either recreational or occupational. Occupational noise exposure is one of the most prevalent, potentially preventable health conditions. It has a slight male predominance and usually affects the middle-aged population.

Etiology/Risk Factors

- Aging with degeneration of nerves leading from the cochlea to the brain
- Congenital syndromes
- Prenatal infections—cytomegalovirus, herpes, rubella, toxoplasmosis
- Fetal exposure to teratogens—thalidomide, retinoic acid
- Long-term exposure to environmental noise (occupational or recreational)
- Long-term playing of loud music at high decibels with/without earphones
- Smoking/second-hand smoke
- Infectious diseases
- Autoimmune disorders
- Ménière's disease

Classification of Hearing Loss

The American National Standards Institute defines hearing loss in terms of decibels lost.

- Slight   16 to 25 dB
- Mild   26 to 40 dB
- Moderate   41 to 54 dB
- Moderately severe   55 to 70 dB
- Severe   71 to 90 dB
- Profound   greater than 90 dB

Historical Data

- Patient may or may not be aware of a hearing loss. In presbycusis, it is a bilateral loss.
- Hears better in quiet settings—Ambient noise increases inability to hear.
- May be associated with tinnitus (noise in affected ears).
- May be associated with vertigo.
- Sudden SNHL—May be viral or an acoustic neuroma. This is a benign slow-growing tumor that develops on the eighth cranial nerve.

*This demands an immediate referral to otolaryngology. Do not assume it is an OME unless you have evidence of fluid in the middle ear.

- In childhood:
  - Problems in school
  - Falling grades
  - Lack of attention to parental directions
  - Language delay

  *All infants are screened for hearing loss before leaving the hospital after birth.

- Thorough history of any known autoimmune or infectious disease.

Physical Assessment
- Patient may speak loudly.
- Otological exam is usually completely within normal limits.
- May fail whispered hearing screening.

Differential Diagnosis
- Conductive hearing loss
- Ménière's disease
- Ototoxicity
- Viral labyrinthitis

Diagnostic Studies
- Assess hearing acuity to whispered voice
- Weber test (see conductive hearing loss) will lateralize to unaffected ear
- Rinne test (see conductive hearing loss) air conduction > bone conduction bilaterally
- Laboratory testing if a known or suspected autoimmune disease
  - Sedimentation rate
  - Lyme titer
  - RPR titer
  - Rheumatoid factor
  - Antinuclear antibody titer
- Vestibular testing if associated with vertigo (see vertigo)

Complications
- Isolation in the older client
- Safety in older people
- Loss of communication
- Long-term tinnitus
- Vertiginous disorders

Management
- Nonpharmacologic:
  - Mandatory ear protection to prevent progressive SNHL
  - Annual hearing tests for persons in occupations with loud noise exposure
  - Smoking cessation
  - Reduce volume on mobile devices—iPods, MP3 players
  - Hearing aids
  - Adaptive measures—lip reading, sign language
- Pharmacologic:
  - Discontinue any ototoxic drugs
  - Sudden SNHL—may respond to systemic steroids—immediate referral
- Surgical:
  - Cochlear implants

Patient Education/Prevention
- Routine screening after age 65 years
- Mandatory newborn screening
- Audiological testing after any intracranial infection
- With children, help parents identify available community resources and refer family to a social worker for specialized assistance
- Hearing aids as soon as possible, if necessary, to increase the possibility of normal speech in children and improved hearing in adults

Indications for Referral
- Otolaryngology, if any hearing loss of unknown etiology or sudden SNHL
- Genetics, if a congenital syndrome is suspected
- Speech therapy, if needed
- Endocrinology, if metabolic disease is suspected
- Rheumatologist, if autoimmune disease is suspected
- Neurotology, if acoustic neuroma is suspected

Expected Course
- Presbycusis and SNHL are usually progressive and irreversible

Clinical Pearls
Presbycusis is usually bilateral, associated with advancing age, and identified by a gradual hearing loss often associated with tinnitus and reduced hearing sensitivity and speech understanding in noisy environments.

Acute Otitis Media/Otitis Media With Effusion

Definition

- AOM is an inflammation of the middle ear often associated with a viral upper respiratory infection. Organisms enter the sterile middle ear through the nasopharynx, creating purulent exudates and increased pressure.
- OME is the presence of an effusion in the middle ear without infection. It can follow an episode of AOM, especially in children.
- OME in adults is associated with ETD.

Incidence

- AOM is less common in adults.
- More than 80 percent of children experience at least one episode of AOM before the age of 2 years, with a peak incidence between 6 and 18 months.
- Respiratory viruses account for most cases of otitis media and are self-limited.
- By age 4 years, 90 percent of children have had at least one episode of OME.

Etiology

AOM

- Follows viral upper respiratory illness causing ETD.
- Viral—includes respiratory syncytial virus (RSV), parainfluenza, influenza, enteroviruses, adenoviruses.
- Bacterial causes:
  - *Streptococcus pneumonia*: 40 to 50 percent
  - *Hemophilus influenza*: 20 to 30 percent
  - *Moraxella catarrhalis*: 10 to 15 percent
  - *Staphylococcus aureus*: 2 to 4 percent

OME

- Residual middle ear fluid s/p AOM
- ETD. The eustachian tube runs from the middle ear to the nasopharynx (**Figure 6-1**). In children, the tubes are short and horizontal, allowing them to become easily edematous or obstructed. Adults have longer eustachian tubes at an angle and are less prone to dysfunction.
- Etiologies include:
  - Allergies
  - Upper respiratory infections and acute sinusitis
  - Excessive mucus and saliva produced during wheezing
  - Infected or hypertrophied adenoids
  - Tobacco smoke

Risk Factors

AOM

- Day care (increased with more than six children present)
- Changes in altitude/climate

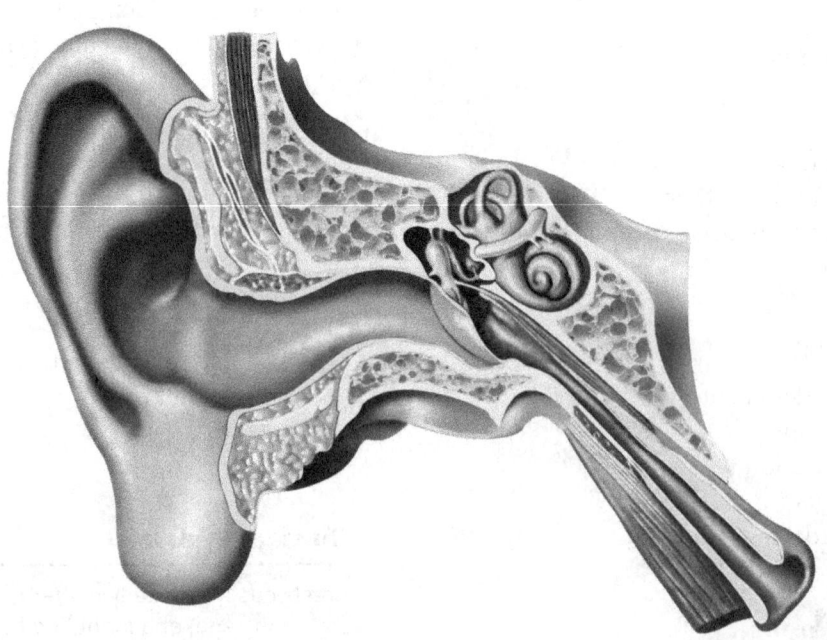

Figure 6-1 Eustachian Tube

- Second-hand smoke
- Family history of AOM
- Bottle feeding in supine position
- Pacifier after age of 6 months
- Low socioeconomic status
- Poor nutrition
- Comorbid ENT problems—hypertrophied adenoids, cleft palate, allergies
- Immunocompromised
- Ethnicity—Native Americans, Eskimos, and Australian aborigines

OME

- Early onset of first episode of AOM (before 3 months of age)
- Nasal allergies
- Recurrent AOM episodes
- Second-hand smoke
- Adenoidal hypertrophy
- Environmental allergies

Historical Data

AOM

- Preverbal children
  - Tugging, rubbing, holding an ear with excessive crying, fever, or change in sleep or behavior pattern
- Older children
  - Rapid onset of otalgia
  - Fever common
  - Fullness in ear
  - Decreased hearing
  - Popping and crackling sensation in affected ear
  - Vomiting, diarrhea

OME

- Asymptomatic in infants and young children
- Decreased conductive hearing
- Usually, no popping or crackling sensation in affected ear
- Sensation of pressure and fullness
- Pain may be present but dull
- May feel lightheaded (adults)

Physical Assessment

Always use a pneumatic otoscope to assess tympanic membrane mobility and thoroughly assess the nose, pharynx, and neck. See (**Figure 6-2**) for an illustration of the tympanic membrane.

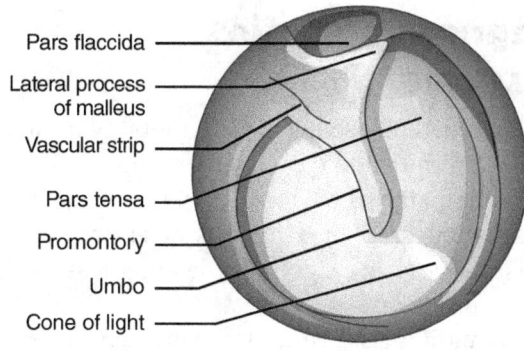

Figure 6-2 Tympanic Membrane

AOM

- Irritated or crying infant or child
- Bulging of the tympanic membrane with inability to identify landmarks
- Erythema of the tympanic membrane with increased vascular markings
- Decreased mobility of tympanic membrane
- May visualize purulent fluid behind the tympanic membrane
- Preauricular or cervical lymphadenopathy with tenderness on affected side
- A normal examination demands looking for comorbidity—acute sinusitis, temporomandibular joint (TMJ) dysfunction, dental problems

OME

- Retraction of the tympanic membrane with diffuse light reflex
- Tympanic membrane is dull and pale with frequent air bubbles present in the middle ear
- Decreased tympanic membrane mobility

Differential Diagnosis

AOM

- Upper respiratory infection
- Crying causing erythema of tympanic membrane
- Referred pain from jaw, teeth, or nasopharynx—more common in adults
- Trauma
- Bullous myringitis—a blister on top of the tympanic membrane that may rupture causing an immediate cessation of otalgia and bloody discharge from the affected ear.

OME

- Hearing loss
- ETD

Diagnostic Studies

AOM/OME

- Pneumatic otoscopy: lack of mobility means fluid within the middle ear or perforation
- Audiometry (if available) when hearing loss persists longer than 3 months or at any time with language delay, significant hearing loss, or learning problems.
- An audiologist can do tympanometry to evaluate hearing loss.
- CBC if complicated or systemic infection is suspected.

Complications

AOM

- Permanent hearing loss (conductive)
- Speech difficulties and delay (children)
- Balance disturbances
- Tympanic membrane perforation
- Facial nerve paralysis
- Otic hydrocephalus
- Mastoiditis
- Cholesteatoma
- Tympanosclerosis
- Intracranial abscess
- Meningitis

OME

- Tympanic membrane atelectasis
- Atrophy of tympanic membrane
- Retraction pockets
- Conductive hearing loss
- Cholesteatoma
- Tympanosclerosis
- Fixation of the ossicles

Management

AOM

Pediatric guidelines:

- For patients ages 6 months to 2 years with unilateral AOM and mild symptoms, a choice between initial antibiotic therapy or initial observation, but only after joint decision-making with the parent(s)/caregiver.
- Amoxicillin remains first-line therapy for children who have not received amoxicillin within the past 30 days.
- Amoxicillin/clavulanate is recommended if amoxicillin has been taken within the past 30 days, if concurrent purulent conjunctivitis is present, or if the child has a history of recurrent AOM unresponsive to amoxicillin.
- For patients allergic to penicillin, cefdinir, cefuroxime, cefpodoxime, or ceftriaxone may be appropriate.
- Prophylactic antibiotics are not recommended to reduce the frequency of recurrent AOM.
- Ibuprofen or acetaminophen in correct doses for age and weight for fever and pain control.
- Antihistamines and decongestants are not effective in AOM.

Clinical Pearls

Use cephalosporins with caution in patients allergic to penicillin because there is a cross-sensitivity greater than 10 percent.

OME

- Nonpharmacologic:
  - Watchful waiting—Most effusions resolve spontaneously. However, an OME persisting for over 3 months has a spontaneous resolution rate of only 10 to 15 percent.
  - Chewing gum
  - Use Valsalva maneuver to facilitate opening of the Eustachian tubes
  - After 3 months, audiometric evaluation is mandatory
  - Appropriate management of nasal allergies if present
- Pharmacologic:
  - Symptom management with oral decongestants/antihistamines
  - Steroid nasal spray may be used if there is the presence of nasal allergies
- Surgical
  - Myringotomy with tube placement may be considered for persistent symptomatic effusions lasting longer than 12 weeks

Acute Otitis Externa

AOE is defined as diffuse inflammation of the external ear canal, which may also involve the pinna or tympanic membrane.

Etiology

- Primary etiology is from water trapped in the ear canal that allows bacteria that normally inhabits

the skin and ear canal to multiply and infect the ear canal.
- Other causes include ears traumatized by Q-tip use, fungal infections, and various dermatological conditions, including eczema, psoriasis, and seborrheic dermatitis.
- Common bacterial causes:
  - *Pseudomonas aeruginosa* (most common)
  - *Proteus mirabilis*
  - *Staphylococcus aureus*
  - *Streptococcus pyogenes*
- Common fungal causes:
  - *Aspergillus* (most common)
  - *Candida albicans*
- Risk Factors:
  - Swimming
  - Foreign body, especially in pediatric patients
  - Cerumen impaction
  - Hot humid weather
  - Prolonged use of earplugs
  - Hearing aid use
  - Dermatological problems
  - Diabetes mellitus
  - Immunosuppression
  - Q-tip use
  - Inadequate drying of ears after showers
  - Use of chemical irritants (hairsprays)
  - Anatomic factors—Narrow ear canals
  - Presence of tympanostomy tubes in middle ear

Clinical Presentation/Assessment Findings

- Rapid onset of unilateral ear pain; tenderness over the tragus, pinna, or both
- Ear canal swelling and erythema, itching, aural fullness, otorrhea.
- Fever, lymphadenopathy—when virulent
- Erythema and edema of the ear canal—rarely the tympanic membrane
- Exudate—color varies from white to gray, yellow, or green
- Hearing loss, if edema severe

Clinical Pearls

Pneumatic otoscopy is the single most specific and clinically useful test for diagnosis.

In uncomplicated presentations (> 6 months of age) without severe illness or otorrhea, consider delaying antibiotics for 24 to 48 hours.

Antibiotics, antihistamines, and steroids are not indicated for OME.

Differential Diagnosis

- AOM, OME, furunculosis
- Perforated tympanic membrane
- Eruption of a wisdom tooth
- Foreign body
- Mastoiditis—tenderness over mastoid bone is present

Diagnostic Studies

- Pneumatic otoscopy
- Tympanometry
- Ear culture

Management

- Pharmacologic
  - **Bacterial causes**
    - Topical (otic) antibiotics
    - Ofloxacin Otic gtts (drops); 3 to 5 gtts bid 2 bid × 7 days
    - Ciprofloxacin and dexamethasone otic gtts 4 bid × 7 days (optimal because it contains both an antibiotic and a steroid)
    - Cortisporin Otic (Neomycin, hydrocortisone, colestin, thonzonium bromide)—5 gtts tid to qid (three to four times a day) × 10 days
  - Oral antibiotics indications include:
    - Patients with diabetes and increased morbidity
    - Patients with HIV/AIDS
    - Suspected malignant OE
    - Concomitant acute otitis media
  - **Fungal Causes:**
    - Topical antifungal agents are not considered a first-line treatment for OE.
    - They are only recommended if fungal etiology is suspected by otoscopic examination or culture results.
    - Fungal infections take much longer to resolve.
- Nonpharmacologic
  - Do **not** irrigate the ear canal.
  - If edema is present and debris is present in the ear canal, attempt to remove debris gently with a curette.
  - Wick placement for 48 to 72 hours is helpful for drawing in ear drops.
  - Place hot water bottle on outer ear for analgesia.
  - No swimming until complete resolution.

Patient Education

- Primary prevention of AOE is aimed at avoidance of risk factors.
- Teach patient the correct use of ear drops: Lie down with their affected side facing upward, apply two to five drops depending on the prescribed drug, and remain in that position for about 3 to 5 minutes.
- Teach earplug precautions for showers and swimming.
- Call if pain or edema increases, fever persists, or lymphadenopathy becomes more pronounced.

> **Clinical Pearls**
>
> Put dry cotton ball in ear canal and put Vaseline over cotton to waterproof ear canal.

Indication for Referral

- Referral to ENT in patients with recurrent AOE
- Presence of facial paralysis
- Erythema and edema over mastoid bone
- Granulation in ear canal
- Unresolved fever and lymphadenopathy following initial management

Evaluation and Follow-Up

- Patients with uncomplicated forms of OE do not usually require long-term monitoring.
- Patients with uncomplicated diffuse OE usually respond to treatment.
- Regardless of the agent used, between 65 and 90 percent of patients have clinical resolution within 7 to 10 days.

> **Clinical Pearls**
>
> Tempomandibular joint dysfunction is the most common etiology for adult ear pain.

Epistaxis

Definition

Epistaxis is any bleeding from the nostril, nasal cavity, or nasopharynx due to the bursting of a vessel within the nose. Nosebleeds are rarely life-threatening and usually resolve spontaneously but may also indicate an underlying health problem. They are classified as anterior (90 percent) or posterior dependent on the bleeding site. Posterior bleeds are an emergency and demand a specialist's attention.

Incidence

Approximately 60 percent of the population will be affected by epistaxis during their lifetime with 6 percent requiring medical attention. They are rare in children younger than 2 years of age.

Etiology/Risk Factors

- Idiopathic
- Direct trauma to nose
- Nose picking
- Foreign body
- Nasal/sinus fracture
- Nasal septal perforation
- Cocaine abuse
- Infection
- Irritant inhalation
- Low humidity in winter months
- Vascular health issues—aging vessels
- Hypertension
- Coagulation defects—Von Willebrand disease, leukemias, blood dyscrasias, platelet dysfunctions
- Medications:
  - Aspirin
  - Warfarin
  - Nonsteroidal anti-inflammatories
  - Clopridogril and other newer anticoagulant medications
- Neoplasm— < 10 percent—consider in unilateral cases

Physical Assessment

- Vital signs: elevated blood pressure (hypertension) or tachycardia (significant blood loss)
- Inspect skin for petechiae/bruising
- Nasal Cavity Exam
  - Gently blow nose to clear nasal cavity.
  - Insert a nasal speculum into the cavity and spread the naris vertically.
  - Assess for obvious bleeding sites on the septum that may be amenable to direct pressure/cautery.
  - **If bleeding is bilateral or there is constant blood dripping in the posterior pharynx, consider a posterior bleed.**
  - Posterior bleeds are more common in older people, can result in a significant hemorrhage, and may be associated with nausea or coffee-ground emesis.
- Massive epistaxis may be confused with hematemesis or hemoptysis.

Differential Diagnosis
- Hematemesis
- Hemoptysis
- Nasal cocaine use
- Isolated event, especially in children

Diagnostic Studies
- Only needed for recurrent or severe cases
  - CBC, platelets, prothrombin time, bleeding time
  - Type and cross match
  - Partial prothrombin time if on anticoagulant
  - CT scan of head
  - Run toxicology screening if drug use is suspected.

Complications
- Nasal septal hematoma/perforation
- External nasal deformity
- Mucosal pressure necrosis
- Vasovagal episode
- Acute rhinosinusitis
- Aspiration

Management
- Nonpharmacologic:
  - Direct pressure to front of nose for up to 20 minutes
  - Upright position
  - Ice packs
  - Nasal saline gel to anterior nose qd (four times a day) for moisturization and prevention of nasal dryness
  - Avoid trauma to nose—no picking or removing scab formations or blowing nose aggressively.
  - For anterior bleeds that do not respond to pressure, place a cotton ball moistened with 1:1,000 epinephrine or a vasoconstrictor nasal drop just inside the affected naris and apply pressure for 5 to 10 minutes or cauterize with a silver nitrate stick applied to the bleeding site.
  - For posterior bleeds, make immediate referral to ENT office.
- Pharmacologic:
  - Vasoconstrictors and topical anesthetics for bleeding cessation and analgesia
  - Epinephrine
  - Antibiotic ointment bid to affected site for 1 week
  - Treatment of any underlying health issue

Patient Education
- Avoid blowing nose for 3 to 4 days, then gentle blowing only.
- Sleep in upright position.
- Apply antibiotic ointment to affected area bid for 1 week.
- Apply icepacks prn to external nose.
- Avoid rubbing site with tissues or fingers.
- Report any new bleeding.

Indications for Referral
- Posterior bleed
- Recurrent epistaxis
- Hematology referral for intractable cases
- Appropriate provider for underlying health issues

Follow-Up
- 1 week to reevaluate bleeding site and check on further episodes

Acute Rhinosinusitis

Definition
Acute rhinosinusitis (ARS) is the symptomatic inflammation of the paranasal sinuses and nasal cavity. The maxillary and frontal sinuses are most affected. Fluid is trapped behind the sinuses causing a secondary viral or bacterial infection. Typically can last up to 4 weeks

Incidence
- Sixteen percent of U.S. adults are diagnosed annually, accounting for 12 million office visits.
- Viral causes account for the majority of cases.

Etiology
- Multiple viruses (See upper respiratory infection)
- *Streptococcus pneumonia*
- *Hemophilus influenza*
- *Moraxella catarrhalis*

Classifications of Rhinosinusitis
- Acute—symptoms lasting less than 4 weeks
- Subacute—symptoms last between 4 and 12 weeks
- Chronic—symptoms lasting more than 12 weeks
- Recurrent—four episodes lasting less than 4 weeks with complete symptom resolution between episodes

History of Present Illness
- The major challenge in correcting the diagnosis is differentiating between viral and bacterial disease.
- The overall symptom duration and trajectory are important factors in differentiating viral from bacterial sinusitis.
- Symptoms of viral infection tend to peak early and gradually resolve.
- Symptoms present for less than 10 days indicate a viral infection.
- Symptoms present for more than 10 days, without an improvement, suggest a bacterial infection.
- History of allergic rhinitis or recent viral URI or "bad cold."

Clinical Presentation/Physical Assessment Findings
- Unilateral facial pain and pressure
- Postnasal pharyngeal secretions or exudate (if bacterial, purulent dark yellow-green)
- Boggy nasal turbinate
- Transillumination of frontal and maxillary sinuses (glow of light absent or duller)
- Maxillary dental pain
- Middle ear effusion, fullness, and pressure
- Headache
- Hyposomnia
- Fever is seen more often in children than adults
  - Predictive symptoms for bacterial disease include:
    - Worsening and persistent symptoms for longer than 10 days
    - Persistent purulent drainage
    - Unilateral dental pain
    - Unilateral maxillary sinus tenderness
    - Persistent fever

Differential Diagnosis
- Viral URI
- Dental disease
- Trauma
- Nasal foreign body
- Tension, migraine headache
- Allergic rhinitis
- Immune disorders, HIV
- Cystic fibrosis

Diagnostic Studies
- Clinical diagnosis
- No labs are indicated in routine evaluations.
- Sinus X-rays, CT scans, and MRIs should be reserved for recurrent infections or failure to respond to medical therapy.

Complications
- Chronic rhinosinusitis
- Asthma exacerbation
- Meningitis when infection spreads to the brain lining
- Brain abscess
- External facial edema, erythema, or cellulitis over an involved sinus
- Vision changes—diplopia
- Impaired external ocular movements
- Proptosis
- Impaired cranial nerve function—drooping face, inability to smile

Management
Uncomplicated acute bacterial rhinosinusitis (ABRS) is generally a self-limiting disease where treatment is geared toward symptom management.

- **Nonpharmacologic:**
  - Hydration
  - Steam inhalation
  - Saline rinses
  - Sleeping with head of bed elevated
  - Avoiding tobacco smoke
  - Avoiding caffeine, alcohol
  - Warm facial packs—Sinus masks are valuable because they can be put in the refrigerator or microwave oven and used for the patient's comfort.
- **Pharmacologic:**
  - Analgesia:
    - Acetaminophen, especially in children
    - Nonsteroidal anti-inflammatories
  - Saline nasal washes
  - Oral decongestants (pseudoephedrine) or pseudoephedrine combined with guaifenesin for drainage (Mucinex D)
  - Topical decongestant Afrin used for a maximum of 3 days to avoid the rebound effect
  - Steroid nasal spray (Flonase) if history of allergic rhinitis
  - Mucolytic (guaifenesin and increased fluids to thin mucus)

Antibiotic Therapy
- If, after 10 days, the patient is still symptomatic, antibiotic treatment should be initiated.

- Choice of treatment is based on the most common bacteria associated with ABRS.
- First-line treatment: Amoxicillin–Clavulinic acid (Augmentin) (XR)—875 mg PO bid for 10 days (adults)
- For penicillin-allergic patients:
  - Doxycycline 100 mg PO bid for 10 days (adults only)
  - Cefpodoximine proxetil, cefuroxamine axetil, cefdinir (caution with cephalosporins because there is a cross-sensitivity with penicillin greater than 10 percent)
- Macrolides and sulfa drugs should not be used in the initial treatment due to the high prevalence of U.S. drug resistance, which may lead to treatment failure.

Treatment Failure
- If the patient's symptoms persist despite treatment (purulent nasal discharge, sinus pain, nasal congestion, and fever), consider switching to a different antibiotic.
- If recurrent sinusitis, refer to otolaryngology.

Patient Education
- Every URI is not a sinus infection. Encourage patients to use watchful waiting for 7 days. Explain the differences between a sinus infection and a URI.
- Discuss your area's antibiotic drug-resistance rates.
- Supportive measures are as important as medications and will enhance treatment success.
- No smoking or exposure to smoke.
- Stress importance of follow-up and contacting the doctor if symptoms worsen.
- Report visual problems or neurological abnormalities immediately.

Indications for Referral
- No treatment success after 3 weeks of antibiotic therapy
- Presence of chronic sinus disease
- Anatomic abnormalities—nasal septal deviation
- Presence of nasal polyps
- Allergy evaluation
- Visual problems
- Neurological impairment

Follow-Up
- See patient in 2 weeks or sooner if there are worsening symptoms or a symptom recurrence after initial improvement.

Allergic Rhinitis

Definition
Allergic rhinitis is an inflammatory condition of the nasal mucosa caused by immunoglobulin E(IgE)-mediated early-phase and late-phase hypersensitivity responses, usually to inhalant allergens, like those in allergic asthma. Increases the risk of sinusitis. May affect sleep and quality of life.

Incidence
- Affects 10 to 30 percent of adults and children in the United States.

Risk Factors
- Family history of atopy (eczema) or allergy
- Asthma
- Pets in house
- Exposure to indoor allergens—dust mites, mold, cockroach dander
- Exposure to outdoor allergens—grasses, ragweed, pollen

Clinical Presentation
- Ocular edema and pruritus
- Ear fullness
- Scratchy throat
- Fatigue
- Nasal pruritus
- Nasal congestion
- Hyposmia
- Headache
- Lightheadedness
- Sneezing

Physical Assessment Findings
- Allergic shiners—circles under eyes
- Allergic salute—transverse line on external nose from frequent rubbing
- Periorbital edema
- Conjunctivitis
- Pale boggy nasal mucosa
- Blue-tinged turbinates
- Serous otitis media
- Pharyngeal cobblestoning
- Postnasal drainage
- Signs of coexisting asthma—wheezing
- Skin—signs of atopic dermatitis

Differential Diagnosis
- Upper respiratory infection
- Vasomotor rhinitis
- Atrophic rhinitis

Diagnostic Studies
- Allergy Testing
  - Skin testing is the most specific screening method for detecting IgE antibodies. Should correlate with the patient's history.
  - Blood testing (RAST or ELISA) is preferable when the patient has severe dermatological problems, takes certain medications, or refuses skin testing. Often done with children.

Management
Strategies to ensure the optimal management of allergic rhinitis:

- Eliminate environmental factors:
  - Dust mite allergies—avoid using ceiling fans
  - No stuffed animals or pets in bed
  - Use HEPA filter for air conditioners
  - Room filters
- Pharmacotherapy:
  - First-line therapy is intranasal steroids for single maintenance therapy (e.g., flonase, nasocort, etc.)
  - With partial relief, consider a topical antihistamine spray once or twice daily (e.g., azelastine)
  - If still no relief, consider a combination of topical antihistamine and steroid nasal spray
  - Mast-cell stabilizers (cromolyn agents) are topical OTC nonsteroid anti-inflammatory agents (less effective than steroids)
  - Decongestants (pseudoephedrine) as needed for short term because tolerance can occur (not for use in children or adults)
  - Second-generation antihistamines (Claritin, Zyrtec) are less sedating.
  - First-generation antihistamines (Benadryl) have sedative side effects that may affect cognition and motor function.

Indications for Referral
- Patient does not respond to first-line medications and environmental control.
- Immunotherapy evaluation
- Chronic comorbid conditions—asthma, rhinosinusitis, middle ear disease, gastroesophageal reflux disease (GERD)
- Severe symptoms

Follow-Up
- Follow-up should occur 3 to 4 weeks after the initial treatment plan for environmental controls and first-line medications.

Aphthous Stomatitis (Canker Sores)

Painful shallow ulcers on the mouth's soft tissue usually heal within 7 to 10 days.

Etiology
- Unknown
- Minor trauma (i.e., biting inside the cheek)
- Acidic foods
- Stress

Treatment
- "Magic mouthwash" (combination of liquid Benadryl, viscous lidocaine, and glucocorticoid): swish, hold, and expectorate every 4 hours prn
- Orabase cream or ointment prn

Oral Candidiasis

- Oral candidiasis (thrush) is a yeast fungal infection of the genus *Candida albicans* that develops on the mucous membranes of the mouth. *Candida glabrata* and *Candida tropicalis* may also cause it. *Moniliasis* refers to adult oral thrush, while "oral thrush" can refer to both adults and babies.
- Oral candidiasis causes thick white or cream-colored deposits, most commonly on the tongue or inner cheeks.
- The lesions can be painful and may bleed slightly when they are scraped.
- The infected mucosa of the mouth may appear inflamed and red.
- Oral thrush can sometimes spread to the roof of the mouth and the back of the throat.

Incidence/Etiology
The condition is generally obtained secondary to immune suppression, which can be local or systemic, including extremes of age (newborns and older adults), immunocompromising diseases such as HIV/AIDS, and chronic systemic steroid and antibiotic use.

Risk Factors
- **People who wear dentures**—especially if not kept clean, do not fit properly, or are not taken out before sleep.
- **Antibiotics**—individuals on antibiotics have a higher risk of developing oral thrush. Antibiotics may destroy the bacteria that prevent candida from reproducing out of control.
- **Excessive mouthwash use**—overuse of antibacterial mouthwashes may also destroy bacteria that keep candida at bay, thus increasing the risk of developing oral candidiasis.
- **Oral or inhaled corticosteroids**—long-term use can increase the risk of oral candidiasis.
- **Oral contraception**
- **Hypothyroidism**
- **Hormonal changes**—pregnancy
- **Other therapies**—medications, chemotherapies, and radiotherapies that cause dry mouth
- **Immunosuppression**—cancer, HIV
- **Organ transplantation**
- **Diabetes**—poorly controlled
- **Stress**
- **Malnutrition**
- **Prematurity**

Clinical Presentation and Assessment Findings
- Redness or soreness in the affected areas
- White coating on tongue, palate, tonsils, posterior pharynx
- Difficulty swallowing
- Cracking at the corners of the mouth (angular cheilitis)
- Fever
- Possible cervical lymphadenopathy
- Inability to suck in infants
- Decreased appetite in adults

Differential Diagnosis
- Exudative pharyngitis
- Leukoplakia in adults
- Lichen planus
- Geographic tongue (normal variant)
- Herpes simplex erythema multiforme
- Pemphigus (rare)
- Baby formula, breast milk

Diagnostic Studies
- Clinical diagnosis through physical examination
- Potassium hydroxide (KOH) preparation for microscopy for persistent cases
- Fungal cultures if first-line treatment fails

Complications
- Dehydration secondary to feeding problems in infants
- Weight loss secondary to appetite loss

Management
- **Nonpharmacologic:**
  - No mouthwash during treatment
  - Bland diet until symptoms resolve
  - Avoid tobacco smoke
  - Soothing cool liquids
- **Pharmacologic:**
  - Topical Nystatin oral suspension 100,000 U/mL, 1 mL on each side of mouth qid × 7 to 14 days
    - Adult dose: 4–6 mL qid
    - Pediatric dose: 2 mL qid
  - Clotrimazole troches 10 mg 5x/day
  - Severe cases: Fluconazole 100–200 mg qd × 7–14 days
  - Pregnancy—Miconazole is safe.

Prevention/Patient Education
- Rinse mouth after meals.
- Brush teeth with a toothpaste that contains fluoride, and floss regularly.
- Regular dental visits
- Remove dentures every night, cleaning them with paste or soap and water before soaking them in water and denture-cleaning tablets.
- Brush the gums, tongue, and inside of the mouth with a soft brush twice a day if the patient has dentures or no or few natural teeth.
- Avoid mouthwashes.
- Smoking cessation
- Rinse mouth with water and spit it out after using a corticosteroid inhaler, and use a spacer (a plastic cylinder that attaches to the inhaler) when using inhaler.
- Judicious use of antibiotics.
- Ensure that any underlying condition, such as diabetes, is well controlled.

Indications for Referral
- Dental consult if dentures do not fit properly.
- If the patient is immunocompromised, refer to the appropriate provider in protracted cases.
- Esophageal infections
- Failure to respond to first-line treatment

Follow-Up
- Simple cases resolve within 7 to 10 days.
- Immunocompromised patients and infants should be seen in 1 week to reevaluate symptoms and weight.

Pharyngitis

- Acute pharyngitis is characterized by the rapid onset of sore throat and pharyngeal inflammation (with or without exudate). It can be caused by viral and bacterial pathogens, including group A *Streptococcus* (GAS), and fungal pathogens (e.g., *Candida albicans*).
- Absence of cough, nasal congestion, and nasal discharge suggests bacterial, rather than viral, etiology.
- In temperate climates, bacterial pharyngitis is more common in winter (or early spring), while enteroviral infection is more common in the summer and fall.

Incidence
- Acute nonbacterial pharyngitis is a common condition in both children and adults, usually arising from noninfectious (i.e., seasonal allergies, postnasal drip, acid reflux) or viral causes
- Bacterial pharyngitis is most often caused by GAS, commonly called strep throat.
- The incubation period of GAS pharyngitis is approximately 2 to 5 days.
- GAS is most prevalent in late fall through early spring.

Etiology
- Common causes of **viral pharyngitis**:
  - Covid 19
    - Rhinovirus
  - Epstein–Barr virus (EBV): mononucleosis is often accompanied by lymphadenopathy and splenomegaly
  - Adenovirus
  - Influenza A and B
  - RSV
- **Bacterial Pharyngitis**
  - The most common and important bacterial cause of pharyngitis is *Streptococcus pyogenes*, GAS in children (20 to 30 percent of episodes) and adults (5 to 15 percent of infections)
  - Bacteria other than GAS that may cause pharyngitis are:
    - Group C and G Streptococci
    - Gonorrhea
    - *Chlamydia trachomatis*
    - *Mycoplasma pneumoniae*
    - *Corynebacterium*

Risk Factors
- Close contact with another person with strep throat is the **most common risk factor** for illness.
- Individuals living and working in crowded conditions (e.g., long-term care centers, day care centers, schools, shelters for the unhoused, prisons, the military)
- 20 to 30 percent of pharyngitis episodes in children
- 5 to 15 percent of pharyngitis infections in adults
- Cold and flu seasons
- Smoking or exposure to second-hand smoke
- Frequent episodes of rhinosinusitis
- Environmental allergies
- Exposure to chemical irritants
- Immunosuppression
  - HIV
  - Diabetes mellitus
- Stress
- Fatigue
- Poor nutrition
- Chemotherapy

Clinical Pearls
Absence of cough, nasal congestion, and nasal discharge suggests a bacterial, rather than viral, etiology.

Bacterial Pharyngitis
Clinical Presentation/Assessment Findings
- Sudden onset of fever, chills, sore throat, and tender anterior cervical adenopathy.
- Purulent tonsillar exudate
- Dark pink to bright red tonsils
- Palatal petechiae
- Trouble swallowing

- Abdominal pain, nausea, and vomiting may be present.
- Sandpapery scarlatiniform rash may be seen in GAS infections.

Viral Pharyngitis

Clinical Presentation/Assessment Findings

- Throat pain, tenderness
- Erythematous tonsils
- Headache
- Ear pain
- Hoarseness or loss of voice
- Loss of appetite
- Mouth breathing
- Cervical lymphadenopathy
- Absence of low-grade fever

Clinical Pearls

Hepatosplenomegaly can be found in an infectious mononucleosis infection.

Differential Diagnosis

- Allergic rhinitis with postnasal drip
- GERD
- Peritonsillar abscess
- Scarlet fever
- Epstein–Barr virus
- Rheumatic fever
- Poststreptococcal glomerulonephritis
- Thyroiditis

Clinical Pearls

Concomitant vesicles on the hands and feet—Coxsackievirus (hand, foot, and mouth disease). See Chapter 19 on Pediatrics.

Diagnostic Studies

To confirm group A strep pharyngitis, use either:

- a rapid antigen detection test (RADT); specificity, high sensitivity varies;
- a throat culture that is 90 to 99 percent sensitive (gold standard);
- a standard throat culture for children older than 3 years with a negative RADT;
- a system to contact the family and initiate antibiotics if the back-up throat culture is positive; or
- antibiotic treatment in children with confirmed group A strep pharyngitis, which can reduce their risk of developing acute rheumatic fever.

Other Diagnostic Considerations Depending on History

- The Modified Centor Criteria helps to guide treatment and testing for adult patients in the ED and urgent care settings; the four-point scale assesses fever, tonsillar exudate, tender anterior cervical lymphadenopathy, and absence of cough. Patients with fewer than three Centor criteria are unlikely to have GAS pharyngitis.
- Monospot test for mononucleosis (Epstein–Barr virus)
- Chlamydia/gonococcal culture if suspecting STI

Complications

- Cervical lymphadenitis
- Mastoiditis
- Peritonsillar abscess
- Retropharyngeal abscess
- Rheumatic fever
- Poststreptococcal glomerulonephritis

Management

- **Nonpharmacologic**
  - Clear fluids
  - Rest
  - Warm saltwater gargles
  - Humidification
  - Judicious use of lozenges
- **Pharmacologic**
  - Antibiotic therapy: All courses should last 10 days (**treatment based on age and weight**)
  - First-line drugs for GAS
    - Penicillin VK
    - Amoxicillin

Treatment for Patients With Allergy to Penicillin

- Azithromycin
- Other alternatives include:
  - erythromycin, and
  - clarithromycin
- Other second-line drugs include:
  - cephalosporins
- Avoid cephalexin and cefadroxil in patients with immediate type hypersensitivity to penicillin.

Patient Education

- Children may return to normal activities and school after fever is gone and they have been on an antibiotic for 24 hours.
- Call with persistent or worsening symptoms after 3 to 5 days of therapy.

Indications for Referral

- Immediate referrals:
  - Airway obstruction—emergency room
  - Peritonsillar abscess/retropharyngeal abscess—otolaryngology or emergency room

Follow-Up

Necessary only with persistent symptoms OR with

- infectious mononucleosis.
- allergies.
- GERD.
- serious viral/bacterial infections.
- See patient in 2 weeks.

Eyes

The FNP in primary care is responsible for assessing vision when a patient presents with any complaint related to the eye and vision. An FNP must be aware of complaints that require prompt referral to an ophthalmologist or ED. Many eye issues require referral to and treatment by an ophthalmologist/specialist. See **Figure 6-3** for a lateral illustration of the eye.

Useful Tips and Terms When Performing an Exam With an Ophthalmoscope

- Use the **right** hand for the **right** eye; **left** hand for **left** eye.
- Check for red reflex and pupillary reactions with light on ophthalmoscope.
- With the room darkened, perform an eye exam, finding blood vessels and following them to the optic disc. Arteries are brighter red and narrower than veins.

Eye Exam

- Visual acuity: Assessed with the Snellen test. A patient with 20/20 vision can see at 20 feet, which is what a "normal" patient can see at 20 feet.
- Observe for symmetry of eyes, eyelids, and eyebrows. Cranial nerves (CN) 3 and 7 control eyelids. The sclera should be white; the conjunctiva is light pink.
- Check confrontation and perform cover/uncover test.
- Check extraocular movements (CN 3, 4, 6) and accommodation.

Common Eye Terminology

- Hyperopia—farsighted (near-vision blurred)
- Myopia—nearsighted (far-vision blurred)
- Presbyopia—hard to maintain clear focus in near vision; common over age 40

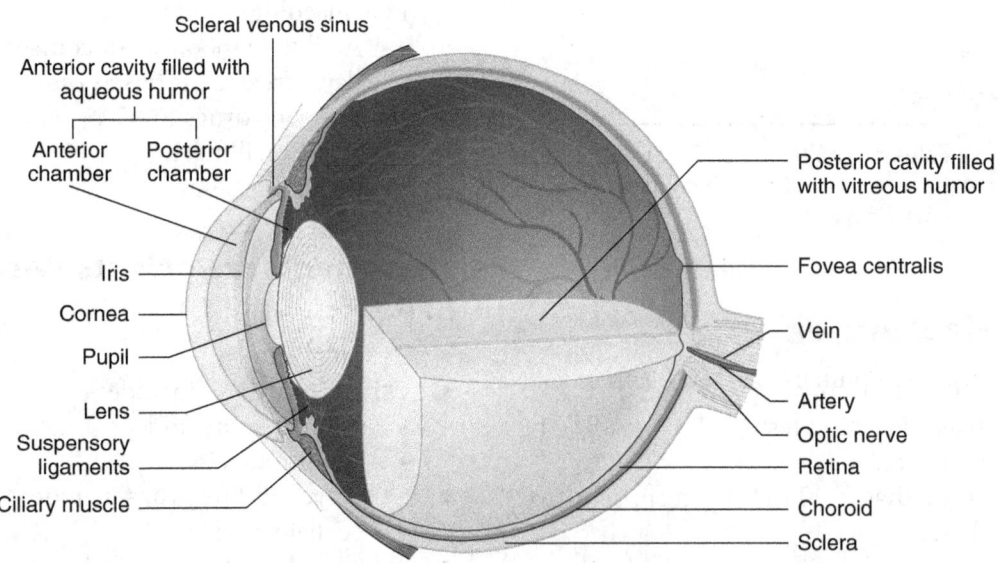

Figure 6-3 Eye

- Amblyopia—"lazy eye" starts in infancy
- Miosis—excessive constriction of the pupil of the eye
- Ptosis—drooping of the upper eyelid
- Disc cupping—Optic nerve cupping is associated with glaucoma and increased intraocular pressure (IOP). As the disease progresses, the disc-to-cup ratio becomes abnormal.
- Ectropion—Eye lid is turned outward, causing irritation and dry eyes.
- Entropion—Commonly seen in older people, the lower eye lid is turned inward and causes irritation, tearing, redness, pain, and foreign body sensation.
- AV Nicking—Refers to retinal arteriolar narrowing, wall thickening, and nicking found in patients with hypertensive retinopathy.
- Papilledema—Optic disc is edematous with blurred borders due to intracranial pressure (ICP) secondary to bleeding, brain tumor, or abscess.
- Nystagmus—Healthy patients will have a few beats of nystagmus on lateral gaze that resolves when the eye moves back to midline. Can also be found in patients with brain lesions.

Common Eye Conditions

Conjunctivitis "Pink Eye"
- Conjunctivitis is the inflammation of the lining of the eyelids and eyeball caused by bacteria, viruses, allergic or immunologic reactions, mechanical irritation, or medications.
- Conjunctivitis commonly affects men, women, and children of all ages.

Etiology
- Eighty percent of acute cases of conjunctivitis are viral with the most common pathogen being adenovirus.
- Other common viral pathogens are herpes simplex, herpes zoster, and enterovirus.
- Bacterial conjunctivitis is far more common in children than adults, and the pathogens responsible for bacterial conjunctivitis are *Pneumococcus*, *Staphylococcus aureus*, *Moraxella catarrhalis*, and *Haemophilus influenzae*.
- Seasonal/perennial allergic conjunctivitis is an acute disorder with a recurrent course, whereas atopic and vernal conjunctivitis are chronic diseases with acute exacerbations.

Bacterial Conjunctivitis
Clinical Presentation/Assessment Findings by Type
Signs and Symptoms
- Normal visual acuity
- Conjunctival redness
- Foreign body sensation in the eye
- Morning matting of the eyes
- White-yellow purulent or mucopurulent discharge
- Conjunctival papillae
- Infrequently preauricular lymphadenopathy

Treatment
- If neither gonococcal nor chlamydial infection is suspected, treat with antibiotic drops (i.e., moxifloxacin 0.5% drops or another fluoroquinolone or trimethoprim/polymyxin B drops)
- Prevent transmission by washing hands frequently, using separate towels, and avoiding close contact with others.
- Avoid wearing contact lenses until healed.
- Safe to return to school or work 24 hours after starting topical antibiotic or when symptoms resolve.

Allergic Conjunctivitis
Signs and Symptoms
- Eye itching and burning
- Watery discharge
- History of allergies/atopy
- Edematous eyelids
- Conjunctival papillae
- No preauricular lymphadenopathy

Treatment
- Cool compresses
- Antihistamine drops or oral antihistamine
- Mast cell stabilizer drops
- Topical nonsteroidal anti-inflammatory drops

Viral Conjunctivitis
Signs and Symptoms
- Eye itching and tearing
- Watery discharge
- History of a recent upper respiratory tract infection
- Inferior palpebral conjunctival follicles
- Tender preauricular lymphadenopathy

Treatment
- Lubricants (artificial tears)
- Topical antihistamine
- May need referral for steroid eye drops to reduce corneal infiltrates associated with photophobia and decreased vision

Subconjunctival Hemorrhage

Etiology
Subconjunctival hemorrhage is bleeding from small blood vessels underneath the conjunctiva and sclera. Can be caused by coughing, sneezing, vomiting, or local trauma (improper contact lens placement). Resolves within 1 to 3 weeks when the blood gets reabsorbed.

Clinical Presentation/Assessment Findings
- Typical presentation is sudden onset of bright-red blood in one eye often associated with extreme coughing, sneezing, or straining.
- Denies vision loss or pain.
- May have a history of trauma, such as a fall.
- Increased risk if patient is on aspirin, anticoagulants, or has hypertension.

Differential Diagnosis
- Consider viral, bacterial, allergic, chemical conjunctivitis, or penetrating trauma

Clinical Management
- Watchful waiting
- Reassurance of the self-limiting nature of the problem and typical time frame for resolution. Most of the time it is not associated with intraocular injury.
- If a concern for traumatic subconjunctival hemorrhage, rule out underlying retinal damage or open globe injury.
- Follow up only if the area does not resolve within 3 weeks.

Pinguecula and Pterygium

Etiology
Pinguecula is a yellowish, raised growth on the conjunctiva. It is usually on the side of the eye nearest to the nose but can also happen on the other side. A pinguecula may contain deposits of protein, fat, or calcium.

Pterygium is a growth of fleshy tissue that extends across the cornea (has blood vessels) that may start as a pinguecula.

Pinguecula and pterygium (surfers' eye) are caused by chronic exposure to ultraviolet (UV) radiation and are worsened by chronic dryness or irritation.

Diagnosis
- A slit-lamp examination can diagnose pinguecula and pterygium.
- A lesion biopsy is needed if it is thought to be a precancerous growth.

Treatment
- In early stages, pinguecula and pterygium can often be treated with artificial lubricating drops for irritation.
- Use of good quality sunglasses (100 percent protection against UV light)
- Excision of pinguecula or pterygium if the growth:
  - becomes thickened and painful.
  - affects how the eye blinks.
  - encroaches on the cornea and affects vision.

Sjogren's Syndrome

Etiology
Chronic autoimmune disorder characterized by decreased lacrimal (dry eyes) and salivary glands (dry mouth) function. May be associated with other autoimmune conditions.

Signs and Symptoms
- Persistent symptoms of dry mouth (xerostoma) and dry eyes for more than 3 months
- Chronic dry eyes with sandy or gritty sensation (keratoconjunctivitis sicca)
- Use of OTC artificial tears several times a day
- Increase in dental caries, and oral exam will show swollen salivary glands

Treatment
- Use OTC tear substitute drops TID
- Saliva substitutes
- Referral to dentist, ophthalmology, and rheumatology for further evaluation and treatment

Diabetic Retinopathy

Etiology
- Microaneurysms and "hard exudates" (leakage of lipid and protein material) are the initial signs of diabetic retinopathy. Neovascularization or the development of new blood vessels results in:
  - hemorrhages,
  - hard exudate,
  - cotton wool spots/soft exudates,
  - macular edema, and
  - tortuous blood vessels.

Risk Factors
- Diabetes
- Hypertension

Treatment
- Referral to ophthalmology for annual eye exams and treatment
  - Control underlying disease

- Use laser on retina to slow the vessel and hemorrhagic changes.
- Make monthly injections into the eye with anti-VEGF or anti-inflammatory agent.

Age-Related Eye Diseases

Glaucoma

Open Angle Glaucoma (Most Common)

Anterior chamber angle is open, but the trabecular meshwork does not drain aqueous fluid well. Can be congenital or steroid induced.

Signs and Symptoms
- Painless, usually no symptoms
- Peripheral vision loss slowly over time
- Increased intraocular pressure
- Optic nerve cupping

Treatment
- Medications
- Usually eye drops
  - Beta-blockers
  - Prostaglandin analogues
  - Alpha-agonists
- Oral medication (carbonic anhydrase inhibitor)
- Surgical options

Angle Closure Glaucoma (Less Common)
- A medical emergency: rapid increase in intraocular pressure due to outflow obstruction of aqueous humor

Signs and Symptoms
- Sudden onset of severe unilateral eye pain or a headache associated with blurred vision, rainbow-colored halos around bright lights, nausea, and vomiting
- Visual acuity reduced
- Fixed ovoid pupil
- Clouded cornea
- Increased intraocular pressure

Treatment
- Make referral ASAP to specialist for the following:
  - IV, oral, or topical medications to lower pressure in the eye
  - Laser iridotomy to improve aqueous release

> **Exam Tip**
>
> Primary closed-angle glaucoma is acute elevated intraocular pressure associated with the closing of the filtration angle or obstruction of the circulation of aqueous humor. **Emergency referral indicated.**

Cataract (Opacity of the Lens)

Etiology
- Congenital
- Disease-related
- Diabetes accelerates cataract formation
- Inflammatory disease (i.e., sarcoid)
- Senile (age related, most common)
- Medication related
- Prednisone can produce a posterior subcapsular cataract after 3 weeks of treatment
- Psychotropic drugs can produce an anterior subcapsular cataract
- Trauma

Signs and Symptoms
- Glare with night driving
- Lights appear to have starbursts
- Seen as a dark opacity in the media of the eye through an ophthalmoscope

Treatment
- In the early stages of cataracts, changing the patient's prescription glasses may help initially.
- Ultimately, the lens must be surgically replaced with a piece of plastic called an intraocular (IOL) implant.
- Referral for surgical removal of the lens.

Age-Related Macular Degeneration (AMD)

Etiology
- Macular degenerative changes involve the central part of the retina, which is the fovea.
- Central vision is affected, resulting in difficulty reading, driving, etc.
- It is the leading cause of blindness worldwide.
- Typically, asymptomatic during the early stages.
- More common in smokers.
- Age-related macular degeneration has been classified into two clinical forms:
  - "dry," or atrophic; and
    - More common and less severe compared to the wet form
  - "wet," or exudative.
    - Responsible for 80 percent of the vision loss

Signs and Symptoms
- Central loss of vision slowly over time.
- Symptoms the patients notice include blurring of vision and distortion, especially for near vision.

- Decreased vision, micropsia, metamorphopsia, or scotoma are other presenting complaints.

Diagnostics
- On fundoscopic examination, pigment epithelial detachment and drusen bodies may be seen
- Amsler grid test (focus eye on center dot and view grid from 12 inches); patients with wet AMD will see the center of the grid as distorted with bent, wavy lines
- Fundus fluorescein angiography (FFA)
- Optical coherence tomography (OCT)

Treatment
- Both wet and dry forms can be treated with ocular supplements recommended by the Age-Related Eye Disease Studies (AREDS), which are a combination of vitamins and minerals.
- Wet AMD can be treated with laser photocoagulation, vascular endothelial growth factor (VEGF) to prevent new blood vessel formation, and surgery in severe cases.
- Educate patient to undergo annual ophthalmologic reassessments to check for progression to intermediate age-related macular degeneration (ARMD)

Corneal Abrasion
Etiology
- Trauma to the eye resulting in a tear in the epithelial surface.
- Acute onset of severe pain with tearing and redness.

Signs and Symptoms
- Foreign body sensation on the surface of the eye
- Visual acuity reduced
- Normal pupil unless traumatic iritis
- Teary discharge
- Corneal florescence after instilling fluorescein drops in eye on Wood's lamp or slit lamp examination

Treatment
- Topical antibiotic drops or ointment to cover pseudomonas (i.e., ciprofloxacin, trimethoprim-polymyxin B to the affected eye for 3 to 5 days)
- Eye patching is not recommended.
- Follow up in 24 hours and consider referral to ophthalmologist.

Chalazion
Chalazion is a common noninfectious inflammatory condition caused by a foreign-body reaction to sebum released by meibomian glands (specialized sweat gland).

Etiology
- Blockage of normal drainage of sebaceous glands, especially at the eyelid margin, by blepharitis, rosacea, or hordeolum (stye) may contribute to development of chalazia
- Contributing factors include poor eyelid hygiene, previous hordeolum, contact lens wearer, application of makeup, etc.
- Associated with acne, seborrhea

Clinical Presentation/Assessment Findings
- Gradual onset of a small superficial nodule on the upper eyelid that feels like a bead
- Superficial nodule is soft and movable
- Painless but may enlarge over time
- Large chalazia can press on the cornea and cause blurred vision
- Lack of constitutional symptoms

Differential Diagnosis
- Hordeolum (stye)
- Blepharitis
- Dacryocystitis

Clinical Management
- Most chalazia respond (within 1 to 2 months) to conservative treatment of warm compresses twice a day to promote drainage.
- Proper lid hygiene (for blepharitis) includes washing the affected eyelid with drops of baby shampoo.
- Keeping the eyelids free of discharge, pus, or crusting also helps to improve the condition.
- Antibiotics are unnecessary.

Indication for Referral
- Referral to an ophthalmologist may be recommended for recurrent, large, or refractory chalazia.

- Persistent chalazia may require more invasive therapies (i.e., corticosteroid injection or incision and curettage).

Hordeolum (Stye)

Etiology

- In 90 to 95 percent of cases of hordeolum, an acute bacterial infection of the eyelid margin is due to *Staphylococcus aureus*, with *Staphylococcus epidermidis* being the second most common cause.
- An external hordeolum represents a localized abscess formation of the follicle of an eyelash, whereas an internal hordeolum is an acute bacterial infection of the meibomian glands of the eyelid.
- A stye is usually a self-limiting condition with resolution occurring spontaneously within a week.

Sign and Symptoms

- Patients present complaining of a confined burning, tender swelling on one eyelid.
- Either the upper or lower lid may be involved.
- In some cases, the complaint may start as generalized edema and erythema of the lid that later becomes localized.
- Patients will frequently have a history of similar prior lesions of the eyelid.
- With external hordeolum, pain, edema, and swelling are localized to a discrete eyelid area that is tender to palpation.
- The stye generally appears as a pustule with mild erythema of the lid margin.
- Pustular exudate may be present.

Diagnostic Testing

- Diagnosing a stye (hordeolum) and chalazion requires only a history and physical exam.
- No diagnostic tests are required or useful in diagnosing a hordeolum or chalazion.

Treatment

- Both internal and external hordeola are treated similarly.
- For sufficient treatment and to hasten recovery and prevent the spread of infection, apply:
  - warm compresses for 15 minutes at least four times a day.
  - erythromycin ophthalmic ointment twice a day for 7 to 10 days.

Complications

- Uncommonly, an untreated stye may evolve into a localized cellulitis of the eyelid and surrounding skin.
- Periorbital, or rarely, orbital cellulitis, may ensue if progression of the infection is allowed to occur.
- Worsening erythema and edema beyond a localized pustule should be monitored closely for cellulitis, which may require systemic antibiotics.
- For very large hordeola in which incision and drainage are considered, referral to an ophthalmologist is appropriate.
- Reevaluation within 2 to 3 days is appropriate to assess response to treatment.

Dangerous Eye Conditions

Herpes Simplex Keratitis (Type I Herpes Simplex)

Etiology

- Herpes simplex keratitis is a common and potentially blinding condition caused by recurrent corneal infections with the herpes simplex virus (HSV). Herpes simplex keratitis remains the leading infectious cause of corneal ulcers and blindness worldwide.
- HSV-1 usually causes infections in the oral, labial, and ocular areas, while HSV-2 primarily causes lesions in the genital region.
- Primary infection with HSV occurs after direct contact inoculation of the mucosal or skin surface. It is often subclinical and goes unnoticed. After the initial HSV infection, the virus becomes latent, traveling to the dorsal root ganglia and remaining there for the person's lifetime. Subsequent infection is caused by viral reactivation in the affected dermatome.

Signs and Symptoms

- Herpes simplex keratitis should be considered in patients complaining of acute, unilateral onset of eye pain, photophobia, foreign body sensation, visual blurring, and watery ocular discharge.
- History of prior episodes, including herpetic lesions in the orofacial or ocular area, should be obtained.
- Other essential clinical history includes contact lens use, prior corneal abrasions, recent stressors, including fever, UV laser treatment or UV light exposure, and topical or systemic corticosteroid use.

Diagnostic Testing
- Herpes simplex keratitis is primarily diagnosed based on clinical features, but laboratory tests can provide definitive evidence of HSV infection.
- Dendrite fluorescein pattern (fernlike and branching) on Wood's lamp or slit lamp examination.
- Serological tests may be used to detect serum HSV IgG and IgM to identify past or recent infections in a comprehensive assessment of the patient's immune status regarding HSV.

Treatment
- Treatments depend on whether the episode is caused by active viral replication or an immune response to past infection.
- For stromal keratitis, topical steroids and antiviral treatments are used.
- Do not use topical steroids for patients with active HSV and epithelial disease present.
- Palliative lubricants (artificial tears and ointments)
- Referral to ophthalmologist

Herpes Zoster Keratitis (Shingles)
Etiology
Herpes zoster involves the ophthalmic division of the trigeminal nerve (CN V).

Signs and Symptoms
- Headache, malaise, fever
- Unilateral involvement along nerve distribution
- Vesicular lesions on one side of the forehead, eyelid, and at tip of the nose indicate ocular involvement.

Treatment
- Potentially sight threatening
- Make referral to ED or ophthalmologist for immediate treatment

Posterior Vitreous Detachment
Etiology
The vitreous gel pulls away from the retina.

Risk Factors
- Age related (above age 40)
- Trauma

Signs and Symptoms
- New onset flashing lights
- New floaters

Treatment
- Make **referral** for a dilated eye exam to confirm diagnosis.

Retinal Detachment
Etiology and Risk Factors
Separation of the retina from the underlying layers of the eye.
- High myopia (nearsightedness)
- Trauma
- Genetic—family history
- Retinal hole or tear
- Diabetes

Signs and Symptoms
- Sudden onset of flashing lights (photopsia) and floaters (black dots)
- Painless with monocular visual field
- "Like a curtain coming down over the vision"

Treatment
- Make **immediate referral** for a dilated eye exam to confirm diagnosis and treatment.

Optic Neuritis
Etiology and Risk Factors
Inflammation of the optic nerve.
- Recent viral illness
- Occurs frequently in patients with multiple sclerosis

Signs and Symptoms
- Decreased color vision in affected eye, especially red color vision
- Decreased pupillary reaction in affected eye
- Pain on eye movement
- Papillitis
- Central scotoma

Treatments
- Referral to neurologist

CASE STUDIES FOR CRITICAL THINKING

Eye Case

A 6-year-old girl with no significant past medical history presents 4 days after developing a red, irritated left eye. Her mother states that she has been wiping thick whitish-yellow discharge from her eye, which is matted shut in the morning. She denies exposure to a sick contact, upper respiratory symptoms, or contact lens use. She also denies any significant pain or light sensitivity. On examination, the patient's pupils are equal and reactive. She does not have a tender preauricular lymph node. Penlight examination reveals no corneal opacity, but thick, whitish discharge is seen.

What other questions should you ask the parent regarding environmental factors?
Child at daycare? Other students with c/o eye discharge?
Would you assess her visual acuity?
What are the treatment options?

Clinical Pearl for Case Study

Conjunctivitis does not alter visual acuity. Topical antibiotics do not significantly alter the course of most types of bacterial conjunctivitis.

Ear Case

A 35-year-old man presents with a 2-day history of rapid-onset severe ear pain and fullness. The patient complains of otorrhea and mild decreased hearing. He reports that his symptoms started after swimming. No fever is reported. On physical exam, the external ear canal is diffusely swollen and erythematous. He has tenderness of the tragus and pain with movement of the auricle. The tympanic membrane was partially visualized because of the swelling. The concha and the pinna look normal. Neck exam fails to reveal any lymphadenopathy.

What other information should you obtain from the patient?
What are some differentials you are considering?

Case Study Sore Throat

A 7-year-old girl presents with an abrupt onset of fever, nausea, vomiting, and sore throat. The child denies cough, rhinorrhea, or nasal congestion. On physical exam, oral temperature is 101°F (38.5°C), and there is exudative pharyngitis with enlarged, tender anterior cervical lymph nodes. A rapid antigen test is positive for group A *Streptococcus* (GAS).

What other questions would you assess from the history of present illness (HPI)?
What is your choice of medication?

Review Questions

1. The most common cause of bacterial pharyngitis is:
   A. gonorrhea.
   B. group C *Streptococcus*.
   C. mycoplasma.
   D. group A *Streptococcus* (GAS).

2. After history and the physical exam, the family nurse practitioner (FNP) suspects a 22-year-old female has infectious mononucleosis (IM). Of the following diagnostic studies that provide the most specific test, the result will be:
   A. a positive heterophile antibody test.
   B. a modest elevation of the white blood count (WBC).
   C. an elevated bilirubin.
   D. a decreased lymphocyte count.

3. The management plan for the patient with infectious mononucleosis will include:
   A. a course of systemic corticosteroids.
   B. bed rest for 3 to 5 days.
   C. avoidance of contact sports for 3 to 5 days.
   D. increased clear fluids.

4. A 67-year-old male presents with a 72-hour history of sore throat associated with nasal congestion, clear rhinorrhea, and slight cough. This is most likely:
   A. Epstein–Barr virus (EBV).
   B. respiratory syncytial virus (RSV).
   C. bacterial pharyngitis.
   D. viral pharyngitis.

5. A 72-year-old male presents with the acute onset of unilateral epistaxis. He has been unable to stop

the bleeding, which is a steady drip from his right naris. He has been coughing up bright red blood. He has hypertension and no history of previous episodes. This is most likely caused by:
   A. a foreign body.
   B. a posterior bleed.
   C. an anterior bleed.
   D. cocaine abuse.

6. After evaluating a 22-year-old female, the FNP diagnoses allergic rhinitis. What treatment will *initially* be prescribed?
   A. Oral antihistamine
   B. Leukotriene receptor antagonist
   C. Oral corticosteroid
   D. Topical decongestant

7. All of the following are risk factors for acute stomatitis **except**:
   A. day care attendance.
   B. vitamin deficiency.
   C. poverty.
   D. intact dentures.

8. First-line treatment for the patient with apthous ulcers would include:
   A. oral corticosteroids.
   B. thalidomide.
   C. valacyclovir.
   D. amlexanox.

9. A 47-year-old female presents to the office with 3 days of nasal congestion with mucoid drainage, a dull frontal headache, and postnasal drip. She is concerned that she has a sinus infection. Treatment will include:
   A. a high dose of amoxicillin for 10 days.
   B. watchful waiting with a backup of antibiotics if her symptoms worsen.
   C. oral corticosteroids to decrease inflammation.
   D. a referral to a neurologist for a headache evaluation.

10. A 50-year-old female patient who was seen 12 days ago and diagnosed with a common cold returns today with worsening nasal congestion and headaches and purulent postnasal drip. She has a low-grade fever. Her exam reveals purulent drainage in the posterior pharynx and an edematous erythematous nasal chamber. Treatment will include:
    A. a high dose of amoxicillin for 10 to 14 days.
    B. a referral to otolaryngology.
    C. ordering a CT scan of the sinuses.
    D. Avelox 400 mg for 14 days.

11. A 4-year-old female patient has otitis media with effusion (OME), following an initial episode of acute otitis media (AOM) 2 months ago. She is experiencing no hearing loss and has no speech problems. Which of the following is the best next step?
    A. Tell the patient's parents that this is within normal limits for resolution and to make a follow-up appointment in 4 weeks.
    B. Refer her to an otolaryngologist.
    C. Place the patient on a decongestant or antihistamine.
    D. Use Augmentin in appropriate doses.

12. A 7-year-old female child is doing poorly in school, and her grades are falling. She has problems concentrating, and her mother is concerned about her ability to hear the teacher. She has a long history of acute and chronic ear infections. A conductive hearing loss is suspected. The FNP expects to find the following:
    A. A Weber test that lateralizes to the unaffected ear
    B. A Rinne test where air conduction = bone conduction
    C. An audiometric test from school showing an "air-bone gap"
    D. A tympanometry test showing no negative pressure

13. A 76-year-old male patient presents with a suspected hearing loss in both ears. He notes that over the past 6 months it is impossible for him to hear anyone when dining in a restaurant, and he is sure that his female partner mumbles all the time. The most likely diagnosis is:
    A. mixed hearing loss.
    B. sensorineural hearing loss (SNHL).
    C. conductive hearing loss.
    D. sudden SNHL.

14. A 29-year-old female patient presents with a 10-hour history of sudden hearing loss in her right ear, accompanied by tinnitus and an echo sensation in the affected ear. The FNP suspects a sudden SNHL. The most appropriate next step is to:
    A. Order a CT scan of her head.
    B. Reassure her that this is temporary and will respond to steroid ear drops.
    C. Immediately refer her to otolaryngology.
    D. Begin her on amoxicillin because this is probably a conductive hearing loss with an effusion of the middle ear.

15. Presyncope is defined as:
    A. a sensation of uneasiness.
    B. a sense of spinning.
    C. a sense of pending loss of consciousness.
    D. a sense of impaired balance.

16. An adolescent male patient is being evaluated for "dizziness" following a concussion. The FNP suspects:
    A. Benign Paroxysmal Positional Vertigo (BPPV).
    B. Ménière's disease.
    C. labyrinthitis.
    D. central vertigo secondary to the concussion.

17. Ms. Hamilton, a 23-year-old female patient, presents with an acute onset of vertigo worsened by head movement and changes in position. She has severe nausea and vomiting and is acutely ill. The most likely diagnosis is:
    A. BPPV.
    B. Ménière's disease.
    C. labyrinthitis.
    D. neuritis.

18. The diagnosis of BPPV will be aided by:
    A. a CBC with differential.
    B. the Dix–Hallpike maneuver.
    C. a CT of the head.
    D. an MRI of the brain.

19. Risk factors for oral candidiasis include all the following **except**:
    A. hyperthyroidism.
    B. denture use.
    C. birth control pills.
    D. stress.

20. A 45-year-old female patient has been on Nystatin Oral Rinse for oral candidiasis for 2 weeks without any symptom relief. She is now having increasing dysphagia and losing weight. The FNP will:
    A. change the medication to Clotrimazole troches.
    B. repeat the Nystatin regime for another course.
    C. refer the patient to infectious disease.
    D. begin an antibiotic.

21. Risk factors for developing acute otitis externa (AOE) include all the following **except**:
    A. swimming in chlorinated pools.
    B. swimming in lakes.
    C. excessive ear cleaning with Q-tips.
    D. frequent upper respiratory infections.

22. The bacteria most responsible for AOE is:
    A. *Staphylococcus aureus*.
    B. *Aspergillus*.
    C. *Pseudomonas aeruginosa*.
    D. *Proteus mirabilis*.

23. A 4-year-old boy is at the office for a preschool physical exam. The FNP performs the cover/uncover test to evaluate for:
    A. strabismus.
    B. presbyopia.
    C. chalazion.
    D. Butler's sign.

24. A 42-year-old female is at the clinic with a complaint of having difficulty focusing on the words in newspapers. The FNP will most likely find that this patient has:
    A. presbyopia.
    B. strabismus.
    C. cataract.
    D. macular degeneration.

25. The FNP is performing a physical examination in a 65-year-old female. Arcus senilis is noted during the examination. The FNP is aware that this finding requires:
    A. a referral to an ophthalmologist for possible surgical intervention.
    B. a referral to a cardiologist for cardiac workup.
    C. no referral because this is a normal finding in this age group.
    D. no referral; however, this finding by itself indicates a need for a lipid profile.

26. A 22-year-old male presents to the walk-in center with the chief complaint of "painful eye swelling." Upon examination, the FNP notes the right eye has a hordeolum. The FNP treats this patient's problem by:
    A. prescribing Tobrex eye drops.
    B. encouraging the patient to use clean, warm soaks to the affected area for 15 minutes four times per day.
    C. referring the patient to an eye surgeon for incision and drainage of the hordeolum.
    D. applying a patch to keep the eye covered and avoid further irritation to the eyelid.

27. A patient complains of sudden vision changes, severe eye pain, and nausea. What ocular emergency should the healthcare provider suspect?
    A. Corneal abrasion
    B. Angle closure glaucoma
    C. Subconjunctival hemorrhage
    D. Bacterial conjunctivitis

Answers and Rationales

1. Answer D is correct. GAS is the most common cause of bacterial pharyngitis, making it the correct answer. The other options are less common causes and do not account for most bacterial pharyngitis cases.

   Answer A is incorrect. Gonorrhea, caused by *Neisseria gonorrhoeae*, is a sexually transmitted infection that can cause pharyngitis, but far less common than GAS as a cause of pharyngitis.

   Answer B is incorrect. Group C *Streptococcus* can cause pharyngitis but is much less common than GAS. Infections caused by Group C *Streptococcus* are relatively rare and are typically associated with specific populations or settings, such as animal exposure or certain occupational environments.

   Answer C is incorrect. Mycoplasma, specifically *Mycoplasma pneumoniae*, is known to cause atypical pneumonia and can sometimes cause pharyngitis, especially in older children and young adults. However, it is not the most common cause of bacterial pharyngitis.

2. Answer A is correct. A positive heterophile antibody test, often called the "monospot test," is the most specific test for diagnosing infectious mononucleosis caused by the EBV. The test detects heterophile antibodies produced in response to an EBV infection. A positive result strongly indicates IM, making this the most specific diagnostic study among the given options.

   Answer B is incorrect. While a modest WBC elevation can be seen in infectious mononucleosis, it is not specific to IM.

   Answer C is incorrect. Elevated bilirubin can occur in IM due to liver involvement, but it is not specific to this condition.

   Answer D is incorrect. IM typically causes an increase, rather than a decrease, in lymphocyte count, often with the presence of atypical lymphocytes. A decreased lymphocyte count is not characteristic of IM and would not be a specific diagnostic indicator for this condition.

3. Answer D is correct. Increased clear fluids are recommended for patients with IM to help maintain hydration, which is essential for recovery.

   Answer A is incorrect. Systemic corticosteroids are not typically recommended for the routine management of infectious mononucleosis.

   Answer B is incorrect. While rest is important, strict bed rest for 3 to 5 days is not a standard recommendation for managing IM.

   Answer C is incorrect. Patients with IM are advised to avoid contact sports for at least 3 to 4 weeks, not just 3 to 5 days, due to the risk of splenic rupture.

4. Answer D is correct. Viral pharyngitis is the most common cause of sore throat associated with nasal congestion, clear rhinorrhea, and slight cough. These symptoms are typical of a viral upper respiratory infection.

   Answer A is incorrect. While EBV can cause pharyngitis, it is typically associated with IM, which presents with additional symptoms, such as significant fatigue, swollen lymph nodes, and sometimes splenomegaly.

   Answer B is incorrect. RSV is more common in young children and infants and typically presents with bronchiolitis or pneumonia in those age groups.

   Answer C is incorrect: Bacterial pharyngitis, usually caused by GAS, typically presents with a sore throat, fever, and tender cervical lymphadenopathy without significant nasal symptoms or cough.

5. Answer B is correct. A posterior bleed is more likely to cause significant and persistent epistaxis that is difficult to control. Posterior nosebleeds typically occur deeper in the nasal cavity and can lead to blood flowing down the back of the throat, causing the patient to cough up blood.

   Answer A is incorrect. A foreign body in the nose is more common in children and might cause unilateral epistaxis. However, it is less likely in an older adult unless there is a specific history of inserting something into the nose.

   Answer C is incorrect. Anterior nosebleeds, which occur in the front part of the nasal septum, are more common and usually less severe. They often occur from the Kiesselbach's plexus and are typically controlled with simple first aid measures.

   Answer D is incorrect. Cocaine abuse can lead to chronic nasal problems and potentially cause nosebleeds due to its vasoconstrictive effects and potential for damaging nasal tissues. However, the patient's age and lack of history of previous episodes make this less likely.

6. Answer A is correct. Oral antihistamines are commonly prescribed as the first-line treatment for allergic rhinitis. They effectively reduce symptoms, such as sneezing, itching, nasal congestion, and runny nose, by blocking histamine receptors.

   Answer B is incorrect. Leukotriene receptor antagonists, such as montelukast, can be used to manage allergic rhinitis, especially in patients with concurrent asthma. However, they are not typically prescribed as the initial treatment. They are often considered as an adjunct therapy if symptoms are not adequately controlled with antihistamines or intranasal corticosteroids.

   Answer C is incorrect. Oral corticosteroids are potent anti-inflammatory agents, but they are generally not recommended for the initial treatment of allergic rhinitis due to their potential for significant side effects with systemic use.

   Answer D is incorrect. Topical decongestants, such as oxymetazoline, can rapidly relieve nasal congestion. However, they are not suitable for long-term use due to the risk of rebound congestion (rhinitis medicamentosa) with prolonged use beyond a few days. They are not typically recommended as the initial treatment for allergic rhinitis.

7. Answer D is correct. Intact dentures are not a risk factor for acute stomatitis. Properly fitting dentures do not typically cause issues in the oral cavity.

   Answer A is incorrect. Daycare attendance is a known risk factor for acute stomatitis, especially in children. It increases exposure to infectious agents like viruses (e.g., herpes simplex virus, coxsackievirus) that can cause stomatitis.

   Answer B is incorrect. Vitamin deficiencies, particularly vitamins B12, folate, and iron, can lead to stomatitis.

   Answer C is incorrect. Poverty is a risk factor for acute stomatitis due to several associated factors, including poor nutrition, limited access to healthcare, and suboptimal living conditions, which can contribute to poor oral hygiene and increased susceptibility to infections.

8. Answer C is correct. Valacyclovir is an antiviral medication commonly used to treat herpes simplex virus infections, including cold sores and genital herpes.

   Answer A is incorrect. Due to their potential systemic side effects, oral corticosteroids are not typically used as a first-line treatment for aphthous ulcers. They are usually reserved for more severe or recalcitrant cases that do not respond to first-line treatments.

   Answer B is incorrect. Thalidomide is not used as a first-line treatment for aphthous ulcers due to its significant side effects and teratogenic potential.

   Answer D is incorrect. Amlexanox is a topical anti-inflammatory and anti-allergic medication specifically used to treat aphthous ulcers.

9. Answer B is correct. Watchful waiting is often recommended for acute sinusitis (sinus infection), especially if symptoms have been present for less than 10 days and are not severe.

   Answer A is incorrect. Immediate antibiotic treatment with high-dose amoxicillin is not typically recommended for initial management of uncomplicated acute sinusitis, particularly if symptoms are mild and have been present for only a few days.

   Answer C is incorrect. Oral corticosteroids are not typically used as a first-line treatment for acute sinusitis. They may be considered in cases of severe inflammation or when there are significant nasal polyps, but their use is not standard for uncomplicated sinusitis.

   Answer D is incorrect. In this scenario, a neurologist's evaluation of the patient's headache is not warranted. The patient's headache is likely related to her sinusitis and is described as dull and frontal, which is consistent with sinus-related headaches.

10. Answer A is correct. High-dose amoxicillin for 10 to 14 days is a standard treatment for acute bacterial sinusitis, particularly when symptoms worsen after an initial period of improvement (a typical "double sickening" pattern) or persist without improvement for more than 10 days.

    Answer B is incorrect. While referral to an otolaryngologist may be considered for chronic or recurrent sinusitis, or if there are complications, it is not typically necessary for initial management of uncomplicated acute bacterial sinusitis.

    Answer C is incorrect. Ordering a CT scan of the sinuses is not indicated for routine cases of acute bacterial sinusitis.

Answer D is incorrect. Avelox (moxifloxacin) is a fluoroquinolone antibiotic that can be used to treat bacterial sinusitis. Still, it is not considered a first-line treatment due to its broader spectrum and higher risk of side effects compared to amoxicillin. Starting with high-dose amoxicillin is more appropriate and follows standard treatment guidelines.

11. Answer A is correct. Tell the patient's parents that this is within normal limits for resolution and to make a follow-up appointment in 4 weeks. OME often resolves itself without treatment. It is common for effusion to persist for a few weeks to several months after an episode of AOM.

    Answer B is incorrect. An otolaryngologist referral is not immediately necessary for a child with OME who is not experiencing hearing loss, speech problems, or other complications.

    Answer C is incorrect. Decongestants and antihistamines are not recommended for the treatment of OME in children. Studies have shown that these medications are ineffective in resolving middle ear effusion and can have potential side effects. The American Academy of Pediatrics does not recommend these treatments for OME.

    Answer D is incorrect. Antibiotics like Augmentin (amoxicillin/clavulanate) are not recommended for OME unless there is an acute infection.

12. Answer C is correct. The Weber test is used to differentiate between conductive and sensorineural hearing loss. In conductive hearing loss, sound will lateralize to the affected ear because the affected ear perceives bone-conducted sound as louder.

    Answer A is incorrect. Lateralization to the unaffected ear with the Weber test indicates sensorineural hearing loss in the affected ear. In sensorineural hearing loss, the inner ear or auditory nerve is damaged, causing the sound to be heard more loudly in the unaffected ear.

    Answer B is incorrect. The Rinne test compares air conduction (AC) to bone conduction (BC). In normal hearing or sensorineural hearing loss, AC is better than BC (positive Rinne test).

    Answer D is incorrect. If sound is equally heard in both ears during the Weber test, it indicates either normal hearing or bilateral symmetrical hearing loss.

13. Answer B is correct. This patient has classic symptoms of sensorineural hearing loss (SNHL) given his age, gradual onset, and bilateral hearing loss.

    Answer A is incorrect since mixed hearing loss would have symptoms of ear pressure and tinnitus.

    Answer C is incorrect because it is usually a unilateral hearing loss.

    Answer D is incorrect because the patient's symptoms have come on gradually.

14. Answer C is correct. SNHL is a medical emergency. Prompt evaluation and treatment by an otolaryngologist (ENT specialist) are crucial because early intervention can significantly improve the chances of hearing recovery.

    Answer A is incorrect. While imaging studies like a CT scan can be helpful in certain cases, they are not the first-line action for sudden SNHL.

    Answer B is incorrect. It is inappropriate to reassure the patient that the condition is temporary and will respond to steroid ear drops. Sudden SNHL is a serious condition that requires urgent medical attention.

    Answer D is incorrect. Starting the patient on amoxicillin is inappropriate because the presentation suggests sudden SNHL rather than conductive hearing loss.

15. Answer C is correct. Presyncope is defined as a sensation of impending loss of consciousness. It often manifests as lightheadedness, dizziness, or feeling faint but does not progress to full syncope (actual fainting).

    Answer A is incorrect. A sensation of uneasiness is too vague and nonspecific to define presyncope. While presyncope can cause discomfort and unease, these feelings alone do not capture the characteristic sense of impending loss of consciousness that defines presyncope.

    Answer B is incorrect. A sense of spinning is characteristic of vertigo, not presyncope. Vertigo is a specific type of dizziness where the patient feels as though they or their surroundings are moving or spinning.

    Answer D is incorrect. A sense of impaired balance may indicate disequilibrium, which refers to unsteadiness or imbalance when walking or standing.

16. Answer D is correct. Concussions are traumatic brain injuries that can affect the central nervous system. Central vertigo arises from dysfunction in the brainstem or cerebellum.

    Answer A is incorrect. BPPV is a common cause of vertigo that occurs when small crystals in the inner ear become dislodged and move into the semicircular canals, causing dizziness with specific head movements.

    Answer B is incorrect. Ménière's disease is a chronic condition related to abnormal fluid balance in the inner ear characterized by episodes of vertigo, tinnitus, hearing loss, and a feeling of fullness in the ear.

    Answer C is incorrect. Labyrinthitis is an inner ear inflammation, often following a viral infection, and can cause sudden vertigo, hearing loss, and balance issues.

17. Answer A is correct. BPPV is characterized by brief episodes of vertigo triggered by changes in head position. The vertigo in BPPV is typically acute in onset and worsens with specific head movements, which matches Ms. Hamilton's symptoms of vertigo worsened by head movement and changes in position.

    Answer B is incorrect. Ménière's disease is characterized by a triad of symptoms: episodic vertigo, tinnitus, fluctuating hearing loss, and a feeling of fullness in the ear.

    Answer C is incorrect. Labyrinthitis, or vestibular neuritis, is an inflammation of the inner ear, often following a viral infection. It typically presents with acute onset of continuous vertigo, hearing loss, and balance issues.

    Answer D is incorrect. Vestibular neuritis (also known as vestibular neuronitis) involves inflammation of the vestibular nerve and typically presents with acute onset of continuous vertigo without hearing loss.

18. Answer B is correct. The Dix–Hallpike maneuver is a clinical test specifically designed to diagnose BPPV. During this test, the patient is rapidly moved from sitting to lying, with the head turned to one side and extended backward. A positive test elicits vertigo and nystagmus (involuntary eye movements), which are characteristic of BPPV. This maneuver helps identify the involvement of the posterior semicircular canal, which is most affected in BPPV.

    Answer A is incorrect. A CBC with differential is a blood test used to evaluate overall health and detect various disorders, including infections and anemia. However, it does not provide information relevant to the diagnosis of BPPV.

    Answer C is incorrect. A head CT scan is used to detect structural abnormalities, such as bleeding, tumors, or fractures. While it is a useful diagnostic tool for various neurological conditions, it is not specific or sensitive for diagnosing BPPV.

    Answer D is incorrect. An MRI of the brain provides detailed images of brain structures and is useful for diagnosing central nervous system disorders, such as multiple sclerosis, tumors, or stroke. While it is more sensitive than a CT scan for detecting certain pathologies, it is not necessary for diagnosing BPPV, which is a peripheral vestibular disorder.

19. Answer A is correct. Hyperthyroidism is not a recognized risk factor for oral candidiasis. Oral candidiasis (thrush) is typically associated with factors that disrupt the normal balance of microorganisms in the mouth or compromise the immune system. Hyperthyroidism, which is an overactive thyroid condition, does not directly impact the balance of oral flora or immune function in a way that would predispose someone to oral candidiasis.

    Answer B is incorrect. Denture use is a well-known risk factor for oral candidiasis. Dentures can create a moist, warm environment ideal for fungal growth. Poorly fitting dentures or inadequate denture hygiene can further increase the risk. Denture wearers are at higher risk of developing oral candidiasis, particularly if the dentures are not cleaned regularly or are worn continuously without proper hygiene measures.

    Answer C is incorrect. Birth control pills are also a recognized risk factor for oral candidiasis. Hormonal changes induced by birth control pills can alter the balance of normal flora in the mouth and may suppress local immune responses, making it easier for Candida to overgrow.

    Answer D is incorrect. Stress is known to have various negative effects on the immune system, which can increase the risk of infections, including oral candidiasis. Chronic stress can suppress immune function, making it easier for opportunistic infections like Candida to take hold.

20. Answer C is correct. Persistent oral candidiasis despite appropriate treatment with Nystatin, coupled with increasing dysphagia and weight loss, suggests a potentially more serious underlying condition. This could indicate a more resistant or systemic fungal infection, immunosuppression, or another underlying disease. Referral to an infectious disease specialist is appropriate for further evaluation and management.

    Answer A is incorrect. Clotrimazole troches are another topical antifungal treatment similar to Nystatin. If the infection has not responded to Nystatin, simply switching to another topical antifungal might not be sufficient, especially if more severe symptoms like dysphagia and weight loss are present.

    Answer B is incorrect. Repeating the same treatment that has already failed is unlikely to provide benefit and could delay necessary investigation and appropriate treatment.

    Answer D is incorrect. Antibiotics are used to treat bacterial infections and would not be effective against a fungal infection like oral candidiasis. Starting an antibiotic would not address the underlying issue and could worsen the condition by further disrupting the normal oral flora and allowing for more fungal overgrowth.

21. Answer D is correct. Frequent upper respiratory infections (URIs) are not a recognized risk factor for AOE. URIs typically affect the upper respiratory tract, including the nose, throat, and sinuses, and can lead to conditions like otitis media (middle ear infection) but not typically otitis externa (OE).

    Answer A is incorrect. Swimming in chlorinated pools is a risk factor for AOE. The moisture from swimming can create a conducive environment for bacterial growth in the ear canal, leading to infection.

    Answer B is incorrect. Swimming in lakes is also a risk factor for AOE. Natural bodies of water like lakes can harbor bacteria and other microorganisms that can enter the ear canal and cause infection, especially when combined with prolonged moisture exposure.

    Answer C is incorrect. Excessive ear cleaning with Q-tips can increase the risk of AOE. Using Q-tips can cause trauma to the delicate skin of the ear canal, remove protective earwax, and potentially introduce bacteria.

22. Answer C is correct. *Pseudomonas aeruginosa* is the most common bacterial cause of AOE, also known as "swimmer's ear."

    Answer A is incorrect. *Staphylococcus aureus* can also cause AOE, but it is not the most common pathogen. It is more typically associated with skin infections, abscesses, and other conditions but is less frequently the primary cause of swimmer's ear than *Pseudomonas aeruginosa*.

    Answer B is incorrect. *Aspergillus* is a genus of fungi, not bacteria.

    Answer D is incorrect. *Proteus mirabilis* is another type of bacteria that can cause infections, including urinary tract infections, but it is not a common cause of AOE.

23. Answer A is correct. The cover/uncover test detects strabismus, a condition where the eyes do not properly align with each other when looking at an object.

    Answer B is incorrect. Presbyopia is an age-related condition where the eye's lens loses its ability to focus on close objects. It typically affects older adults, not children.

    Answer C is incorrect. A chalazion is a chronic inflammatory lesion caused by blockage of a meibomian gland in the eyelid. It presents as a painless swelling in the eyelid.

    Answer D is incorrect. Butler's sign is not a recognized medical term or diagnostic test in ophthalmology or general medicine. Therefore, it is irrelevant to the cover/uncover test or the evaluation of eye conditions.

24. Answer A is correct. Presbyopia is an age-related condition in which the lens of the eye loses its flexibility, making it difficult to focus on close objects. It typically begins to affect people in their early to mid-40s. The classic symptom is difficulty reading small print, such as words in newspapers, which perfectly aligns with the patient's complaint. This condition is commonly corrected with reading glasses or bifocals.

    Answer B is incorrect. Strabismus is a condition in which the eyes do not align properly and point in different directions. It is usually diagnosed in childhood and can cause issues with depth perception and double vision, but it does not typically present as difficulty focusing on near objects in adults.

Answer C is incorrect. Cataracts cloud the eye's natural lens, leading to blurred vision, glare, and difficulty with night vision.

Answer D is incorrect. Macular degeneration affects the macula, the central part of the retina, leading to loss of central vision. This condition is more common in individuals over 50 and typically presents with symptoms such as a blurry or blind spot in the central vision, making it difficult to see fine details up close and at a distance.

25. Answer C is correct. Arcus senilis is a common and benign finding in older adults, characterized by a white, gray, or blue opaque ring in the corneal margin. It is due to lipid deposits in the cornea that do not affect vision. In individuals over 60, it is considered a normal age-related change and does not require any treatment or referral.

    Answer A is incorrect. Arcus senilis does not require surgical intervention, as it is a benign condition that does not affect vision. Referral to an ophthalmologist is unnecessary unless there are other eye symptoms or conditions present that need evaluation.

    Answer B is incorrect. While arcus senilis can be associated with hyperlipidemia in younger individuals, in older adults, it is generally considered a normal aging change and not specifically linked to cardiac issues.

    Answer D is incorrect. Arcus senilis is a common and typically benign finding in older adults, but it is not necessarily associated with abnormal lipid levels. While a lipid profile might be considered based on the patient's overall cardiovascular risk factors and history, arcus senilis alone in this age group does not mandate one.

26. Answer B is correct. The standard first-line treatment for a hordeolum (stye) is warm compresses. These soaks help reduce pain and swelling and can facilitate the drainage of the blocked gland causing the hordeolum.

    Answer A is incorrect. Tobrex (tobramycin) eye drops are antibiotic drops that are not typically necessary for the initial treatment of a hordeolum.

    Answer C is incorrect. Referral to an eye surgeon for incision and drainage is not usually necessary for an uncomplicated hordeolum. Most hordeola resolve with conservative treatment, such as warm compresses.

    Answer D is incorrect. Applying an eye patch is not recommended for a hordeolum. Patching the eye can create a moist environment that may promote bacterial growth and worsen the condition. Warm compresses are the preferred method to alleviate symptoms and promote drainage.

27. Answer B is correct. Angle closure glaucoma (also known as acute angle-closure glaucoma) is an ocular emergency characterized by sudden onset of severe eye pain, vision changes (such as halos around lights or blurred vision), headache, nausea, and vomiting.

    Answer A is incorrect. A corneal abrasion typically presents with eye pain, a sensation of a foreign body in the eye, tearing, and photophobia (sensitivity to light). While it can cause discomfort and vision changes, it does not usually cause severe eye pain accompanied by nausea and is not typically an ocular emergency.

    Answer C is incorrect. A subconjunctival hemorrhage is characterized by a bright red patch on the white part of the eye (sclera) due to a burst blood vessel. It is usually painless and does not affect vision.

    Answer D is incorrect. Bacterial conjunctivitis typically presents with redness, swelling, and purulent discharge from the eye. While it can cause discomfort and affect vision due to discharge, it does not cause severe eye pain, sudden vision changes, or systemic symptoms like nausea.

Resources

Ahmad, B., Gurnani, B., Patel, B. C. (2024, March 10). Herpes simplex keratitis. In: *StatPearls* [Internet]. StatPearls Publishing. https://www.ncbi.nlm.nih.gov/books/NBK545278/

CDC. (2024, March 1). *Clinical guidance for group A Streptococcal pharyngitis*. https://www.cdc.gov/group-a-strep/hcp/clinical-guidance/strep-throat.html

Centers for Disease Control (CDC). (2017). *Outpatient clinical care for pediatric populations*. https://www.cdc.gov/antibiotic-use/hcp/clinical-care/pediatric-outpatient.html?CDC_AAref_Val=https://www.cdc.gov/antibiotic-use/clinicians/pediatric-treatment-rec.html

Centor, R. M., & McIsaac, W. (n.d.). *Centor score (Modified/McIsaac) for strep pharyngitis*. https://www.mdcalc.com/calc/104/centor-score-modified-mcisaac-strep-pharyngitis)

DeBoer, D. L., & Kwon, E. (2023, August 7). Acute sinusitis. In: *StatPearls* [Internet]. StatPearls Publishing. https://www.ncbi.nlm.nih.gov/books/NBK547701/

Emeryk, A., Emeryk-Maksymiuk, J., & Janeczek, K. (2019). New guidelines for the treatment of seasonal allergic rhinitis. *Postepy dermatologii i alergologii*, *36*(3), 255–260. https://doi.org/10.5114/ada.2018.75749

Harberger, S., & Graber, M. (2023, July 3). Bacterial pharyngitis. In: *StatPearls* [Internet]. StatPearls Publishing. https://www.ncbi.nlm.nih.gov/books/NBK559007/

Hashmi, M. F., Gurnani, B., & Benson, S. (2024, January 26). Conjunctivitis. In: *StatPearls* [Internet]. StatPearls Publishing. https://www.ncbi.nlm.nih.gov/books/NBK541034/

Khazaeni, B., Zeppieri, M., & Khazaeni, L. (2023, November 26). Acute angle-closure glaucoma. In: *StatPearls* [Internet]. StatPearls Publishing. https://www.ncbi.nlm.nih.gov/books/NBK430857/

Leik, M. (2021). *Family nurse practitioner certification intensive review* (4th ed.). Springer Publishing Company.

Medina-Blasini, Y., & Sharman, T. (2023, July 31). Otitis externa. In: *StatPearls* [Internet]. StatPearls Publishing. https://www.ncbi.nlm.nih.gov/books/NBK556055/

Ruia, S., & Kaufman, E. J. (2023, July 31). Macular degeneration. In: *StatPearls* [Internet]. StatPearls Publishing. https://www.ncbi.nlm.nih.gov/books/NBK560778/

Seidman, M. D., Gurgel, R. K., Lin, S. Y., et al. (2015). Clinical practice guideline: allergic rhinitis. *Otolaryngology–Head and Neck Surgery*, *152*(1_suppl):S1–S43. doi:10.1177/0194599814561600

Shukla, U. V., & Tripathy, K. (2023, August 25). Diabetic retinopathy. In: *StatPearls* [Internet]. StatPearls Publishing. https://www.ncbi.nlm.nih.gov/books/NBK560805/

Smolinski, N. E., Antonelli, P. J., & Winterstein, A. G. (2022). Watchful waiting for acute otitis media. *Pediatrics*, *150*(1):e2021055613.

Solano, D., Fu, L., & Czyz, C. N. (2023, August 28). Viral conjunctivitis. In: *StatPearls* [Internet]. StatPearls Publishing. https://www.ncbi.nlm.nih.gov/books/NBK470271/

Taylor, M., Brizuela, M., & Raja, A. (2023, July 4). Oral candidiasis. In: *StatPearls* [Internet]. StatPearls Publishing. https://www.ncbi.nlm.nih.gov/books/NBK545282/

Willmann, D., Guier, C. P., Patel, B. C., et al. (2023, August 8). Hordeolum (stye). In: *StatPearls* [Internet]. StatPearls Publishing. https://www.ncbi.nlm.nih.gov/books/NBK459349/

CHAPTER 7

Respiratory System

Susan M. DeNisco, DNP, APRN, FNP-BC, FAANP

Review Basic Anatomy of the Respiratory System

- Functions of the respiratory system include gas exchange, acid–base balance, phonation, pulmonary defense, and metabolism.
- The respiratory system comprises the lungs, conducting airways, and the chest wall.
- The apex of the lung is slightly above the clavicle.
- The bases of the lungs extend to the diaphragm.
- The right lung consists of three lobes and is positioned in a more horizontal plane.
- The left lung has upper and lower lobes, separated by an oblique fissure.

Gas Exchange

- The intrathoracic (inferior) airway includes the trachea, the mainstem bronchi, and multiple bronchial generations.
- The actual exchange of gases occurs in the respiratory bronchioles, alveolar ducts and sacs, and alveoli.
- Lung compliance determines the rate and force of expiration.
- Thoracic compliance determines the elastic load during inspiration.

> **Clinical Pearls**
>
> Adults and children differ in airway anatomy and physiology. At approximately 8 years old, the pediatric airway anatomy and physiology become similar to the adult airway.

- Structural changes to the thoracic cage due to aging cause a reduction in chest wall compliance.

Assessment of the Respiratory System

History and Physical Examination

Tables 7-1 and **7-2** provide the components of obtaining a comprehensive respiratory medical history and physical examination.

Diseases of the Respiratory System

Asthma

Asthma is a chronic heterogeneous disorder of the lungs characterized by chronic airflow inflammation, including:

- variable and recurring symptoms;
- bronchospasm (bronchial hyperresponsiveness);
- inflammatory cell infiltration, eosinophils, neutrophils, lymphocytes, epithelial cell injury, and mast cell activation;
- the development of asthma appears to involve the interplay between host factors, primarily genetics and environmental exposures;
- genetic predisposition with family history of allergies, eczema, and allergic rhinitis (atopic history and an immunoglobulin E (IgE)-mediated response to common aeroallergens); and
- exacerbations can be life-threatening (**Table 7-3**).

Table 7-1 Obtaining a Respiratory History

Chief Complaint	Reason your patient is seeking care	

History of Present Illness	Presenting problem:
	- Systematic symptoms (night sweats, weight loss, fatigue)
	- Frequency of daytime and nocturnal symptoms
	- Frequency of rescue inhaler use (albuterol)
	- Cough characteristics:
	  - Productive
	  - Nonproductive (dry)
	  - Bronchospastic
	  - Secondary to medications?
	- Wheeze, dyspnea
	- Shortness of breath on exertion and/or at rest
	- Exercise tolerance and limitations
	- Orthopnea
	- Chest pain—characteristics
		For each symptom describe:
		- Onset
		- Location/radiation
		- Duration
		- Character
		- Aggravating factors
		- Relieving factors
		- Temporal/timing
		- Severity (quantitative value)
		
		Important Questions:
		- What questions or concerns?
		- What does the patient want the provider to know or answer?
		- Management of disease(s)
		- Adherence to medical treatment regiment
		- Environmental exposures
		- Barriers to medical care

Other Subjective Data	Activities of Daily Living Functional Status Developmental Status	
Past Medical History	Review for any conditions that have the potential for respiratory manifestations or atopic components (eczema) Environmental allergy evaluation (including allergy testing), food allergy, anaphylaxis, hospital or emergency room admissions, ICU admission, and intubations or noninvasive ventilation Include comorbid conditions (gastroesophageal reflux disease, obesity, sleep apnea, allergic diseases, food allergy, anaphylaxis, urticaria/angioedema, vocal cord dysfunction, diabetes mellitus, anxiety, or depression) History of COVID-19 Lung cancer Pulmonary embolism Recurrent respiratory infections Injuries/chest trauma/head injury Other chronic illnesses Childhood disease or illnesses	Current and past disease management Adherence to medical treatment regimen
Past Surgical History	Tonsil and adenoidectomy Chest surgery Cardiac surgery	
Past Diagnostic Studies	Chest or sinus radiograph Pulmonary function testing Allergy testing Bronchoscopy or laryngoscopy Tuberculin and/or fungal skin testing	
Immunizations	Influenza (month/year) Pneumococcal (month/year) Adult immunizations Childhood immunizations	

Medications	Short-acting beta agonist (SABA) Inhaled corticosteroids (ICS) Long-acting beta agonist (LABA) Combination of ICS/LABA Leukotriene receptor antagonists/inhibitors Mast cell stabilizers Methylxanthines Anti-immunoglobin E antibodies Short-acting muscarinic antagonist (SAMA; i.e., Ipratropium bromide) Long-acting muscarinic antagonist (LAMA) Long-acting anticholinergics Phosphodiesterase-4 inhibitors Oral corticosteroids (prednisone) Home oxygen Herbal therapy Over-the-counter therapy Other	Barriers to medication adherence Technique using respiratory devices Knowledge of medical treatment regimen
Allergies	Medications such as aspirin (ASA) Food Environmental	Type of reaction
Family History	History of asthma, eczema, aspirin allergy, cystic fibrosis, chronic obstructive pulmonary disease (COPD), lung cancer	
Social History	Home, work, and school environment Occupation Environmental hazards Use of protective devices Use of heater, air conditioner, humidifiers Exercise habits Diet/nutrition Low socioeconomic status or inner-city residence Past and present illicit drug use, tobacco or marijuana use, alcohol use Second- or third-hand tobacco smoke exposure Travel outside the United States	

Asthma Triggers

- Viral infections
- Airborne allergens (e.g., grass, pollen, dust mites, mold, cockroach and animal dander)
- Food allergies (e.g., seafood, nuts, sulfites, food dye)
- Irritants (e.g., pollution, cold air, humid air, smoke exposure, chemical exposure, tobacco use, illicit drug use)
- Exercise-induced asthma
- Emotional stress
- GERD (acid reflux into the esophagus irritates airways)
- Medications (e.g., ASA, NSAIDs, ACE-I, beta blockers)

Asthma Physical Examination Findings

- A classic physical examination finding in asthma is wheezing intermittently associated with cough or dyspnea.
  - Wheezing with prolonged expiratory phase
  - Wheezing typically has a high-pitched and musical sound
  - Worsening attack will include both inspiratory and expiratory wheezing
  - Severe bronchoconstrictive breath sounds are faint or inaudible
  - Signs of severe or life-threatening asthma include tachycardia (heart rate > 120 beats per minute), tachypnea (respiratory rate

Table 7-2 Physical Examination

Inspection	Palpation	Percussion	Auscultation
General appearance Diaphoresis Cough or audible wheeze Use of accessory muscles Pursed lip breathing Dyspnea Tachypnea Nasal flaring Inability to speak in complete sentences Cyanosis Shape of the chest (barrel chest) Paradoxical chest movement Nail clubbing (< 160 degree)	Trachea Use index finger to determine central alignment or deviation Thoracic expansion Adult is 4–5 cm Symmetrical Tactile fremitus "99" normal vibrations are on upper lobes and softer vibrations on lower lobes	Diaphragmatic excursion Assessment of diaphragmatic excursion provides a method for evaluating the degree of muscle deterioration in neuromuscular and respiratory diseases. Ask patient to breathe deeply and hold breath. Percuss downward along scapular line, just below the scapula on one side until tone changes from resonant to dull. Mark the location on the skin. Allow patient to breathe normally 2–3 breaths, then ask the patient to exhale completely and hold. Percuss upward, starting just below the mark, observing for dull to resonant. Measure distance. Repeat on the opposite side. Ask patient to resume breathing comfortably. EXPECTED: 3–5 cm (higher on right than left) Percussion—over all lobes of the lungs, comparing right and left. **Resonant sounds** are low-pitched, hollow sounds heard over normal lung tissue. **Flat or extremely dull sounds** are normally heard over solid areas. **Dull sounds** are normally heard over dense areas such as the heart or liver. Dullness replaces resonance when fluid or solid tissue replaces air-containing lung tissues, such as occurs with pneumonia, pleural effusions, or tumors. **Hyperresonant sounds** are louder and lower pitched than resonant sounds and are normally heard when percussing the chests of children and very thin adults. May also be heard when percussing lungs hyperinflated with air. **Tympanic sounds** are hollow, high, drum-like sounds. Tympany is normally heard over the stomach. Tympanic sounds heard over the chest indicate excessive air in the chest, such as may occur with pneumothorax.	**Normal Lung Sounds** **Vesicular**: I > E low-pitch soft intensity; turbulent flow of air throughout the airways of nondiseased lungs **Bronchovesicular**: I = E moderate pitch and intensity, turbulent, heard over bronchi **Bronchial/Tracheal**: I < E high-pitched, loud, less harsh, easily heard in central airways **Whispered Pectoriloquy "99" or "1,2,3"**: normal whispered voice test will be distant and muffled **Egophony "eee" test**: normally sounds like "eee" clearly and not "bah" **Adventitious Sounds** **Wheeze**: continuous, high-pitched, musical, usually expiratory, but can be inspiratory or both; sounds produced by air flowing through narrowed bronchi **Rhonchi**: low-pitched, loud, often gurgling, generally heard on inspiration, snore-like sounds, often clears with cough; characterized by secretions within the large airways; can be heard in a wide variety of pathologies **Crackles**: discontinuous, explosive, "popping" sounds that originate within the airways

Table 7-3 Risk Factors for Asthma-Related Death

Previous severe exacerbation (e.g., intubation or ICU admission for asthma)
Two or more hospitalizations or > three emergency department (ED) visits in the past year
Use of > two canisters of SABA per month
Difficulty perceiving airway obstruction or the severity of worsening asthma
Low socioeconomic status or inner-city residence
Illicit drug use
Major psychosocial problems or psychiatric disease
Comorbid diseases (e.g., cardiovascular disease or other chronic lung disease)

Data from National Heart Lung and Blood Institute. (2020). Focused Updates to Asthma Management Guidelines. Retrieved from https://www.nhlbi.nih.gov/resources/2020-focused-updates-asthma-management-guidelines

---

Table 7-4 Diagnostic Criteria for Asthma in Adults, Adolescents, and Children 6–11 years

Consider a diagnosis of asthma and perform spirometry if any of these indicators are present:

- Symptoms of dyspnea, cough, and/or wheezing, especially nocturnal, difficulty breathing, or chest tightness
- With acute episodes: hyperinflation of thorax, decreased breath sounds, high-pitched wheezing, and use of accessory muscles
- Symptoms worse in presence of exercise, viral infections, inhaled allergens, irritants, changes in weather, strong emotional expression, stress, menstrual cycles
- Reversible airflow obstruction: FEV1 > 12% from baseline, or increase in FEV1 > 10% of predicted after inhalation of a bronchodilator, if able to perform spirometry
- Alternative diagnoses are excluded

Data from National Heart Lung and Blood Institute. (2020). Focused Updates to Asthma Management Guidelines. Retrieved from https://www.nhlbi.nih.gov/resources/2020-focused-updates-asthma-management-guidelines

---

> 30 breaths per minute), pulsus paradoxus > 18 mmHg, use of accessory muscles, nasal flaring, evidence of a hyperinflated chest, cyanosis, difficulty speaking, and silent chest (Table 7-3) describes patients at risk for fatal asthma)

Diagnostic Testing

- Spirometry (pulmonary function testing) is the gold standard for evaluating airflow obstruction.
- Measure the FVC (forced vital capacity) and FEV1 (forced expiratory volume in one second before and after inhalation of a short-acting bronchodilator).
- Peak flow measurements are not a substitute for spirometry but are good for monitoring treatment.
- Pulse oximetry measurement in patients with acute asthma to exclude hypoxemia.
- Chest X-ray only for a compelling reason or to rule out an alternate diagnosis.
- Complete blood cell count (CBC) to check for infection and/or eosinophilia.
- Allergy testing for children with persistent symptoms.
- Exercise challenge is the standard method for assessing patients with exercise-induced bronchospasm.

Table 7-4 provides key indicators for diagnosing asthma, and **Table 7-5** lists recommendations for referring patients to an asthma specialist.

Table 7-5 Recommendations for Referral to an Asthma Specialist

Not meeting the goals of asthma therapy after 3–6 months of treatment.
Comorbid conditions complicate asthma (e.g., sinusitis, nasal polyps, allergic bronchopulmonary aspergillosis [ABPA], severe rhinitis, vocal cord dysfunction [VCD], gastroesophageal reflux disease [GERD], chronic obstructive pulmonary disease [COPD]).
Additional diagnostic testing is indicated (e.g., allergy skin testing, rhinoscopy, complete pulmonary function studies, provocative challenge, bronchoscopy).
Patient requires additional education and guidance on complications of therapy, problems with adherence, or allergen avoidance.
Patient is being considered for immunotherapy.
Patient requires step 4 care or higher (step 3 for children 0–4 years of age). Consider referral if patient requires step 3 care (step 2 for children 0–4 years of age).
Prescribed more than two bursts of oral corticosteroids in 1 year.
Exacerbation requiring hospitalization.
Occupational or environmental inhalant or ingested substance contributing to asthma.

Data from National Heart Lung and Blood Institute. (2020). Focused Updates to Asthma Management Guidelines. Retrieved from https://www.nhlbi.nih.gov/resources/2020-focused-updates-asthma-management-guidelines

Asthma Treatment Goals

- Perform all usual symptom-free activities (i.e., attend school, play without limitation, work full time, no absence of work due to asthma symptoms).
- Prevent symptom exacerbation.
- Minimize the use of rescue inhalers to < 2 times per week.
- Avoid ED visits or hospitalization.
- Maintain normal pulmonary function tests (PFTs).
- Minimize permanent lung damage and prevent loss of lung function.
- Reduce adverse medication effects.

Treatment

Pharmacologic treatment is the mainstay of asthma therapy and is recommended at all levels of asthma severity. Asthma treatment classifies asthma symptoms and lung function and takes a stepwise approach to treatment (Steps 1–6, NAEPP, 2020; Steps 1–5, GINA, 2023).

A comprehensive review of asthma guidelines can be read at:

- National Asthma Education and Prevention Program: Expert Panel Working Group (NAEPP, 2020), which provides the most recent asthma management guidelines; and
- the Global Initiative for Asthma (2023) report.

A synopsis comparing the guidelines can be found in **Table 7-6**.

Medications for treating asthma and chronic obstructive pulmonary disease (COPD) are described in **Table 7-7**.

Table 7-6 Asthma Classifications and Therapy Approaches

NAEPP (2020)		Global Initiative for Asthma (2023)	
Asthma Symptoms/Lung Function	Treatment	Asthma Symptoms	Treatment
Step 1: Intermittent Asthma		**Step 1**	
Symptoms: 2x week or less Nighttime waking: 2 times or less per month Normal FEV1 Exacerbations: 1x or less per year	SABA prn	Infrequent asthma symptoms < 2x/week	Low-dose ICS with rapid onset LABA Or Low-dose ICS daily and SABA prn
Step 2: Mild Persistent Asthma		**Step 2**	
Symptoms: more than 2x/week but not daily Nighttime waking: 3–4x/month Interference in activities Normal FEV1 Exacerbations: 2x or more/year	Low-dose ICS daily and SABA prn or Low-dose ICS-SABA or ICS plus SABA given together prn	Asthma symptoms or need for rescue inhaler more than 2x/week	Low-dose ICS prn Or Low-dose ICS daily and SABA prn
Step 3: Moderate Persistent Asthma		**Step 3**	
Symptoms: Daily nighttime waking: every night Uses SABA several times daily Extreme limitation in activities FEV1 60–80% predicted Exacerbations: 2x or more/year	Combination low dose ICS 1–2 inhalations prn (maximum 12 inhalations/day)	Most days have troublesome asthma symptoms Nighttime awakenings ≥ 1x/month Risk factors for exacerbations	Low-dose ICS as maintenance and rescue therapy Or Medium-dose ICS-LABA daily and SABA prn

Steps 4–6: Severe Persistent Asthma		Steps 4 and 5	
Symptoms: all day Nightly awakenings Uses SABA several times daily Extreme limitation in activities FEV1 < 60% predicted Exacerbations: 2x or more/year	Step 4 Combination low-dose ICS 1–2 inhalations prn (maximum 12 inhalations/day)	Severely uncontrolled asthma with ≥ 3 of the following: Daytime asthma symptoms ≥ 2x/week Nighttime awakenings daily Rescue inhaler ≥ 2x/week Severe activity limitation Or An acute exacerbation	Step 4: Medium-dose ICS as maintenance and rescue therapy Or Medium-dose ICS-LABA daily and SABA prn
	Step 5 Medium-to-high dose ICS-LABA plus LAMA daily and SABA prn		Medium-dose ICS as maintenance and rescue therapy plus LAMA daily Or Medium-dose ICS-LABA plus LAMA daily and SABA prn Assess asthma phenotype and evaluate for asthma biologics
	Step 6 High-dose ICS-LABA daily; consider LAMA as substitute or add-on therapy Oral steroids Possible addition of asthma biologics		

Table 7-7 Medications Used for Asthma and COPD

Drug Classification	Generic Name (Trade Name)
Short-acting beta agonist (SABA)	Albuterol (Proventil HFA, Ventolin HFA, ProAir HFA Albuterol nebulizer solution) Levalbuterol (Xoponex HFA, Xoponex nebulizer solution)
Long-acting beta2 agonists	Salmeterol (Serevent) Formoterol (Foradil)
Inhaled corticosteroid (ICS)	Fluticasone (Flovent) Budesonide (Pulmicort) Beclomethasone (Q-var) Mometasone (Asmanex)
Combined inhaled corticosteroid (ICS) + Long-acting beta2 agonist (LABA)	Budesonide/Formoterol (Symbicort) Fluticasone/Salmeterol (Advair) Mometasone/Formoterol (Dulera) Fluticasone Furoate/Vilanterol (Breo Ellipta)
Leukotriene receptor antagonists/inhibitors (LTRAs)	Montelukast (Singular) Zafirlukast (Accolate) Zileuton (Zyflo)

(continues)

Table 7-7 Medications Used for Asthma and COPD (continued)

Drug Classification	Generic Name (Trade Name)
Methylxanthines	Theophylline
Mast cell stabilizers	Cromolyn for nebulizer treatments in the United States
Anti-immunoglobulin E antibodies	Dupilumab (Dupixent) Omalizumab (Xolair)
Oral corticosteroids ("Short Burst")	Prednisone Prednisolone Methylprednisolone
PDE4 (Approved for COPD)	Roflumilast (Dairesp) Cilomilast (Ariflo)
Anticholinergics (Approved for COPD)	Ipratropium (Atrovent) *Ipratropium + Albuterol (Duoneb) Tiotropium (Spiriva)

Clinical Pearls

Newly available biologics include dupilumab for severe eosinophilic/type 2 asthma in adults and children over 6. Consider for severe asthma, test results for perennial allergens, and an IgE level between 30 IU/mL and 700 IU/mL.

Assessment of Control

Poor asthma control can increase future risks of asthma, including exacerbation, accelerated decrease in lung function, and side effects of treatment.

The goals of treatment include:

- minimal or no symptoms during the day or night;
- full physical activity, including exertion;
- prevention of exacerbations;
- maintenance of (near) normal pulmonary function;
- decreased use of rescue (reliever) medication (i.e., short-acting beta agonist [SABA]); and
- minimal or no adverse effects from medications.

Reliable assessment of asthma control is essential to managing asthma effectively and initiating or changing pharmacotherapy.

- Regular follow-up visits will be held at 1- to 6-month intervals, depending on the level of control.
- Asthma control should be assessed at every patient encounter using a standardized, validated self-administered questionnaire, such as the Asthma Control Test (ACT) and the Asthma Control Questionnaire (ACQ), or the Test for Respiratory and Asthma Control in Kids (TRACK).
- Assessment of asthma control is identified by the patient and/or parent or caregiver's perception and provides information for asthma management.
- An Asthma Action Plan is recommended for all patients with asthma (**Table 7-8**)
  - Medications reconciliation
  - Daily self-management behaviors for worsening asthma
  - Poor inhaler technique
  - Avoidance of triggers
- When asthma is well-controlled and maintained for at least 3 months, a step-down or reduction in pharmacologic therapy may be implemented.

Clinical Pearls

Asthma education is the cornerstone of achieving asthma control.

Chronic Obstructive Pulmonary Disease

- COPD is characterized by the presence of progressive airflow limitation.
- COPD is associated with enhanced chronic inflammatory response to noxious particles or gases in the airways.
- Tobacco use is the most prevalent cause of COPD in the United States.

Table 7-8 Asthma Action Plans

Asthma Zones	Self-Assessment
Green Zone: Doing Well	Symptoms: - Breathing is good - No coughing or wheezing - Can work and play - Sleeps well at night Peak Flow Meter > 80% of personal best
Yellow Zone: Caution	Symptoms: - Some problems breathing - Coughing, wheezing, or tight chest - Problems working or playing - Wake at night Peak Flow Meter between 50–79% of personal best
Red Zone: Get Help Now!	Symptoms: - Lots of problems breathing - Cannot work or play - Gets worse instead of better - Medicine is not helping Peak Flow Meter < 50% of personal best

Table 7-9 Comparison of Presentation of Chronic Bronchitis and Emphysema

Chronic Bronchitis	Emphysema
Middle age to older patient	Weight loss
May be of higher body weight	"Barrel chest" (increased anterior/posterior [A/P] diameter)
History of many years of smoking	Pursed lip breathing and use of accessory muscles
Dyspnea on exertion	Tripod sitting position
Chronic productive cough with large amounts of thick sputum	Acute exacerbation, worsening dyspnea, increased sputum production, and sputum purulence
Use of accessory muscles of respiration is common	Decreased breath and very distant heart sounds
Coarse rhonchi crackles and expiratory wheezing may be heard on auscultation	Prolonged expiratory phase
Hyperresonance	Chest X-ray with flattened diagram, hyperinflation, and sometimes presence of bullae
Decreased tactile fremitus and egophony	
Patients may have signs of right-sided heart failure, such as edema and cyanosis.	

- Risk factors for COPD
  - History of smoking
  - Asthma and increased airway responsiveness to allergens, antioxidant deficiency, and tuberculosis
  - Environmental and occupational exposure
  - Alpha-1-antitrypsin deficiency
- COPD is subdivided into two major groups based on clinical symptoms:
  - Chronic bronchitis
  - Emphysema
  - Most patients have a mixture of both, but one may dominate.

Emphysema
- Abnormal, irreversible enlargement of the air spaces distal to the terminal bronchioles
- Loss of elastic recoil
- Chronic hyperinflation of the lungs
- Expiratory phase is markedly prolonged
- Use of accessory muscles
- "Pink puffers"

Exam Clue
"Gold standard" is pulmonary function testing for evaluating asthma and COPD.

Chronic Bronchitis
- Clinically defined as the presence of a chronic productive cough for 3 months during each of 2 consecutive years
- Large amounts of sputum with cough
- Airway hypersecretion and inflammation, with other causes of cough being excluded
- "Blue bloaters" secondary to chronic hypoxemia and hypercapnia
- Peripheral edema from cor pulmonale

Table 7-9 describes the clinical presentation of chronic bronchitis and emphysema, and **Table 7-10** highlights the Global Initiative for Chronic Obstructive Lung Disease (GOLD) Guidelines criteria to base the severity of COPD.

Table 7-10 Classification of COPD Severity GOLD Guidelines, 2024

Classification of Severity of Airflow Limitations in COPD
(Based on postbronchodilator FEV1)
In patients with FEV1/FVC < 0.70

Gold 1:	Mild	FEV1 ≥ 80% predicted
Gold 2:	Moderate	50% ≤ FEV1 < 80% predicted
Gold 3:	Severe	30% ≤ FEV1 < 50% predicted
Gold 4:	Very Severe	FEV1 < 30% predicted

Modified from Global Initiative for Chronic Obstructive Lung Disease. (2024). Global Strategy for Diagnosis, Management and Prevention of COPD 2024. https://goldcopd.org/2024-gold-report/

Clinical Pearl

COPD may be difficult to distinguish from congestive heart failure (CHF). Peak expiratory flow is a crude point of care test for distinguishing COPD from CHF. Patients who blow 150 to 200 mL or less indicate a COPD exacerbation; higher flows indicate a probable CHF exacerbation.

COPD Pharmacologic Treatment Plan

- Management and treatment of COPD are based on current GOLD guidelines (Global Initiative for Chronic Obstructive Lung Disease, 2024).
- GOLD guidelines classify patients into one of three groups (i.e., A, B, or E) to guide pharmacologic treatment (refer to GOLD guidelines)
- The COPD Assessment Test (GlaxoSmithKline, n.d.) is an eight-item questionnaire that measures symptoms. The prevalence of respiratory symptoms is determined by a score ranging from 0 to 40.
- The Modified Medical Research Council (mMRC) Dyspnea Scale (Mahler, n.d.) is used to assess the degree of baseline functional impairment due to dyspnea.
- SABA and long-acting bronchodilators (LABAs) are used for all patients with COPD and are prescribed for relief of dyspnea and early treatment of exacerbations (Group A patients; CAT score < 10).
- Long-acting muscarinic (LAMA) and LABAs are used for more symptomatic patients who are at a low risk of exacerbation (Group B patients; CAT score ≥ 2).
- LAMA and LABAs for patients with a high risk of exacerbation, with more than two exacerbations per year or one hospitalization (Group E patients).
- If the eosinophil count is greater than 300 cells/mcL, consider inhaled corticosteroids (ICS); they can be used in Group E patients in combination with LAMAS and LABAs.
- Long-term treatment with oral corticosteroids is not recommended for monotherapy in COPD.
- Roflumilast (Daliresp), a selective phosphodiesterase-4 inhibitor, can be used to reduce the risk of COPD exacerbations in patients with severe asthma.

COPD Education and Follow-Up

- Close follow-up and education imperative for patients with COPD
- Discussion of smoking cessation modalities at each visit
- Adherence to the pharmacologic treatment regimen
- Review the correct use of inhaler and nebulizer treatments, if applicable.
- Pulmonary hygiene and rehabilitation
- Physical activity to improve exercise tolerance
- Selection of antibiotic treatments with coverage for *Haemophilus* and *Streptococcus pneumoniae*
- Administer pneumococcal, annual influenza, and COVID-19 vaccines according to the current Advisory Committee on Immunization Practices (ACIP) recommendations.
- Comorbidities of COPD must be identified and appropriately managed.

Clinical Pearl

Patients with normal spirometry values may report respiratory symptoms, whereas patients with severe airflow obstruction by spirometry may report no symptoms.

Pneumonia

- Pneumonia is a serious, life-threatening lower respiratory tract infection and is a leading cause of increased morbidity and mortality and costly medical utilization.
- Pneumonia can result from viral or bacterial infections and is associated with an acute inflammation of the pulmonary parenchyma and consolidation of the alveoli.

- Bacteria is the common cause of lower respiratory tract infections.
- *Streptococcus pneumoniae* is the most common source of bacterial pneumonia.
- Symptoms generally include cough, dyspnea, fever, chills, and pleuritic chest pain.
- Objective findings of pneumonia include fever; tachycardia; tachypnea; asynchronous breathing; and dull percussion notes over the consolidations, bronchophony, and vocal fremitus.
- Diagnostic tests may include chest radiology, CBC count, ultrasonography, sputum and blood cultures, or serology. **Table 7-11** describes the signs and symptoms of bacterial pneumonia.

Clinical Pearl

Antibiotic therapy is the mainstay of treatment of bacterial pneumonia.

Pediatric Considerations

- Viral infections tend to be resolved within 1 to 3 weeks with symptomatic treatment.
- Viral infections are the most common cause of pneumonia in children under 5 years old.

Table 7-11 Signs and Symptoms of Bacterial Pneumonia

Streptococcus Pneumoniae: rust-colored sputum
Pseudomonas, Haemophilus, and pneumococcal species: may produce green sputum
Klebsiella species pneumonia: red currant-jelly sputum
Anaerobic infections: foul-smelling sputum

Signs of bacterial pneumonia
Hyperthermia (fever, typically > 38°C) or hypothermia (< 35°C)
Tachypnea (> 18 respirations/min)
Use of accessory respiratory muscles
Tachycardia (> 100 beats per minute [bpm]) or bradycardia (< 60 bpm)
Central cyanosis
Altered mental status
Physical exam findings may include the following:
Adventitious breath sounds—rales/crackles, rhonchi, or wheezes
Decreased intensity of breath sounds
Egophony
Whispering pectoriloquy
Dullness to percussion
Tracheal deviation
Lymphadenopathy
Pleural friction rub

- Most cases of viral pneumonia are mild.
- Some cases may be more serious and require hospitalization.

Community-Acquired Pneumonia

- Community-acquired pneumonia (CAP) is an acute infection of the pulmonary parenchyma that causes inflammatory changes and lung damage.
- It is acquired in the community setting and is a common presenting condition seen in primary care.
- Risk factors for CAP:
  - Older age
  - Malnutrition
  - Chronic comorbid conditions (e.g., COPD, heart failure [HF], diabetes mellitus [DM], alcoholism)
  - Viral respiratory infection
  - Dysphagia and aspiration
  - Smoking
  - Prematurity
  - Crowded conditions (e.g., daycare, prisons, dormitories)
  - Indoor pollutants from cooking or heating wood
  - Lack of immunizations
  - Medications (e.g., immunosuppressives, oral steroids, proton pump inhibitors (PPIs) and histamine H2 receptor antagonists
- Most forms of CAP are treatable, and defining the pathogen significantly simplifies the selection of antimicrobial agents.
- *Streptococcus pneumoniae* (gram-positive) is the most common pathogen causing CAP.
- Hemophilus influenza (gram-negative)
- Atypical bacteria (i.e., *Mycoplasma pneumoniae, Chlamydophila pneumoniae*)
- Viral respiratory pathogens include influenza, respiratory syncytial virus (RSV), and COVID-19.
- *Legionella pneumoniae* is found in areas with moisture, air conditioning, and hospital settings.
  - Fatality rate is 5 to 10 percent.

Diagnosing CAP

- CAP is diagnosed by clinical presentation, including pleuritic chest pain, cough, and fever, and infiltrates seen on chest radiography (CXR).
- **CXR is the gold standard test for diagnosing CAP.**
  - Common focal infiltrate pattern is typical on CXR (lobar pneumonia).
  - Repeat CXR in 4 to 6 weeks in adult smokers older than 60.

- No need to repeat CXR in patients younger than 60, nonsmokers, and those who feel well at 6 weeks.
- Labs
  - Sputum for culture and sensitivity and gram stain are not required.
  - CBC is used to assess for leukocytosis with positive left shift (↑band forms).
- Physical examination findings may include crackles upon auscultation, dullness to chest percussion, bronchial breath sounds, tactile fremitus, and egophony.
- Tachypnea may be present but is more common in older patients with CAP.

> **Clinical Pearl**
>
> Consolidation is seen on CXR with *Streptococcus pneumoniae*.

CURB-65 Score for Pneumonia Severity in Adult Patients

The CURB-65 score estimates the mortality of CAP to help determine inpatient versus outpatient treatment (MDCALC, n.d.)

- The CURB-65 calculator can be used in the emergency department (ED) setting to risk stratify a patient's CAP.
  - **CURB Scoring**
    Confusion = 1 point
    Urea (Blood urea nitrogen) > 19 mg/dL = 1 point
    Respiratory Rate: > 30/minute = 1 point
    Blood Pressure: Systolic < 90 mmHg or Diastolic < 60 mmHg = 1 point
    Age: ≥ 65 years = 1 point
  - **Interpretation:**
    - Score of 0 or 1 suggests that the patient may be appropriate for outpatient therapy
    - Score of 2 or higher indicates a higher mortality, and these patients should usually be admitted to the hospital for monitoring and therapy
    - Score of 3 or higher indicates that the patient should be considered for admission to an intensive care unit, particularly for patients with a score of 4 or 5

Table 7-12 describes the treatment regimen for CAP.

Table 7-12 Community-Acquired Pneumonia (CAP)

Outpatient Treatment
CURB Score ≤ 1 No comorbidities/previously healthy. No risk factors for drug-resistant *S. pneumoniae*.   First-line monotherapy: Amoxicillin 1 gram PO three times daily for 5–7 days **or**   Azithromycin 500 mg PO one dose, then 250 mg PO daily for 4 d or extended release 2 g PO as a single dose **or**   Clarithromycin 500 mg PO bid or extended release 1,000 mg PO q24h **or**   Doxycycline 100 mg PO bid 5–7 days
If received prior antibiotic within 3 months: Azithromycin or clarithromycin **plus** amoxicillin 1 g PO q8h **or** amoxicillin-clavulanate 2 g PO q12h **or**   Fluoroquinolone (e.g., levofloxacin 750 mg PO daily **or** moxifloxacin 400 mg PO daily)
Comorbidities present (e.g., alcoholism, bronchiectasis/cystic fibrosis, COPD, IV drug user, postinfluenza, asplenia, DM, lung/liver/renal diseases):   Levofloxacin 750 mg PO q24h **or**   Moxifloxacin 400 mg PO q24h **or**   Combination of a beta-lactam (amoxicillin 1 g PO q8h **or** amoxicillin-clavulanate 2 g PO q12h **or** ceftriaxone 1g IV/IM q24h **or** cefuroxime 500 mg PO BID **plus** a macrolide (azithromycin **or** clarithromycin)   Duration of therapy: minimum of 5 days, should be afebrile for 48–72 hours, or until afebrile for 3 days; longer duration of therapy may be needed if initial therapy was not active against the identified pathogen, or if it was complicated by extrapulmonary infections.

Atypical Pneumoniae

- *Mycoplasma pneumoniae* is a common cause of CAP, usually affecting young adults, school-aged children, military recruits, and those living or working in crowded places (e.g., schools, prisons, shelters for the unhoused).
- Symptomatology includes cough, rhinorrhea, pharyngitis, headache, fever, diaphoretic, and chills.
- Treatment for *M. pneumonia* includes macrolides (azithromycin, clarithromycin, erythromycin), doxycycline, and fluoroquinolones.
- *Mycoplasma pneumoniae* symptoms are generally mild and respond well to antibiotic therapy.
- *Pneumocystis jirovecii* pneumonia (formerly PCP) in patients with human immunodeficiency virus (HIV).

> **Clinical pearl**
>
> Alert: Amoxicillin plus Macrolide or Doxycycline to target atypical pathogens and patients with comorbidities

Viral Pneumonia and Pediatrics

- Most cases of viral pneumonia are mild.
- Viral infections are the most common cause of pneumonia in children younger than 5.
- Pneumonia in children under 5 years old generally has an etiology of a virus.
- Viral infections tend to be resolved within 1 to 3 weeks with symptomatic treatment.

Prevention Guidelines

Center for Disease Control and Prevention (CDC)
Influenza vaccine for all persons
CDC recommends **PCV15 or PCV20** (pneumococcal conjugate vaccines) for: ■ children younger than 5 years old, ■ people 5–64 years old with certain risk conditions who never received a PCV, and ■ Adults 65 years or older who never received a PCV. People previously recommended to get both PCV13 and PPSV23 who already received PCV13 can complete the recommended series with: ■ PCV20, **or** ■ PPSV23.
CDC recommends **PPSV23 (pneumococcal polysaccharide vaccines)** for: ■ Children 2–18 years old with certain risk conditions who get PCV15 ■ Adults 19 years or older who get PCV15 People previously recommended to get both PCV13 and PPSV23 who already received PCV13 can complete the recommended series with: ■ PCV20, **or** ■ PPSV23
Pediatric Immunizations Haemophilus influenzae type b (HIB) Pneumococcus Measles Whooping cough (pertussis) RSV (respiratory syncytial virus)

> **Clinical Pearl**
>
> Routine administration of the pneumococcal conjugate vaccine has resulted in an overall reduction in invasive disease and pneumonia rates.

Lung Cancer

- A primary lung neoplasm is a malignancy arising from lung tissue.
- The major types of neoplasm are large-cell carcinoma, small-cell carcinoma, nonsmall-cell, squamous-cell carcinoma, and adenocarcinoma.
- Approximately 85 percent of lung cancer cases are nonsmall-cell lung cancer.
- Cigarette smoking is responsible for approximately 90 percent of cases of lung cancer.
- Smoking cessation or never smoking is the most important method to decrease the morbidity and mortality associated with this disease.
- Lung cancer is often insidious, producing no symptoms until the disease has advanced.
- Many patients with lung cancer have advanced disease when metastatic disease is present.
- Risk factors include older age, current or history of tobacco abuse, hemoptysis, and the presence of a previous malignancy.
- Cough, pain, or hemoptysis may present in patients with hilar involvement, particularly when the metastases adjoin or invade the bronchi.
- **Table 7-13** describes common signs and symptoms of lung cancer.

Screening Recommendations for Lung Cancer

Effective screening is imperative for high-risk patients. **Table 7-14** displays the American Cancer Society (ACS)

> **Clinical Pearls**
>
> Prevention and cessation of smoking offer the most important route to decreasing the morbidity and mortality associated with lung cancer.

Table 7-13 Common Signs and Symptoms of Lung Cancer

Cough, wheezing, dyspnea
Hemoptysis, hoarseness, dysphagia
Recurring infections, such as bronchitis and pneumonia
Weight loss, fever, fatigue, anorexia
Metastatic signs and symptoms
Bone pain
Spinal cord impingement
Neurologic problems such as headache, weakness or numbness of limbs, dizziness, and seizures

Table 7-14 Lung Cancer Screening Guidelines

American Cancer Society (2023)	USPTF (2021)

Recommends annual lung cancer screening with low-dose computed tomography (LDCT) in people who meet all these criteria:
▪ Persons aged 50–80 years who currently smoke or formerly smoked
▪ Accumulated a ≥ 20 pack-year smoking history
▪ Years since quitting smoking among individuals who formerly smoked is not an inclusion or exclusion criteria for lung cancer screening
▪ Other exclusions:
  • Health conditions that may increase harm or hinder further evaluation, surgery, or treatment for lung cancer
  • Comorbid conditions that limit life expectancy < 5 years; not willing to accept treatment for screen-detected cancer
	Recommends annual lung cancer screening with LDCT in people who meet all these criteria:
	▪ Are ages 50–80 years
	▪ Have a 20 pack-year smoking history
	▪ Currently smoke cigarettes or quit within the past 15 years
	▪ End screening for people in this group who develop a health problem that seriously limits their life expectancy or who aren't willing to have lung surgery if needed

Table 7-15 Comparison of Latent Versus Active TB

Latent Tuberculosis Infection	Active Tuberculosis Disease

▪ Has no symptoms
▪ Does not feel sick
▪ Cannot spread TB bacteria to others
▪ Has a positive skin test or blood test result indicating TB infection
▪ Has a normal chest x-ray and a negative sputum smear
▪ Needs treatment for latent TB infection to prevent TB disease
	▪ Has symptoms that may include:
	  • productive cough that lasts ≥ 3 weeks
	  • chest pain
	  • hemoptysis
	  • weakness or fatigue
	  • weight loss
	  • no appetite
	  • chills
	  • fever
	  • night sweats
	  • spreading TB bacteria to others
	  • a skin test or blood test result indicating TB infection
	  • an abnormal chest x-ray or positive sputum smear or culture
	▪ Needs pharmacologic treatment

and U.S. Preventive Services Task Force (USPSTF) guidelines for screening.

Tuberculosis

- Tuberculosis (TB) is a common infectious, granulomatous disease and a leading cause of morbidity and mortality worldwide, particularly in developing countries.
- Approximately 1.5 million people worldwide die of TB each year, and 9 million become infected.
- TB is a leading cause of death in people who are infected with HIV.
- TB is a reportable infectious disease to the public health department.
- Pulmonary TB is caused by the bacterium *Mycobacterium tuberculosis* (*M. tuberculosis*).
- *M. tuberculosis* is transmitted via airborne droplets (droplet nuclei) expelled by coughing, sneezing, or talking with pulmonary or laryngeal tuberculosis.
- Extrapulmonary tuberculosis can result from *M. tuberculosis* spreading to other organs, including bone, joints, meninges, lymphatics, pleura, pericardium, and perihilar lymph nodes.
- Not everyone infected with TB bacteria becomes sick. As a result, two TB-related conditions exist: latent TB infection (LTBI) and active TB disease.
- If not treated properly, TB disease can be fatal. (Refer to **Table 7-15** for a comparison of latent versus active TB.)

Risk Factors for TB

- Exposure to someone with an active disease
- High-risk groups:
  - Minorities
  - Children under 5 years old
  - Elderly
  - Foreign-born people
  - Prisoners

- Nursing home residents
- Teachers
- Homeless population
- Migrant workers
- Healthcare providers
- People with HIV infection
- Patients undergoing steroid therapy, chemotherapy, and hematologic malignancies
- People treated with tumor-necrosis alpha-factor (TNF-alpha) antagonists for autoimmune diseases
- Measles, mumps, and pertussis may reactivate TB
- Smokers
- People with malnutrition
- People with alcoholism
- Intravenous drug users
- Congenital TB (rare)

Tuberculosis Tests

- Mantoux Tuberculin Skin Test (TST) measures the delayed hypersensitivity reaction to the purified protein derivative (PPD), a heat-inactivated tubercle bacilli protein precipitate.
  - Measure intradermal reaction within 48 to 72 hours after placement (see **Box 7-1** for interpretation of TST)
- Interferon-gamma release assay (IGRA) blood test: QuantiFERON-TB Gold Plus (QFT-Plus) test
  - Results are not affected by patients who had prior BCG (bacillus Calmette–Guerin) vaccination.
  - Consider for patients who may not return for skin test interpretation or need results within 24 hours.

> **Box 7-1 Interpretation of Tuberculin Skin Testing**
>
> An **induration of ≥ 5 mm** is considered positive in people:
> - living with HIV.
> - who have had recent contact with a person with infectious TB disease.
> - with chest x-ray findings suggestive of previous TB disease.
> - with organ transplants.
> - who are immunosuppressed (e.g., patients on prolonged therapy with corticosteroids ≥ 15 mg per day of prednisone or those taking TNF-a antagonists).
>
> An **induration of ≥ 10 mm** is considered positive in people:
> - born in countries where TB disease is common, including Mexico, the Philippines, Vietnam, India, China, Haiti, and Guatemala, or other countries with high rates of TB.
> - who abuse drugs.
> - working in mycobacteriology laboratories.
> - who live or work in high-risk congregate settings (e.g., nursing homes, homeless shelters, or prisons).
> - with certain medical conditions that place them at high risk for TB (e.g., silicosis, diabetes mellitus, severe kidney disease, certain types of cancer, and certain intestinal conditions).
> - with a low body weight (< 90% of ideal body weight)
> - < 5 years of age
> - who are infants, children, and adolescents exposed to adults in high-risk categories
>
> An **induration of 15 ≥ mm** is considered positive in low-risk patients.

> **Test Taking Strategy**
>
> Be able to differentiate between the 5 mm and 10 mm results of a TST.

Other Diagnostic Tests

- Mycobacterium tuberculosis (MTB) isolation from clinical specimens is the standard for TB diagnosis:
  - Acid-fast bacilli (AFB) smear microscopy
  - False-positive culture rates are reported to be approximately 2 to 4 percent.
- Chest X-ray (may be suggestive of TB but not diagnostic; assess for upper- and middle-lobe cavitations and mediastinal lymphadenopathy

See **Table 7-16** for chest X-ray findings of common respiratory conditions.

> **Clinical pearl**
>
> Check baseline liver function tests and monitor when patients are taking PZA and IRF; educate on alcohol abstinence.

Table 7-16 Common Chest X-Ray Findings by Respiratory Condition

COPD	Asthma	Lobar Pneumonia	TB
■ hyperlucency of the lungs ■ increased anterior-posterior (A-P) diameter of the chest ■ bullae contain no bronchovascular markings ■ flattened diaphragm	■ bronchial thickening ■ hyperinflation ■ focal atelectasis	■ focal dense opacification of most of an entire lobe ■ relative sparing of the large airways ■ -ground-glass opacity in a lobar or segmental pattern ■ possible atelectasis	■ infiltrates cavitation ■ pleural effusion ■ lymphadenopathy-miliary pattern

Data from Sait, S., & Tombs, M. (2021). Teaching Medical Students How to Interpret Chest X-Rays: The Design and Development of an e-Learning Resource. *Advances in medical education and practice*, 12, 123–132. https://doi.org/10.2147/AMEP.S280941

Treatment of Latent TB Infection and Active TB Disease

- All patients with TB should be checked for HIV.
- Untreated LTBI and HIV are more likely to develop active TB.
- The CDC recommends four treatment regimens for LTBI with a preference for short-term treatment.
- Duration of treatment for active TB can be 4, 6, or 9 months, depending on drug susceptibility, comorbid medical conditions, and potential drug interactions.
- Directly observed treatment (DOT) is mandatory for nonadherent patients.
- Please consult with infectious disease experts regarding drug-resistant TB and/or recurrent TB.
- Current TB treatment guidelines are provided by the CDC (2025).
- See **Box 7-2** for treatment of latent and active tuberculosis.

Adverse Drug Considerations

- Isoniazid (INH): give with pyridoxine (Vitamin B6) to decrease risk of peripheral neuritis, neuropathy, hepatitis, and seizures.
- Ethambutol (ETH): causes optic neuritis and rash. Get a baseline ophthalmologic exam and avoid in patients with eye problems.
- Pyrazinamide (PZA): causes hepatitis, hyperuricemia, arthralgias, and rash.
- Rifampin (RIF): causes hepatitis, thrombocytopenia, and orange-colored tears, saliva, and urine (normal).
- INH increases blood levels of phenytoin (Dilantin) and disulfiram (Antabuse).

Box 7-2 Treatment of Latent TB Infection and Active Disease

Latent TB	Active TB Disease
Rifapentine (RPT) (3 months) Rifampin (RIF) (4 months) Isoniazid (INH) (6–9 months)	Treated by taking several different agents for 6–9 months. First-line pharmacologic agents include: Isoniazid (INH) Rifampin (RIF) Ethambutol (ETH) Pyrazinamide (PZA)

- RIF and Rifapentine (RPT) decrease blood levels of many drugs, including oral contraceptives, warfarin and some other anticoagulants ("blood thinners"), sulfonylureas (used for diabetes), and methadone.
- RIF and RPT are contraindicated in HIV-infected individuals being treated with protease inhibitors (PIs) and most nonnucleoside reverse transcriptase inhibitors (NNRTIs).

Clinical Pearl

The TST is valid and safe to use during pregnancy; the TB blood test is also safe in pregnancy but is not validated in diagnosing TB in this population. Pregnant women with TB should be treated immediately, but pharmacologic treatment must be carefully selected for safety in the fetus.

Table 7-17 Causes of Cough

Common
Asthma
COVID-19
GERD
Upper airway inflammatory diseases (e.g., allergic rhinitis, sinusitis)
Postnasal drip
Chronic bronchitis
Upper airway cough syndrome
Bronchiectasis
Nonasthmatic eosinophilic bronchitis

Other Causes
Angiotensin-converting enzyme inhibitor (ACEI)
Bronchogenic carcinoma
Chronic aspiration
Congestive heart failure (CHF)
Interstitial lung disease
Neuromuscular disorders
Pertussis
Psychogenic cough
Sarcoidosis
Tracheoesophageal fistula
Tuberculosis

Cough

- Cough is one of the most common complaints that prompts a patient to seek health care.
- Patients may report cough as the only complaint, or other nonspecific symptoms, such as pharyngitis, malaise, or low-grade temperature that may accompany the cough.
- The cough reflex is a physiologic function that protects the pulmonary tract from aspiration, inhaled irritants, particulates, and pathogens.
- Cough can be characterized as:
  - acute, less than 3 weeks;
  - subacute, lasting 3 to 8 weeks; or
  - chronic, lasting more than 8 weeks.

Table 7-17 describes the causes of chronic cough.

Management of Cough

- A detailed history must be performed in all patients, including assessing health status, cough severity, chronic illnesses, tobacco use, environmental irritants, and medications, including ACE inhibitors (ACE-I) and oxymetazoline (Afrin).
- Managing acute cough includes evaluating and treating the likely causes of cough, using diagnostic tests, appropriate empiric therapy, and short-term medication trials.
- Vagal-mediated esophageal reflux stimulated by acid or nonacid volume reflux should be considered in patients with chronic cough.
- Inflammatory mediators in the lower airways are elevated in patients with cough variant asthma, GERD, and upper airway cough syndrome (UACS), also known as postnasal drip.
- Chronic cough is a multifactorial symptom that may require referral to allergy and asthma, pulmonology, and/or gastrointestinal specialists for consultation.
- In chronic cough, a heightened cough reflex may be the primary etiology.
- If a cough does not subside within 3 weeks, a chest radiograph should be obtained to exclude tuberculosis, carcinoma, or other serious pulmonary diseases.
- Expectorants, such as guaifenesin, may be therapeutic in cases of excessive mucus production. They increase the volume of mucus and facilitate the removal of secretions by ciliary transport and/or cough.
- Antitussives, such as codeine and dextromethorphan, have been shown to be limited or ineffective in treating chronic cough. Any beneficial effect is largely due to the placebo effect.

Clinical Pearl

After discontinuing ACEI, the cough generally resolves within 1 to 4 days but can take up to 4 weeks.

Test Taking Tip

If the cough persists, empirical treatment for GERD with a proton pump inhibitor, with appropriate lifestyle and dietary modifications, should be considered.

Acute Bronchitis

- Acute bronchitis is a self-limited infection with the primary symptom of cough lasting 10 to 20 days.
- Etiology of acute bronchitis is most often viral and is generally associated with an upper respiratory infection.
- Wheezing may be present, along with chest wall tenderness that is generally related to muscle strain from coughing.

- The appearance of the sputum cannot be used to distinguish between viral and bacterial bronchitis.
- Acute bronchitis should be differentiated from other respiratory complications.
- Cough accompanied by fever, sputum production, and constitutional symptoms is typically a complication of influenza or pneumonia.
- Antimicrobial agents are not recommended in most cases of acute bronchitis.
- Symptomatic treatment may include NSAIDs or acetaminophen directed toward presenting symptoms.
- Bronchodilators can help to relieve the cough in people who show evidence of bronchospasm.
- Antitussives (dextromethorphan) may be carefully considered in patients age 6 and older.
- No data supports the use of oral corticosteroids in patients with acute bronchitis and no asthma.

Clinical Pearl

Acute bronchitis is one of the most common causes of antibiotic misuse.

COVID-19 Infection

- COVID-19 (Coronavirus disease 2019) is a disease caused by a virus named SARS-CoV-2.
- Over one million people have died from COVID-19 in the United States.
- It can be very contagious and spreads quickly.
- Symptoms typically appear 2 to 14 days after exposure.
- COVID-19 most often causes respiratory symptoms that resemble a cold, the flu, or pneumonia (e.g., fever, chills, headache, myalgia, cough, shortness of breath (SOB), rhinitis, diarrhea, nausea and vomiting, loss of taste and smell, etc.).
- Most people with COVID-19 have mild symptoms, but some people become severely ill.
- To prevent COVID-19, the vaccination is recommended for everyone aged 6 months and older in the United States.
- There is currently no FDA-approved or FDA-authorized COVID-19 vaccine for children younger than 6 months.
- The CDC guidelines for the COVID-19 vaccine apply to all age groups and patients who are moderately to severely immunocompromised (CDC, 2024b).
- There is strong scientific evidence that antiviral treatment of mild-to-moderate illness in persons who are at risk for severe COVID-19 reduces their risk of hospitalization and death.
- The antiviral drugs ritonavir-boosted nirmatrelvir (Paxlovid) and remdesivir (Veklury) are the preferred treatments in eligible adult and pediatric patients who are at high risk for progression to severe COVID-19.
- Consider COVID-19 treatment in patients with mild-to-moderate COVID-19 who have one or more risk factors for severe COVID-19.
- Treatment must be started as soon as possible and within 5 to 7 days of symptom onset. Refer to the CDC (2024a) for more information on treatment of COVID-19.

Respiratory Syncytial Virus

- RSV is a common cause of severe lower respiratory tract diseases, including bronchiolitis, pneumonia, and acute respiratory failure, generally seen in infants and young children.
- Older people and adults with chronic cardiac or lung disease or weakened immune systems are at high risk.
- Annual epidemics occur in winter and early spring.
- Household members should be immunized against influenza and practice good hand and cough hygiene.
- RSV preventative measures are an ideal priority for patients with the highest risk of complications.
- Symptomatic RSV infections may occur in adults, primarily in healthcare workers or caretakers of small children.
- Clinical symptoms are usually consistent with an upper respiratory tract infection and last approximately 5 days.
- The CDC recommends that adults 60 and older get the RSV vaccine, which is available as a single dose, in late summer and early fall, before RSV usually starts to spread in the community.

For comprehensive information on RSV in infants and children, see Chapter 19, "Pediatrics."

Clinical Pearl

RSV is an enveloped, nonsegmented, negative-stranded RNA virus and a member of the *Paramyxoviridae* family. Adult vaccines are **recombinant protein vaccines** that cause the immune system to produce RSV antibodies.

Test Taking Tip

Antibiotics are not indicated for RSV infection unless there is a secondary bacterial infection.

Review Questions

1. When you teach clients about using steroid inhalers for asthma or COPD, what information is essential?
   A. Keep the inhaler in the refrigerator.
   B. Do not use another inhaler for 10 minutes after the steroid inhaler.
   C. Rinse your mouth after using the inhaler.
   D. Be careful not to shake the container before using.

2. The Curb-65 criteria may be used to help assess whether a patient needs to be treated in the hospital or can be effectively treated at home. The R in curb stands for:
   A. respiratory rate.
   B. rapid pulse rate.
   C. C retractions.
   D. recent use of antibiotics.

3. Community acquired bacterial pneumonia is most commonly caused by:
   A. *Streptococcus pneumonia*.
   B. *Mycoplasma pneumonia*.
   C. *Hemophilus influenza*.
   D. *Staphylococcus aureus*.

4. A 53-year-old male with a 45 pack-year smoking history presents to the nurse practitioner's (NP) office for a follow-up visit. This patient had a recent emergency department (ED) admission for exertional dyspnea that has progressed to dyspnea at rest and a cough for 2 months. The chest radiograph report showed a suspicious nodule in the right hilar region. What should the NP order at this visit?
   A. Sputum culture
   B. Confirmatory chest X-ray
   C. CT scan of the chest
   D. Bronchoscopy

5. HIV coinfection is the most potent immunosuppressive risk factor for which of the following?
   A. Distal acinar emphysema
   B. Active tuberculosis (TB) disease
   C. Diabetes mellitus (DM)
   D. Paraseptal emphysema

6. Screening for latent tuberculosis infection (LTBI) is recommended in:
   A. persons at risk of recent infection and patients infected with HIV.
   B. groups with an increased flow of progression to active disease.
   C. persons with nocturnal coughing.
   D. persons whose CD4 cell count increases to more than 600 cells/µL.

7. According to the GINA guidelines, poor asthma control can increase risks of asthma exacerbations, including all the following (select all that apply):
   A. Airway remodeling
   B. Accelerated decrease in lung function
   C. Generally, no side effects of treatment
   D. Fatal asthma

8. Empiric treatment for suspected mycoplasma pneumonia involves which of the following?
   A. Five-day course of oral azithromycin (500 mg for the first dose, then 250 mg daily for the next 4 days)
   B. Dexilant 60 mg 1 tablet twice daily for 14 days
   C. Treat symptomatically
   D. Palivizumab according to weight for 14 days

9. According to the GINA guidelines for asthma treatment, at what step should a rescue course of an inhaled corticosteroid be initiated for asthma symptoms?
   A. When the client is in step 1, intermittent stage
   B. When the client is in Step 2, mild persistent stage
   C. When the client is in Step 4, severe persistent stage.
   D. Whenever the client needs it, at any time and any step

10. The NP orders a chest radiograph on a 28-year-old Caucasian female who presents to the office for uncontrolled asthma with symptoms of cough, wheezing throughout all lung fields, and shortness of breath. Which clinical finding on the chest radiograph is not suggestive of asthma?
    A. Bronchial thickening
    B. Nodules
    C. Hyperinflation
    D. Focal atelectasis

11. A 62-year-old Black male with mild chronic obstructive pulmonary disease (COPD) presents to the clinic with a chief complaint of cough. The NP understands pharmacological treatment is based upon (check all that apply):
    A. adherence to medical treatment regimen.
    B. the CAT score, breathlessness, and wheezing.
    C. diet.
    D. airflow limitations.

12. A mother brings her 3 year old son to the clinic for an urgent visit. She states he has a 2 day history of coughing, sneezing, runny nose and sore throat.

The NP obtained a laboratory diagnosis of respiratory syncytial virus (RSV), which was made by analyzing respiratory secretions. The NP understands that:
- A. RSV infection usually is a self-limited process, but it is associated with recurrent wheezing in some patients.
- B. Infection with RSV requires direct admission to the ED.
- C. Adolescents are most severely affected by RSV.
- D. A prescription for Synagis (palivizumab) should be ordered for this patient.

13. Vesicular breath sounds:
    - A. are high-pitched, musical sounds heard throughout the lung.
    - B. are loud, hollow, harsh sounds, and are heard best over the manubrium.
    - C. are low-pitched sounds that can be heard over the periphery of both lung fields.
    - D. have an expiratory phase that is longer than their inspiratory phase.

14. The standard short-course anti-TB regimen includes which of the following?
    - A. Enablex, Myrbetriq, and Ditropan
    - B. Isoniazid, rifampicin, pyrazinamide, and ethambutol
    - C. Linezolid and Sutezolid
    - D. Panobinostat, palbociclib, and lenvatinib

15. Chest radiographs showing new consolidations or infiltrates suggest which of the following?
    - A. Emphysema
    - B. Acute respiratory distress syndrome (ARDS)
    - C. Interstitial pulmonary edema
    - D. Pneumonia

16. A 48-year-old Black male comes to the family nurse practitioner's (FNP) office for a follow-up visit complaining of shortness of breath, coughing, and dyspnea on exertion. The FNP identifies the findings of COPD as:
    - A. appearance of Kerley lines on chest X-ray.
    - B. FEV1/FVC < 0.70.
    - C. hypotension and tachycardia.
    - D. low serum glucose level and elevated serum lactate level.

17. According to the National Asthma Education Prevention Program Expert Panel Report 4 (EPR-4), the risk factors for fatal asthma include the following (select all that apply):
    - A. Two or more hospitalizations in the past year for severe exacerbation requiring admission for asthma into an intensive care unit or intubation
    - B. Perceiving an airway obstruction or the severity of worsening
    - C. Comorbid conditions
    - D. Higher income with varying sociodemographic groups

18. Clinical features that suggest malignancy on initial evaluation include:
    - A. older age, a current or past abuse of tobacco, hemoptysis, and the presence of a previous malignancy.
    - B. cough, chest pain, bloody sputum, night sweats, fatigue, and weight loss.
    - C. tobacco use, hemoptysis, chest congestion, and shortness of breath.
    - D. persistent cough or wheezing with white or pink blood-tinged mucus and fatigue.

19. A 76-year-old male with COPD presents to a clinic. Pulmonary function testing reveals an FEV1 of 69 percent. According to the Global Initiative for Lung Disease (GOLD), which of the following is the severity classification?
    - A. Mild
    - B. Moderate
    - C. Severe
    - D. Very severe

20. A 20-year-old patient has been taking albuterol via a metered dose inhaler for the past 2 months and remains in the yellow zone. Which of the following statements is true?
    - A. Medication should be decreased to produce desired effects.
    - B. The patient is 50 to 80 percent of their personal best.
    - C. The patient is 80 to 100 percent of their personal best.
    - D. Current medication dosage places the patient at risk for hypoxia.

21. When a normal lung transmits a palpable vibratory sensation to the chest wall, this is known as:
    - A. whispered pectoriloquy.
    - B. bronchophony.
    - C. tactile fremitus.
    - D. egophony.

22. Which of the following antihypertensive agents should the NP avoid prescribing to patients with emphysema?
    - A. Calcium channel blockers
    - B. Angiotensin-converting enzymes inhibitors (ACEI)
    - C. Beta blockers
    - D. Diuretics

23. When initially treating an adult for uncomplicated bronchitis, which of the following is the NP most likely to prescribe?
    A. Antivirals
    B. Antibiotics
    C. Oral steroids
    D. Antitussives

24. Chronic use of high-dose inhaled corticosteroids can cause which of the following? Select all that apply.
    A. Hypokalemia
    B. Osteoporosis
    C. Glaucoma
    D. Cataracts

25. A patient from India has an appointment for follow-up of TB exposure. The health history revealed that the patient received the Bacillus Calmette–Guerin (BCG) vaccine as a child. What is the best method to determine if the patient was exposed to TB?
    A. Purified protein derivative (PPD) skin test
    B. Interferon gamma release assay (IGRA) blood test
    C. Chest X-ray
    D. Sputum culture

Answers and Rationales

1. Answer C is correct. After using a steroid inhaler, the client should always rinse their mouth to prevent oral candidiasis or thrush. Brushing their teeth will also remove any bad taste.

   Answer A is incorrect because steroid inhalers do not need refrigeration

   Answer B is incorrect. If the client is taking a beta-2 agonist, tell them to take it first. Doing so will open the airway, allowing more steroid medication to be administered.

   Answer D is incorrect. The inhaler should be shaken first.

2. Answer A is correct. The 'R' in CURB stands for a respiratory rate of 30 or more breaths per minute. The CURB 65 criteria is an objective tool to determine the severity of community-acquired pneumonia (CAP). A point is given for each of the following that is present: The 'C' is for confusion. The 'U' is for a BUN greater than 19 mg/dL. The 'R' is for respiratory rate of 30 or more breaths per minute. The 'B' is for a systolic blood pressure less than 90/60. A point is also given if the patient is 65 years or older. A score of 1 is low risk, and the patient may be treated at home. With a score of 2, there should be a short period of hospitalization or closely monitored outpatient treatment. A score of 3 or greater indicates severe pneumonia, and the patient should be hospitalized with consideration of ICU placement.

   Answers B, C, and D are incorrect. These are not included in the CURB criteria.

3. Answer A is correct. *Streptococcus pneumonia* causes 30 to 75 percent of all community-acquired bacterial pneumonia cases.

   Answer B is incorrect. *Mycoplasma pneumonia* causes 5 to 35 percent of cases.

   Answer C is incorrect. *Hemophilus influenza* causes 6 to 12 percent of cases.

   Answer D is incorrect. *Staphylococcus aureus* causes 3 to 10 percent of cases.

4. Answer C is correct. Given the suspicious finding on the recent chest X-ray, a chest CT scan will be the next step. Following the CT scan results, the patient may be referred to a pulmonologist for additional assessment, bronchoscopy, and a possible lung biopsy.

   Answer A is incorrect. A sputum culture may be ordered if TB is suspected.

   Answer B is incorrect. A repeat chest X-ray would give no further information.

   Answer D is incorrect. A bronchoscopy would be considered as additional testing depending on CT scan results and consultation with a pulmonologist.

5. Answer B is correct. People living with HIV are more likely than others to become sick with TB if they are exposed and become infected. According to the CDC, TB remains a serious threat in the United States, especially for people living with HIV.

   Answers A and D are incorrect. Patients with emphysema are at risk for bacterial pneumonia with typical infectious organisms (*S. pneumoniae, Hemophilus,* Pseudomonas, Staph species, and Klebsiella and not co-infection with patients with HIV.

   Answer C is incorrect. Chronic inflammation (ongoing activation of the immune system) in response to HIV infection may also raise the risk of diabetes but is not as prevalent as TB.

6. Answer A is correct. According to the CDC, screening for LTBI is recommended for people

living with HIV and those at risk of recent LTBI infection. The diagnosis of LTBI is based on information gathered from the medical history, a tuberculin skin test (TST) or interferon gamma release assay (IGRA) result, chest radiographs, physical examination, and, in certain circumstances, sputum examinations. The presence of TB must be excluded before treatment for LTBI is initiated because failure to do so may result in inadequate treatment and development of drug resistance. A TST reaction of more than 5 mm of induration is considered positive in patients with HIV.

Answer B is incorrect. The increased progression of the disease does not apply to screening, as it is assumed that LTBI is already present.

Answer C is incorrect. Noctural coughing may indicate heart failure, so screening for LTBI doesn't apply here.

Answer D is incorrect. The CD4 cell count of a person who does not have HIV can be anything between 500 and 1,500.

7. Answers A, B, and D are correct. Poor asthma control can increase future risks of asthma, including exacerbation, accelerated decrease in lung function, and side effects of treatment. Increased risk for fatal asthma includes poor asthma control.

Answer C is incorrect. There are several side effects from medications to treat asthma. Inhaled glucocorticoid medication may sometimes cause hoarseness, a sore throat, or oral thrush.

8. Answer A is correct. CAP may be treated with monotherapy or combination therapy. Effective monotherapy antibiotics include combination therapy, which usually consists of ceftriaxone plus doxycycline, amoxicillin, azithromycin, doxycycline, and respiratory quinolones. Immunocompromised hosts who present with CAP are treated in the same manner as otherwise healthy hosts but may require a longer duration of therapy.

Answer B is incorrect. Dexilant is a proton pump inhibitor (PPI) to treat GERD.

Answer C is incorrect. A bacterial infection commonly causes CAP, and antibiotic treatment is warranted.

Answer D is incorrect. Palivizumab is used to treat children 24 months and younger with certain conditions that place them at high risk for severe RSV disease.

9. Answer D is correct. A rescue course of an inhaled corticosteroid should be initiated for an attack of asthma whenever the client needs it, at any time, and any step. Attempts should be made to use systemic corticosteroids in an acute or rescue fashion—a short burst followed by tapering to the lowest dose possible and preferably discontinued—with inhaled steroids prescribed for chronic or maintenance therapy.

Answers A, B and C are incorrect. Please review the GINA guidelines for the role of other pharmacologic regimens for all steps and severity as well as modifiable risk factors.

10. Answer B is correct. Nodules are diagnostic for cancer.

Answers A, C, and D are incorrect. Bronchial thickening, hyperinflation, and focal atelectasis are clinical findings on chest X-ray of exacerbated asthma.

11. Answers A, B, and D are correct. Validated tools, such as the CAT, can assess symptoms. Adherence is important and can be improved with an individualized approach. Pharmacological treatment is also based on airflow limitations, symptoms, and exacerbations.

Answer C is incorrect. Diet may be considered, but other options have a higher ranking.

12. Answer A is correct. RSV infection usually is a self-limited process, but it is associated with recurrent wheezing in some patients.

Answer B is incorrect. Patients usually have mild symptoms that can be treated symptomatically at home.

Answer C is incorrect. RSV can cause severe infection in some people, including babies 12 months and younger (infants), especially premature infants, older adults, people with heart and lung disease, or anyone with a weakened immune system (immunocompromised).

Answer D is incorrect. Synagis (palivizumab) is used to prevent RSV in premature infants and children with certain severe heart and lung conditions.

13. Answer C is correct. Vesicular breath sounds are soft, low-pitched sounds that can be heard over the periphery of both lung fields.

Answer A is incorrect. Wheezing is a high-pitched, musical sound heard throughout the lungs.

Answer B is incorrect. Bronchial breath sounds are loud, hollow, harsh sounds heard best over the manubrium.

Answer D is incorrect. Airflow limitation during the expiratory phase in airway obstructive disease causes prolonged expiration.

14. Answer B is correct. The standard short-course anti-TB regimen includes isoniazid, rifampicin, pyrazinamide, and ethambutol.

    Answer A is incorrect. Enablex, Myrbetriq, and Ditropan are prescribed for overactive bladder.

    Answer C is incorrect. Linezolid and Sutezolid are oxazolidinones, a class of antibacterials used for multidrug-resistant tuberculosis in evolving countries.

    Answer D is incorrect. Panobinostat, palbociclib, and lenvatinib are agents targeted to treat advanced forms of cancer.

15. Answer D is correct. Chest radiographs showing new consolidations or infiltrates are definitive in helping to establish a diagnosis of pneumonia.

    Answer A is incorrect. Emphysema manifests as lung hyperinflation with flattened hemidiaphragms, a small heart, and possible bullous changes.

    Answer B is incorrect. Common ARDS chest radiograph findings are bilateral, predominantly peripheral, and somewhat asymmetrical consolidation with air bronchograms.

    Answer C is incorrect. Plain chest radiographs can be normal in up to 75 percent of patients with asthma; other findings may include pulmonary hyperinflation, bronchial wall thickening, and nonspecific peribronchial cuffing.

16. Answer B is correct. Airflow obstruction is determined by spirometry, where the ratio of forced expiratory volume in the first second to forced vital capacity (FEV1/FVC) after bronchodilation is less than 0.70.

    Answer A is incorrect. Kerley lines on a chest radiograph are usually consistent with interstitial pulmonary edema.

    Answer C is incorrect. Hypotension and tachycardia together are not consistent with COPD; the NP should consider other causes, such as dehydration, heart failure, pregnancy, arrhythmias, shock, and so on.

    Answer D is incorrect. A high lactate level combined with low glucose is associated with the highest risk of acute kidney injury (AKI), liver dysfunction, dehydration from blood loss, and so on.

17. Answers A, B, C are correct. According to the EPR-4, risk factors for asthma-related death include previous severe exacerbation, two or more hospitalizations, or more than three ED visits in the past year, use of more than two canisters of short-acting beta agonist (SABA) per month, difficulty perceiving airway obstructions or the severity of worsening asthma, low socioeconomic status or inner-city residence, illicit drug use, major psychosocial problems or psychiatric disease, and comorbidities such as cardiovascular disease or other chronic lung disease.

    Answer D is incorrect. Risk factors for asthma fatality are typically found in lower income households.

18. Answer A is correct. Clinical features that suggest malignancy on initial evaluation include older age, current or past abuse of tobacco, hemoptysis, and the presence of a previous malignancy.

    Answer B is incorrect. Cough, chest pain, bloody sputum, night sweats, fatigue, and weight loss may indicate active TB.

    Answer C is incorrect. Tobacco use, hemoptysis, chest congestion, and shortness of breath can be associated with acute and chronic bronchitis, pneumonia, tuberculosis, and late stages of lung cancer.

    Answer D is incorrect. Persistent cough or wheezing with white or pink blood-tinged mucus and fatigue can indicate heart failure from fluid collecting in the lungs.

19. Answer B is correct. Moderate since the FEV1 is 69 percent.

    According to the GOLD 2024 Guidelines:

    Classification of Severity of Airflow Limitations in COPD in patients with FEV1/FVC < 0.70

    | Gold 1: | Mild | FEV1 ≥ 80% predicted |
    | Gold 2: | Moderate | 50% ≤ FEV1 < 80% predicted |
    | Gold 3: | Severe | 30% ≤ FEV1 < 50% predicted |
    | Gold 4: | Very Severe | FEV1 < 30% predicted |

20. Answer B is correct. The patient is at 50 to 80 percent of their personal best. Spirometry readings are used to assess a patient's personal best.

    Answer A is incorrect. The medication must be adjusted and not decreased to produce desired effects.

    Answer C is incorrect. The green zone ranges from 80 to 100 percent expected lung volume.

Answer D is incorrect. The red zone is below 50 percent of expected lung volume, which would place the patient at risk of hypoxia.

21. Answer C is correct. A normal lung transmits a palpable vibratory sensation to the chest wall. This is known as tactile fremitus. Increased tactile fremitus is generally present in conditions that increase lung tissue density, such as pneumonia. Other conditions, such as emphysema, crepitus, and pneumothorax, typically decrease tactile fremitus.

    Answer A is incorrect. In areas of the lung where there is lung consolidation, whispered pectoriloquy, or spoken sounds said by the patient (such as "99"), will be clearly heard through the stethoscope.

    Answer B is incorrect. Bronchophony is a test for lung consolidation. If the test is negative, when the patient says "99," the lungs will muffle the words. In a positive test, the words sound clear through the stethoscope.

    Incorrect D. Egophony is an increased resonance of voice sounds heard when auscultating the lungs, often caused by lung consolidation and fibrosis. A positive test will make a hard 'E' sound like an 'A.'

22. Answer C is correct. Beta blockers should be avoided in patients with a history of emphysema. Research shows that a reduction in FEV1 increases airway hyper-responsiveness and bronchoconstriction.

    Answer A is incorrect. Calcium channel blockers stop calcium from entering the cells of the heart and arteries which relaxes the blood vessels and slows the heart rate; it does not have broncho constrictive side effects.

    Answers B and D are incorrect. ACEIs and diuretics do not have this bronchoconstrictive effect.

23. Answer D is correct. Acute bronchitis is a viral infection, so treatment is typically symptomatic and involves rest, expectorants, and antitussives.

    Answer A is incorrect. Antivirals are not typically prescribed.

    Answer B is incorrect. Antibiotics are not effective against viral infections.

    Answer C is incorrect. A bronchodilator may be prescribed for wheezing, but oral steroids are recommended for severe wheezing.

24. Answers B, C, and D are correct. Evidence shows the prolonged use of corticosteroids can cause loss of bone mineral density or osteoporosis and ophthalmologic problems like glaucoma or cataracts.

    Answer A is incorrect. Hypokalemia is attributed to loop diuretics.

25. Answer B is correct. If a patient has been vaccinated with BCG, the IGRA blood test is the gold standard for evaluating their exposure to TB.

    Answer A is incorrect. PPD test may cause a false-positive reaction.

    Answers C and D are incorrect. A chest X-ray or sputum culture is unnecessary until positive symptoms or a positive test are present.

Resources

American Lung Association. (2024, October 23). *Create an asthma action plan.* https://www.lung.org/lung-health-diseases/lung-disease-lookup/asthma/managing-asthma/create-an-asthma-action-plan

Center for Disease Control (CDC). (2025, January 6). *Clinical guidelines.* https://www.cdc.gov/tb/hcp/clinical-guidance/?CDC_AAref_Val=https://www.cdc.gov/tb/publications/guidelines/default.htm

Center for Disease Control (CDC). (2024a, December 20). *COVID-19 treatment clinical care for outpatients.* https://www.cdc.gov/covid/hcp/clinical-care/outpatient-treatment.html?CDC_AAref_Val=https://www.cdc.gov/coronavirus/2019-ncov/hcp/clinical-care/outpatient-treatment-overview.html

Center for Disease Control (CDC). (2024b, October 31). *Interim clinical considerations for COVID-19 in the United States.* https://www.cdc.gov/vaccines/covid-19/clinical-considerations/interim-considerations-us.html#covid-vaccines

Center for Disease Control (CDC). (2024c, October 26). *Pneumococcal vaccinations.* https://www.cdc.gov/pneumococcal/vaccines/index.html

GlaxoSmithKline Services Unlimited. (n.d.). *COPD assessment test.* https://www.catestonline.org/

Global Initiative for Asthma. (2023). *2023 GINA report, Global strategy for asthma management and prevention.* https://ginasthma.org/2023-gina-main-report/

Global Initiative for Chronic Obstructive Lung Disease. (2024). *Global strategy for the diagnosis, management, and prevention of COPD: 2024 report.* https://goldcopd.org/2024-gold-report/

Macfarlane, J. (n.d.). *Curb-65 score for pneumonia severity.* MD Calc. https://www.mdcalc.com/calc/324/curb-65-score-pneumonia-severity#when-to-use

Mahler, D. A. (n.d.). *mMRC (Modified Medical Research Council) dyspnea scale.* https://www.mdcalc.com/calc/4006/mmrc-modified-medical-research-council-dyspnea-scale

Mahler, D. A., & Wells, C. K. (1988). Evaluation of clinical methods for rating dyspnea. *Chest*, *93*(3), 580–586. https://doi.org/10.1378/chest.93.3.580

National Heart, Lung, and Blood Institute. (2020). *2020 focused updates to asthma management guidelines*. https://www.nhlbi.nih.gov/resources/2020-focused-updates-asthma-management-guidelines

Rajala, K., Lehto, J. T., Sutinen, E., Kautiainen, H., Myllärniemi, M., & Saarto, T. (2017). mMRC dyspnoea scale indicates impaired quality of life and increased pain in patients with idiopathic pulmonary fibrosis. *ERJ Open Research*, *3*(4). https://doi.org/10.1183/23120541.00084-2017

Sait, S., & Tombs, M. (2021, February 5). Teaching medical students how to interpret chest x-rays: the design and development of an e-learning resource. *Advances in Medical Education and Practice*, *12*, 123–132. https://doi.org/10.2147/AMEP.S280941

U.S. Preventive Services Task Force. (2021, March 9). Final recommendation statement: lung cancer: screening. *JAMA*. *325*(10). https://www.uspreventiveservicestaskforce.org/uspstf/recommendation/lung-cancer-screening

Wolf, A. M. D., Oeffinger, K. C., Shih, T. Y-C, Walter, L. C., Church, T., Fontham, E. T. H., Elkin, E. B., Etzoni, R. D., Guerra, C. E., Perkins, R.B., Kondo, K.K., Kratzer, T. B., Mamassaram-Baptiste, D., Dahut, W. L., Smith, R. A. (2023, November 1). Screening for lung cancer: 2023 guideline update from the American Cancer Society. *CA: A Cancer Journal for Clinicians*, *74*(1), 50–81. https://acsjournals.onlinelibrary.wiley.com/doi/10.3322/caac.21811

CHAPTER 8

Cardiovascular Disorders in Primary Care

Heather Ferrillo, PhD, APRN, FNP-BC, CNE

Murmurs

Basics of auscultating murmurs:

- Auscultate the patient supine, in the left lateral position, and leaning forward
- Auscultate with both the bell and the diaphragm
  - Right sternal border—second intercostal space (aortic area)
  - Left sternal border—second intercostal space (pulmonic area)
  - Along the left sternal border at each intercostal space
  - Lower left sternal border—(tricuspid area)
  - Apex—(mitral area)
- Murmurs should be characterized by:
  - Timing (systolic or diastolic)
  - Loudness (1 to 6 for systolic, 1 to 4 for diastolic)
  - Pitch (high, medium, or low)
  - Pattern (i.e., crescendo-decrescendo)
  - Quality (blowing, harsh, rumbling)
  - Location (where the loudest)
  - Radiation
  - Changes with position
- Identification of murmurs
- Systolic
  - Innocent/physiologic murmur
  - Mitral regurgitation
  - Tricuspid regurgitation
  - Ventricular septal defect (VSD)
  - Aortic stenosis (AS)
  - Hypertrophic cardiomyopathy
  - Pulmonic stenosis
- Diastolic—Diastolic murmurs are always pathologic
  - Aortic regurgitation
  - Mitral stenosis

(Jarvis, 2024)

Valvular Heart Disease

Identifying valvular abnormalities is an important role of the family nurse practitioner (FNP), along with close collaboration with a cardiologist for treatment and ongoing monitoring. Valvular heart disease (VHD) is classified into stages (**Figure 8-1**), which consider symptoms, valve anatomy, severity, and overall response of the cardiac circulation to the valvular disorder. Treatment is specific to the valve affected and severity.

Initial assessment of valve disorders should include a correlation between history and physical findings and noninvasive testing.

- Diagnostics
  - Detailed history and physical
  - Electrocardiogram
  - Chest X-ray
  - Transthoracic echocardiography (with doppler)

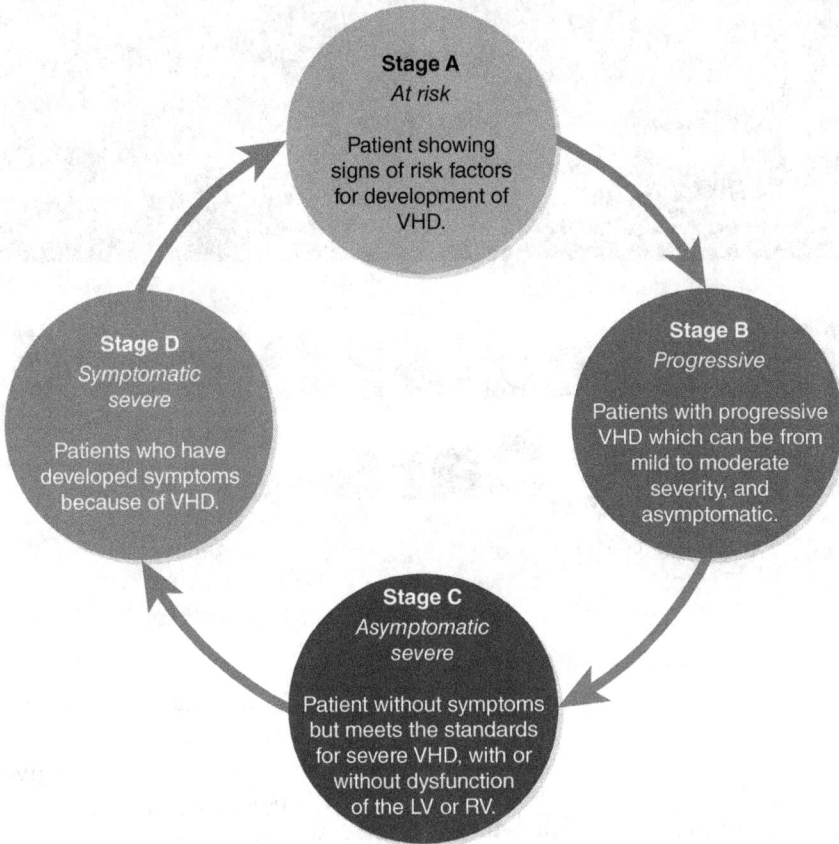

Figure 8-1 Stages of Valvular Heart Disease

Common Valvular Disorders

Aortic Stenosis
- Most common causes
  - Bicuspid valve (congenital)
  - Calcification
  - Rheumatic heart disease (RHD)
- Clinical presentation
  - Angina
  - Syncope
  - Heart failure (HF)
  - Decreased blood pressure (BP)
  - Narrowed pulse pressure
- Diagnosis
  - Murmur—harsh, midsystolic, crescendo-decrescendo, diffusely radiating
  - Echocardiogram
  - Cardiac catheterization
- Medical management
  - Control hypertension (HTN) using low dose and gradual titration of medications
  - Calcific aortic stenosis (AS) should be treated with statin therapy.
- Surgical management—timing based on symptoms and severity of stenosis
  - Surgical valve replacement
  - Transcatheter aortic valve replacement
  - Balloon valvuloplasty—short-term option

Mitral Regurgitation
- Most common causes
  - Mitral valve prolapse (MVP)
  - Rheumatic heart disease (RHD)
  - In ST-segment elevation myocardial infarction (MI), acute mitral regurgitation (MR) can be caused by infectious endocarditis and papillary muscle rupture.
- Clinical presentation
  - Few symptoms until severe, then HF results.
- Diagnosis
  - Murmur—pansystolic, high-pitched, blowing, radiating to axilla
  - Echocardiogram

- Medical management
  - Serial echocardiograms
  - BP control with vasodilators
  - Medical therapy for LV dysfunction in secondary MR or nonsurgical candidates
- Surgical management
  - Mitral valve repair or replacement

Aortic Regurgitation

- Common causes
  - Congenital (bicuspid valve)
  - Acquired (RHD [HTN], endocarditis)
  - A significant portion is idiopathic.
- Clinical presentation
  - Widened pulse pressure
  - HF symptoms
- Complications
  - Arrhythmias
  - Endocarditis
- Diagnosis
  - Murmur—soft diastolic, high-pitched, blowing, heard best leaning forward
  - Echocardiogram
- Medical management
  - Serial echocardiograms
  - BP control with vasodilators
- Surgical management—symptomatic and severe dysfunction
  - Aortic valve replacement or repair

Mitral Valve Prolapse

- Common causes
  - Myxomatous degeneration of the valve
  - Genetic link
- Clinical presentation
  - Mostly asymptomatic
  - Tachycardia
  - Palpitations
  - Lightheadedness
  - Atypical chest pain
  - Lethargy
- Complications
  - Mitral regurgitation
  - Atrial fibrillation (AF)
  - Rare endocarditis, stroke, and sudden death
- Diagnosis
  - Murmur of MR and midsystolic click
  - Echocardiogram
- Medical management
  - Beta blocker may control symptoms.
  - If a patient presents with MR, they will need afterload reduction, diuresis, and anticoagulation.

(McCance and Heuther, 2014; Jarvis, 2024; Otto et al., 2020)

Subacute Bacterial Endocarditis Prophylaxis

The guidelines revised in 2007 reflect the small likelihood of developing subacute bacterial endocarditis (SBE) after a dental procedure, the success rate of premedication in preventing SBE, and the increased incidence of antibiotic resistance. Research has been reviewed since these guidelines were revised, and the American Heart Association (AHA) has not recommended any changes.

Procedures warranting prophylaxis:

- Dental procedures
- Invasive respiratory tract procedures
- Procedures of infected skin, skin structures, or musculoskeletal tissue

Diagnosis requiring SBE prophylaxis for dental procedures (not recommended in others):

- Prosthetic heart valves
- History of bacterial endocarditis
- Congenital heart disease (specific types)
- Heart transplant with valvulopathy

Recommended agents for dental procedures (given 30 to 60 minutes before procedure):

- First line
  - Amoxicillin, 2 grams
- For patient allergic to penicillin (PCN):
  - Cephalexin, 2 grams,
  - Azithromycin or clarithromycin, 500 mg, or
  - Doxycycline, 100 mg.
  - Clindamycin is no longer recommended as an option due to adverse effects.

(Wilson et al., 2007, 2021)

Heart Failure

- HF is a state of decreased cardiac output due to the failure of the ventricles to pump sufficient blood to meet the body's demands.
- Can be left or right or biventricular
- Etiology
  - Right-sided (failure of right ventricle)
    - Most common is a disorder that increases pulmonary pressures
      - COPD
      - Pulmonary embolism
    - Left ventricular failure
    - RV infarct (least common)
  - Left-sided (failure of the left ventricle) (systolic or diastolic)
    - Most common is LV infarct

- HTN
- AS
- Clinical presentation
  - Forward effects (both sides) due to decreased cardiac output
    - Fatigue
    - Shortness of breath with exertions
    - Decreased peripheral perfusions
  - Right-sided (backward effects due to fluid buildup)
    - Jugular venous distention
    - Peripheral edema
    - Ascites
    - Hepatosplenomegaly
  - Left-sided
    - Crackles in the lungs
    - Dyspnea on exertion (DOE)
    - Paroxysmal nocturnal dyspnea (PND)
    - Orthopnea
    - Pulmonary edema
    - Diminished ejection fraction (EF) on echocardiogram, normal is 55 percent +/- 10
  - Diastolic—nonspecific
    - Dyspnea
    - Exercise intolerance
    - Fatigue
- Differential diagnosis
- Right versus left HF
- VHD
- Chronic lung disease
- Coronary artery disease
  - Ischemia versus infarct
- Diagnostics
  - Laboratory testing
  - Natriuretic peptide
    - N-Terminal Pro-B-Type Natriuretic Peptide (NT-pro BNP) > 125 pg/mL
    - BNP > 35 pg/mLA
  - Noninvasive cardiac imaging
    - Right-sided
      - Echocardiogram—Increased pulmonary pressures, dilated RV
    - Left-sided
      - Echocardiogram—Left ventricular size and function, left ventricular hypertrophy (LVH), valvular disorders
      - MUGA (multi-gated acquisition scan)—Nuclear determination of ejection fraction
    - Nuclear stress test—Determine infarct, ischemia, dilation of LV, ejection fraction
    - Grading/classification (2 scales)—Treatment based on both systems

- The New York Heart Association (NYHA) classification is dynamic and changes depending on the patient's current functional ability. It is a good indicator of treatment success.

The AHA, American College of Cardiology (ACC)/Heart Failure Society of America (HFSA) Classification of HF (see **Figure 8-2**) differs from functional classification because regression to prior stages is impossible, even if symptoms temporarily reside.

Both the AHA and the NYHA use four classifications based on symptoms (**Figure 8-3**).

Treatment

Stage A

- BP control to prevent symptomatic HF
- Diabetics should be treated with Sodium Glucose Cotransporter 2 inhibitor (SGLT2i)
- Healthy lifestyle habits to reduce HF, including physical activity, diet, weight management, and avoiding smoking

Stage B

- Patients with EF < 40 percent should receive an angiotensin enzyme inhibitor (ACEI) to prevent symptoms and reduce mortality.
  - Angiotensin receptor blocker (ARB) can be used if ACE intolerant and recent MI.
- Patients with a history of MI should receive a statin.
- Patients with a history of MI/ acute coronary syndrome (ACS) and EF < 40 percent should receive beta blockers to reduce mortality.
- Evaluation for implantable cardioverter/defibrillator (ICD) in patients with EF < 30 percent.

Stage C and D

- Multidisciplinary team approach
- Avoiding excessive sodium
- Fluid volume management
- Considerations for ICD and biventricular pacing.
- See (**Table 8-1**).

Follow-Up

- Routine visits for vital signs, symptoms, and fluid management
- Continued evaluation for factors contributing to adherence to clinical plan
- EF monitoring with serial echocardiography
- Renal function and electrolyte monitoring
- Consider telemonitoring

Heart Failure   **147**

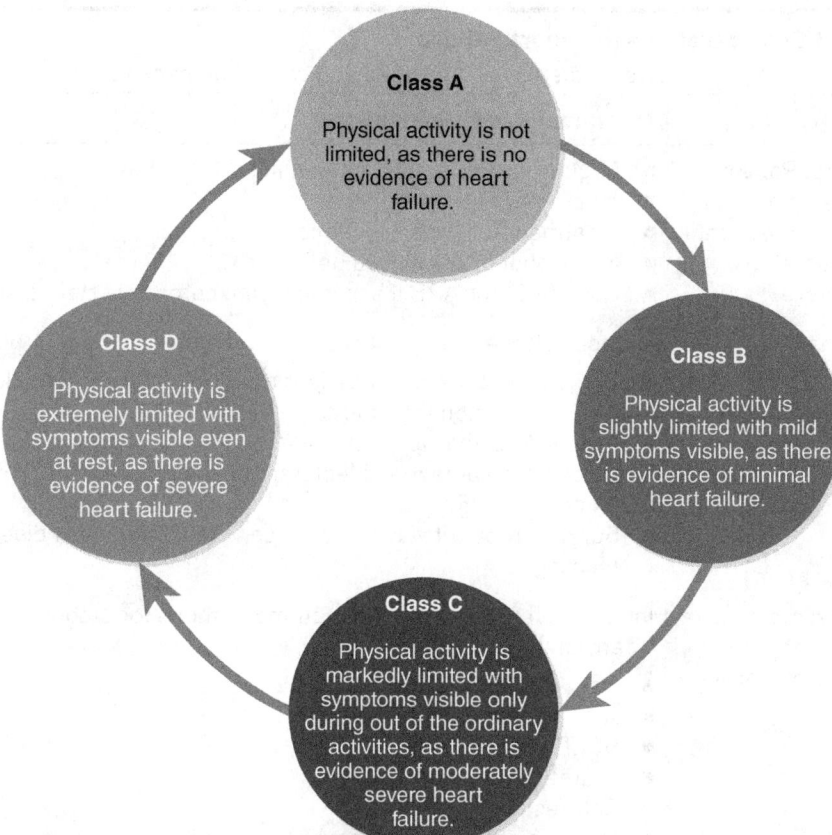

Figure 8-2 AHA/ACC, HFSA Grading and Classification

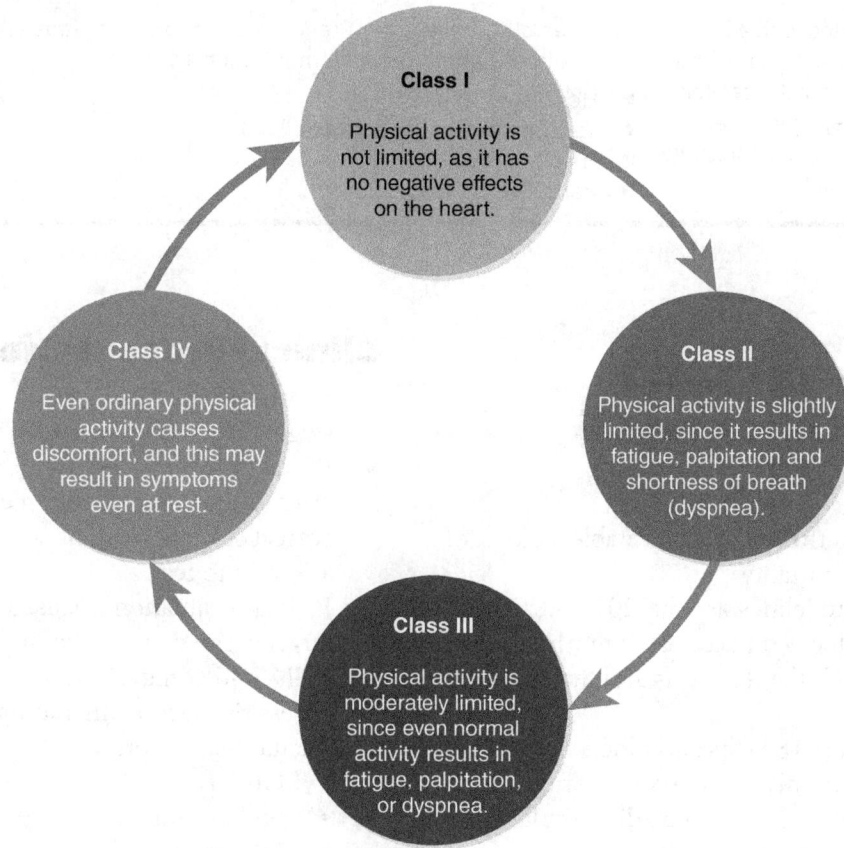

Figure 8-3 Patient Symptoms

Table 8-1 Treatment Considerations for Heart Failure
(Keep in mind, heart failure is progressive, and stages go forward and cannot go backwards.)

Heart Failure Stage	Treatment Recommendations
Stage A. Preheart failure. Patients are at high risk for developing heart failure. The goal of treatment is to slow down or prevent the progression of heart failure.	<ul><li>Regular exercise such as walking</li><li>Treatment of hypertension</li><li>Treatment for hyperlipidemia</li><li>No alcohol or illicit drug use</li><li>Use of ACE or ARB if accompanying coronary artery disease, diabetes, HTN</li></ul>
Stage B. Patient remains asymptomatic, but the left ventricle is not pumping normally due to left ventricular hypertrophy or structural abnormality.	Includes all the treatment recommendations for stage A plus:<ul><li>Beta blocker therapy if patient has had a myocardial infarction (MI) and ejection fraction (EF) <40%</li><li>ACE or ARB therapy if EF <40%</li><li>Aldosterone antagonist (eplerenone, spironolactone) if patient has had an MI or if EF <35%</li><li>Surgical repair if valvular disease, congenital heart disease, or CAD with blockage.</li></ul>
Stage C. Patients have symptoms of heart failure and have an established heart failure diagnosis.	Includes all the treatment recommendations for stages A and B and includes any of the following:<ul><li>Beta blocker therapy</li><li>Aldosterone antagonist</li><li>SGLT2 inhibitors</li><li>Diuretics</li><li>Salt restriction</li><li>Daily weights (report if gain >4 pounds)</li><li>May need fluid restriction</li><li>May need a biventricular pacemaker</li><li>May need an implantable cardiac defibrillator (ICD)</li></ul>
Stage D. It is associated with a high risk of complications and death. The patient is frequently hospitalized for management. Their symptoms are persistent and severe and significantly impacts their quality of life.	Includes all the treatment recommendations for stages A, B, and C and may require more advanced treatment such as:<ul><li>Heart transplant</li><li>Ventricular assistive device (VAD)</li><li>Heart surgery</li><li>Palliative or hospice care</li></ul>

Hypertension (2017 ACC/AHA Guidelines)

Overview

- HTN is one of the most preventable causes of morbidity and mortality.
- Most current guidelines are the 2017 ACC/AHA guidelines and focus on decreasing morbidity and mortality through the diagnosis and management of HTN.
- Focuses on adults 18 years and older.
- Studies included only those who reported effects on hard outcomes, including cardiovascular (CV) disease, MI, HF, stroke, coronary revascularization, and end-stage renal disease.

Clinical Presentation

- BP categorized as normal, elevated, stage 1, or stage 2 HTN (**Figure 8-4**).
- BP taken on at least two different visits in both arms, and ensure proper measurement, including correct cuff size, patient positioning, and following a 5-minute rest.
- Patient evaluation focused on identification of target organ damage, possible causes of secondary HTN, and comorbid risk.
- Assess risk factors, including genetic and environmental risk factors
  - Obesity
  - Sodium intake
  - Potassium
  - Physical activity

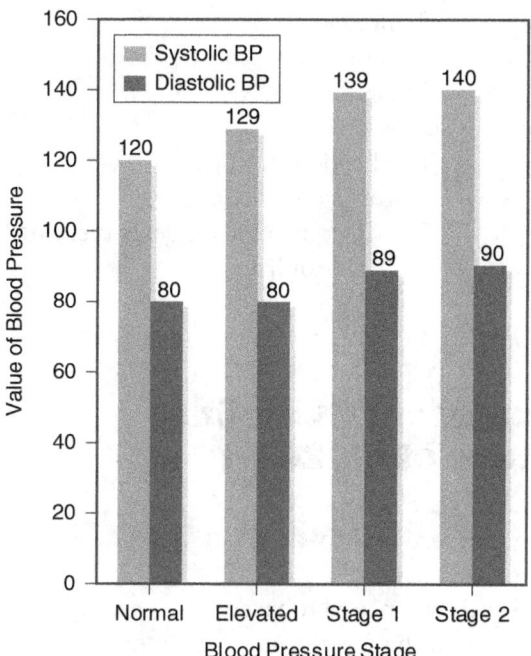

Figure 8-4 Clinical Presentation of Blood Pressure

- Alcohol use
- Baseline diagnostics
- Electrocardiogram/echocardiogram
- Urinalysis
- Complete blood count (CBC), renal function, electrolytes, cholesterol screening, thyroid function
- Ophthalmologic exam

Goals for Treatment

130/80 mmHg

Treatment Recommendations

The diagnosis of HTN is based on two separate BP readings obtained at two separate visits.

Treatment based on stage and risk factors.

- Stage 1 and less than 10 percent CV risk—nonpharmacologic, and follow up in 3 to 6 months
- Stage 1 and greater than 10 percent CV risk—combination of pharmacologic and nonpharmacologic, and follow up in 1 month
- Stage 2—combination of pharmacologic (with two classes of agents) and nonpharmacologic, and follow up in 1 month
- SBP > 180 or DBP > 110—prompt initiation of pharmacologic treatment to avoid target organ damage

Nonpharmacological:

- Weight management
- Heart healthy diet
- Sodium reduction
- Potassium supplementation unless contraindicated due to renal function
- Increased physical activity
- Limit alcohol use to 2 drinks per day for men, and 1 drink per day for women.

Pharmacologic Treatment:

- Patients with coronary artery disease (CAD) history or 10-year cardiovascular risk of 10 percent or higher should start pharmacologic treatment for SBP 130 mmHg or higher or DBP of 80 mmHg or higher.
- Patients with no CAD history and 10-year cardiovascular risk less than 10 percent should start pharmacologic treatment for SBP 140 mmHg or higher and DBP 90 mmHg or higher.
- First-line agents in all patients—consider comorbidities when choosing agents.
  - Thiazide diuretic
  - Calcium channel blocker
  - ACEI
  - ARB
    - Per the American Diabetes Association (ADA), ACEI or ARB is preferred for renal protection in patients with DM.

Follow-Up

- Monthly until goal BP is achieved
  - Monitor BP and response to treatment
  - Adverse medication effects

Cholesterol Management

Based on the current ACC/AHA guidelines on managing blood cholesterol (2018).

Goals

- Lowering cholesterol lowers atherosclerotic cardiovascular disease (ASCVD) risk.
- Relationship between low density lipoprotein (LDL) and coronary and atherosclerotic disease.

Assessment

- Presence of clinical ASCVD
  - Acute coronary syndrome
  - History of MI
  - Stable or unstable angina
  - Coronary or other arterial revascularization

- Stroke
- TIA
- Peripheral arterial disease
- Calculated 10-year risk of ASCVD using Pooled Cohort Equation
- Secondary causes of elevated LDL (Stone et al., 2014)
  - Diet
    - Saturated fats
    - Weight gain
  - Drugs
    - Diuretics
    - Steroids
    - Amiodarone
    - Cyclosporine
  - Diseases
    - Biliary obstruction
    - Nephrotic syndrome
    - Hypothyroidism
    - Obesity
    - Pregnancy
- Secondary causes of elevated triglycerides (Stone et al., 2014)
  - Diet
    - Weight gain
    - Very-low-fat diets
    - High intake of refined carbs
    - Excessive alcohol
  - Drugs
    - Estrogens
    - Glucocorticoids
    - Bile acid sequestrants
    - Protease inhibitors
    - Tamoxifen
    - Beta blockers
    - Thiazides
  - Diseases
    - Nephrotic syndrome
    - Chronic renal failure
    - Poorly controlled diabetes mellitus (DM)
    - Hypothyroidism
    - Obesity
    - Pregnancy

Treatment Guidelines (Stone et al., 2014)

- Lifestyle changes
  - Heart-healthy diet
  - Exercise
  - Avoidance of tobacco
  - Healthy weight
- Focus is on LDL cholesterol.
- Triglyceride is a priority if more than 500.
- Evidence supports using fixed-dose statins (**Table 8-2** for statin doses).
- Secondary prevention—managed in close collaboration with lipid/cardiac specialist.
- Primary prevention—see **Table 8-3**.

Follow-Up

- Monitoring for success of treatment
  - Initial fasting lipid panel
  - Second panel in 4 to 12 weeks to assess adherence
  - Then, every 3 to 12 months as clinically warranted

Table 8-2 High-, Moderate-, and Low-Intensity Statin Therapy (used in the randomized control trials [RCTs]; reviewed by the expert panel)

High-Intensity Statin Therapy	Moderate-Intensity Statin Therapy	Low-Intensity Statin Therapy
Daily dose lowers LDL-C, on average, by approximately ≥ 50%	Daily dose lowers LDL-C, on average, by approximately 30% to < 50%	Daily dose lowers LDL-C, on average, by < 30%
Atorvastatin (40[†])–80 mg Rosuvastatin 20 (40) mg	Atorvastatin 10 (20) mg Rosuvastatin (5) 10 mg Simvastatin 20–40 mg[‡] Pravastatin 40 (80) mg Lovastatin 40 mg *Fluvastatin XL 80 mg* **Fluvastatin 40 mg BID** *Pitavastatin 2–4 mg*	*Simvastatin 10 mg* **Pravastatin 10–20 mg** **Lovastatin 20 mg** *Fluvastatin 20–40 mg* *Pitavastatin 1 mg*

Reproduced from Stone, N. J., Robinson, J. G., Lichtenstein, A. H., Merz, C. N. B., Blum, C. B., Eckel, R. H., . . . Wilson, P. W. F., et al. (2014). 2013 ACC/AHA Guideline on the Treatment of Blood Cholesterol to Reduce Atherosclerotic Cardiovascular Risk in Adults: A Report of the American College of Cardiology/American Heart Association Task Force on Practice Guidelines. *Circulation, 129*(25 suppl 2), S1–S45. http://doi.org/10.1161/01.cir.0000437738.63853.7a

Table 8-3 Primary Prevention of Atherosclerotic Cardiovascular Disease (ASCVD)

All decisions for preventative changes should be made using shared decision-making.

Age	Lifestyle	Risk Factor Considerations	Medications
0–19 years	Healthy diet, minimizing trans fats, sugary drinks, refined carbs. Age-appropriate, moderate to vigorous exercise at least 150 minutes per week. Avoid smoking and exposure to secondhand smoke.	Assess for risk factors: Weight gain; Low activity; Poor dietary habits; Tobacco use or exposure; Exposure to or use of illicit drugs or vaping	Generally, no preventative medications are recommended for this age group, but this needs to be individualized to the patient.
20–39 years	Same lifestyle recommendations as earlier age group.	■ Same risk factors as earlier group. Additionally: ■ Assess for hypertension ■ Assess for elevated cholesterol, especially LDL and triglycerides ■ Consider sociodemographic characteristics ■ Consider family history of premature ASCVD ■ Assess ASCVD risk using tools online that help determine 10-year ASCVD risk ■ Assess for persistently elevated triglycerides	■ Statin therapy is recommended for those with LDL > 160 mg/dl. ■ Antihypertensive therapy for persistent BP > 130/80 ■ Aspirin (ASA) no longer recommended for primary prevention due to bleeding risk. ■ For persistent hypertriglyceridemia (greater than 175 mg/dl), consider statins, fibrates, and omega-3 fatty acids.
40–75 years	Same lifestyle recommendations as previous age groups.	■ Same assessments and considerations as previous age groups.	■ Recommend all patients with DM2 age 40–75 to be on statin therapy regardless of cholesterol levels. ■ Medication recommendations are the same as for previous age group.
>75 years	■ Age appropriate recommendations for activity. ■ All other lifestyle recommendations remain the same as previous age groups.	Same assessments as previous age group as it relates to ASCVD. If patient does not have ASCVD, statin therapy does not provide additional benefit for this age group.	■ Statin therapy does not seem to provide a benefit to patients over age 75 **without** ASCVD. ■ Antihypertensive therapy for patients with BP > 130/80. ■ ASA therapy not used for primary prevention.

- Monitor for adherence and intolerance if less than anticipated therapeutic response
- Evaluate need for increased intensity of statin
- Safety and monitoring
  - Consider decreasing statin dose if two consecutive LDL levels are less than 40.
  - Doses of simvastatin 80 mg may be harmful.
  - Monitor for new onset DM in patients on statin therapy.
- Closely monitor patients on multiple drugs, especially those that interfere with the metabolism of statins.
- For patients presenting with confusional state or memory impairment, evaluate for nonstatin cause, and adverse statin effects.
- Management of muscle symptoms:
  - Obtain a good baseline before initiating statin to avoid unnecessary discontinuation of statin.

- Unexplained severe muscle symptoms
- Discontinue statin.
- Evaluate for rhabdomyolysis
  - serum creatine kinase (CK)
  - Urine
- Mild to moderate symptoms
  - Discontinue statin until evaluation.
  - Evaluate for conditions that may increase risk.
  - If symptoms resolve, reinstitute statin therapy to establish causal relationship.
  - If a causal relationship, discontinue statin and use a low dose of a different statin when symptoms resolve.
  - Once low dose is tolerated, gradually increase dose.
  - If symptoms do not resolve after 2 months without statins or elevated CK does not resolve, consider the other cause of the symptoms.
  - If persistent symptoms are determined to be from another condition, resume statin therapy at the original dose.

Evaluation of Chest Pain

Pathogenesis

- Cardiac
- Musculoskeletal
- Neurologic
- Gastrointestinal (GI)
- Pleural
- Psychogenic

Clinical Presentation

- Location of the pain:
  - Ischemic pain is diffuse and usually difficult to localize.
  - Levine sign (fist in center of chest) + predictive value.
- Quality of the pain: Not often "pain"

> **Clinical Pearl**
>
> Be sure to be specific when asking about pain, as often patients do not equate ischemic symptoms with "pain" but rather as heaviness, tightness, burning.

- Myocardial ischemia usually feels like squeezing, tightness, fullness, knot, ache, heavy weight, toothache, bra too tight.
- Quantity/severity of the pain: Rate intensity on 0 to 10 pain scale (not useful in ACS)
- Radiation:
  - Myocardial ischemia can radiate to the neck, jaw, teeth, throat, shoulder (radiation to **both** arms is very predictive of MI).
  - Pain radiating to right shoulder with epigastric pain indicative of cholecystitis.
  - Pain that radiates between scapulae may be aortic dissection.
  - Pericarditis pain usually radiates to one or both trapezius ridges.
- Timing: including onset, duration, and frequency (quick and sharp, recurring or one-time, duration of each episode).
  - Gradual onset associated with myocardial ischemia.
  - Abrupt with great intensity is more often dissection or pulmonary embolism (PE).
  - Myocardial ischemia is more often in the morning (increased sympathetic tone r/t circadian rhythm).
  - Chest pain that only lasts for a few seconds or that is constant over weeks is most likely not due to ischemia.
- Setting where/when the pain occurs:
  - At rest—nonischemic or unstable angina
  - With exertion—indicative of ischemia
  - With stressful situations—consider ischemia or psychogenic cause
- Aggravating factors:
  - Occurs with eating, more suggestive of GI, although postprandial chest pain could be ischemic
  - Provoked by exercise, more likely cardiac
  - Cold, stress, meals, and intercourse can aggravate cardiac ischemia
  - Worsens with swallowing = esophageal
- Alleviating factors:
  - Pain that goes away or is lessened with sublingual nitroglycerin
    - Cardiac
    - Esophageal

> **Clinical Pearl**
>
> Sublingual nitroglycerin (SL NTG) can relieve symptoms of esophageal spasms, so symptom relief with NTG does not always mean ischemic cause.

- Improves with change of body position = musculoskeletal origin likely

- Pain that abates with cessation of physical activity frequently is of cardiac origin
- Pain that improves with sitting upright and leaning forward = pericarditis likely
- Associated symptoms:
  - Dyspnea, especially in people with diabetes; more atypical presentation of ischemia
  - Older people most often present with fatigue, confusion, and dyspnea with chest pain
  - Cough—include infection, congestive heart failure (CHF), PE, neoplasm in differentials
  - Syncope—patients with ACS may have presyncope, but syncope raises suspicion of aortic dissection, PE, or ruptured abdominal aortic aneurysm
  - Belching, bad taste, dysphagia, consistent with esophageal disease
  - Vomiting is common in MI in addition to peptic ulcer disease (PUD), cholecystitis, pancreatitis, and diabetic ketoacidosis (DKA)
  - Diaphoresis more common in MI
  - Palpitations—ventricular ectopy
  - New onset of AF with chest pain, consider PE
- Past medical history:
  - Any prior history of CAD, percutaneous coronary intervention (PCI), coronary artery bypass graft (CABG), peripheral vascular disease
  - PUD, gastroesophageal reflux disease (GERD), gallstones
  - Panic disorder
  - Bronchospasm
  - Neoplasm
- Cardiac risk factors:
  - Age (40+) in men
  - Postmenopausal state for women
  - HTN (risk for MI and aortic dissection)
  - Dyslipidemia
  - Family history
  - DM
  - Abdominal aortic aneurysm, cerebrovascular accident (CVA), peripheral vascular disease (PVD), renal artery stenosis (RAS)
  - Obesity
  - Metabolic syndrome
  - Cigarette use (prior or current use)
  - Stress
  - Sedentary lifestyle
  - Cocaine use
- Differential diagnosis
  - Life-threatening conditions:
    - ACS
    - Stress-induced cardiomyopathy
    - Tension pneumothorax
    - Gastric perforation
    - Aortic dissection
    - Pulmonary embolus
  - Other nonischemic and noncardiac conditions
    - CHF
    - Chronic stable angina
    - New arrhythmia
    - HTN
    - Infectious/bacterial process (i.e., pericarditis, myocarditis)
    - Musculoskeletal pain
    - Anxiety
    - GERD
- Diagnostics:
  - EKG—Compare to previous EKG that the patient had done in the past
    - Arrhythmias (atrial/ventricular)
    - ST-T abnormalities (depression/elevation)
    - New left bundle branch block (LBBB)
    - Cannot interpret with baseline LBBB, paced rhythm, LVH with strain
  - Chest X-Ray (CXR)
    - CHF
    - Infiltrates
    - Widened mediastinum
  - Blood work—Troponins, CBC, thyroid function tests (TFTs), basic metabolic panel (BMP)
  - Echocardiogram
  - Stress test
  - Cardiac catheter
  - Endoscopy

Coronary Artery Disease
Etiology
- MI—Complete occlusion of coronary artery
- Angina—Partial occlusion of coronary artery; supply versus demand problem
  - Stable—Occurs with exertion or other precipitating event
  - Unstable—Occurs at rest
  - Vasospastic—Not related to activity, often at night

Treatment
- Acute MI/Acute Coronary Syndrome
  - Call 911
  - Aspirin—Chew 325 mg of a chewable form of aspirin (not enteric coated)
  - SL nitroglycerin (NTG)—Important safety information—before giving NTG, ensure patient has not taken any phosphodiesterase

inhibitors in the previous 24 to 48 hours to avoid profound hypotension
- Oxygen
- Early revascularization shows most benefit and less mortality
- Ongoing care
  - Percutaneous angioplasty with stenting
  - CABG
  - Meds
    - Aspirin (ASA)/antiplatelet drugs
    - Beta-blockers—mortality benefit and prevention of second MI
    - ACE inhibitors—prevents remodeling
    - For significant, persistent LV dysfunction: HF management and consider defibrillator
- Angina
  - Revascularization via PTCA or CABG if feasible
  - Meds
    - ASA
    - NTG for acute angina attacks
      **see safety note above regarding NTG
    - 1 tab SL q 5 min × 3, if no relief, go to ED
    - Long-acting nitrates
    - Calcium channel blockers

Atrial Fibrillation

Etiology

The incidence and prevalence of AF are increasing worldwide and associated with increased healthcare visits and high healthcare costs. AF is associated with a 1.5 to 2 times higher risk of death as well as significant morbidity risk. Risk factors are multifactorial, including cardiac and noncardiac factors and lifestyle impacts (Joglar et al., 2024).

Staging: The progression of AF is identified through staging, which informs treatment guidelines (**Table 8-4**).

Clinical Presentation

- CHA2DS2-VASc Score—quantifies risk of thromboembolic event
  - Low risk— <1 percent per year
  - Intermediate risk—1 to 2 percent per year
  - high risk— >2 percent per year
- Assess for increased risk for bleeding
- Assess for reversible causes
  - Thyroid disease
  - Anemia
  - HF
  - Obstructive sleep apnea (OSA)

Table 8-4 Stages of Atrial Fibrillation (A-fib) with Treatment Recommendations

Stage 1 Risk for A-fib	Stage 2 Pre-A-fib	Stage 3 Substages of A-fib	Stage 4 Permanent A-fib
Modifiable factors that increase risk: ■ Obesity ■ Sleep apnea ■ Hypertension ■ Alcohol use ■ Diabetes ■ Sedentary lifestyle Nonmodifiable factors: ■ Male ■ Older age ■ Genetic predisposition	Electrical or structural changes that predispose patient to A-fib: ■ Atrial enlargement ■ Atrial flutter ■ Occasional runs of atrial tachycardia ■ Occasional atrial ectopy	Patient has A-fib but may transition through different stages. **3A**—Intermittent A-fib <7 days **3B**—Sustained A-fib for >7 days and requires intervention **3C**—Sustained A-fib for >12 months **3D**—Resolved A-fib after surgical intervention with ablation	Patient has a permanent A-fib condition. No further attempts at rhythm control if this is decided between patient and cardiologist.
Recommendation	**Recommendation**	**Recommendation**	**Recommendation**
1. Treat modifiable risk factors.	1. Treat modifiable risk factors. 2. More frequent surveillance.	1. Treat modifiable risk factors. 2. Ongoing monitoring as clinically appropriate. 3. Assessment of stroke risk with anticoagulation if appropriate. 4. Treat symptoms. 5. Assess for pathological changes.	1. Treat modifiable risk factors. 2. Assessment of stroke risk with anticoagulation if appropriate. 3. Treat symptoms. 4. Assess for pathological changes.

Diagnostics in New/Suspected AF

- Electrocardiogram
  - Echocardiogram for cardiac structure
  - CBC, metabolic panel, thyroid function

Treatment (Based on 2023 AHA/ACC/HRS Guidelines for the Management of AF)

- **Goals of management**
  - Assess and treat stroke risk
  - Optimize modifiable risk factors
  - Symptom management through rhythm and rate control
- **Nonpharmacological management**
  - Management of obesity
  - Physical activity
  - Smoking cessation
  - Alcohol moderation
  - Control of HTN and other comorbidities
- **Pharmacological/nonpharmacological management**
- **Antithrombotic therapy**
  - Indications
    - Should be shared decision based on risks of stroke and bleeding.
    - Decisions regarding antithrombotic therapy should be made regardless of whether the AF is paroxysmal, persistent, or permanent and regardless of whether rhythm or rate control strategies are utilized.
    - For patients with AF and a greater than 2 percent risk, anticoagulation is recommended to prevent stroke and systemic thromboembolism.
    - Anticoagulation is reasonable for patients with a greater than 1 percent but less than 2 percent risk and should be considered based on risk/benefit analysis.
    - Direct oral anticoagulant (DOAC) is recommended over warfarin in patients without rheumatic mitral stenosis or a mechanical heart valve.
    - An International Normalization Ratio (INR) of 2 to 3 is recommended for patients receiving warfarin for stroke prevention.
    - Antiplatelets should not be used as stroke prevention in patients with AF.
    - In patients with moderate to high risk of stroke with contraindication to anticoagulation, percutaneous occlusion of the left atrial appendage can be considered.

> **Clinical Pearl**
>
> Rate versus rhythm control has similar clinical outcomes in many patients with AF. The strategy of rate versus rhythm should be discussed with the patient considering symptoms, comorbidities, medications, and patient preference.

- Rate control
  - Control of ventricular rate to resting heart rate (HR) less than 100 beats per minute (bpm).
  - Resting HR less than 110 bpm is reasonable without symptoms and with normal ventricular function.
  - Beta blockers or nondihydropyridine calcium channel blockers are recommended for rate control.
  - Digoxin can be considered when calcium channel blockers/beta blockers (CCB/BB) are ineffective or contraindicated.
  - In patients with EF less than 40 percent, nondihydropyridine CCB should not be administered due to the risk for HF exacerbations.
  - Symptoms during exercise should be evaluated to ensure HR control with exercise.
- Rhythm control
  - Patients with reduced LV function who are in AF should be considered for rhythm control to evaluate whether AF is contributing to LV function.
  - Rhythm control can be useful in symptomatic AF.
  - Patients with AF for more than 48 hours should have at least 3 weeks of anticoagulation or transesophageal echocardiogram (TEE) to rule out left atrium (LA) thrombus before cardioversion (chemical or electrical).
  - Referral to cardiologist warranted.
  - Options
    - Cardioversion
    - Antiarrhythmic therapy
    - Catheter ablation

Prevention

- Data suggests ACE or ARB is useful for preventing AF in patients with ventricular dysfunction.
- ACE or ARB therapy may be warranted to prevent AF in the presence of HTN.
- Statin therapy may be useful in preventing AFib after coronary artery surgery.

(January et al., 2014)

Peripheral Vascular Disease—Atherosclerosis (PAD)

- Disease in arteries outside the heart
- Increased incidence with DM
- Most common sites
  - Abdominal aorta
  - Carotid arteries
  - Femoral and iliac arteries

Clinical Presentation

- Increasing fatigue and weakness in the legs
- Intermittent claudication
  - Muscle ischemia
  - Sensory impairment—tingling, burning, numbness
  - Peripheral pulses distal to occlusion become weak
  - Appearance of the skin of the feet and legs:
    - Marked pallor or cyanosis
    - Skin dry and hairless
    - Toenails thick and hard

Clinical Management

- Revascularization
- Blood sugar control in DM
- Weight loss
- Cholesterol management
- Platelet inhibitors
- Cessation of smoking
- Increase activity and exercise—ambulation through pain increases collateral development
- Maintain dependent position for legs—improves arterial perfusion

Peripheral Vascular Disease—Venous Disorders

- **Venous Insufficiency**
  - Clinical presentation
    - Edema
    - Skin friable, weeping, open wounds
    - Chronic skin changes include brown and thick skin from hemosiderin deposits
    - Diminished pulses only if edema is affecting arterial circulation
  - Differential diagnosis
  - Deep vein thrombosis (DVT)
  - Right-sided HF
  - Clinical management
    - Leg position—elevated
    - Monitor for signs and symptoms (s/s) of infection
    - Compression—need to rule out arterial involvement first
- DVT
  - Clinical presentation
    - Maybe asymptomatic
    - Heaviness in extremities—dull ache
    - Unilateral edema
    - Redness, warmth, if a superficial vein involved
- Risk factors
  - Virchow's triad
    - Stasis
      - Immobility
  - Hypercoagulable state
    - Cancer
    - Pregnancy
    - Clotting disorders
  - Intimal changes
    - Inflammation
    - Trauma
- Differential diagnosis
  - Venous insufficiency
  - Right-sided HF
  - Superficial thrombophlebitis
  - Baker's cyst
- Diagnostic
  - Doppler ultrasound of the extremity
  - D-Dimer—not specific
  - CT scan if inconclusive
  - Workup for clotting disorders if no apparent cause
- Complications
  - Goal is to avoid PE.
  - Can have chronic venous insufficiency as a sequela.
- Clinical management (Patel, 2015)
  - Anticoagulation—first episode 3 to 6 months, recurrent 1 year
    - Low molecular weight heparin (LMWH) or unfractionated heparin with bridge to warfarin
    - DOACs :
      - Rivaroxaban
      - Apixaban
      - Dabigatran
  - Bed rest—controversial
    - Studies show no increase in PE with ambulation

- Recommendation is early ambulation (day 2 after initiation of anticoagulation)
- Invasive treatments
  - Thrombectomy (if extensive and flow limiting)
  - Placement of inferior vena cava (IVC) filter
    - High risk for PE
    - Not a candidate for anticoagulation
    - Risk of reoccurrence
- Evaluate for familial clotting disorders if no obvious reason for DVT or in the presence of recurrence

Varicose Veins

Risk Factors
- Prolonged standing
- Obesity
- Pregnancy
- Family history
- Weightlifting

Clinical Presentation
- Complaints of aching and fullness
- Presence of engorged, tortuous superficial leg veins
- Edema may be present if venous flow is limited

Differential Diagnosis
- DVT
- Venous insufficiency
- Baker's cyst
- Superficial thrombophlebitis

Clinical Management
- Elevation
- Exercise
- Compression
- Weight loss
- Avoid restrictive clothing
- Surgical intervention if symptoms warrant

Review Questions

1. A 62-year-old male patient presents with complaints of dyspnea on exertion, presyncope, and mild exertional chest pain. Exam reveals a harsh 3/6 late peaking systolic murmur loudest at the right sternal border that radiates to the carotids. Which disorder does the family nurse practitioner (FNP) suspect?
   A. Mitral valve prolapse (MVP)
   B. Unstable angina
   C. Aortic stenosis
   D. Mitral regurgitation (MR)

2. A patient with a history of type 2 diabetes and coronary disease has the following lipid panel: LDL 128, HDL 30, and Trig 208. What should the preferred first-line treatment be?
   A. Lifestyle modification with diet and exercise
   B. Atorvastatin 20 mg daily
   C. Atorvastatin 80 mg daily
   D. Fenofibrate

3. The FNP is performing a routine physical exam on a 60-year-old male who is a new patient and has been lost to medical follow-up for 20 years. The patient denies any past medical history and has a family history of hypertension (HTN) and coronary artery disease (CAD). BP today is 158/92. What would be the appropriate next step?
   A. Start Lisinopril 10 mg daily.
   B. Have the patient return in 2 weeks to recheck the blood pressure (BP).
   C. Start hydrochlorothiazide (HCTZ) 12.5 mg daily.
   D. Teach the patient lifestyle modification and have him return in 1 year for a follow-up.

4. A patient with a history of systolic heart failure (HF) presents for a routine follow-up. His medication list consists of an ACE inhibitor (ACEI), aspirin, and a statin. Which medication should be added for decreased mortality?
   A. Metoprolol XR
   B. Furosemide
   C. Digoxin
   D. Irbesartan

5. A 45-year-old male presents with chest tightness with exertion that resolves with rest over the past 2 weeks. He is pain free at the office. He has a past medical history of HTN and high cholesterol. Based on the presentation, which diagnostic test would help identify the likely etiology of these symptoms?
   A. EKG
   B. Exercise stress test
   C. Cardiac catheterization
   D. Troponin levels

6. A patient with a history of a mitral valve prolapse (MVP) and a penicillin allergy (PCN) asks about risk for subacute endocarditis prevention in dental care. What does the patient need to know?
   A. No prophylaxis is needed in MVP.
   B. Take clindamycin 600 mg BID for 3 days before the treatment.
   C. Take amoxicillin 2 g one hour before treatment.
   D. You should not have dental care if you have MVP.

7. A patient presents for a routine physical exam, and the nurse practitioner identifies that the patient has a 2/4 diastolic murmur located at the midaxillary line. What would be the next step in the treatment plan?
   A. Assure the patient that it is likely a physiologic murmur.
   B. Order an echocardiogram.
   C. Order a stress test.
   D. Educate the patient on identification of symptoms of aortic stenosis (AS).

8. During the routine physical exam of a new 30-year-old male patient, he states his father died of sudden cardiac death at the age of 40. What diagnostic test would be a priority in the treatment plan?
   A. Echocardiogram
   B. Lipid panel
   C. Genetic testing
   D. Exercise stress test

9. A 38-year-old woman presents to the office with complaints of chest pain that started this morning. The pain is described as sharp and worsening on inspiration. The patient's heart rate (HR) is 108 and BP 100/70. What question is important to ask to support the most likely diagnosis in this patient?
   A. Does the patient have a family history of coronary disease?
   B. What is her normal BP?
   C. What medications is the patient on?
   D. Does she have diabetes?

10. On a routine visit, a 78-year-old male is found to be in atrial fibrillation (AF) on an EKG. The patient has a history of CAD and congestive heart failure (CHF) and is asymptomatic. Vitals include BP of 118/70, pulse of 90 and irregular, respiratory rate (RR) 18. The rest of the physical exam is normal. What is most important to include in the patient's treatment plan?
    A. Immediate cardioversion
    B. Anticoagulation
    C. Beta blocker therapy
    D. Stress test

11. While doing a cardiovascular exam on a patient, the FNP identifies that the point of maximum impulse (PMI) is 11 cm lateral to the midsternal border. What is the appropriate next step?
    A. Document the findings as this is normal
    B. Get an EKG
    C. Refer patient directly to a cardiologist
    D. Start the patient on an ACEI

12. What should be included in the plan for a patient with HF taking an ACEI, a beta blocker, and spironolactone?
    A. Monitor potassium and renal function
    B. Echocardiograms every 3 months
    C. Encourage a diet high in bananas, orange juice, and salmon
    D. Discontinuation of all other diuretics

13. A 45-year-old female with obesity with a history of type 2 diabetes asks if she could start an aerobic exercise plan. How should the NP respond?
    A. "Absolutely, you may begin immediately."
    B. "You should have a stress test before you begin intense exercise."
    C. "Aerobic exercise is not safe in a patient with diabetes."
    D. "Once your blood sugar is under control, you can start exercising."

14. A 65-year-old male patient with a history of DM and asthma is diagnosed with HTN. Which medication would be appropriate for the patient to start at this time?
    A. Lisinopril
    B. Amlodipine
    C. Hydrochlorothiazide
    D. Atenolol

15. A 54-year-old female with no significant past medical history (PMH) presents to the FNP for yearly follow-up. Her LDL cholesterol is 130 mg/dl and triglycerides of 90 mg/dl. The FNP calculates her 10-year risk of vascular disease as 4 percent. What recommendations would the FNP make to the patient for treatment? Select all that apply.
    A. Weight training three times a week
    B. Begin low-dose statin therapy
    C. High-fiber diet
    D. Maintain a normal body mass index (BMI)

16. Which condition requires prophylaxis before dental work to prevent bacterial endocarditis?
    A. Mitral valve prolapse
    B. Previous episode of endocarditis
    C. Mitral valve repair
    D. Presence of a pacemaker

17. The FNP is seeing a 70-year-old male patient who has not seen a primary care physician (PCP) in several years. He is not on any medications but states that his nurse at the congregation told him his BP was "high." His BP today is 148/92. The FNP knows that the main goal for treatment of HTN is what?
    A. Maintain cerebral perfusion
    B. Prevent target organ damage
    C. Lower lipids
    D. Prevent obesity

18. A patient presents with complaints of a "fast heartbeat." An EKG reveals sinus tachycardia 122 bpm at rest. What would be the next appropriate step?
    A. Start a beta blocker to lower the heart rate.
    B. Assess for the underlying cause of the tachycardia.
    C. Discuss anxiety treatments.
    D. Explain to the patient that this is a normal variant.

19. A patient with a history of CAD presents to the office for a follow up visit of systolic HF with an ejection fraction (EF) of 29 percent. His medications are a beta-blocker, an ACE inhibitor and a baby aspirin daily. He is New York Heart Association (NYHA) class III. What should be included in the plan of care? (select all that apply)
    A. Add spiranolactone 12.5 mg daily
    B. Refer to a cardiologist. Patients with EF of 30 percent or less may need implantable defibrillator
    C. Discontinue aspirin
    D. Limit activity

20. A 42-year-old male presents with signs and symptoms of a deep vein thrombosis (DVT), which an ultrasound confirms. He has no PMH, is active, and is not on any medications. He has not traveled recently, and his job is very active. The patient is placed on anticoagulation to treat the DVT. What would the FNP do next?
    A. Continue anticoagulation indefinitely since there is no known cause.
    B. Evaluate the presence of familial clotting disorders.
    C. Plan for insertion of an inferior vena cava (IVC) filter.
    D. Since the patient does not have risk factors, anticoagulation is unnecessary.

21. A 45-year-old female with no medical history presents to the office with complaints of dull, intermittent chest discomfort over the past week. The discomfort does not occur with exertion or stress but rather occurs when she is cleaning the house. During a physical exam, the FNP can reproduce the pain by palpating the chest wall. The EKG is unchanged from the previous one. What should the FNP do next?
    A. Order an NSAID for musculoskeletal chest pain.
    B. Order an exercise stress test for the presence of CAD.
    C. Send the patient to the ER immediately.
    D. Start the patient on a proton pump inhibitor.

22. A patient with known peripheral vascular disease—atherosclerosis (PAD) presents to the office with complaints of increasing leg pain at rest. What does the NP think may be occurring?
    A. Progression of the arterial disease
    B. Development of a DVT
    C. Normal PAD symptoms
    D. A clotting disorder

23. A 42-year-old female presents to the office with bulging and painful superficial leg veins. What risk factors would the nurse assess for to support the suspected diagnosis?
    A. A desk job
    B. Obesity
    C. HTN
    D. High cholesterol

24. In evaluating a patient with chest pain, it is noted that the pain is resolved with sublingual nitroglycerin (NTG). What does this information indicate?
    A. The pain is ischemic in nature.
    B. The patient's BP is too high.
    C. The pain may be ischemic or esophageal in nature.
    D. No further workup is necessary.

25. A 75-year-old patient with a history of HTN and PVD presents with dyspnea on exertion and palpitations over the past 2 weeks. An EKG shows AF with a HR of 155 bpm. Other than the palpitations, the patient is asymptomatic. Vitals include BP of 120/78, HR of 155 and irregular, and RR of 20. What would the initial treatment plan include?
    A. Anticoagulation and rate control
    B. Initiation of an antiarrhythmic drug
    C. Immediate hospitalization
    D. Immediate stress test

Answers and Enhanced Rationales

1. Answer C is correct. The hallmark symptoms of AS are exertional chest pain, dyspnea, and syncope. The typical murmur is a systolic murmur, loudest at the aortic area radiating to the carotid. The severity of AS is related to how late it peaks and whether it obliterates the second heart sound. Loudness does not correlate with severity.

   Answer A is incorrect. MVP would present with a midsystolic click. If the patient has developed MR, the murmur would be pansystolic, blowing, and best heard at the apex with radiation to the axilla.

   Answer B is incorrect. It would be in the differential, but the presence of murmur and inclusion of dyspnea and syncope would point more to AS.

   Answer D is incorrect. The murmur of MR would be pansystolic, blowing, and best heard at the apex with radiation to the axilla and would present with fatigue and orthopnea.

2. Answer C is correct. A patient with known coronary disease and DM is at high risk for a cardiac event. Per the ACC/AHA cholesterol management guidelines, the patient will need high-dose statin therapy, such as Atorvastatin 80, as first-line treatment. Atorvastatin will also lower the triglycerides and raise the high density lipoproteins (HDL) somewhat in this patient.

   Answer A is incorrect. It is not the priority treatment but would be included in the patient's plan in addition to the high-dose atorvastatin.

   Answer B is incorrect. The dose of atorvastatin is too low to treat this lipid panel.

   Answer D is incorrect. The fenofibrate would target triglycerides, which would be a secondary target after LDL.

3. Answer B is correct. Two measurements must be made on different occasions to diagnose HTN. Per HTN guidelines, the BP is considered elevated and will need medication if it is elevated when he returns. Either Lisinopril or HCTZ will be appropriate as first-line treatment.

   Answer A is incorrect. The repeat BP would need to be taken first.

   Answer C is incorrect. The patient has DM; therefore, an ACEI would be the first line to protect renal function.

   Answer D is incorrect. The patient will need medication for the elevated BP and follow-up until the BP is controlled.

4. Answer A is correct. Patients with systolic HF should be on certain beta blockers for their mortality benefits. Carvedilol and sustained-release Metoprolol are indicated for this. Other beta blockers do not have the mortality data and should not be used in HF.

   Answers B and C are incorrect. Furosemide and digoxin are effective in symptom management in HF, but do not have mortality benefits.

   Answer D is incorrect. ARBs do have mortality data, but they are not indicated if a patient is already on an ACEI. In HF, ARBs are used as an alternative to ACEIs.

5. Answer B is correct. The patient is likely experiencing stable angina, which is characterized by exertional chest pain resolved with rest. The patient has risk factors such as sex, HTN, and high cholesterol. An exercise stress test is the first-line test for diagnosing CAD.

   Answer C is incorrect. A cardiac catheterization is an invasive test that would be ordered as confirmatory if the stress test were positive.

   Answers A and D are incorrect. An EKG or troponins will only be helpful in the setting of current chest pain, a previous MI, or a current MI.

6. Answer A is correct. The most current guidelines for bacterial endocarditis prophylaxis do not include MVP as a condition that warrants prophylaxis. Based on the old guidelines, MVP was treated with prophylaxis, and patients may be used to this. The NP should educate the patient on the new guidelines.

   Answer B is incorrect. The patient does not require prophylaxis, and guidelines recommend not using clindamycin as an option due to side effects. Additionally, prophylaxis is given 30 to 60 minutes before dental care, not 3 days before.

   Answer C is incorrect. This is the correct dosage/timing for a patient who qualifies for prophylaxis, but this patient does not qualify.

   Answer D is incorrect. The patient should not withhold dental work, as mouth and dental infections are a risk factor for subacute bacterial endocarditis (SBE).

7. Answer B is correct. A diastolic murmur is never physiologic and should be evaluated by an echocardiogram to determine the cause.

   Answer A is incorrect. A diastolic murmur is not physiologic.

   Answer C is incorrect. A stress test will not give information on the type of the murmur but would rather give information on ischemic risk and exercise capacity.

   Answer D is incorrect. AS is a systolic murmur.

8. Answer A is correct. This is a priority question. Patients with a family history of early sudden cardiac death should be evaluated for hypertrophic cardiomyopathy. An echocardiogram is the most accurate means to identify this condition.

   Answer B is not incorrect. The lipid panel would not predict sudden cardiac death.

   Answer C is incorrect. Genetic testing would be undertaken later if the patient had an indication of obstructive cardiomyopathy.

   Answer D is incorrect. An exercise test would be part of the workup. However, the echocardiogram would need to be done first to rule out any structural abnormalities that would pose a risk for high-intensity exercise on the treadmill.

9. Answer C is correct. The patient presents typical signs and symptoms of a pulmonary embolism (PE). In a young patient, the most likely culprit would be the use of oral contraceptives, which could be ascertained with a medication history.

   Answer A is incorrect. The situation described does not support a diagnosis of CAD.

   Answer B is incorrect. The information about previous BP does not assist in making the diagnosis.

   Answer D is incorrect. The description of the pain does not support a diagnosis of coronary artery disease/angina for which DM is a risk factor. DM is not a risk factor for PE.

10. Answer B is correct. A CHADS (Congestive heart failure; Hypertension; Age >75 years; Diabetes; previous Stroke) score should be calculated to determine the patient's risk of stroke and the need for anticoagulation. This patient's score is 3 (age over 75, history of CHF, and history of HTN). A CHADS score greater than 2 indicates a high risk of CVA and that the patient needs to be anticoagulated.

    Answer A is incorrect. A patient with AF of unknown duration is not a candidate for immediate cardioversion without identifying if a clot is present in the LA.

    Answer C is incorrect. Beta blockers are only indicated if a patient has a fast ventricular rate, which is not indicated in this scenario.

    Answer D is incorrect. A stress test would not be indicated until the patient's rates were identified as controlled (via Holter monitor) and fully anticoagulated.

11. Answer B is correct. A 12 lead EKG can reveal if there is an abnormality in the electrical pathway of the heart and can reveal left ventricular hypertrophy.

    Answer A is incorrect. A PMI greater than 11 cm from the midsternal border is considered displaced and abnormal. It likely represents LVH.

    Answer C is incorrect. A cardiology referral is not immediately necessary.

    Answer D is incorrect. While the patient will likely need an echocardiogram and an ACEI, the EKG should be performed first.

12. Answer A is correct. Patients with renal dysfunction are at risk for hyperkalemia on spironolactone, and ACEIs also increase potassium levels. Therefore, renal function and potassium should be closely monitored, and consideration should be given to discontinuing spironolactone in patients with renal insufficiency.

    Answer B is incorrect. Echocardiograms are not warranted every 3 months.

    Answer C is incorrect. Patients should follow a low-potassium diet.

    Answer D is incorrect. Spiranolactone dosage in HF is aimed at neurohormonal effects and is not sufficient to cause diuresis. Loop diuretics are still warranted for fluid management.

13. Answer B is correct. Patients with type 2 DM have the same risk of an MI as a patient with a previous MI. In addition, neuropathy from diabetes can mask the typical angina symptoms. A patient with DM should have a screening stress test before beginning an intense exercise program.

    Answer A is incorrect. The patient should be screened for CAD before beginning exercise.

    Answer C is incorrect. Aerobic exercise is good for DM if the patient is screened for risk first.

    Answer D is incorrect. Although aerobic exercise can help control blood sugar, the patient will still need a stress test first.

14. Answer A is correct. Diabetic patients with HTN should be treated with an ACEI or ARBs for renal protection, as well as for BP control.

    Answer B is incorrect. The patient is not on an ACEI yet. CCB can be used as a second line as needed.

    Answer C is incorrect. The patient is not on an ACEI yet. Thiazides can be used as a second line as needed.

    Answer D is incorrect. Beta blockers (BBs) are not the first-line medication for BP control as they are not as effective as other medications. Additionally, the patient is asthmatic, and BBs should be used with care to avoid bronchospasms.

15. Answers C and D are correct. Therapeutic lifestyle changes for high cholesterol include changing to a low-saturated-fat and high-fiber diet. Maintaining a healthy weight is important.

    Answer A is incorrect. Exercise should consist of aerobic exercise, not necessarily weight training.

    Answer B is incorrect. The patient does not warrant a statin currently due to her very low 10-year risk of CAD.

16. Answer B is correct. According to the updated guidelines, prophylaxis is only warranted in high-risk conditions. Previous endocarditis is considered high risk for developing infectious endocarditis (IE) again.

    Answer A is incorrect. MVP is no longer an indication.

    Answer C is incorrect. Valve replacement would be an indication but not repair of a valve.

    Answer D is incorrect. A pacemaker or implantable cardioverter/defibrillator (ICD) does not necessitate SBE prophylaxis.

17. Answer B is correct. The goal of treating HTN is to prevent target organ damage.

    Answer A is incorrect. Avoiding hypotension will maintain perfusion.

    Answers C and D are incorrect. Lipid levels and obesity are not affected by HTN, but both are comorbidities that can contribute to cardiovascular complications.

18. Answer B is correct. Sinus tachycardia is a sign of an underlying cause, and treatment is focused on finding and treating the cause.

    Answer A is incorrect. Beta blockers would suppress and mask the underlying cause.

    Answer C is incorrect. There is no indication of anxiety from the case, but a workup to determine if this is a factor is warranted.

    Answer D is incorrect. The HR is not a normal variant and needs to be explored.

19. Both A and B are correct. Patients with EFs of less than 35 percent are at risk for sudden cardiac death from ventricular arrhythmias. Prophylactic placement of ICDs is indicated in this population. Spirinolactone is only indicated in class II, III, and IV HF.

    Answer C is incorrect. The patient has CAD; therefore, ASA is indicated for secondary-event prevention.

    Answer D is incorrect. HF treatment should focus on maximizing function, and activity should not be limited.

20. Answer B is correct. Without obvious risk factors or cause for the DVT, the provider should evaluate the patient for the presence of familial clotting disorders. Once the presence or absence of these disorders is identified, the time frame for anticoagulation can be determined.

    Answer A is incorrect. We need more information to make that determination.

    Answer C is incorrect. IVC filters are used to prevent PE in patients with contraindicated or high-risk anticoagulation.

    Answer D is incorrect. Regardless of the risk factors, the patient needs anticoagulation to treat the existing DVT and prevent PE.

21. Answer A is correct. Chest discomfort that is localized, reproducible, and not associated with exertion is likely musculoskeletal, and NSAIDs would help in this situation.

    Answer B is incorrect. Chest discomfort in a patient with exertional risk factors is likely ischemic in nature, but the patient does not show those signs.

    Answer C is incorrect. The patient does not exhibit acute coronary signs, so a trip to the ER is unnecessary.

    Answer D is incorrect. The symptoms do not indicate GERD, which would warrant a PPI. GERD symptoms would include pain after eating or at night, no exertional activity, and belching or a sour taste in the mouth would also be likely.

22. Answer A is correct. Patients with PAD experience intermittent claudication. Progression to rest pain means that the disease is worsening.

Answer B is incorrect. A DVT often does not cause significant pain but rather swelling and heaviness.

Answer C is incorrect. The question notes that the pain is increased.

Answer D is incorrect. There is no indication of a clotting disorder in this patient.

23. Answer B is correct. The symptoms described likely indicate varicose veins. Predisposing factors include standing for long periods, obesity, pregnancy, and family history.

    Answer A is incorrect. A patient working a desk job is not at risk for varicose veins because sitting at a desk does not increase the venous pressure.

    Answer C is incorrect. HTN is arterial, and varicose veins are a venous disorder.

    Answer D is incorrect. High cholesterol causes arterial plaque in the arteries.

24. Answer C is correct. The fact that pain is relieved with nitroglycerin (NTG) does not necessarily point to an ischemic cause for the pain. NTG can also be effective at relieving the pain or esophageal spasm.

    Answer A is incorrect. Additional assessment would need to be completed to support ischemia.

    Answer B is incorrect. There is no note of BP in the question.

    Answer D is incorrect. Further assessment and workup are essential to determining the actual cause of this pain.

25. Answer A is correct. The patient has likely had AF with rapid response for the past 2 weeks. To decrease his symptoms, he needs to be started on anticoagulation and his rate controlled.

    Answer B is incorrect. An antiarrhythmic drug would not be a first-line treatment and could not be considered until the patient has been adequately anticoagulated for 3 to 4 weeks.

    Answer C is incorrect. The patient does not need to be hospitalized unless they are unstable.

    Answer D is incorrect. A stress test would be indicated once the rate was controlled, but if it were performed without rate control, it would likely worsen symptoms.

CASE STUDY

A 78-year-old female presents to the FNP as a new patient with new onset shortness of breath, which started over the last several weeks and is exacerbated by exertion. The patient has a history of HTN and type 2 diabetes. Her medications include metformin 500 mg BID, ASA 81 mg, and amlodipine 5 mg daily. In the review of systems, she denies chest pain or palpitations, complains of some mild bilateral nonpitting edema, and has no other concerns. Her vitals are BP 140/90, pulse 88, RR 20. Oxygen saturation is 95 percent. Clinical assessment includes lung sound diminished bilaterally, mild nonpitting edema bilaterally, and otherwise unremarkable PE.

Considerations for the clinician:

- Patient has several risk factors for CAD and CHF, including HTN, DM, and age.
- Patients with DM are at the same risk for MI as a patient with a previous MI.
- Hyperglycemia increases the risk of CAD in patients with DM. To assess this risk, it is important to explore her BS control.
- Further risk factor analysis should be pursued, including cholesterol assessment.
- Shortness of breath (SOB) can be an ischemic equivalent to chest pain, especially in a patient with DM who may not have chest discomfort due to neuropathies. Further exploration of her exertional SOB should be conducted considering the potential ischemic component, and an EKG should be performed.
- If the EKG is unremarkable, the FNP should consider stress testing with imaging to assess for ischemia due to exertional symptoms and significant risk factors.
- BP is uncontrolled, and target organ assessment should be explored, including echocardiogram and blood work.
- Patient is at risk for HF, but other than the SOB and some mild edema, there are no overt signs of HF. An echocardiogram will provide more information about LV function.
- A common side effect of amlodipine is nonpitting edema; this could explain the edema.
- Patients with HTN and DM should be on ACE or ARB for renal protection. Because of her uncontrolled BP, one of these should be started.
- A urinalysis should be ordered to screen for microalbuminuria as she has DM with unknown control and not on ACE/ARB.
- ASA use for cardiac event prevention in patients over 60 without evidence of previous CAD is no longer indicated due to lack of benefit in the setting of increased risk for bleeding. If her cardiac work up is negative, the FNP should consider discontinuing the aspirin.

Resources

American Heart Association. (2015). *Classes of heart failure.* http://www.heart.org/HEARTORG/Conditions/HeartFailure/AboutHeartFailure/Classes-of-Heart-Failure_UCM_306328_Article.jsp#.Vu6lcxEUWpo

Grundy, S. M. et al. (2019). 2018 AHA/ACC Guideline on the management of blood cholesterol: Executive summary. *Circulation, 139*, e1046–e1081.

Heidenreich, P. A., Bozkurt, B., Aguilar, D., Allen, L. A., Byun, J. J., Colvin, M. M., Deswal, A., Drazner, M. H., Dunlay, S. M., Evers, L. R., Fang, J. C., Fedson, S. E., Fonarow, G. C., Hayek, S. S., Hernandez, A. F., Khazanie, P., Kittleson, M. M., Lee, C. S., Link, M. S., Milano, C. A., . . . ACC/AHA Joint Committee Members (2022). 2022 AHA/ACC/HFSA Guideline for the Management of Heart Failure: A Report of the American College of Cardiology/American Heart Association Joint Committee on Clinical Practice Guidelines. *Circulation, 145*(18), e895–e1032. https://doi.org/10.1161/CIR.0000000000001063

January, C. T., Wann, L. S., Alpert, J. S., Calkins, H., Cigarroa, J. E., Cleveland, J. C., . . . Yancy, C. W. (2014). 2014 AHA/ACC/HRS guideline for the management of patients with atrial fibrillation: Executive summary. A report of the American College of Cardiology/American Heart Association Task Force on practice guidelines and the Heart Rhythm Society. *Circulation, 130*(23), 2071–2104.

Jarvis C., & Eckhardt, A. (2024). *Physical examination and health assessment.* Elsevier.

Joglar, J. A., et al. (2024). 2023 ACC/AHA/ACCP/HRS Guideline for the diagnosis and management of atrial fibrillation: A report of the American College of Cardiology/American Heart Association Joint Committee on clinical practice guidelines. *Circulation, 149*(1), e1–e156.

McCance, K. L., & Huether, S. E. (2014). *Pathophysiology: The biological basis for disease in adults and children.* Elsevier.

Otto, C., et al. (2020). ACC/AHA Guidelines for the management of patients with valvular heart disease: A report of the American College of Cardiology/American Heart Association joint committee clinical practice guidelines. *Circulation, 143*(5), e72-e227.

Patel, K. (2015). *Deep venous thrombosis treatment & management: Approach considerations, general principles of anticoagulation, heparin use in deep venous thrombosis.* https://emedicine.medscape.com/article/1911303-treatment

Stone, N. J., Robinson, J. G., Lichtenstein, A. H., Merz, C. N. B., Blum, C. B., Eckel, R. H., . . . Wilson, P. W. F. (2014). 2013 ACC/AHA guideline on the treatment of blood cholesterol to reduce atherosclerotic cardiovascular risk in adults: A report of the American College of Cardiology/American Heart Association Task Force on practice guidelines. *Circulation, 129*(25 suppl 2), S1–S45. http://doi.org/10.1161/01.cir.0000437738.63853.7a

Whelton, P. K., et al. (2017). ACC/AHA guideline for prevention, detection, evaluation and management of high blood pressure in adults: A report of the American College of Cardiology/American Heart Association Task Force on Clinical Practice Guidelines. *Hypertension, 71*(6), e13-e115.

Wilson, W., Taubert, K. A., Gewitz, M., Lockhart, P. B., Baddour, L. M., Levison, M., . . . Quality of Care and Outcomes Research Interdisciplinary Working Group (2007). Prevention of infective endocarditis: guidelines from the American Heart Association: A guideline from the American Heart Association Rheumatic Fever, Endocarditis, and Kawasaki Disease Committee, Council on Cardiovascular Disease in the Young, and the Council on Clinical Cardiology, Council on Cardiovascular Surgery and Anesthesia, and the Quality of Care and Outcomes Research Interdisciplinary Working Group. *Circulation, 116*(15), 1736–1754. http://doi.org/10.1161/CIRCULATIONAHA.106.183095

Wilson, W. R., et al. (2021). Prevention of viridans group streptococcal infective endocarditis: A scientific statement from the American Heart Association. *Circulation, 143*, e963-e978.

VanMeter, K. C., & Huber, R. J. (2014). *Gould's pathophysiology for the health professions.* Elsevier.

Yancy, C. W., Jessup, M., Bozkurt, B., Butler, J., Casey, D. E., Drazner, M. H., . . . Wilkoff, B. L. (2013). 2013 ACCF/AHA guideline for the management of heart failure: Executive summary. A report of the American College of Cardiology Foundation/American Heart Association Task Force on Practice Guidelines. *Circulation, 128*(16), 1810–1852. http://doi.org/10.1161/CIR.0b013e31829e8807

CHAPTER 9

Gastrointestinal System

Sylvie Rosenbloom, DNP, APRN, FNP-BC, CDCES
Nancy L. Dennert, MS, MSN, FNP-BC, CDCES, BC-ADM

Patients who present with abdominal pain require prompt and comprehensive evaluation. Obtaining an appropriate history and an accurate physical examination is key to rapid referral in acute situations. Acute abdominal pain may be related to obstruction, vascular injury, peritoneal irritation, among other conditions, and may require immediate surgical intervention. Patients who present with fever, chills, and rebound tenderness should be sent to the closest emergency department for evaluation. Most often, in outpatient settings, the family nurse practitioner (FNP) will encounter a wide variety of nonacute abdominal complaints that may or may not require consultation and/or referral. An accurate history of abdominal discomfort or pain must ascertain the following eight attributes of a symptom:

- Onset
- Location
- Duration
- Character
- Aggravating/relieving
- Radiation
- Timing
- Severity

Physical Examination

1. Inspection: Examine abdomen and report any scars, rashes, striae, symmetry, contour, masses, pulsations, peristalsis, hernias, and skin discoloration. Divide the abdomen into four quadrants and know the location of the abdominal organs.
2. Auscultation: Done before palpation. Listen over all four quadrants for bowel sounds and bruits over the aorta, iliac, renal, and femoral arteries.
3. Percussion: Note areas of dullness indicative of solid or fluid-filled masses rather than air. Percuss for the liver span and spleen to assess for organomegaly.
4. Palpation: Start with light palpation in nontender areas and then move on to deep palpation to assess for distention and tenderness, including rebound, guarding, rigidity, organomegaly, and masses.
5. Rectal Examination: Examine perianal area for hemorrhoids. Insert gloved finger into the anus and note sphincter tone, assess for internal hemorrhoids, fissures, masses, and tenderness.

Abdominal Content

Area	Organs
Right upper quadrant (RUQ)	Liver, gallbladder, ascending colon, right kidney, pancreas (small portion) Note: The right kidney is lower than the left because of liver displacement.
Left upper quadrant (LUQ)	Stomach, pancreas, descending colon, left kidney
Right lower quadrant (RLQ)	Appendix, ileum, cecum, right ovary
Left lower quadrant (LLQ)	Sigmoid colon, left ovary
Suprapubic area	Bladder, uterus, rectum

Special Maneuvers

- Rebound tenderness: Increased pain intensity when quickly releasing the abdomen during palpation. Rebound pain is indicative of peritonitis, an inflammation of the peritoneal cavity. An alternative is to ask the patient to jump in place—if they experience pain or refuse because of pain, consider it positive for rebound tenderness.
- Involuntary guarding: As the nurse practitioner (NP) palpates the abdomen, the patient tenses the abdomen reflexively or the abdomen becomes "board-like."
- Rovsing's sign: This can indicate appendicitis. When the LLQ is palpated, the patient has pain in the right lower quadrant (RLQ).
- Obturator sign: With the knee slightly bent, have the patient rotate their hip inwardly, stretching the obturator internus muscle. Pain may signify appendicitis.
- Psoas sign: Have the patient lift their leg while your hand is placed on their thigh, creating resistance. In appendicitis, the psoas contraction produces pain.
- McBurney's point: The area between the superior iliac crest and umbilicus in the RLQ. Tenderness in this area can indicate possible acute appendicitis.
- Murphy's sign: As the patient takes a deep breath, palpate under the rib cage. Mid-inspiratory arrest indicates a positive finding commonly elicited in cholecystitis.
- Cullen's sign: Periumbilical ecchymosis associated with retroperitoneal bleeding.
- Grey Turner's sign: Ecchymosis/blueish discoloration to flank area can indicate retroperitoneal hemorrhage.
- Hepatojugular reflux: As firm pressure is applied in the epigastrium, observe the neck for an elevation in jugular venous pressure (JVP). Note the drop in JVP as you release the abdomen.
- Scratch test: Position the diaphragm of your stethoscope over the liver and scratch with your finger or tongue depressor parallel to the costal margin until the intensity of the sound drops off, indicating the liver's edge.
- Shifting dullness: With the patient lying on their side, percuss for dullness on the dependent side of the abdomen to assess for ascites.

Liver Enzymes

- Liver enzymes often provide information for the clinician about how well the liver is functioning.
- Gamma-glutamic transpeptidase (GGT)—Marker of liver cell function; used to detect alcohol-induced liver disease; can also be elevated in patients with marked jaundice, liver disease, and acute pancreatitis.
- Alanine aminotransferase (ALT)—Specific indicator for liver function (think A, L = liver, T). More specific for hepatic inflammation than aspartate aminotransferase (AST). Normal range: 0 to 40 mg/dL.
- AST—Not specific to liver. Can also be found in muscles, brain, kidneys, pancreas, and lungs. Normal range: 0 to 45 mg/dL.
- Alkaline phosphatase—Derived from bone, liver, gallbladder, kidneys, gastrointestinal (GI) tract, and placenta. Tends to be higher during growth spurts in children and teens. Can also be elevated in patients with healing fractures, osteomalacia, bone malignancy, vitamin D deficiency.
- Elevation in both ALT and AST indicate liver inflammation and damage. Levels over 500 likely indicate some form of drug-related injury, viral hepatitis, or ischemia.

Other tests that may indicate issues with liver function include alkaline phosphatase (indicate bile flow issues and/or bone diseases). In actual liver disease, the liver will have true function issues, such as alteration in prothrombin time (elevated), albumin (low), and inability to break down bilirubin, which leads to jaundice as the bilirubin levels rise. The ratio of AST/ALT may be greater than 2 in alcoholic liver disease. A ratio of less than 1 may indicate fatty liver disease.

Cholecystitis

Cholecystitis refers to an inflammation of the gallbladder. Acute cholecystitis occurs primarily as a complication of gallstones. Risk factors include obesity, elevated cholesterol, pregnancy, rapid weight loss, female gender, and being over the age of 50.

A patient with cholecystitis is likely to present with RUQ or epigastric pain, which can radiate to the right shoulder and occurs 1 hour (or more) after consuming a fatty meal. Often accompanied by fever, chills, nausea, vomiting, and anorexia.

The physical exam will likely include RUQ and/or epigastric pain with palpation. A positive Murphy's sign may be a strong indicator of cholecystitis. If the common bile duct is obstructed, the patient may present with jaundice.

Ultrasonography is often performed to assess for the presence of cholelithiasis. A more sensitive and specific imaging study called cholescintigraphy (HIDA scan) can also be performed to confirm the diagnosis. Laboratory studies include a complete blood count (CBC) (elevated white blood count [WBC] and bands—left shift) and ALT and AST, which may be greater than 300 IU/L. The amylase and lipase may also both be elevated. The GGT, serum total bilirubin, and alkaline phosphatase can be elevated when the bile duct is obstructed and jaundice develops but are usually within normal limits in uncomplicated acute cholecystitis.

Differential Diagnoses

- Acute pancreatitis
- Acute hepatitis
- Biliary colic
- Peptic ulcer disease (PUD)
- Gastroesophageal reflux
- Right-sided pneumonia
- Abdominal abscess
- Fitz-Hugh-Curtis disease (perihepatitis caused by gonococcal infection)

Treatment

- Low-fat diet
- Clear liquids
- Pain management
- Surgical referral for gallbladder removal

Patient Education

- Teach patients to avoid fatty meals.

Referral

- Signs of peritonitis
- Patient is unable to tolerate fluids or appears dehydrated

Constipation

Constipation is passing bowel movements that are less frequent than usual or passing stool that is dry/harder than usual. It can be chronic or acute. Constipation is a common complaint among all individuals but more frequently with older adults. It is often the result of inactivity and/or inadequate water and fiber intake. It can also be seen in individuals resisting the urge to have a bowel movement.

Differential Diagnosis

- Colon cancer
- Diabetes
- Diverticulosis
- Parkinson's disease
- Bowel obstruction

Triggers

- Medical conditions: hypothyroidism, stress, chronic kidney failure, pregnancy
- Medications: narcotics, beta blockers, antihistamines, muscle relaxants, diuretics, iron preparations, and tricyclic antidepressants

Management

- Dietary changes: increased fiber and fluids; low-fat diet
- Behavioral approaches, such as biofeedback, may help decrease involuntary pelvic muscle contractions and those of the external anal sphincter during bowel movements.
- Medications
  - Fiber: The recommended daily allowance of fiber is 20 to 35 g. It can be taken in natural (food) or supplement form.
  - Bulk-forming laxatives: Laxatives, such as Metamucil, Citrucel, FiberCon, and Benefiber, work by absorbing water in the colon, increasing fecal mass, and softening the consistency of stools.
  - Osmotic laxatives: Laxatives, such as Miralax (polyethylene glycol) and lactulose, pull water into the intestine.
  - Stimulant laxatives: Laxatives, such as senna or bisacodyl, change the intestinal wall's electrolyte transport, thereby increasing intestinal motility.
  - Surfactants: stool softeners, such as Colace, help to decrease the stool's surface tension, thereby increasing the water absorption of the stool.

Complications

- Bowel obstruction
- Chronic constipation
- Hemorrhoids
- Anal fissures
- Hernia
- Laxative dependency

Treatment and Follow-Up

- Prompt medical attention should be given to the individual who complains that they have not had a bowel movement in 5 or more days.

- Educate patients about therapeutic lifestyle changes, such as increasing activity, water, and fiber intake.
- Advise patient to try to defecate after meals, especially in the morning when bowel motility is optimal.

Gastroesophageal Reflux Disease

Gastroesophageal reflux disease (GERD) occurs when the gastric contents ascend to the esophagus and cause symptoms such as burning, discomfort, or pain. It can lead to erosive esophagitis. Chronic GERD can damage the esophageal epithelium leading to Barrett's esophagus, a precancerous condition, and esophageal cancer. Patient with 5 or more years of GERD symptoms should be referred to a gastroenterologist.

Triggers

- Many medications, foods, and beverages can decrease the control of the lower esophageal sphincter.
  - Drugs
    - Theophylline
    - Dopamine
    - Diazepam
    - Calcium-channel blockers
    - nonsteroidal anti-inflammatory drugs (NSAIDs)
  - Foods/beverages
    - Caffeine
    - Alcohol
    - Fatty foods
    - Gassy foods
    - Peppermint
    - Spicy and acidic foods/drinks
- Obesity
- Overeating
- Tight clothing (increases intra-abdominal pressure)
- Tobacco
- Lying down shortly after a meal

> **Red Flag**
> - Dysphagia (difficulty swallowing) and/or odynophagia (painful swallowing)
> - Weight loss
> - GI bleeding
> - Anemia

Clinical Manifestations

Heartburn after a meal is the most common symptom. It is often relieved with antacids. The patient may also experience burping, regurgitation, or waking up with acid or a bad taste in their mouth. The increased reflux of acidity to the throat most often occurs at night and can lead to coughing, wheezing, hoarseness, and aspiration. Risk factors include chronic use of NSAIDs, aspirin, or alcohol.

Diagnostic Studies

The diagnosis of GERD is most often made by history. However, an upper endoscopy with possible biopsy may be performed if the patient experiences dysphagia, odynophagia, gastrointestinal bleeding, anemia, weight loss, or recurrent vomiting.

Treatment

- Medications:
  - Antacids
    - Usually taken after meals
    - Provide 1 to 2 hours of relief.
    - Examples
      - *Calcium carbonate* antacids, such as Tums, also provide an additional source of calcium.
      - *Antacids with alginic acid*, such as Gaviscon, form a barrier at the top of the stomach contents, thus decreasing stomach acid reflux to the esophagus.
      - *Antacids with simethicone*, such as Maalox and Mylanta, reduce gas in the stomach and prevent reflux from ascending to the esophagus.
  - H_2 blockers (H2B), such as ranitidine and famotidine, decrease stomach acid production.
  - Proton-pump inhibitors (PPIs), such as omeprazole, pantoprazole, rabeprazole, esomeprazole, and lansoprazole, work by blocking stomach acid production.
- Treatment Principles
  - Start patient on H2B or PPI and reassess symptoms at 4 to 6 weeks.
  - If partial resolution and the patient was started on H2B, switch to PPI; if the patient was started on PPI, try another PPI or use same PPI. Twice daily rather than once a day.
  - Reassess in 4 weeks. If symptoms persist, referring to gastroenterology for endoscopy could be necessary.

Follow-Up and Education
- Maintain optimal body mass index
- Avoid triggers
- Avoid eating before bedtime
- Elevate the head of the bed

Complications
- Barrett's esophagus
- Esophageal cancer

Peptic Ulcer Disease, Gastric Ulcer, and Duodenal Ulcer Disease

PUD is a lesion affecting the lining of the stomach or duodenum (more common). If untreated, PUD can lead to hemorrhage and perforation. *Helicobacter pylori* infection and chronic use of NSAIDs, the two most often implicated factors in PUD, should be ruled out. Duodenal ulcers are more common than gastric ulcers, but gastric ulcers are more likely to be malignant than duodenal ulcers.

Clinical Manifestations

Up to 70 percent of patients with PUD will be asymptomatic. Hematemesis (bright red or coffee ground–like vomit) or melena (dark tarry stool) can occur and lead to bleeding, anemia, and hypovolemia. If untreated, this can result in the patient becoming hemodynamically compromised (hypovolemic shock). Epigastric pain is common.

Gastric ulcer disease causes pain when eating, and duodenal ulcer pain is more common on an empty stomach and may awaken the patient late at night. The pain is often described as burning or gnawing and may radiate to the back. Associated symptoms may include burping, bloating, nausea, and anorexia.

Differential Diagnosis
- Neoplasm of the stomach
- Pancreatitis
- Pancreatic cancer
- Diverticulitis
- Ischemic bowel disease
- Nonulcer dyspepsia (also called functional dyspepsia)
- Cholecystitis
- Gastritis
- Gastroparesis
- GERD
- myocardial infarction (MI) or coronary artery disease (CAD), not to be missed if having chest pain

Diagnostic Studies
- Stool for guaiac (low sensitivity for upper GI bleed).
- *H. Pylori* testing
  - Urea breath test: The patient is given a labeled carbon isotope by mouth, allowing the tagged CO released by the *H. pylori* bacteria to be detected. Test sensitivity and specificity are about 88 to 95 percent and 95 to 100 percent, respectively.
  - Stool antigen test: This test detects the presence of *H. pylori* in the stool. Its sensitivity is 94 percent, and its specificity is 86 percent.
  - Serologic test: A blood test to detect immunoglobulin G (IgG). Sensitivity is 90 to 100 percent, and specificity is 76 to 96 percent.
- Upper endoscopy with biopsy is the gold standard.
- Barium swallow (less often done).
- CBC and iron studies rule out anemia.

Treatment of *H. Pylori*
- **Triple Therapy:**
  - Clarithromycin Triple Therapy: PPI (omeprazole 20 mg PO BID, lansoprazole 30 mg PO BID, esomeprazole 40 mg PO QD, pantoprazole 40 mg PO QD, rabeprazole 20 mg PO BID) **plus** clarithromycin 500 mg PO BID **plus** amoxicillin 1 g PO BID **or** metronidazole 500 mg PO BID x 14 days.
  - Clarithromycin Concomitant Therapy: PPI PO BID **plus** metronidazole 500 mg PO BID or tinidazole 500 mg PO BID **plus** clarithromycin 500 mg PO BID **plus** amoxicillin 1G PO BID x 10 to 14 days.
  - Clarithromycin-Based Sequential Therapy: PPI PO BID **plus** amoxicillin 1 g PO BID x 5 days followed by PPI PO BID **plus** metronidazole **or** tinidazole 500 mg PO BID x 5 days.
  - Clarithromycin Hybrid Therapy: PPI PO BID **plus** amoxicillin 1 g PO BID x 7 days followed by PPI PO BID **plus** amoxicillin 1 g PO BID **plus** clarithromycin 500 mg PO BID **plus** metronidazole **or** tinidazole 500 mg PO BID x 7 days
- **Quadruple Therapy:** PPI PO BID **plus** bismuth subsalicylate 525 mg PO QID **plus** metronidazole 250 to 500 mg PO TID to QID **plus** Tetracycline 500 mg QID x 10 to 14 days (14-day treatment highly recommended)

Follow-Up and Education

- Confirming eradication after treatment is highly recommended. (See testing methods mentioned earlier.)
- Avoid NSAIDs.
- Adhere to medication regimen.
- Encourage weight loss if obesity is present.
- Encourage smoking cessation.

Red Flags (Referral for Endoscopy)
Symptoms > age 55
Dysphagia or odynophagia
Anemia
Weight loss
GI Bleeding (stool positive for occult blood)

Clinical Pearls

- Any patient with more than 5 years of heartburn or GERD symptoms should be referred to a gastroenterologist for endoscopy to rule out Barrett's esophagus.
- Patients with Barrett's esophagus have up to a 30 times higher risk of esophageal adenocarcinoma.
- PPIs are recommended over H2B if esophagitis or ulcers (heal faster).
- High rate of clarithromycin *H. pylori* resistance in the United States.

Gastroenteritis

Acute viral gastroenteritis is an increase in bowel movements or the passing of watery/loose stool, usually accompanied by nausea, vomiting, abdominal pain, and fever. Both vomiting and diarrhea are usually present; however, they can sometimes occur alone.

Etiology

- Norovirus
- Rotavirus
- Enteric adenovirus
- Astrovirus

Clinical Manifestations

- Nausea/vomiting
- Diarrhea
- Abdominal pain
- Fever

Red Flag

- Dehydration
- Fluid/electrolyte imbalances
- Rectal bleeding/bloody stools
- Severe abdominal pain
- Antibiotic use within the last 3 to 6 months
- Pregnancy
- Older people
- Immunocompromised individuals
- Prolonged symptoms (over 1 week).

Differential Diagnosis

- Other infectious or noninfectious causes of diarrhea
  - *Clostridium difficile* infection in patients with recent hospitalization or antibiotic use
  - Protozoal infection, such as giardia or cryptosporidium, in patients with recent travel
  - Inflammatory bowel disease
  - Irritable bowel syndrome
  - Malabsorption syndrome
  - Laxative abuse

Treatment and Follow-Up

- Acute viral gastroenteritis is usually self-limiting, and no treatment is recommended.
- Fluids and electrolyte replacements in volume-depleted patients.
- Small frequent bland meals, such as the B.R.A.T. diet (banana, rice, apple sauce, and toast); resume regular diet slowly as tolerated.
- Avoid greasy or spicy foods, caffeine, alcohol, and nicotine.
- Avoid NSAIDs because they may further irritate the gastric mucosa.
- Discuss hand hygiene.
- Antimotility agents, such as loperamide (Imodium-AD), and anti-emetic medications, such as ondansetron (Zofran) or prochlorperazine, may be used cautiously.
- Laboratory studies may be warranted if dehydration or parasitic or bacterial infection is suspected: CBC, complete metabolic panel (CMP), stool culture, stool for ova and parasites, stool for *C. difficile*.
- Hospitalization may be required in very young and older patients or if there are signs of volume depletion or electrolyte imbalances.

Appendicitis

Inflammation resulting from the accumulation of fecaliths in the vermiform appendix located at the base of the cecum. It is most frequently seen between 20 to 30 years of age. If left untreated, peritonitis can ensue—most frequent reason for emergent abdominal surgery.

Most patients present with acute onset of periumbilical pain which worsens over time. After 12 to 24 hours, the pain moves toward McBurney's point. Patient often develops anorexia and may also have low-grade fever and RLQ pain on palpation. The psoas and obturator signs are positive.

Clinical Manifestations

- Abdominal pain: Can be periumbilical or epigastric initially and then may shift toward the RLQ region. Pain usually worsens with movement, coughing, and walking (peritoneal irritation). Rebound tenderness is a common finding. Positive Rosving's, heel strike, psoas, and obturator signs.
- Anorexia
- Nausea, vomiting (later signs), diarrhea may be present
- Fever
- Leukocytosis: (10,000 to 16,000 cells/mm^3) with a shift to the left (neutrophilia/bandemia)

Diagnostic Testing

- Ultrasonography and abdominal CT. Abdominal X-rays do not aid in the diagnosis of appendicitis.

Differential Diagnosis

- Gynecologic
  - Pelvic inflammatory disease
  - Ectopic pregnancy
  - Ovarian tumor
  - Ovarian torsion
  - Mittelschmerz
  - Endometriosis
- Gastrointestinal
  - Irritable bowel syndrome
  - Inflammatory bowel disease
  - Colitis
  - Diverticulitis
- Renal
  - Nephrolithiasis
  - Pyelonephritis

Treatment and Follow-Up

- Urgent surgical referral for appendectomy required.
- Some candidates without signs of peritonitis may benefit from nonoperative management with antibiotics.

Diverticulitis

When uncomplicated, acute diverticulitis is usually self-limiting and does not involve abscess, perforation, and/or peritonitis. When the latter are involved, prompt referral and hospitalization are required. This acute stage involves further diagnostic testing, such as CT scans, to rule out other causes of acute abdominal pain.

Older patients typically present with acute onset of LLQ pain and possibly fever, anorexia, and nausea/vomiting. LLQ tenderness present on palpation with or without signs of peritonitis.

Clinical Manifestations

- LLQ pain
- Nausea/vomiting
- Low-grade fever
- Diarrhea
- When acute
  - Signs of an acute abdomen ensue, such as a positive Rosving's sign, rebound tenderness, and abdominal rigidity (a "board"-like abdomen).
  - CBC with leukocytosis, neutrophilia, and a left shift.
  - Bands usually indicate severe bacterial infection.
  - Referral to emergency department for evaluation and possible hospital admission is necessary.

Differential Diagnosis

- Gynecologic
  - Pelvic inflammatory disease
  - Ectopic pregnancy
  - Ovarian tumor
  - Ovarian torsion
  - Mittleschmerz
  - Endometriosis
- Gastrointestinal
  - Constipation
  - Inflammatory bowel disease
  - Colitis
- Renal
  - Nephrolithiasis
  - Pyelonephritis
  - Urinary tract infection (UTI)

Outpatient Treatment and Follow-Up

Initial outpatient management of diverticulitis includes pain control with analgesics, such as acetaminophen, ibuprofen, or oxycodone and a liquid diet with reassessment of symptoms in 2 to 3 days after initial visit and then weekly until complete resolution of symptoms. There is no longer a recommendation for avoidance of nuts, seeds, and corn. If the patient improves, there is no indication for imaging studies. However, the American Gastroenterological Association and the American Society of Colon and Rectal Surgeons suggest using antibiotics to treat uncomplicated diverticulitis.

- Antibiotic therapy (mild/outpatient setting):
  - Ciprofloxacin 500 mg PO BID **plus** metronidazole 500 mg PO q8h **OR** levofloxacin 750 mg PO QD **plus** metronidazole 500 mg PO q8h **OR** Bactrim DS 800/100 mg q12h **plus** metronidazole 500 mg PO q8h **OR** amoxicillin-clavulanate 825/125 mg PO q12h **OR** moxifloxacin 400 mg PO QD for patient intolerant of both metronidazole and beta-lactam agents. Therapy should be for 10 to 14 days
- Anti-inflammatory agents, such as mesalamine, may be utilized.

Guidelines for Outpatient Management

1. Compliance with medical regimen
2. Able to tolerate PO intake
3. Abdominal pain is not severe
4. No fever/or low-grade fever
5. No or minimal comorbidities
6. Able to return for follow-up
7. Support system available

Colon Cancer

Cancer of the lower intestinal tract ranks as the third most common cause of death in the United States for both males and females. The median age of diagnosis is 69 years.

Typical presentation includes gradual (years) vague GI symptoms. The patient can develop anemia. Oftentimes, the patient will have changes in bowel habits or stool (bloody/black stools).

Clinical Manifestations

Most often dependent upon the location and stage of the disease:

- Change in bowel habit
- Hematochezia
- Iron-deficiency anemia—usually from unknown etiology
- Abdominal pain
- Tenesmus, bright red blood per rectum, rectal pain, and changes in stool caliber can be seen with rectal cancer.

Differential Diagnosis

- Diverticulitis
- Ulcerative colitis
- Crohn's disease
- Appendicitis
- Thrombosed hemorrhoids

Treatment and Follow-Up

- Treatment will depend upon the disease's staging but often includes surgery, chemotherapy, and radiation. The patient will then undergo routine colonoscopy, often yearly at first.
- Screening should begin at age 45 in asymptomatic individuals or those without a family history.
  - American Cancer Society recommends:
    - Regular screening should occur between ages 45 and 75. Fecal occult blood testing, fecal immunochemical testing (FIT), or stool DNA should be tested every three years. If these tests are positive, a colonoscopy should be performed.
    - Every 5 years, a flexible sigmoidoscopy should be performed to detect polyps and cancer. A colonoscopy is conducted every 10 years, and a double contrast barium enema or CT colonography (virtual colonoscopy) every five years.
    - Patients aged 76 and 85 should discuss the pros of finding a precancerous polyp vs the cons of having an invasive test with their providers, considering patient preferences, overall health, and past screening history.
    - Colorectal cancer screening is no longer recommended for individuals younger than 85.
- In patients with a strong family history of polyposis or who have first-degree relatives with colon cancer, patients will see a gastroenterologist who will recommend colonoscopies every 3 to 5 years.
- In patients with colon cancer, a colonoscopy will be performed 1 year after resection.
- To detect polyps and cancer, the American Cancer Society guidelines for colorectal

cancer screening recommends the following screening options, which should begin at age 45, for those with average risk:
- Flexible sigmoidoscopy every 5 years
- Colonoscopy every 10 years
- Double-contrast barium enema every 5 years
- CT colonography (virtual colonoscopy) every 5 years
• Tests that mainly detect cancer include:
- guaiac-based fecal occult blood test (gFOBT) every year
- fecal immunochemical test (FIT) every year
- stool DNA test (sDNA) every 3 years*

Hepatitis

Hepatitis is a liver inflammation arising from an autoimmune disorder (rare) or viral infection.

History

- Ask about alcohol use/abuse (CAGE questionnaire), IV drug use
- Tactfully obtain the patient's sexual history
- Ask about usage of potentially hepatotoxic medications (acetaminophen) or environmental toxins
- Assess for potential high-risk work environments, such as HIV or sexually transmitted infection (STI) clinics

Clinical Manifestations

- Jaundice
- Fatigue
- Anorexia, nausea, vomiting, diarrhea
- Abdominal pain
- Headache
- Fever
- Dark-colored urine and pale-looking stool

Liver Function Tests

- Serum aspartate aminotransferase (AST)—also known as glutamic oxaloacetic transaminase (SGOT)
  - Normal: 0 to 45 mg/dL
  - Found in liver, heart muscle, skeletal muscle, and kidney
  - Low specificity for liver injury because it is found in other organs and can be elevated in other conditions, such as acute myocardial infarction
- Serum alanine aminotransferase (ALT)—also known as serum glutamic pyruvic transaminase (SGPT)
  - Normal: 0 to 40 mg/dL
  - Found mainly in the liver. An elevated value signifies liver inflammation.
  - ALT is a more specific marker of hepatic inflammation than AST.
- AST/ALT (aspartate aminotransferase/alanine aminotransferase) ratio (SGOT/SGPT ratio)
  - A ratio greater than 2.0 is often found with alcohol misuse.
- Alkaline phosphatase enzyme
  - is found in bone, liver, gallbladder, kidneys, GI tract, and placenta.
  - elevation is often seen during children's growth spurts, healing fractures, malignancy, and osteomalacia.
- Serum GGT
  - Normal: 0 to 51 IU/L
  - Indicator of alcohol misuse
  - Elevated in liver disease and acute pancreatitis
  - Can be affected by other drugs: alcohol, phenytoin, and phenobarbital can increase GGT levels, whereas birth control pills and clofibrate can decrease GGT levels.

Hepatitis A

- Causative agent is an RNA picornavirus, which is a single serotype worldwide.
- Transmission: via fecal or oral route
- Incubation period: 15 to 20 days. The highest incidence rates are between the ages of 5 and 14. Hepatitis A is an acute condition (as opposed to hepatitis B, which is chronic) and may lead to fulminant hepatitis.
- Antibodies resulting from infection will provide lifelong immunity.
- Self-limiting infection with symptomatic treatment.
- Educate patient to avoid the use of oral contraception, hormone replacement therapy, and alcohol use.
- Hepatitis A is a reportable disease to the public health department.
- Hepatitis A vaccination is available.

Hepatitis B

- A small DNA virus of the *Hepadnaviridae* family is the causative agent of hepatitis B. This virus has an inner core and an outer shell and has an incubation period of 60 to 90 days.

- Transmission can occur through blood and mucosal tissues being exposed to blood or other bodily fluids (sexual contact), via drug use (parenteral), and perinatal (mother to child).
- Chronic infection can occur in 10 percent of infected adults, 30 to 50 percent of exposed children, and 90 percent of infants exposed to the virus. Hepatitis B–infected patients can also have a hepatitis D coinfection. Vaccination is encouraged.
- First-line treatment: pegylated interferon alfa (PEG-IFN-a), entecavir (ETV), tenofovir disoproxil fumarate (TFD).
- See **Table 9-1** for the interpretation of the hepatitis B serologic panel.

Hepatitis C

- Transmitted through blood products, especially with blood transfusions or organ transplants before 1992 or transfusion of clotting factors before 1987. It is often seen in IV drug users. Hepatitis C infection is four times more likely to occur in IV drug users than HIV infection. Sexual transmission has been known to occur, especially in individuals with multiple partners or with males having intercourse with other males.
- Hepatitis C has an incubation period of 6 to 7 weeks.
- Up to 85 percent of infected individuals will become chronically infected.
- Factors associated with increased progression and severity are as follows:
    - Older than 40 years at the time of infection
    - HIV coinfection
    - Chronic HBV coinfection
    - Increased alcohol intake
    - Male
- There are no vaccinations available against hepatitis C. However, current therapies have shown great success rates in treating and curing hepatitis C infections. A patient with chronic hepatitis C should be vaccinated against hepatitis A and B if not immune.
- Hepatitis C is a reportable disease to the public health department.
- The CDC (CDC, 2025b) clinical screening and diagnosis for hepatitis C recommends once in a lifetime screening for hepatitis C in all individuals over the age of 18.

See the Hepatitis A, B, and C Summary Table for health care professionals from the CDC (2020) for a comprehensive review.

Table 9-1 Interpretation of the Hepatitis B Serologic Panel

Tests	Results	Interpretation
HBsAg	Negative	Susceptible
anti-HBc	Negative	
anti-HBs	Negative	
HBsAg	Negative	Immune due to natural infection
anti-HBc	Positive	
anti-HBs	Positive	
HBsAg	Negative	Immune due to hepatitis B vaccination*
anti-HBc	Negative	
anti-HBs	Positive	
HBsAg	Positive	Acutely infected
anti-HBc	Positive	
IgM anti-HBc	Positive	
anti-HBs	Negative	
HBsAg	Positive	Chronically infected
anti-HBc	Positive	
IgM anti-HBc	Negative	
anti-HBs	Negative	
HBsAg	Negative	Four interpretations possible¶
anti-HBc	Positive	
anti-HBs	Negative	

HBsAg: hepatitis B surface antigen; anti-HBc: hepatitis B core antibody; anti-HBs: hepatitis B surface antibody; IgM: immunoglobulin M; HBV: hepatitis B virus.
*Antibody response (anti-HBs) can be measured quantitatively or qualitatively. A protective antibody response is reported quantitatively as 10 or more milli-international units (≥10 mIU/mL) or qualitatively as positive. Postvaccination testing should be completed 1 to 2 months after the third vaccine dose for results to be meaningful.
¶ Four interpretations:
1. Might be recovering from acute HBV infection
2. Might be distantly immune and test not sensitive enough to detect very low level of anti-HBs in serum
3. Might be susceptible with a false positive anti-HBc
4. Might be undetectable level of HBsAg present in the serum and the person is actually chronically infected.

Modified from Centers for Disease Control and Prevention. (2023). Interpretation of Hepatitis B serologic test results. Retrieved from https://www.cdc.gov/hepatitis/hbv/interpretationOfHepBSerologicResults.htm

Nonalcoholic Steatohepatitis

Commonly known as nonalcoholic fatty liver disease (NAFLD), nonalcoholic steatohepatitis (NASH) increases an individual's risk of cardiovascular disease, diabetes, cirrhosis, and liver-related deaths. A liver biopsy is done to confirm diagnosis.

Risk Factors

- Obesity, especially in individuals with increased waist circumference
- Diabetes mellitus
- Hypertriglyceridemia
- Elevated liver function tests (LFTs) (twice the upper limit of normal)

Treatment and Follow-Up

- Encourage patients with obesity to lose weight and maintain a healthy BMI.
- Optimize cardiovascular risk factors. Patients with NASH often have multiple cardiovascular risk factors and will benefit from therapeutic lifestyle changes to decrease their cardiovascular risk factors.
- Avoid alcohol and hepatotoxic medications that can worsen disease progression.
- Patients with NASH should undergo screening for hepatocellular carcinoma.
- Individuals should receive immunizations for hepatitis A and hepatitis B.
- Patients should be referred to a hepatologist.
- Use insulin-sensitizing agents, such as Metformin (glucophage) and thiazolidinediones (in individuals with diabetes mellitus).

Clinical Pearl

Beginning in 2023 more than 200 experts in liver disease formalized their decision to rename nonalcoholic fatty liver disease (NAFLD) to metabolic dysfunction-associated steatotic liver disease (MASLD) which requires the presence of at least one of five cardiometabolic risk factors in the context of hepatic steatosis. For detailed information refer to American Association for the Study of Liver Diseases practice guidance on nonalcoholic fatty liver disease.

Irritable Bowel Syndrome

Irritable bowel syndrome (IBS) is a chronic disorder of the brain–gut interaction characterized by chronic recurrent abdominal pain in the absence of organic disease and with symptoms lasting at least 3 days per month. It is associated with two or more of the following:

- Abdominal pain improved with bowel movement
- Diarrhea or constipation (stool frequency)
- Change in stool appearance
- Cramping, flatulence, and bloating may also be present.

Additional testing may be needed to rule out other potential malignant causes. Triggers can be foods (chocolate, spices, fats, carbonated beverages, alcohol), stress, or hormones. There is an increased prevalence of IBS in females (about twice as many as men), individuals under age 40, those with a family history, and individuals with psychiatric disorders (anxiety, depression, personality disorder, history of childhood sexual abuse, or domestic abuse in women).

Typical presentation: Young to middle-aged female reporting intermittent episodes of moderate to severe abdominal cramping pain in the lower abdomen (often LLQ), bloating, and flatulence. Pain typically improves after defecation. Bowel habits can range from diarrhea to constipation or include both.

Clinical Manifestations

- Vital signs are usually stable.
- Abdominal exam: pain with palpation to LLQ during acute exacerbation.
- Rectal exam: stool is normal (no blood or pus). Stool is negative for occult blood.

Differential Diagnosis

- Crohn's disease
- Inflammatory bowel disease
- Lactose intolerance
- Gluten intolerance
- Malignancy

Management

Therapy aims to minimize flare-ups and symptoms and optimize quality of life. Initially, the management should focus on lifestyle changes rather than specific pharmacological agents.

- Dietary modification:
  - A diet low in fermentable oligo-, di-, and monosaccharides and polyols (FODMAPs); in certain cases, avoidance of lactose and gluten
  - Avoidance of gas-producing foods
  - Adequate fiber intake
- Food allergy testing may be needed
- Physical activity
- Medical management:
  - Constipation—fiber or osmotic laxative, such as lactulose or polyethylene glycol (Miralax), lubiprostone, linaclotide, plecanatide (guanylate cyclase agonists), or tenapanor, if fiber fails
  - Diarrhea: Antidiarrheal agent, such as loperamide, eluxadoline, and bile sequestrants (cholestyramine, colestipol, colesevelam), can be

utilized if antidiarrheals are ineffective. Alosetron can be used in severe diarrhea-prominent IBS.
- Antispasmodic agents (dicyclomine, hyoscyamine) can be used to temporarily relieve abdominal pain and bloating.
- Psychiatric disorders (anxiety, depression) should be treated with antidepressants or anxiolytics as needed.
- The role of probiotics is uncertain, but improvements in symptoms have been seen.

Patient Education
- Teach patients to keep a food/symptoms diary to help identify potential triggers and to avoid these triggers.
- Teach patients about FODMAPs foods.
- Teach patients to seek medical attention if there is rectal bleeding, weight loss, or abdominal pain that progresses or occurs at night.

> **Red Flags**
> - More than minimal rectal bleeding
> - Unexplained weight loss
> - Unexplained iron deficiency anemia
> - Symptoms at night
> - Family history of colorectal cancer, inflammatory bowel disease, or celiac sprue

Acute Pancreatitis

Acute pancreatitis is an acute inflammation of the pancreas secondary to alcohol misuse, cholelithiasis, elevated triglycerides (often seen in patients with diabetes), and infection. The pancreatic enzymes get activated and cause autodigestion of the pancreas. The condition can be severe and become life-threatening. Triglycerides greater than 500 mg/dL increase the risk for pancreatitis. Patients usually require prompt referral to the emergency department.

Typical presentation: Patient presents with acute onset of epigastric and/or right upper abdominal pain, fever, nausea, and vomiting. The pain may radiate to the back.

Clinical Manifestations
- Hypoactive bowel sounds
- Epigastric/RUQ pain with palpation, rebound, guarding, or board-like abdomen may be present.
- Positive Cullen's and/or Grey Turner's sign
- Jaundice

Diagnostics
- Elevated amylase, lipase, and trypsin
- Elevated ALT, AST, GGT, bilirubin
- Elevated WBC
- Abdominal CT scan or ultrasound may show ileus.

Complications
- Ileus
- Sepsis
- Shock
- Death

Clostridium Difficile Colitis

Clostridioides difficile is a gram-positive bacterium that is spore-forming and toxin-producing and can cause antibiotic-associated colitis.

Presenting Symptoms
- History of recent antibiotic use—mainly fluoroquinolones, clindamycin, cephalosporins, and penicillins.
- Watery diarrhea (more than 3 loose stools/24 hours), which can be associated with mucus and/or occult blood. Melena or hematochezia are rare.
- Low abdominal pain and cramping
- Low-grade fever
- Nausea and anorexia

Clinical Presentation
- May have hyperactive bowel sounds
- May have some low abdominal tenderness with palpation
- If severe, may have symptoms of dehydration or hypovolemia

Diagnostics
- Positive nucleic acid amplification test (NAAT) for C. difficile toxin gene
- Positive stool test for C. difficile toxin
- CBC with leukocytosis (> 15,000 cells/mL)

Treatment
- If the condition is severe (WBC > 15,000 cells/mL and serum creatinine ≥ 1.5 mg/dL), hospitalization is required.
- Outpatient treatment:

- Fidaxomicin 200 mg PO BID x 10 days
- Vancomycin 125 mg PO QID x 10 days
- If the above regimens are not available: metronidazole 500 mg PO TID x 10 to 14 days

Inflammatory Bowel Disease

Ulcerative colitis (UC) is a chronic inflammatory illness leading to ulcerations of the colon mucosa. It can occur anywhere from the rectum to the colon. Commonly seen between the ages of 20 and 40. In UC, the primary lesions are continuous (no skip lesions) and usually involve only the mucosa of the GI tract. The disease is usually most severe in the rectum and sigmoid colon. In severe inflammatory cases, the small erosions can lead to ulcers, and abscess formation can ensue. Up to 10 percent of persons affected with UC can present with extraintestinal manifestations such as episcleritis, arthritis, erythema nodosum, fatty liver, and autoimmune diseases. Chronic complications can lead to strictures. Patients with UC have an increased risk of venous and arterial thromboembolism and colon cancer.

Risk Factors

- Family history or Jewish descent
- More prevalent in White people and Northern Europeans
- Less common in smokers

Etiology

Unknown, but diet, genetics, infections, and immunologic causes are known to be associated with the disease.

Clinical Manifestations

- Characterized by periods of exacerbation and remission
- Diarrhea and bloody stool (common)
- Abdominal pain (occasional)
- Fever
- Weight loss
- Fatigue
- Tenesmus (sudden urge to move bowels)
- Characterized by remissions and exacerbations

Differential Diagnosis

- Crohn's disease
- Colitis
- Infectious
- Radiation
- Medication associated, especially NSAIDs

Diagnostic Testing

- Stool cultures for *Clostridium difficile*, *Salmonella*, *Shigella*, *Campylobacter*, *Yersinia* and *E. coli O157:H7*
- Stool for ova and parasites
- Giardia stool antigen
- Serologic testing for STIs such as *Neisseria gonorrhea*, HSV, *Treponema pallidum*
- CBC, electrolytes, albumin, ESR, CRP
- Endoscopy and biopsy

Treatment and Follow-Up

- The severity of UC needs to be assessed, and a prompt referral should be given to GI when UC is moderate or severe.
- Mild UC: Topical 5-aminosalicylic acids, mesalamine, steroids such as beclomethasone, enemas, or oral prednisone.
- Moderate–severe UC (usually managed by gastroenterologist): Anti-TNF antibodies, cyclosporine, tacrolimus. In severe cases, surgery may be needed.
- Symptomatic treatment: In mild UC, loperamide can be given for diarrhea, and anticholinergic preparations, such as dycosamine and hyoscyamine, can be given for abdominal discomfort.
- Immunizations: Routine immunizations are highly recommended because patients are more susceptible to infectious conditions.
- Colon cancer screening: Patients with UC have an increased risk for colorectal cancer and should be screened. (See American Cancer Society [2023] guidelines for the early detection of cancer.)
- Pap smear: Women with UC have an increased risk of dysplasia.
- Skin cancer screening: Patients with UC have an increased risk of nonmelanoma skin cancers.
- Osteoporosis screening: Patients have an increased risk of osteoporosis, especially with increased corticosteroid use.
- Laboratory screening: Routine labs should be done to monitor for developing electrolyte imbalances resulting from severe diarrhea and CBC to monitor for anemia.

Complications

- Severe bleeding
- Fulminant colitis

- Toxic megacolon
- Perforations and strictures requiring prompt referral for surgery
- Development of colorectal cancer and cervical dysplasia

Crohn's Disease

Crohn's disease (CD) is an idiopathic inflammatory gastrointestinal disorder that can affect all portions of the GI tract from the mouth to the anus. The disease begins in the submucosa of the intestine and then extends to the intestinal wall, involving both the intestinal mucosa and serosa. The most affected sites are the distal small intestine and proximal large colon, with the ileocolon being the most frequently involved site. CD tends to affect the GI tract in some segments but not others, a pattern called "skip lesions." Patients may develop extraintestinal symptoms such as arthritis, eye involvement (uveitis, episcleritis, iritis), skin disorders (erythema nodosum), cholangitis, secondary amyloidosis, renal lithiasis, increased incidence of venous and arterial thromboembolism, osteoporosis, and vitamin B12 deficiency. It is slightly more prevalent in females than males and tends to develop under the age of 40. As many as 20 to 40 percent may require a colectomy.

Risk Factors
- Smoking
- Jewish descent
- Family history

Etiology
- Genetic mutation

Clinical Manifestations
- Can be difficult to differentiate from UC
- Abdominal pain and diarrhea (common)
- Bloody stool (less common)
- Fever, fatigue, and weight loss may be present
- Abdominal mass, steatorrhea, malabsorption syndrome (common)
- Characterized by remissions and exacerbations

Differential Diagnosis
- Ulcerative colitis
- Colitis (infectious, radiation, diversion, medication associated, especially NSAIDs)
- Rectal ulcer
- Lactose intolerance

Diagnostic Testing
- Laboratory testing
  - CBC
  - Blood chemistry, including blood glucose, electrolytes, kidney tests and LFTs, erythrocyte sedimentation rate (ESR), C-reactive protein (CRP), vitamin B12 levels, and iron studies
- Stool culture for *Clostridium difficile*, ova, and parasites
- Colonoscopy is the preferred study for examination of the colon.
- Barium enemas can also be used if colonoscopy is not indicated.
- MRIs are utilized for assessment of perianal fistulas.

Treatment and Follow-Up
- Moderate or severe disease will require hospital admission and prompt referral.
- For mild disease, CD without systemic symptoms is treated with glucocorticoids, immunomodulator, and biologic therapies, utilizing either a "step-up" or "top-down" approach.

Complications
- Severe bleeding
- Toxic megacolon
- Abscesses, perforations, fistulae, obstructions, and strictures that may require prompt referral for surgery
- Development of colorectal cancer and cervical dysplasia

Hemorrhoids

Hemorrhoids are swollen and inflamed vascular structures located in the anal canal. They result from arteriovenous connective tissues draining into the superior and inferior hemorrhoidal veins. Hemorrhoids can be classified as external (found distally to the dentate line), internal (situated proximally to the dentate line), or mixed (found both distally and proximally to the dentate line). Internal hemorrhoids can be classified depending on the degree of prolapse from the anal canal:

Grade I: May bulge into the lumen but not prolapse distally to the dentate line. Can visualize with the anoscope.

Grade II: Can prolapse out of the anal canal with straining and defecation but reduces spontaneously.

Grade III: Also prolapses out of the anal canal with straining/defecation but needs to be manually reduced.

Grade IV: Hemorrhoids cannot be reduced and may strangulate.

Prompt referral is recommended in patients with bright red blood per rectum, orthostatic changes, or symptoms suggestive of malignancy (anemia, changes in bowel habits, or stool caliber or consistency). Patients with colon cancer or familial polyposis should also be referred for colonoscopy.

Clinical Manifestations

- Pruritus
- Rectal bleeding—stool is usually bright red; can be copious amounts. May lead to anemia or other associated symptoms such as weakness, dizziness, fatigue, exercise intolerance, and headaches.
- Prolapse
- Anal swelling
- Rectal pain resulting from thrombosis
- Mild fecal incontinence, wetness, fullness feeling in perianal area

Differential Diagnosis

- Malignancy, chronic infection, or inflammation (usually associated with systemic symptoms such as night sweats, fever, weight loss, and abdominal pain)
- Colorectal cancer or polyps
- Inflammatory bowel disease

Diagnostic Testing

- Perineal/anal inspection
- Digital rectal exam
- Anoscopy
- Colonoscopy
- Laboratory testing (CBC and iron studies) to rule out anemia or iron deficiency if complaints of bleeding or bleeding present during physical examination.

Treatment

- Initial approach: Conservative medical management aimed at prevention and symptomatic treatment.
  - Constipation: Increase PO fiber and fluid intake to decrease the risk of constipation/straining, including the use of bulk-forming laxatives such as methylcellulose (Citrucel), polycarbophil (FiberCon, Konsyl), psyllium (Metamucil), and wheat dextrin (Benefiber).
- Pain relievers and anti-pruritus: Benzocaine 5 to 20% rectal ointment (Americaine), dibucaine 1% rectal ointment (Nupercainal), pramoxine 1% rectal foam, ointment, or wipes (Proctofoam, Pramox).
- Pain relievers and anti-inflammatory: hydrocortisone rectal creams 1 to 2.5% (Anusol–HC, Preparation H, Proctosol), hydrocortisone rectal suppository 25 to 30 mg (Anusol-HC).
- Stool softeners: Ducosate sodium (Colace)
- Pain associated with anal sphincter spasm: Nitroglycerin 0.2 to 0.5% ointment, phenylephrine 0.25% (Preparation-H, Rectacaine)

Patient Education

Teach patients the importance of prevention and avoidance of constipation/straining.

Anal Fissures

Perianal/anal fissures are the result of increased anal pressure and may be acute or chronic. They are usually caused by anal trauma (hard stool) or can be the result of an underlying medical/surgical condition, often attributed to symptomatic hemorrhoids. They can be primary (local trauma) or secondary (malignancy or resulting from IBD), depending on their etiology. Commonly seen in middle-aged adults and infants.

All patients with rectal bleeding should have a sigmoidoscopy or colonoscopy, especially with a family history of colorectal cancers.

Clinical Manifestations

- Tearing pain, worse with bowel movements
- Burning
- Bright rectal bleeding, usually only a small amount on toilet paper or on stool surface.
- Perianal pruritus or irritation
- On exam: Anal fissures are most commonly located in the posterior anal midline. May be superficial excoriation, shallow laceration, or deep wound that extends into the external sphincter.

Differential Diagnosis

- Perianal ulcers/sores
- Anorectal fistula

Treatment

- Referral to proctologist
- Conservative: Local wound care such as sitz bath, relief of constipation

- Medical management (more severe cases):
  - Topical vasodilators: nifedipine or nitroglycerin cream/ointment
  - Stool softeners/laxative (bulk-forming) to relieve constipation
  - Topical analgesics without Xylocaine
- With more chronic cases, botulinum toxin type A injection or lateral sphincterotomy may be considered. Surgery is considered as a last resort treatment.

Follow-Up

- Increase fiber and fluid intake to avoid constipation
- Laxatives
- Keep anal area dry by wiping with soft cotton—keep cotton ball between buttocks
- Used moistened wipes/cloths

Exam Tips

- Barrett's esophagus is a precursor to esophageal cancer diagnosed by upper endoscopy with biopsy.
- Know lifestyle changes to teach patients with PUD and GERD.
- Know Cullen's, Grey Turner's, Rovsing's, psoas, and obturator signs.
- Be aware of presentation of acute appendicitis (positive psoas and/or obturator signs).
- With PUD, first determine if *H. pylori* positive, and if so, know 14-day treatment.
- High risk for cirrhosis and liver cancer in a patient with hepatitis C.
- GGT can be elevated in patients with liver disease and biliary obstruction. "Lone" elevation can indicate possible alcohol misuse.
- ALP can be elevated in children and teens secondary to growth spurt (bone growth). It may also be elevated in conditions such as vitamin D deficiency, Paget's disease, and bone cancer. Ordering a GGT can help differentiate the source of ALP elevation. The GGT is elevated with liver disease.
- ALT is more likely to indicate liver disease than AST because AST is also found in the skeletal system and the heart. Elevated ALT and AST indicate acute liver inflammation or injury. However, they can also be elevated in chronic liver disease such as cirrhosis.
- Know hepatitis serology. You will likely need to figure out if the patient has hepatitis A, B, or C. With hepatitis B, HbsAg-positive means the patient has an infection (new or chronic).
- A patient needs to have hepatitis B to become infected with hepatitis D. No vaccination exists against hepatitis D, but the hepatitis B vaccination may help prevent it.
- When screening for hepatitis C, start with HCV antibody (HCV Ab). If positive, then order HCV RNA. If positive, then the patient has hepatitis C.
- Amylase and lipase are useful tests to assess for pancreatitis.

CASE STUDY 1

The NP is seeing a 37-year-old female who states that she has had some epigastric tenderness for the past few weeks. She reports that pain tends to occur after meals but is uncertain of food triggers. She denies having any changes in appetite or bowel habits or having bloody or black stools. She denies any pain at present. On examination, the patient has stable vital signs, including no changes in weight, and the only positive finding is some epigastric and right upper quadrant tenderness upon palpation.

1. What are the differential diagnoses?
2. What initial diagnostic testing does the NP consider?

The NP asks the patient to keep a food/symptom diary, and the patient returns 2 weeks later stating that the pain seems to happen more in the evening when she lays down on the couch to watch television and when she eats pasta with tomato sauce or pizza or drinks a glass of wine with dinner.

Laboratory findings include:
- CBC: normal
- CMP: normal
- Urea breath test: positive for *Helicobacter pylori*
- Abdominal ultrasound without abnormalities

The patient has no known allergies and has not been on antibiotics in the last 2 months. Her last menstrual period was a week ago, and she denies pregnancy.

3. What is the pharmacological treatment plan for this patient?

CASE STUDY 2

The NP is seeing a 32-year-old female who states that for the last 4 to 5 days she has had a low-grade fever and LLQ pain. She reports that her bowel movements have been slightly more difficult to pass. The patient denies any changes in appetite, nausea, vomiting, or diarrhea. She is sexually active but reports that she has been with the same male partner for over 2 years and no longer uses condoms. She denies any new vaginal discharge and reports no urinary symptoms. On examination, there is tenderness over the LLQ, but no rebound, guarding, or rigidity. A pelvic exam reveals tenderness over the left ovary, but no masses are palpated, and there is no cervical motion tenderness.

1. What are the differentials?
2. What initial diagnostics will the NP order?
   The NP suspects a most likely diagnosis of diverticulitis. The patient is stable and can be treated on an outpatient basis.
3. What is the gold standard diagnostic testing that the NP would order to rule out a suspected diagnosis of diverticulitis?
4. What is the treatment plan for this patient?

Review Questions

1. A 33-year-old male patient is new to the family nurse practitioner's (FNP) practice. During the health history, he mentions he was told he had hepatitis. The FNP orders bloodwork for this new patient. To evaluate which hepatitis the patient was previously diagnosed with, the **initial** laboratory testing will include:
   A. HAV viral load, HBV viral load, and immunoglobulin G (IgG).
   B. HCV Ag, HBV eAg, and HAV viral load.
   C. HAV total Ab, HCV Ab, anti-HBc, and anti-HBs.
   D. HAV, immunoglobulin M (IgM), and HBV viral load.

2. The 33-year-old male patient with history of unknown type of hepatitis has the following results. What do these results indicate?
   HBsAg = positive
   HBsAb = negative
   IgM HbcAB = negative
   HAV Ab total = positive
   HCV Ab = nonreactive
   A. Acute hepatitis C infection, past hepatitis A infection
   B. Chronic hepatitis B infection, acute hepatitis A infection
   C. Past hepatitis A infection, chronic hepatitis B infection
   D. Past hepatitis B infection, past hepatitis A infection

3. A 19-year-old male college football player has suffered an injury during the game. The patient is pale, anxious, and complaining of left upper quadrant (LUQ) pain that radiates to the left shoulder. The FNP recognizes that this most likely indicates:
   A. a ruptured spleen.
   B. an acute pancreatitis.
   C. a right-sided pneumothorax.
   D. a gastrointestinal bleed.

4. A 50-year-old male acquired HCV+ from intravenous drug use (IVDU) many years ago. He has not used street drugs for over 15 years and works long hours as a train conductor. He is asking about his routine health maintenance regarding HCV. Which of the following yearly exams are recommended by the FNP?
   A. CT scan, liver biopsy, HCV viral load, and liver enzymes
   B. Liver ultrasound, liver enzymes, AFP, HCV viral load
   C. Liver biopsy, liver ultrasound, liver enzymes, CBC
   D. HCV viral load, genotype, and CT scan

5. A 62-year-old female patient has come to the FNP's office with complaints of constipation for the past few months. She has tried to increase her water and fiber intake without much success. A yearly physical exam and colonoscopy were negative for

any significant findings 6 months before this visit. Which of the following options would be most appropriate to recommend for the next step?
   A. Daily Dulcolax use as an addition to the fiber and water.
   B. Increasing exercise, such as walking, and daily Miralax use for 2 weeks, then have her return for evaluation in 1 month.
   C. Daily fleet enema use upon arising in addition to current approach. Refer to GI specialist if no improvement.
   D. CT scan of abdomen to rule out malignancy.

6. A 42-year-old female patient with a BMI of 31 has a chief complaint of intermittent abdominal pain for about 2 months. The pain is generally in the right upper quadrant (RUQ) and is described as "stabbing," ranging from a 4 to 9 on the 1-to-10 pain scale. Nothing seems to help it go away, but it only lasts about 20 to 30 minutes. Upon further interview, it is uncovered that the patient often eats fried foods. When discussing the past 24-hour food intake, she recalls she felt nauseated and had slight RUQ discomfort after eating a cheeseburger and french fries the night before. Which of the following signs is most likely to be found on physical exam?
   A. Cullen's sign
   B. Rosvig's sign
   C. Murphy's sign
   D. Psoas sign

7. The FNP orders an abdominal ultrasound for a patient with right-sided and mid-epigastric pain. The patient has type 2 diabetes mellitus (DM) and is currently taking a weekly dose of GLP-1RA. The FNP orders a complete metabolic panel and complete blood count (CBC). What other bloodwork should be ordered?
   A. Homocysteine and amylase
   B. HbA1c and amylase
   C. Amylase and lipase
   D. Lipase and homocysteine

8. Which of the following medications may reduce the motility of the lower esophageal sphincter (LES) and thereby decrease its effective function?
   A. Ibuprofen
   B. Pseudoephedrine
   C. Furosemide
   D. ACE inhibitors

9. An 80-year-old male patient comes to the clinic with complaints of diarrhea for 2 days. The FNP notes that the patient had been hospitalized 2 weeks ago for pneumonia. What is the most appropriate next question to ask the patient?
   A. What type of antibiotic were you given in the hospital?
   B. How many days were you hospitalized?
   C. How many times per day are you passing stool?
   D. What over-the-counter medications are you taking for the diarrhea?

10. A patient with generalized lower abdominal pain and nausea is being evaluated. The patient has a low-grade fever (100.4°F). Which of the following signs, if found upon physical examination, would suggest appendicitis?
    A. Mittelschmerz
    B. Psoas
    C. Murphy's
    D. Kernig

11. Crohn's disease differs from ulcerative colitis (UC) because:
    A. Crohn's disease causes more severe abdominal cramping.
    B. Crohn's disease may affect any part of the gastrointestinal (GI) tract. UC is limited to the large intestine.
    C. UC symptoms tend to flare up more often around menses.
    D. UC is a chronic condition, whereas Crohn's disease may occur once, and no further flare-ups happen.

12. A 47-year-old male patient is in the office for a physical examination. He has not been seen in 3 years. The FNP discusses three screening options for detecting colon cancer with the patient. What are appropriate colorectal screening options for this patient?
    A. Yearly fecal immunochemical testing (FIT), colonoscopy every 10 years, FIT every year along with flexible sigmoidoscopy every 5 years
    B. Colonoscopy every 5 years, FIT annually
    C. Annual FIT along with flexible sigmoidoscopy or colonoscopy every 3 years
    D. Yearly colonoscopy and FIT for those with genetic predisposition to colon cancer

13. A 28-year-old man with a long-standing history of IV drug use presents with malaise, nausea, fatigue, and "yellow eyes" for the past week. After ordering diagnostic tests, you confirm the diagnosis of acute hepatitis B. Anticipated laboratory results include:
    A. positive hepatitis B surface antibody (HBsAB).
    B. eosinophilia.
    C. lymphopenia.
    D. positive hepatitis B surface antigen HBsAG.

14. Which of the following is true concerning the hepatitis B vaccine?
    A. The vaccine contains live hepatitis B virus.
    B. The nurse practitioner (NP) should consider postvaccination HBsAB titers for those at the highest risk of infection.
    C. The vaccine is contraindicated in the presence of HIV infection.
    D. Post-vaccine arthralgias are often reported.

15. Serologic features of acute hepatitis B are:
    A. HBsAg reactive and high titer of IgM.
    B. HBsAg reactive and high titer of IgG.
    C. HBeAg and HBsAg negative.
    D. IgM anti-HBc (high titer) HBsAg-nonreactive.

16. Monitoring for hepatocellular carcinoma in a patient with chronic hepatitis B or C often includes the periodic evaluation of which of the following?
    A. Erythrocyte sedimentation rate (ESR)
    B. HBsAB
    C. Alpha-fetoprotein (AFP)
    D. Serum creatinine level

17. Which factors predict the severity of chronic liver disease in a patient with chronic hepatitis C?
    A. Female, younger than 30 years old
    B. Genotype, viral load, and daily alcohol use
    C. Acquisition of the virus through IV drug use and a history of hepatitis A infection
    D. ALT and AST levels

18. What is the *most common* source for hepatitis A infection?
    A. Needle sharing
    B. Raw shellfish
    C. Contaminated water supplies
    D. Intimate person-to-person contact

19. Effective treatment of *H. pylori* can be expected to result in the following:
    A. Treatment of the initial episode, which may recur with stress
    B. A protective mucosal barrier to gastric acid
    C. The need to repeat the same triple therapy if symptoms persist
    D. Eradication of the bacteria

20. A 67-year-old male presents to the office with a chief complaint of a chronic cough for 3 years that has worsened in the past 2 months. The cough keeps him awake at night and is nonproductive, but he denies any wheezing, fever, chills, hemoptysis, dyspnea or shortness of breath, night sweats, or sick contacts. He has a history of chronic obstructive pulmonary disease (COPD) and stopped smoking 10 years ago. His physical exam is negative except for a BMI of 32 and his respiratory exam reveals slight bibasilar crackles, which do not clear with cough, but no rales, rhonchi, and wheezing. With the information you now have, what are the differential diagnoses?
    A. Lung cancer, chronic bronchitis, and gastroesophageal reflux disease (GERD)
    B. Postnasal drip, tuberculosis (TB), upper respiratory infection
    C. COPD, gastroesophageal reflux disease, and allergic rhinitis
    D. Possible TB, pneumonia, GERD

21. Which of the following diagnostics would be *most* helpful in initial clinical decision-making for the patient in question 20?
    A. Posterior/anterior (PA) and lateral chest X-ray (CXR), endoscopy
    B. Pulmonary function tests (PFT), CBC, and erythrocyte sedimentation rate (ESR)
    C. Sputum smear and culture for acid-fast bacilli
    D. CBC, complete metabolic panel (CMP), *H. pylori* breath test

22. A 55-year-old schoolteacher with type 2 DM presents to your office with complaints of a low-grade fever for 3 days and cramping pain in their RUQ, radiating to the right scapula. Laboratory diagnostics indicate:

WBC	13,000	(NL 4.5–11,000)
SGOT (AST)	55	(NL 5–40)
SGPT (ALT)	65	(NL 5–55)
BUN	25	(NL 6–25)
Alk. Phos.	140	(NL 35–110)
Amylase	130	(NL 20–90)

    The physical exam reveals epigastric tenderness, guarding, and a positive Murphy's sign. The FNP suspects:
    A. acute cholecystitis.
    B. acute appendicitis.
    C. hepatitis.
    D. peptic ulcer disease (PUD).

23. The most important contributing factor to the development of a PUD is:
    A. eating spicy/acidic foods.
    B. using nonsteroidal anti-inflammatory drugs (NSAIDs).
    C. stress.
    D. drinking alcohol.

24. A 78-year-old male patient walks into the office complaining of feeling lightheaded for a few hours. He appears pale and anxious. Past medical history includes controlled atrial fibrillation, hypertension, and hyperlipidemia. The patient's vital signs include:
    - Temp. 98.2°F
    - BP 100/58
    - heart rate 92
    - resp. rate 16
    - O_2 sat 94%

    Which of the following findings from the physical exam are most concerning?
    A. Obturator sign
    B. Cohen's sign
    C. Jacob's sign
    D. Cullen's sign

25. A 19-year-old male football player was injured during the game. The patient is pale, anxious, and complains of LUQ abdominal pain radiating to the left shoulder. The FNP recognizes that this most likely indicates:
    A. a ruptured spleen
    B. an acute pancreatitis
    C. a right-sided pneumothorax
    D. a testicular torsion

Answers With Enhanced Rationales

1. Answer C is correct. HAV total Ab, HCV Ab, anti-HBc, and anti-HBS. HAV total AB and HCV Ab will detect antibodies against hepatitis A and B, respectively, indicating a previous infection. If anti-HBc and anti-HBs are both positive, this would indicate a past hepatitis B infection. HAV viral load and HBV viral load assess the amount of virus in a currently infected person with hepatitis A and B, respectively.

    Answer A is incorrect. HAV viral load and HBV viral load assess the amount of virus in a currently infected person with hepatitis A and hepatitis B, respectively. This patient states he has a history of hepatitis. IgG levels are a nonspecific indicator of infection or autoimmune disease.

    Answer B is incorrect. HCV Ag is a screening test for early hepatitis C, not chronic hepatitis C.

    Answer D is incorrect. HAV IgM indicates an active HAV infection. HBV viral load is an appropriate test for a currently infected person.

2. Answer C is correct. Past hepatitis A infection, chronic hepatitis B infection. Positive HAV Ab total indicates past hepatitis A infection. HBsAg positive, HBsAb negative indicate chronic hepatitis B infection.

    Answer A is incorrect. HCV Ab is nonreactive and indicates no prior hepatitis C infection.

    Answer B is incorrect. HbsAb negative indicates no immunity to hepatitis B.

    Answer D is incorrect. Patient does have a past hepatitis A infection, but lab tests indicate a chronic hepatitis B infection.

3. Answer A is correct. The history of injury during physical contact along with left-sided pain and referred pain to the left shoulder is likely a ruptured spleen.

    Answer B is incorrect. Acute pancreatitis usually manifests as mid-epigastric abdominal pain along with nausea, vomiting, and anorexia. The pain more commonly radiates to the back.

    Answer C is incorrect. A right-sided pneumothorax would manifest symptoms on the right side of the chest.

    Answer D is incorrect. An upper GI bleed is most related to a peptic ulcer. The patient would typically be vomiting blood.

4. Answer B is correct. Liver ultrasound, liver enzymes, AFP, and HCV viral load are all appropriate annual monitoring tests.

    Answer A is incorrect. An annual CT scan is not appropriate and exposes the patient to large amounts of radiation, so a liver biopsy is not warranted.

    Answer C is incorrect. A liver biopsy is not a routine procedure and would be performed only when necessary to look for malignancy or other pathology.

    Answer D is incorrect. An annual abdominal CT scan is not an appropriate routine test for an asymptomatic patient with a history of HCV.

5. Answer B is correct. An increase in exercise, such as walking may stimulate bowel movements, and

daily medications, such as magnesium hydroxide or polyethylene glycol (Mirlax) will draw water into the intestines, softening stools. Having the patient return for evaluation in 1 month is a realistic plan.

Answer A is incorrect. The patient should not be instructed to take daily Dulcolax, as this leads to laxative dependence and electrolyte disturbances. Dulcolax may be used on occasion.

Answer C is incorrect. Using a fleet enema daily leads to dependence on enemas to evacuate the bowels and electrolyte imbalance.

Answer D is incorrect. A CT scan of the abdomen is not warranted. If other interventions are not effective, the patient may need this in the future and should then be referred to a GI specialist.

6. Answer C is correct. Murphy's sign involves pain in the upper right abdomen when the examiner palpates the abdominal area just under the ribcage during inspiration.

Answer A is incorrect. Cullen's sign indicates ecchymosis around the umbilicus, which may indicate intraperitoneal or retroperitoneal bleeding.

Answer B is incorrect. A positive Rosvig's sign indicates a likely appendicitis when the examiner palpates the left side of the abdomen and the patient experiences pain on the right side of the abdomen.

Answer D is incorrect. The psoas sign indicates an inflamed appendix, and the pain is elicited by the patient lying on the left side and flexing the right thigh backwards.

7. Answer C is correct. Amylase and lipase will help the NP rule out pancreatitis. Amylase has the greater sensitivity and specificity of the two tests.

Answer A is incorrect. Homocysteine levels are used to diagnose vitamin B deficiencies.

Answer B is incorrect. An HbA1C level does not help determine the source of epigastric pain. It is an indicator of blood glucose average over the previous 3 months.

Answer D is incorrect. Amylase is the better choice when suspecting pancreatitis. Homocysteine levels are not diagnostic for pancreatitis.

8. Answer A is correct. NSAIDs, such as ibuprofen, are known to affect and worsen GERD and PUD and can irritate the stomach lining, causing gastritis. Some studies have shown that it also relaxes the LES.

Answer B is incorrect. Pseudoephedrine commonly causes nervousness, tachycardia, headache, and nausea.

Answer C is incorrect. Furosemide does not affect the LES.

Answer D is incorrect. ACE inhibitors do not affect the LES. Be aware that beta blockers and calcium channel blockers may reduce the motility of the LES and lead to GERD.

9. Answer C is correct. The FNP needs to assess the severity of the diarrhea and inquire about the frequency, quality, and amount of diarrhea. Individual perception of constipation or diarrhea can vary greatly.

Answer A is incorrect. All antibiotics may potentially cause diarrhea. A patient who has been hospitalized for pneumonia will likely have received antibiotic therapy.

Answer B is incorrect. The length of time a patient spends in the hospital will not help to determine the etiology of the patient's diarrhea.

Answer D is incorrect. Ascertaining what OTC medications the patient has used to control the diarrhea may help determine the effectiveness of treatment, but the FNP first needs to determine the degree of diarrhea the patient is experiencing.

10. Answer B is the correct answer. Positive psoas can indicate appendicitis.

Answer A is incorrect. Mittelschmerz is low abdominal pain experienced during ovulation.

Answer C is incorrect. A positive Murphy's sign is an indicator of cholecystitis.

Answer D is incorrect. A positive Kernig sign can indicate meningeal irritation.

11. Answer B is correct. Crohn's disease differs from ulcerative colitis in that Crohn's may affect any part of the gastrointestinal (GI) tract. UC is limited to the large intestine.

Answer A is incorrect. Both conditions may cause severe abdominal cramping.

Answer C is incorrect. UC is a chronic condition that has flare-ups and periods of remission that are not associated with menses.

Answer D is incorrect. Both conditions are chronic with periods of remission and exacerbation.

12. Answer A is correct. Yearly FIT, colonoscopy every 10 years, FIT every year, and flexible sigmoidoscopy every 5 years. The United States Preventative Services Task Force (USPSTF)

recommends the following for all adults between the ages of 45 and 75:
- High-sensitivity guaiac fecal occult blood test (HSgFOBT) or FIT every year
- Stool DNA-FIT every 1 to 3 years
- Computed tomography colonography every 5 years
- Flexible sigmoidoscopy every 5 years
- Flexible sigmoidoscopy every 10 years + annual FIT
- Colonoscopy screening every 10 years

Answer B is incorrect. A colonoscopy is recommended every 10 years unless there is a concern by the gastroenterologist that more frequent monitoring is necessary.

Answer C is incorrect. An annual FIT is appropriate; however, sigmoidoscopy or colonoscopy every three years are not standard screening recommendations.

Answer D is incorrect. A yearly colonoscopy is unnecessary unless recommended by a GI specialist. This patient was not identified as a high-risk patient in the question.

13. Answer D is correct. Positive HBsAG indicates acute infection.

    Answer A is incorrect. A positive hepatitis B surface antibody indicates a prior infection.

    Answer B is incorrect. Eosinophilia is a result of the bone marrow making too many eosinophils. This is mostly caused by allergies, parasitic or fungal infections, or autoimmune disorders.

    Answer C is incorrect. Lymphopenia is an abnormally low level of lymphocytes. It may be seen in HIV+ infections and is most commonly due to a recent infection, such as a common cold, flu, or other viruses.

14. Answer B is correct. The FNP should consider postvaccination HBsAB titers for those at the highest risk of infection.

    Answer A is incorrect. The hepatitis B vaccine is not a live vaccine and is often recommended in persons with HIV and other conditions affecting the immune system.

    Answer C is incorrect. The hepatitis B vaccine should be offered to those persons who are HIV+.

    Answer D is incorrect. The hepatitis B vaccine is not a live vaccine and is well tolerated. The most common symptoms after vaccination are redness, swelling, or soreness at the injection site.

15. Answer A is correct. The presence of HBsAg indicates HBV infection, either acute or chronic, except when it might be transiently positive shortly after a dose of HepB vaccine. IgM anti-HBc is a hallmark of acute HBV infection and is typically detectable at the onset of symptoms, persisting for 6 to 9 months following infection.

    Answer B is incorrect. A high titer of IgG indicates previous infection.

    Answer C is incorrect. A negative HbeAg would indicate that the person is no longer acutely infected with the e-antigen. Acute hepatitis would have a positive HbsAg (Hepatitis B surface antigen)

    Answer D is incorrect. An anti-HBc (hepatitis B core antibody) indicates that the patient was likely infected with the hepatitis B in the past. A nonreactive hepatitis B surface antigen indicates no active infection.

16. Answer C is correct. AFP is made by a fetus's liver and is found in low levels in adults unless they have certain cancers, particularly hepatocellular cancer.

    Answer A is incorrect. An ESR is only an indicator of an inflammatory response by the body.

    Answer B is incorrect. The HBsAB will always be positive because it indicates a prior infection.

    Answer D is incorrect. Serum creatinine level reflects kidney function.

17. Answer B is correct. Genotype, viral load, and daily alcohol use predict the severity of chronic liver disease in a patient with hepatitis C. Male gender and HIV coinfection are risk factors for more progressive, severe HCV disease.

    Answer A is incorrect. Female sex is not a predictor of severity.

    Answer C is incorrect. Hepatitis C is mainly transmitted through contact with infected blood. How it is acquired is not a determinant of the severity of the liver disease.

    Answer D is incorrect. While elevations in liver function tests (LFTs) may help look for disease states that affect the liver, severe liver disease that results in liver cirrhosis can reduce the liver's ability to release these enzymes. Therefore, elevations in ALT and AST values are not always a valid predictor of the extent of liver disease.

18. Answer C is correct. Contaminated water supplies are the most common source of hepatitis A transmission.

    Answer A is incorrect. Sharing of needles is a more common way of transmitting hepatitis B and C.

Answer B is incorrect. Raw shellfish harvested from a contaminated water supply may cause hepatitis A, but it is not the most common source.

Answer D is incorrect. Intimate person-to-person contact may cause transmission of hepatitis B or C. It is possible to transmit hepatitis A between persons through inadequate sanitation, poor personal hygiene, and anal-oral sex, but this is not the most common mode of transmission.

19. Answer D is correct. Eradication of the bacteria. The goal of therapy for a person infected with *H. pylori* is to eradicate the bacteria to prevent complications.

    Answer A is incorrect. *H. pylori* is not stress induced.

    Answer B is incorrect. *H. pylori* treatment consists of typically two antibiotics and a proton-pump inhibitor (PPI). The PPI may reduce gastric acid, but it does not provide a protective mucosal barrier and is not the goal of therapy. While bismuth subsalicylate (commonly known as Pepto Bismol) may protect the stomach from acid, it does not eradicate the *H. pylori* bacteria.

    Answer C is incorrect. Testing for eradication of *H. pylori* is done approximately 4 weeks after therapy is completed. If *H. pylori* is still present, a different regimen of antibiotics may be needed. Repeating the same triple therapy would not be effective.

20. Answer A is correct. Lung cancer, chronic bronchitis, and GERD are the differentials for this patient.

    Answer B is incorrect. He is currently not experiencing any symptoms of TB (night sweats, weight loss)

    Answer C is incorrect. No evidence of allergic rhinitis (no boggy or pale nasal turbinates) exists.

    Answer D is incorrect. The patient is not experiencing symptoms consistent with TB. His symptoms have lasted longer than 2 months without fever, chills, or sick contacts. Therefore, it is unlikely that he has pneumonia.

21. Answer A is correct. The CXR will rule out pneumonia, pleural effusion, and/or congestive heart failure, although it should not be used to assess for lung cancer. Low-dose radiation CT scan will assist in the diagnosis of lung cancer. The endoscopy will evaluate for any erythema or ulcers related to GERD.

    Answer B is incorrect. PFTs will only help identify worsening symptoms if compared with the patient's baseline PFT. CBC and SED rates may indicate infection but are nonspecific tests and would not help identify lung cancer, GERD, or chronic bronchitis.

    Answer C is incorrect. A sputum smear and culture for acid fast bacilli are tests done to assess for TB. This patient does not exhibit TB symptoms.

    Answer D is incorrect. A CBC and CMP would not be specific enough to assist in the diagnosis, and the *H. pylori* test specifically looks for peptic ulcers. The patient does not exhibit symptoms of peptic ulcers.

22. Answer A is correct. Mild elevation of white blood cells, liver enzymes, and amylase are found in patients with acute cholecystitis.

    Answer B is incorrect. The patient would have been expected to have some tenderness in the right lower quadrant. Additionally, the amylase would not be elevated.

    Answer C is incorrect. Although hepatitis is a possible differential diagnosis, the patient's subjective symptoms of colicky RUQ pain with radiation are more consistent with cholecystitis.

    Answer D is incorrect. Patients with PUD commonly experience pain in the LUQ over the stomach area. The pain may be worse between meals and at night. Patients with PUD may experience a feeling of fullness, bloating, nausea, and heartburn.

23. Answer B is correct. Overuse of NSAIDS or infection with *H. pylori* are risk factors for the development of PUD.

    Answer A is incorrect. Eating spicy or acidic foods may worsen the symptoms of PUD, but it is not a contributing factor to the development of the disease.

    Answer C is incorrect. Stress may worsen the symptoms, but it is not the cause of PUD.

    Answer D is incorrect. Drinking alcohol may increase stomach acid and worsen symptoms, but in and of itself, it does not cause stomach ulcers. However, alcohol and smoking may make the ulcers worse, and therefore, it will take longer to heal.

24. Answer D is correct. Cullen's sign causes a bluish discoloration in the periumbilical area that may indicate retroperitoneal bleeding, which can occur in patients on warfarin or anticoagulants. The patient is showing early signs of hypovolemia.

    Answer A is incorrect. Obturator sign occurs when the right knee is flexed and passively internally rotated. It is an indicator of an inflamed appendix.

Answer B is incorrect. Cohen's sign is a developmental abnormality characterized by hypotonia, intellectual impairment, delayed milestones, microcephaly, neutropenia, joint laxity, characteristic facial features, overly friendly behavior, and truncal obesity.

Answer C is incorrect. Jacob's sign is a genetic condition in which the male child has an extra y chromosome (XYY). It may go undiagnosed or the patient may exhibit mild learning disabilities and behavioral disturbances.

25. Answer A. is correct. Traumatic injuries are the most common cause of splenic rupture, which is a life-threatening condition. The pain is commonly in the LUQ of the abdomen and radiating to the left shoulder. This is known as Kehr's sign.

Answer B is incorrect. The primary symptom of acute pancreatitis is abdominal pain that often causes nausea, vomiting, and fever. The most common causes of acute pancreatitis are cholelithiasis and heavy drinking.

Answer C is incorrect. A right-sided pneumothorax would cause pain in the RUQ accompanied by shortness of breath.

Answer D is incorrect. Testicular torsion causes severe pain in the scrotum as well as lower abdominal pain, nausea and vomiting.

Resources

Alexandraki, I., & Smetana, G. (2024). *Acute viral gastroenteritis in adults*. https://www.uptodate.com/contents/acute-viral-gastroenteritis-in-adults?search=acute%20viral%20gastroenteritis%20in%20adults&source=search_result&selectedTitle=1~150&usage_type=default&display_rank=1

American Cancer Society. (2023). *American Cancer Society guidelines for the early detection of cancer*. https://www.cancer.org/cancer/screening/american-cancer-society-guidelines-for-the-early-detection-of-cancer.html

Berman, J. (2023). *Gamma-glutamyl transferase (GGT) blood test*. Medline Plus. https://www.nlm.nih.gov/medlineplus/ency/article/003458.htm

Bleday, R. (2023). *Anal fissure: Medical management*. https://www.uptodate.com/contents/anal-fissure-medical-management?search=anal%20fissure&source=search_result&selectedTitle=1~92&usage_type=default&display_rank=1

Bleday, R., & Breen, E. (2023a). *Hemorrhoids: Clinical manifestations and diagnosis*. https://www.uptodate.com/contents/hemorrhoids-clinical-manifestations-and-diagnosis?search=hemorrhoids%20management&source=search_result&selectedTitle=3~150&usage_type=default&display_rank=3

Bleday, R., & Breen, E. (2023b). *Home and office treatment of symptomatic hemorrhoids*. https://www.uptodate.com/contents/home-and-office-treatment-of-symptomatic-hemorrhoids?search=hemorrhoid%20treatment&source=search_result&selectedTitle=1~150&usage_type=default&display_rank=1

Cartwright, S. L. & Knudson, M. P. (2008). Evaluation of acute abdominal pain in adults. *American Family Physician, 77*(7): 971–978. http://www.aafp.org/afp/2008/0401/p971.html

Centers for Disease Control and Prevention. (2025a). *Clinical testing and diagnosis for hepatitis B*. https://www.cdc.gov/hepatitis-b/hcp/diagnosis-testing/?CDC_AAref_Val=https://www.cdc.gov/hepatitis/hbv/interpretationOfHepBSerologicResults.htm

Centers for Disease Control and Prevention. (2025b). *Clinical screening and diagnosis for hepatitis C*. https://www.cdc.gov/hepatitis-c/hcp/diagnosis-testing/?CDC_AAref_Val=https://www.cdc.gov/hepatitis/hcv/guidelinesc.htm

Centers for Disease Control and Prevention. (2020). The ABCs of hepatitis—for health professionals. https://www.cdc.gov/hepatitis/resources/professionals/pdfs/ABCTable.pdf

Chopra, S., & Lai, M. (2024). *Management of metabolic dysfunction-associated steatotic liver disease (nonalcoholic fatty liver disease) in adults*. https://www.uptodate.com/contents/management-of-nonalcoholic-fatty-liver-disease-in-adults?search=nonalcoholic%20steatohepatitis&source=search_result&selectedTitle=1~104&usage_type=default&display_rank=1

Gilbert, D., Chambers, H., Eliopoulos, G., Saag, M., Black, D., Freedman, D., Pavia, A., & Schwartz, B. (2023). *The Sanford guide to antimicrobial therapy 2023* (53rd ed.). Antimicrobial Therapy, Inc.

GlobalRPh. (n.d.). *Diverticulitis*. https://globalrph.com/antibiotic/diverticulitis/

Goolsby, M. J., & Grubbs, L. (2022). *Advanced assessment: Interpreting findings and formulating differential diagnoses* (5th ed.). F.A. Davis.

Hall, J., Hardiman, K., Lee, S., Lightner, A., Stocchi, L., Paquette, I. M., Steele, S. R., Feingold, D. L., & Prepared on behalf of the Clinical Practice Guidelines Committee of the American Society of Colon and Rectal Surgeons (2020). The American Society of Colon and Rectal Surgeons Clinical Practice Guidelines for the Treatment of Left-Sided Colonic Diverticulitis. *Diseases of the Colon and Rectum, 63*(6), 728–747. https://doi.org/10.1097/DCR.0000000000001679

Hashash, J., & Regueiro, M. (2025). *Medical management of moderate to severe Crohn disease in adults*. UpToDate. https://www.uptodate.com/contents/medical-management-of-moderate-to-severe-crohn-disease-in-adults?search=crohns%20treatment&source=search_result&selectedTitle=2~150&usage_type=default&display_rank=2

Hashash, J., & Regueiro, M. (2023). *Medical management of low-risk adult patients with mild to moderate ulcerative colitis*. UpToDate. https://www.uptodate.com/contents/medical-management-of-low-risk-adult-patients-with-mild-to-moderate-ulcerative-colitis?search=ulcerative%20colitis%20treatment&sectionRank=2&usage_type=default&anchor=H27&source=machineLearning&selectedTitle=1~150&display_rank=1#H1226801754

Kahrilas, P. (2025). *Initial management of gastroesophageal reflux disease in adults*. UpToDate. https://www.uptodate.com/contents/medical-management-of-gastroesophageal-reflux-disease-in-adults?search=GERD&source=search_result&selectedTitle=3~150&usage_type=default&display_rank=3

Kelly, C. P., Lamont, J. T., & Bakken, J. S. (2025). *Clostridioides difficile infection in adults: treatment and prevention*. UpToDate. https://

www.uptodate.com/contents/clostridioides-difficile-infection-in-adults-treatment-and-prevention?search=c%20diff%20colitis%20treatment&sectionRank=3&usage_type=default&anchor=H35&source=machineLearning&selectedTitle=1~150&display_rank=1#H35

Lamont, T., Kelly, C. P., & Bakken, J. S. (2025). *Clostridioides difficile infection in adults: Clinical manifestations and diagnosis.* UpToDate. https://www.uptodate.com/contents/clostridioides-difficile-infection-in-adults-clinical-manifestations-and-diagnosis?search=c%20diff%20colitis&source=search_result&selectedTitle=1~150&usage_type=default&display_rank=1

Macrae, F. A., Parikh, A. R., Ricciardi, R. (2025). *Clinical presentation, diagnosis, and staging of colorectal cancer.* UpToDate. https://www.uptodate.com/contents/clinical-presentation-diagnosis-and-staging-of-colorectal-cancer?search=colon%20cancer%20staging&source=search_result&selectedTitle=1~150&usage_type=default&display_rank=1

Martin, R. F. (2024). *Acute appendicitis in adults: Clinical manifestations and differential diagnosis.* UpToDate. https://www.uptodate.com/contents/acute-appendicitis-in-adults-clinical-manifestations-and-differential-diagnosis?search=acute%20appendicitis%20adult&source=search_result&selectedTitle=2~150&usage_type=default&display_rank=2

Mayo Clinic Staff. (2022). *Viral gastroenteritis (stomach flu).* Mayo Clinic. http://www.mayoclinic.org/diseases-conditions/viral-gastroenteritis/basics/definition/con-20019350

Peery, A. F., Shaukat, A., & Strate, L. L. (2021). AGA clinical practice update on medical management of colonic diverticulitis: Expert review. *Gastroenterology, 160*(3), 906–911.e1.

Peppercorn, M. A., & Kane, S. V. (2024). *Clinical manifestations, diagnosis, and prognosis of ulcerative colitis in adults.* UpToDate. https://www.uptodate.com/contents/clinical-manifestations-diagnosis-and-prognosis-of-ulcerative-colitis-in-adults?search=ulcerative%20colitis&source=search_result&selectedTitle=1~150&usage_type=default&display_rank=1

Raghavendran, K. (2025). *Acute colonic diverticulitis: Triage and inpatient management.* UpToDate. https://www.uptodate.com/contents/acute-colonic-diverticulitis-medical-management?search=diverticulitis%20treatment%20outpatient&sectionRank=1&usage_type=default&anchor=H667444990&source=machineLearning&selectedTitle=2~150&display_rank=2#H667444990

Regueiro, M., & Hashash, J. (2024). *Overview of the medical management of mild (low risk) Crohn disease in adults.* UpToDate. https://www.uptodate.com/contents/overview-of-the-medical-management-of-mild-low-risk-crohn-disease-in-adults?search=crohns%20treatment&source=search_result&selectedTitle=1~150&usage_type=default&display_rank=1

Rinella, M. E., & Sookoian, S. (2024). From NAFLD to MASLD: Updated naming and diagnosis criteria for fatty liver disease. *Journal of Lipid Research, 65*(1), 100485. https://doi.org/10.1016/j.jlr.2023.100485

Smink, D., & Soybel, D. I. (2024). *Management of acute appendicitis in adults.* UpToDate. https://www.uptodate.com/contents/management-of-acute-appendicitis-in-adults?search=appendicitis&source=search_result&selectedTitle=1~150&usage_type=default&display_rank=1

Vakil, N. B. (2024a). *Peptic ulcer disease: Clinical manifestation and diagnosis.* UpToDate. https://www.uptodate.com/contents/peptic-ulcer-disease-clinical-manifestations-and-diagnosis?search=pud&source=search_result&selectedTitle=2~150&usage_type=default&display_rank=2

Vakil, N. B. (2024b). *Peptic ulcer disease: Treatment and secondary prevention.* Uptodate. https://www.uptodate.com/contents/peptic-ulcer-disease-treatment-and-secondary-prevention?search=pud%20treatment&sectionRank=3&usage_type=default&anchor=H19&source=machineLearning&selectedTitle=1~150&display_rank=1#H368390202

Wald, A. (2025). *Treatment of irritable bowel syndrome in adults.* UpToDate. https://www.uptodate.com/contents/treatment-of-irritable-bowel-syndrome-in-adults?search=irritable%20bowel%20syndrome&source=search_result&selectedTitle=1~150&usage_type=default&display_rank=1

Wald, A., & Rao, S. (2025). *Management of chronic constipation in adults.* UpToDate. https://www.uptodate.com/contents/management-of-chronic-constipation-in-adults?search=constipation&source=search_result&selectedTitle=1~150&usage_type=default&display_rank=1

Zakko, S. (2024). *Clinical manifestation and evaluation of gallstone disease in adults.* UpToDate. https://www.uptodate.com/contents/overview-of-gallstone-disease-in-adults?search=calculus%20cholecystitis&source=search_result&selectedTitle=1~150&usage_type=default&display_rank=1

CHAPTER 10

Musculoskeletal Review

Nancy L. Dennert, MS, MSN, FNP-BC, CDCES, BC-ADM

In the primary care setting, 10 to 20 percent of outpatient primary care visits are for musculoskeletal (MS) injuries. These injuries may be traumatic (injury related) or atraumatic (i.e., overuse or degenerative syndromes) as well as acute or chronic.

- Sprains and strains are the most common.
- Injuries to ligaments occur secondary to sudden stress on an affected joint.
- Ankle (inversion) sprains are the most common and may be sports related or occur during normal daily activities such as stepping off a curb or into a hole.

Assessment of the injury in the primary care setting:

- Chief complaint
- History of present illness (HPI): Onset history and location—typically pain, instability, or dysfunction—ask patient to "point to pain." Remember the seven attributes of a symptom OLD-CART: Onset, Location, Duration, Characteristic, Aggravating or Alleviating factors, and Timing.
- Review of systems (ROS): Assess the MS system and the patient's injury, including safety and mobility considerations.
- Physical Exam: Inspection (swelling, erythema, atrophy, deformity, surgical scars), palpation, range of motion (ROM), and neurovascular status
- Tests that can be done in the primary care setting by the practitioner:
  - Provocative: Recreate mechanism of injury to reproduce pain
  - Stress: Apply load to ligament of concern
  - Functional: Simple tasks performed with activities of daily living

Imaging Considerations:

- Standard (2 planes/views—Anterior/posterior (AP) and lateral or both obliques—mortise) radiographs for bony pathology assessment.
- CT can visualize bony pathology and morphology of fractures.
- Nuclear bone scans identify stress fractures, infection, malignancy, or multisite pathology.
- MRI visualizes ligaments, cartilage, and soft tissues.
- Ultrasound identifies superficial tissue problems, including tendinopathies and synovial problems.

Foot and Ankle

Morton (Interdigital) Neuroma

- Morton neuroma is a nonneoplastic perineural fibrous proliferation involving the plantar digital nerve usually between the 3 and 4 toes, or less commonly the 2 and 3 toes, and affecting women more than men.
- Symptoms include pain in the involved web space that often radiates to the toes. Numbness, burning, and tingling may also be present.

Clinical Presentation

- Clinical exam
- Mulder's sign
- Magnetic resonance imaging (MRI) or ultrasound (US)
- Rule out metatarsal fracture

Treatment
- Shoe wear modification
  - Orthotics with a possible metatarsal pad
  - Rocker bottom shoes.

Plantar Fasciitis
- The most common cause of plantar heel pain.
- Characterized by heel pain with the first steps in the morning or when standing up after prolonged sitting and tenderness at the calcaneal tuberosity that is increased with passive dorsiflexion of the toes. There is often a history of prolonged WB (weight-bearing) activity either recreationally or occupationally resulting in repetitive microtrauma to the heel. Can occur in isolation or be a manifestation of systemic disease such as RA (rheumatoid arthritis) or other spondyloarthropathy.

Clinical Presentation
- Clinical exam
- Possibly MRI, US, or bone scintigraphy

Treatment
- Analgesics
- Stretching
- Exercise
- Orthotics
- Night splints
- Taping
- Physical therapy (PT)
- Corticosteroid injections
- A plantar fasciotomy can be performed in severe cases.

Bilateral Heel Pain
Bilateral heel pain has several causes, including plantar fasciitis; Achilles tendinopathy (pain is usually more posterior heel); Achilles bursitis; calcaneal stress fractures; tarsal tunnel syndrome (consider if pain is accompanied by tingling, burning, or numbness in the heel, which may radiate into the sole of the foot and worsens with ankle dorsiflexion and eversion); heel pad atrophy, especially in older individuals and patients with obesity; osteomyelitis (signs of infection, especially in those with vascular compromise); peripheral nerve entrapment (especially if there are sensory changes); and as a result of rheumatologic disorders or malignancy.

Achilles Tendinopathy
Achilles tendinopathy causes pain in the posterior ankle and heel, which worsens with running, jumping, and quick motions. Risk factors include abnormal ankle dorsiflexion motion, increased foot pronation, obesity, hypertension (HTN), hyperlipidemia, diabetes mellitus (DM), and training errors.

Clinical Presentation
- Subjective pain reports with local pain, swelling, and stiffness in the Achilles tendon region, especially following a period of inactivity.
- Initially, these symptoms may lessen with activity and then increase again after activity.
- Clinical tests include tenderness to palpation over the tendon or posterior calcaneus, a positive arc sign and positive Royal London Hospital Test, and pain with resisted plantar flexion.
- US and MRI can aid diagnosis.

Treatment
- Modalities
  - Laser
  - Iontophoresis
- Stretching
- Foot orthoses
- Manual therapy
- PT
- Taping
- Heel lifts
- Night splints

Charcot Neuropathic Osteoarthropathy (Charcot Foot)
Charcot Foot is a foot pathology that occurs in the presence of a peripheral neuropathy (usually diabetic), where inflammation leads to osteolysis, subluxation, dislocation, and foot deformity. Due to a loss of pain sensation, WB activities may continue to cause further repetitive trauma.

Clinical Presentation
- The hallmark sign is mid-foot collapse, described as a "rocker-bottom foot".
- There is neuropathy with reduced pain sensation, swelling, warmth, erythematous foot with mild to moderate pain.

- Radiographs for fracture and subluxation, as well as MRIs, aid in clinical diagnosis.
- Cellulitis, deep vein thrombosis (DVT), and gout should be ruled out.

Treatment
- Offloading the foot to arrest progression of the deformity.
- Immobilization with cast and assistive devices, such as crutches or wheelchair, may be used initially until swelling resolves.
- Transition to a walking boot and maybe eventually custom footwear.
- Surgery may be required to resect any infection or bony prominences that cannot be accommodated.
- Achilles tendon lengthening and arthrodesis may be last-resort surgeries.
- Pharmacologically, anti-resorption bone therapy, such as calcitonin, may be initiated.

For any MS injury to a limb, the general rule of initial management is:

P.R.I.C.E

P–Protection from further injury

R–Rest

I–Ice

C–Compression

E–Elevation

Ankle Sprain Lateral/Medial
- Lateral and medial ankle sprains are due to trauma involving inversion for a lateral ankle sprain or eversion for a medial ankle sprain.
- An ankle sprain is diagnosed primarily through a physical assessment of the foot and ankle as well as the ability to bear weight. The Ottowa Ankle rules help to determine if a foot and ankle X-ray is needed.

Clinical Presentation
- Tenderness over the involved ligaments
- Swelling
- Limited motion
- Pain
- Possible bruising or discoloration
- Decreased strength
- Altered gait and balance, depending on the severity

Risk Factors
- Previous ankle sprain
- Improper warm up
- Decreased ankle dorsiflexion motion

Treatment
- Initial external support and assistive gait device
- PT, consisting of manual therapy, physical agents, therapeutic exercise, and eventual return to sports training

Compartment Syndrome

Clinical Pearl

The 5 Ps of compartment syndrome:
1. Pain (worsening)
2. Parasthesia (neurologic changes)
3. Pallor (vascular compromise)
4. Paralysis
5. Pulselessness or cyanosis (vascular compromise)

**Acute compartment syndrome is a surgical emergency.

Compartment syndrome results in severe uncontrolled pain, swelling, and pain due to the complication of a foot crush injury, fracture, surgery, vascular injury, and rarely, ankle sprain. Compartment syndrome can be acute or chronic.

Clinical Presentation
- Pain with motion of the foot and toes, which increases with exertion.
- Compartment pressure may be measured by using an intra-compartment pressure monitor.
- Long-term sequelae may include contracture, deformity, weakness, paralysis, and sensory neuropathy.

Treatment
- Acute compartment syndrome is a medical emergency, while chronic compartment syndrome typically is not.
- In severe cases, surgery may be necessary to decompress the limb.

Ottawa Ankle Rules
- X-rays indicate if there is trauma to the foot or ankle, bony pain in the malleolar zone, and any one of the following:
  - Tenderness at the distal 6 cm of the posterior edge of the tibia or tip of medial malleolus
  - Tenderness at the distal 6 cm of posterior edge of the fibula or tip of the lateral malleolus
  - Inability to bear weight both immediately after the injury and in the emergency department (ED) for four steps.

Ottawa Foot/Ankle Rules

- X-rays indicate if there is trauma to the foot or ankle, bony pain in the mid-foot zone, and any one of the following:
  - Tenderness at the base of the fifth metatarsal
  - Tenderness at the navicular bone
  - Inability to bear weight both immediately after the injury and in the ED for four steps

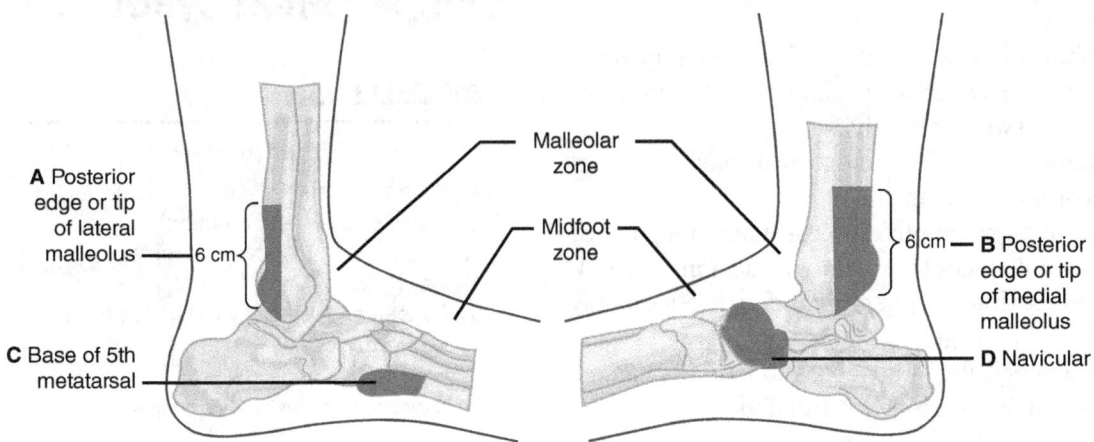

Modified from Stiell, I. G., McKnight, R. D., Greenberg, G. H., McDowell, I., Nair, R. C., Wells, G. A., Johns, C., & Worthington, J. R. (1994). Implementation of the Ottawa ankle rules. *JAMA, 271*(11), 827–832. doi:10.1001/jama.1994.03510350037034.

Knee

Osgood Schlatter Disease

Osgood Schlatter disease is a traction injury of the tibial tuberosity by the quadriceps, affecting children involved in sports (boys more often than girls) between 11 and 15 years old. Usually occurs unilaterally but may be bilateral and often during a growth spurt.

Clinical Presentation
- Pain
- Swelling
- Enlargement of the proximal tibia where the patellar tendon inserts

Treatment
- Over-the-counter (OTC) pain relievers
- PT for stretching, strengthening, and modalities
- Activity modification
- Patellar tendon straps
- The condition is usually self-limiting with good long-term outcomes.

Meniscus Tear

A meniscus tear is a traumatic or degenerative condition of the knee's medial and/or lateral meniscus. Traumatic injuries usually include a WB and rotation mechanism.

Clinical Presentation
- History of mechanical catching or locking in the knee
- Joint line tenderness
- Pain with knee hyperextension
- Maximum passive knee flexion
- Pain or clicking
- Possible stiffness, swelling, and a sensation of the knee giving way
- X-ray and MRI can assist diagnosis.

Treatment
- PT
- Possible arthroscopic surgery

Patellar Fracture

A patellar fracture is an injury to the patella caused by a direct blow, such as a fall or motor vehicle accident (MVA). It is an uncommon fracture comprising only 1 percent of all fractures. The fracture can be classified as stable, displaced, comminuted (three or more pieces) or open.

Clinical Presentation
- Pain and swelling in the anterior knee with bruising and an inability to straighten the knee fully or walk
- X-ray used to confirm diagnosis.

Treatment
- If the fracture is nondisplaced, surgery may be unnecessary with treatment, including casting and splinting and a period of nonweight-bearing (NWB) with crutch use followed by PT.
- If displaced, the usual intervention is surgery followed by PT.

Knee Osteoarthritis

Knee osteoarthritis (OA) is a degenerative condition of the knee joint characterized by progressive loss of motion, strength, and pain.

Clinical Presentation
- Plain radiographs can aid diagnosis.
- Altman Criteria for knee degenerative joint disease (DJD) includes three or more of the following positives:
  - Older than 50 years
  - Morning stiffness lasting less than 30 minutes
  - Crepitus with active knee motion
  - Bony tenderness
  - Bony enlargement
  - No palpable warmth

Treatment
- Acetaminophen
- Capsaicin
- Corticosteroids for pain relief
- PT provides therapeutic exercise, manual therapy, and weight management for patients who have excess weight or obesity (BMI > 25 kg/m^2) with a goal of losing 5 percent of their body weight.
- Aquatic therapy and assistive devices to aid ambulation.
- In severe cases, joint replacement surgery may be indicated, followed by PT and rehabilitation.

Medial Tibial Stress Syndrome (MTSS) (Shin Splints)

Medial tibial stress syndrome (MTSS) is an overuse injury caused by repetitive stress and injury to the anterior shin area. It is multifactorial and may involve tendinopathy, periostitis, tibia stress reaction, tibialis posterior dysfunction, tibialis anterior and/or soleus muscles.

Clinical Presentation
- Vague and diffuse pain and tenderness to palpation along the middle and distal tibia are associated with exertion and activity.
- Seen commonly in runners who log more than 20 miles per week.
- Stress fractures may need to be ruled out if symptoms persist using X-ray, bone scan, or MRI.

Treatment
- Activity modification
- Assessment of possible training errors, as well as muscle imbalances, inflexibility, foot pronation, and weakness

Ottawa Knee Rules
- With a history of recent trauma, the presence of one positive finding indicates the need to order radiographs:
  - Age is 55 years and older
  - Isolated tenderness of the patella
  - Tenderness of the fibular head
  - Inability to flex the knee to 90°
  - Inability to bear weight both immediately after injury and in the ED for 4 steps

Hip
Legg-Calve-Perthes Disease

Legg-Calve-Perthes disease results in osteonecrosis of the femoral head epiphysis in children younger than 15 years of age, with boys being affected four times more than girls. Etiology is not completely understood but there is an association with passive smoking, small stature, skeletal retardation, and low birth weight.

Clinical Presentation
- Limping
- Pain
- Stiffness in the hip, groin, thigh, or knee, with limited hip ROM.
- Diagnosis is confirmed with X-ray, MRI, and bone scan.

Treatment
- PT is especially important for stretching, activity limitation, and gait training in children under 6 years of age, with an emphasis on avoiding WB.
- If pain is severe, bed rest and traction may be indicated, as well as leg casting.
- Surgery may be recommended for individuals greater than 6 to 8 years of age. This may include

contracture release, joint realignment, and excess bone or loose body removal.
- Pain medication and PT, when cleared by the physician, are provided.

Intertrochanteric Fracture

An intertrochanteric fracture occurs between the greater and lesser trochanters of the femur. There are 252,000 hip fractures in the United States each year. The fractures affect women twice as often as men, especially in those older than 60 years. The typical mechanism is a fall with a history of osteoporosis. There is a 20 to 30 percent mortality rate in the first year after a fracture in older adults. It can also occur in younger male patients in high-force injuries.

Clinical Presentation
- Pain
- Decreased ability to bear weight and move the involved limb
- AP radiographs of the pelvis and hip, frog lateral views, traction AP, or CT will confirm diagnosis.

Treatment
- Open reduction and internal fixation (ORIF), followed by rehabilitation unless severe arthritis is present, in which case a total hip replacement (THR) may be recommended.
- In the younger population, surgery will be followed by a course of PT.

Hip Dislocation
- Traumatic injury to the hip such as an MVA or fall.

Clinical Presentation
- Posterior dislocations occur 90 percent of the time when the patient presents with the knee and foot medially rotated.
- Patient presents in extreme pain with an inability to move the leg.
- If a nerve has been injured, there may also be a loss of sensation.

Treatment
- In the ED, the MD will administer an anesthetic and manipulate or reduce the hip.
- Another set of X-rays or CT will follow this to rule out fracture.

- Osteonecrosis is also a complication.
- Normally, there is a 2- to 3-month recovery period, during which PT focuses on assisted walking, hip motion, and strengthening.

Hip Impingement

Hip impingement causes pain in the hip or groin. It can stem from multiple causes, including intra-articular loose bodies, labral injuries, or bony anomalies (cam or pincer deformity). It is usually seen in younger to middle-aged individuals and athletes.

Clinical Presentation
- Groin and/or hip pain, which worsens with hip flexion and medial rotation and may be worse with walking
- Sharp pinching pain when twisting and squatting, and sometimes a dull ache
- X-rays, CT, and MRI can identify lesions in the hip contributing to the impingement.

Treatement
- Activity changes
- NSAID
- PT to address muscle imbalances and provide modalities
- If conservative treatment fails, arthroscopic debridement may be performed, followed by PT.

Shoulder

Labrum Tear
- Labrum tears represent 4 to 8 percent of all shoulder injuries. There are several ways that a labrum tear can occur. The most common occurrence is from a sports injury. This is especially true for sports that require a lot of overhead movement of the arm and shoulder. A labrum tear may also occur when a person tries to block a fall with an outstretched arm or if they use a jerking movement to lift a heavy object.

Clinical Presentation
- Shoulder pain—often catching, locking, popping, grinding, occasional night pain
- A sense of instability
- Limited ROM and strength.
- CT or MRI with contrast can aid diagnosis, with the gold standard being arthroscopic surgery.

Treatment

- Anti-inflammatory medication
- Rest
- Activity modification
- PT for mobility and strengthening
- With a lack of improvement, arthroscopic surgery may be recommended, followed by a period of immobilization and PT.

Acromioclavicular (AC) Joint Injury/Dislocation

An AC joint injury, sustained by direct force to the acromioclavicular joint, is usually caused by a fall directly onto the point of the shoulder or an outstretched hand. Five times more common in men than women.

Clinical Presentation

- Pain at the superior-anterior aspect of the shoulder with swelling and point tenderness
- Possible loss of motion and pain with resisted testing of the muscles around the shoulder
- Depending on the severity of the injury, there may be a displacement between the clavicle and acromion. Diagnosis is aided with standard GH radiographs, which also rule out coracoid fracture.

Treatment

- Usually nonoperative for 3 months, except in severe cases, with brief immobilization, ice, and oral analgesics, followed by PT for mobility exercise and strengthening over the next 6 to 12 weeks.
- Surgery may be indicated if symptoms persist, including instrumentation, distal clavicle excision, reconstruction, or suture fixation.

Rotator Cuff Injury

The rotator cuff (RTC) is the primary stabilizer of the glenohumeral joint. When injured, there is little potential for spontaneous healing. The RTC can be injured through trauma or from repetitive overuse and gradual degradation.

Clinical Presentation

- Shoulder pain that may radiate down the lateral aspect of the arm, usually not past the elbow
- Limited and painful ROM
- Pain may be particularly intense at night when lying on the affected shoulder.
- Weakness, with or without crepitus, and snapping. Plain radiographs, US, MRI, and MRI-arthrography aid in diagnosis.

Treatment

- PT
- Activity modification
- Strengthening
- Steroid injections
- Acute or chronic partial-thickness tears often improve with conservative management.
- If symptoms persist, surgery may be indicated, followed by a lengthy rehabilitation course.
- At 5 years, RTC repairs have a high failure rate.

Adhesive Capsulitis (Frozen Shoulder)

Frozen shoulder is a disease process that causes glenohumeral capsular thickening. It is classified as either primary, which has an unknown cause, or secondary, which is often caused by immobilization after an injury or mastectomy. It is more likely in women over 40 who have been immobilized and have DM, cardiovascular disease, a thyroid condition, TB, or Parkinson's disease.

Clinical Presentation

- Varies depending on which of the three stages the patient is within:
  - Stage 1: Lasts 1 to 3 months and is characterized by progressive pain with little to no motion loss and is often misdiagnosed.
  - Stage 2: Lasts 3 to 9 months and is characterized by less pain but diminishing shoulder motion and increased stiffness.
  - Stage 3: Occurs from 9 to 14 months, and ROM improves. It is primarily a clinical diagnosis, but X-rays and MRI may help rule out other diagnoses.

Treatment

- OTC pain medications
- Anti-inflammatory medications
- Steroid injections
- Joint distension
- PT
- Shoulder manipulation under anesthesia
- TENs
- Rarely surgery to remove scar tissue

Wrist and Hand

Distal Radius Fracture

The distal radius is the most often fractured bone in the body. It is usually caused by a fall onto an outstretched hand. Fractures can be intra-articular, extra-articular, open, comminuted, or Colles. Risk factors include osteoporosis and age older than 60, but they can occur in healthy bones with enough force.

Clinical Presentation
- Immediate pain
- Tenderness
- Bruising
- Swelling
- Possible deformity
- X-ray is diagnostic.

Treatment
- Casting up to 6 weeks if bony alignment is preserved.
- If the fracture is displaced, it must be reduced and then cast.
- If the damage is severe enough, surgery is recommended with instrumentation or an external fixator.
- After immobilization, PT is prescribed to restore motion, strength, and function.
- Full recovery may take more than 1 year.

Ligament Strain

Ligament strain usually occurs when someone falls onto an outstretched hand. Up to 2 percent of patients diagnosed with a sprained wrist have a more significant injury.

Clinical Presentation
- Swelling
- Pain with movement
- Possible bruising or discoloration, tenderness, popping, and warmth over the injured ligament.
- X-rays and CT may be used to rule out fracture.

Treatment
- Grade I sprains may require rest and splinting for approximately 1 week, followed by a gradual return to activity.
- For moderate to severe strains, treatment includes immobilization, followed by rehabilitation.
- In very severe cases, surgery may be required to repair the torn ligament, followed by rehabilitation, which may take several months.

Carpal Tunnel Syndrome

Carpal tunnel syndrome occurs due to increased pressure in the carpal tunnel, resulting in mechanical compression and ischemia of the median nerve. It is more common in women and those with DM; inflammatory conditions, such as RA; pregnancy; thyroid disorders; kidney failure; obesity; menopause; and workplace factors, such as repetitive wrist and hand movements. There is eventual hand weakness. Diagnosis is aided by nerve conduction velocity (NCV) and electromyography (EMG).

Clinical Presentation
- Pain
- Numbness
- Tingling in the median nerve distribution of the hand
- Symptoms often increase with upper limb tension testing, as well as the Phalen's and the reverse Phalen's tests.
- There is often a positive flick sign.

Treatment
- Splinting
- Therapy for exercise
- Modalities
- Corticosteroid injections
- Therapeutic US
- Nocturnal hand braces
- Ergonomic workstation modifications
- Surgery may be necessary in severe cases, followed by PT or occupational therapy (OT).

Deformities: Boutonniere Deformity, Mallet Finger, and Swan Neck Deformity

Boutonniere Deformity

Boutonniere deformity is caused by damage to the central slip of the extensor tendon and rheumatoid arthritis.

Clinical Presentation

It is characterized by disfigurement and impaired function due to hyperextension of the distal interphalangeal joint (DIP) and flexion of the proximal interphalangeal joint (PIP).

Treatment
- Splinting initially (within 6 weeks) and then surgery to reconstruct the proximal and distal joints.
- Therapy is beneficial both before and after surgery.

Mallet Finger
Mallet finger disrupts the terminal extensor tendon, usually from a forceful blow to the tip of the finger. Often seen in athletes. Fracture must be ruled out in the DIP.

Clinical Presentation
Patient presents with an extensor lag of the distal IP joint.

Treatment
- Splinting in hyperextension for approximately 6 weeks.
- Surgery is controversial but may be the only option with open injuries and with large avulsion fragments.

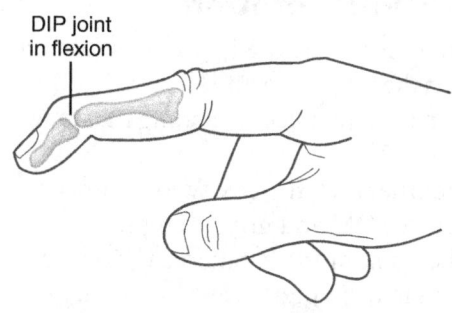

Swan Neck
Swan neck is a deformity that consists of hyperextension of the PIP and flexion of the DIP joints. A common cause of swan neck deformity is RA. It can also result from excessive extension force, posttraumatic wrist or MP joint flexion contractures, tightness of intrinsic muscles, chronic volar subluxation, or degeneration of the volar structures of PIP joint. There is usually a history of prior injury.

Treatment
- If inflammatory arthritis or RA is suspected, the patient is referred to a rheumatologist.
- Radiography is performed to rule out fracture.
- If only a mild deformity is present, a splint can be used. Otherwise, surgery is indicated.

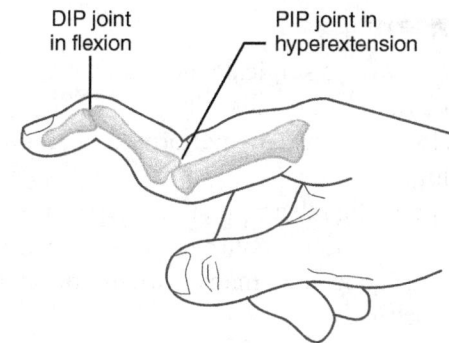

Trigger Finger (Stenosing Tenosynovitis)
The etiology of stenosing tenosynovitis is unclear, but the condition is more common in women, those with DM, and those whose work requires repetitive gripping.

Clinical Presentation
- Stiffness that worsens in the morning
- Painful snapping of the affected finger with movement
- Tenderness.
- Inability to straighten the finger or locking.

Treatment
- Splinting
- NSAIDs
- Corticosteroids
- Injections
- Rest
- Ice or heat
- Stretching
- In severe cases, percutaneous or open surgery is indicated, followed by rehabilitation.

Dupuytren's Contracture
Dupuytren's contracture is a fibroproliferative condition of the hand that affects older patients, causing a digital flexion contracture. The prevalence varies but typically affects older men of Northern European descent.

Clinical Presentation
- Thickening of the palmar skin and a nodule in the early stages.
- As the condition progresses, a cord develops that gradually contracts and pulls the metacarpophalangeal (MCP) and PIP joint into flexion.
- Commonly affects the ring and little fingers and can be bilateral.

Treatment

- Almost always surgical when function is impeded or the deformity is disabling.
- Fasciotomy is usually performed in an outpatient setting.
- Rarely, a digital amputation is performed if an irreversible joint contracture is present. Prognosis is good and many patients never develop contracture.

Degenerative Joint Disease (DJD)

Degenerative joint disease (DJD) causes inflammation and degradation of the distal and proximal IP joints. Predominantly affects postmenopausal women and older people.

Clinical Presentation

- Pain
- Stiffness
- Heat, redness, and swelling
- A loss of motion
- Eventual loss of function in the involved fingers and hand
- There is decreased grip strength, and Heberden (DIP) or Bouchard nodes (PIP) may be present.
- X-ray is the gold standard, but MRI and US can be used as well as lab values.

Treatment

- Controlling pain and inflammation
- Activity modification
- Splinting
- Ice and heat
- Joint injection
- If symptoms are persistent, referral to a hand surgeon is indicated.
- Surgery is usually reconstructive, followed by rest and splinting for 4 to 6 weeks, followed by therapy for 4 to 8 weeks.

Osteomyelitis

Osteomyelitis is a pyogenic bone infection (frequently *Staphylococcus aureus*) that can occur in any bone, usually after penetrating trauma. Risk factors include DM, sickle cell disease, HIV, RA, intravenous drug use, alcoholism, long-term steroid use, hemodialysis, poor circulation, and recent injury.

Clinical Presentation

- Redness, warmth, and inflammation
- Stiffness
- Pus drainage
- Loss of ROM
- Fever or chills may or may not be present.
- The gold standard for diagnosis is bone biopsy, but X-ray, MRI, and CT may be used.

Treatment

- Antibiotic therapy
- Possible need to drain the infection or debride the dead bone or other surrounding tissue
- Therapy may be beneficial once cleared by the MD.

Ganglion Cyst

- Ganglion cysts are 1 to 2 cm cystic structures that are more commonly seen on the dorsal aspect of the wrist, particularly over the scapholunate ligament. The origin is unknown but may theoretically be related to acute or chronic stress, allowing leakage of synovial fluid.

Clinical Presentation

- Firm cystic structure in the wrist with no warmth or erythema
- Often accompanied by aching that may radiate up the arm
- Tenderness with activity or palpation and decreased ROM and grip strength
- If the ulnar or median nerve is compressed, paresthesia may be present.
- X-rays are usually not indicated.

Treatment

- Interventions with variable success include:
  - repeated pressure on the cyst, or
  - cyst removal with an incision or aspiration.

Raynaud's Phenomenon

Raynaud's phenomenon is a recurrent, long-lasting, and episodic vasospasm of the fingers and toes, often associated with exposure to cold. Risk factors include associated diseases, such as scleroderma and lupus; occupations with vibration; exposure to smoking; and medications that affect blood vessels. Prevalence increases in women, cold climates, and those with a family history. Age, thin body type, and underlying cardiovascular disease may also be associated with this disease.

Clinical Presentation
- Typical episodes of pallor in the digits followed by rubor (cyanosis may be present in severe disease).
- Cold or throbbing in the digits
- Capillaroscopy aids in diagnosis.
- An antinuclear antibody or erythrocyte sedimentation rate (ESR) test may be performed if a secondary disease process is suspected.

Treatment
- Pharmacological medications that promote vasodilation (calcium channel antagonists)
- Smoking cessation
- Avoidance and coping of emotional stress
- Decreasing cold exposure
- Improved clothing and measures to protect the skin

Pelvis and Sacrum

Ankylosing Spondylitis

Ankylosing spondylitis is inflammatory arthritis primarily affecting the spine and sacroiliac (SI) joints. It affects men more than women and usually begins in early adulthood. Hereditary and genetic factors, such as HLA-B27, may be risk factors. Complications may include uveitis, compression fractures, and spinal vertebrae fusing.

Clinical Presentation
- Progressive stiffening of spine and thorax
- Pain in the lower back and hips, especially in the morning and after activity
- A rigid thoracolumbar kyphosis and stooped posture may be noticed as the disease progresses.
- X-rays, showing a "bamboo spine," and lab tests, may aid diagnosis.

Treatment
- Medications such as tumor necrosis factor
- PT for stretching and strengthening

Lumbar Spine

Degenerative Lumbar Disc Disease

Degenerative lumbar disc disease causes discogenic low back pain (LBP), which is the most common type of chronic LBP.

Clinical Presentation
- Deep and dull low-grade midline backache that may radiate into the gluteal area and rarely to the knees and lower legs.
- The pain worsens with prolonged sitting, axial loading, and sometimes with prolonged standing.
- Symptoms increase with bending, twisting, and lifting.
- There is usually no sensory or motor loss, but there may be numbness and tingling in severe cases or during acute exacerbations.
- MRI is the most used method of diagnosis, but discography is the gold standard.

Treatment
- Activity modification
- Heat and ice
- Patient education
- PT for flexibility
- Lumbar stabilization exercises
- Medications
  - NSAIDs
  - Epidural steroid injections
- If symptoms fail to improve, lumbar fusion is the most common surgical intervention, but lumbar disc replacements are becoming more popular.
- Rehabilitation follows the surgical interventions.

Radiculopathy

Radiculopathy causes pain secondary to compression or inflammation of a spinal nerve(s). It may be referred to as sciatic pain. A herniated lumbar disc, stenosis, or trauma can cause radiculopathy.

Clinical Presentation
- Pain that often radiates from the back into the lower limb and may include numbness, electric-type symptoms, paresthesia, and myotomal muscle weakness
- Pain may increase with coughing, sneezing, or straining.
- Clinical examination may reveal a positive straight leg raise (SLR) test, altered reflexes, and sensory deficits.
- Diagnostic tests include radiographs, EMGs, MRIs, and CT scans.

Treatment
- PT
- Pain and anti-inflammatory medication, as well as spinal injections

- If there is a lack of improvement after 6 to 8 weeks, surgical intervention, such as a laminectomy, discectomy, or micro-discectomy, may be considered. These procedures have high success rates and are generally followed by a healing period and progressive rehabilitation.

Abdominal Aortic Aneurysm

Abdominal aortic aneurysm (AAA) is a dilation of the abdominal aorta. It is classified by size:

- Small: 4 cm or less and usually observed by MD
- Medium: 4 to 5.3 cm, and if so, the physician may continue to observe the aneurysm or perform surgery
- Large: 5.6 cm or growing more than 0.5 cm every 6 months. This is treated surgically.

A ruptured abdominal aorta carries an 80 percent mortality rate. Risk factors include men older than 60, smoking, and family history of AAA and atherosclerosis.

Clinical Presentation

- This is a rare finding in the orthopedic setting; most patients do not have symptoms.
- Some people present with a pulsating feeling near their navel, deep and constant pain in the abdomen or the side of the abdomen, or with back pain.
- Clinically, there may be an alteration of pulse that can be detected with a stethoscope.
- Diagnosis is confirmed with abdominal US, CT scan, or MRI.

Treatment

Intervention is a medical referral to a cardiologist.

Spinal Stenosis

Spinal stenosis involves the narrowing of the spinal canal or nerve root foramen. The narrowing can be congenital or part of a degenerative joint condition surrounding the spine and transverse foramen. The symptoms may intensify if there is a concomitant disc herniation, further narrowing the foramen for the nerves. It can mimic vascular insufficiency. This is the most common cause of lumbar surgery in the United States.

Clinical Presentation

- Pain in the lower back, buttock, and thigh, which may be unilateral or bilateral
- The pain may be claudicating in nature and usually worsens with extension activities, such as standing and walking, and is relieved with sitting or lying down in a hook-lying position.
- Paresthesia and lower extremity (LE) weakness may accompany the pain.

Treatment

- Pain and anti-inflammatory medication (NSAIDs)
- Referral for PT for education, flexibility, and lumbar stabilization training.
- If conservative measures fail, lumbar surgery may be indicated, with the most popular being a decompressive laminectomy.

Spondylolisthesis

Spondylolisthesis occurs when a superior vertebra slides forward over the vertebra below it. It may be caused by disc degeneration, which results in a loss of intervertebral disc height; traumatic fracture or stress fracture to the pars interarticularis; an anatomic anomaly; or joint damage, resulting from infection or arthritis. In the aging adult population, the overall incidence is 8.7 percent, with the L4–5 level being the most affected. In the older adult, the symptoms are similar to spinal stenosis.

Clinical Presentation

- In degenerative conditions, the patient is older, but the typical presentation is a child or teenager who is active in sports.
- Lower back pain with sharp pain, +/− paresthesia, and neurogenic claudication into one or both LEs
- Worsening pain with walking, standing, bending over, twisting, and playing sports
- In rare cases, bowel and bladder function may become impaired.
- X-ray, MRI, and CT scan are common diagnostically.

Treatment

- Pain medication
- NSAIDs
- Steroid injections
- PT, which includes hamstring stretching and lumbar flexibility, strengthening exercises, and a bracing/lumbar corset
- Conservative measures are usually successful, but if they fail, surgical options include laminectomy and spinal fusion, followed by rehabilitation.

Cauda Equina Syndrome

Cauda equina syndrome is the most frequent cause of a neurologic disability syndrome. It involves urinary, defecation, and sexual function. It is caused by the compression of the sacral nerve roots inside the lumbosacral vertebral canal from tumor, infection, fracture, or stenosis. Overall incidence is 1 in 33,000 to 1 in 100,000. It occurs in 2 percent of all lumbar disc herniations.

Clinical Presentation
- LBP with bilateral sciatica, saddle anesthesia, and bilateral LE motor weakness, and often gait abnormalities.
- There are variable rectal and urinary tract complaints.

Treatment
Interventions include medical referral and usually surgery (laminectomy) to decompress the nerve roots, followed by rehabilitation when cleared by the physician.

Clinical Lumbar Instability

Clinical lumbar instability is a benign joint hypermobility syndrome, characterized by an inability to control the lumbar spine at a segmental level.

Clinical Presentation
- Younger individual (up to age 40)
- Clicking, crunching, or clunking in the low back
- The pain usually remains in the lumbar region and is intermittent and mild to moderate.
- Exam is clinically based and includes joint mobility and ROM testing (Gower's sign). A Gower's sign is observed when the patient flexes forward and then pushes themselves upright using their hands on their thighs.
- X-rays are usually negative but may be used with MRI to rule out other diagnoses.

Treatment
- PT, with emphasis on education, ergonomics, and lumbar stabilization
- Anti-inflammatory and pain medication may be used during exacerbations.
- Depending on the degree of instability, outcomes of conservative treatment are generally good.

Thoracic Spine

Rib Dysfunction: Costochondritis

Costochondritis refers to inflammation of the cartilage connecting the ribs to the sternum, most often the second to fifth ribs. The condition usually affects people older than 40; in most cases, more than one site is affected. Women have a higher incidence than men. Due to the chest wall pain, heart conditions are a differential diagnosis.

Clinical Presentation
- Chest wall pain with an insidious onset but may have a history of an injury to the chest, physical strain using the pectoralis muscles, arthritis, or infection, including tuberculosis.
- The pain may be sharp or aching or give a feeling of pressure that worsens with deep breathing or coughing.
- Tenderness to palpation over the sternocostal junction, and swelling may be present.
- The diagnosis is clinical, but imaging may be performed to rule out other conditions.

Treatment
- NSAIDs
- Corticosteroid injections
- Narcotics
- Antidepressants, such as amitriptyline
- Antiseizure drugs, such as gabapentin
- PT provides stretching and modalities, such as TENS, heat, and ice.
- The condition often improves over several weeks.

Thoracic Disc Herniation

Thoracic disc herniation results in the bulging or extrusion of the thoracic disc, which incites an inflammatory reaction and may compress thoracic nerve roots and inflame the dura.

- Sharp pain in the thoracic spine, which is exacerbated with coughing or sneezing
- Pain may radiate around the chest or into the belly.
- If the disc herniation is central and encroaches on the spinal canal, there may be signs and symptoms of myelopathy with sensory disturbances at the level of compression, difficulty walking/ataxic gait, abnormal reflexes, decreased proprioception,

multi-segmental LE weakness, or bowel and bladder dysfunction.
- Usually, X-ray is the first imaging procedure performed; however, depending on the severity of myelopathy, an MRI, CT, or myelogram may be performed.

Treatment
- Rest
- Narcotic and nonnarcotic analgesic medications
- Epidural injections
- Ice packs
- PT for gentle exercise, manual therapy, and back strengthening
- If conservative treatment fails, surgery is indicated and includes dorsal laminectomy.
- In the case of thoracic myelopathy, surgery is the preferred and immediate treatment, and a thoracotomy or costotransversectomy may be performed.

Stress Fracture Ribs

Stress fractures of the ribs are a common pathology in rowers and other sports with repetitive and vigorous shoulder motion, such as baseball. Risk factors include low bone mineral density, poor diet, amenorrhea, poor mechanics during athletics, and changes in training. They occur most frequently with the first rib and can also occur traumatically.

Clinical Presentation
- Gradual onset of pain in the side of the neck and upper back or back of the shoulder
- Pain worsens with activity, deep breathing, coughing, and overhead activity and improves with rest.
- Possible popping, snapping, or grinding sensation and tenderness around the involved rib.
- Diagnosis is confirmed with X-ray, bone scan, MRI, or CT scan.

Treatment
- The preferred treatment is rest for 4-6 weeks. No physical activity should be undertaken that causes or aggravates the pain.
- Ice packs may be used to help alleviate pain.
- NSAIDs may help with pain and add an anti-inflammatory effect.
- Supplements of Vitamin D and calcium may be taken and a correction of any nutritional deficiencies.

Shingles

Varicella zoster virus (VZV) is a neurotropic herpes virus that infects nearly all humans. The primary infection causes chickenpox, after which the virus becomes dormant in the cranial nerve ganglia, dorsal root ganglia, and autonomic ganglia. Risk factors include individuals older than 50 years, those with diseases that weaken the immune system (HIV, cancer), those undergoing radiation or chemotherapy, and those taking medications that weaken the immune system, such as after an organ transplant.

Clinical Presentation
- Pain, burning, numbness, tingling, and sensitivity to touch, followed by a red rash that begins a few days after the pain and may follow a single dermatome around the right or left torso.
- Fluid-filled blisters break open and crust over, causing itching.
- Some patients will also experience fever, headache, fatigue, and sensitivity to light.
- Skin lesions may resolve in a week, but the pain can last up to 6 weeks.
- Complications include postherpetic neuralgia, vision loss, neurologic issues, and skin infections.

Treatment
- Preventative interventions include vaccines.
- This disease is particularly dangerous for anyone with a weak immune system, newborns, and pregnant women.
- Treatment includes antiviral medication and pain medication:
  - Capsaicin cream
  - Lidocaine gel
  - Gabapentin
  - Tricyclic antidepressants
  - Codeine
  - Corticosteroids
  - Local anesthetics
- Modalities, such as TENS, may provide temporary relief.

Scoliosis

Scoliosis is a three-dimensional deformation of the spine. The cause is multifactorial, including genetic predisposition, abnormal spinal growth, connective tissue disease, cerebral palsy (CP), muscular dystrophy (MD), and congenital disabilities. Scoliosis can also be acquired by habitually maintaining poor posture. It affects 3 percent of the population, and the girl–boy ratio is 8:1. Symptoms usually occur in the 9 to 15 age bracket. The curvature can be in the shape of a "C," or if a compensatory curve is present, in the shape of an "S." In severe scoliosis, the rib cage may press on the lungs and heart.

Clinical Presentation
- Back pain, which may be intermittent or constant and is usually dull and achy
- Asymmetry in the shoulders and waist height, usually with a leg length discrepancy. A rib hump is present, with forward flexion of the trunk.

Treatment
- Conservative treatment is generally successful and includes outpatient PT, exercise, electrical stimulation, traction, postural training, manual therapy, and bracing (Milwaukee brace).
- In severe cases, a spinal fusion with instrumentation may be performed, followed by a course of PT.
- Support groups may be beneficial for the altered appearance of the spine and asymmetry in shoulders and hips.

Cervical Spine

Torticollis

Torticollis shortens the sternocleidomastoid muscle (SCM) on one side, leading to ipsilateral side flexion and contralateral rotation of the head. Nonmuscular causes contribute to over 18 percent of torticollis cases. These causes include tumor, syringomyelia, Klippel-Feil syndrome, ocular deficiency, and infection. It affects 1 out of 250 live births.

Clinical Presentation
- Abnormal head posture with pain, stiffness, and tightness in the SCM muscle
- Myofascial pain may radiate into the cranium, producing a headache.
- Limited ROM in contralateral side flexion and ipsilateral rotation
- Decreased flexibility in the SCM muscle
- Medical referral is indicated to ensure that the cause is muscular.

Treatment
- Pain medication
- Muscle relaxers
- Anti-inflammatory medications
- Medications with PT for postural education, possible bracing, modalities, stretching, manual therapy, and exercise.
- The underlying condition is treated medically if a nonmuscular cause of torticollis is found.
- PT and bracing may occur simultaneously.

Acute Cervical Disc Herniation/Radiculopathy

Acute Cervical Disc Herniation/Radiculopathy is the bulging or extrusion of the cervical disc, which incites an inflammatory reaction and may provide compression on cervical nerve roots and inflame the dura. It can occur over time from cervical degeneration or habitually poor posture, or more acutely from an injury such as whiplash.

Clinical Presentation
- Neck pain that is sharp initially but may become dull over time.
- Tingling and paresthesia in the fingers or hand, with upper extremity (UE) weakness and a loss of sensation.
- The pain worsens with certain neck motions, especially quick motions, but is better at rest.
- Radiographs are typically performed, but MRIs and CT scans are more diagnostic, and an EMG is used if neural involvement in the UE is suspected.

Treatment
- NSAIDs
- Corticosteroids
- Steroid injections
- Soft cervical collars
- PT for modalities, including traction, stretching, and neck strengthening
- Conservative treatment is often successful, but surgery may be indicated in severe cases (laminectomy and fusion).

Spinal Stenosis

Spinal stenosis narrows the spinal canal or nerve root foramen. The narrowing can be congenital or part of a degenerative condition (such as OA) of the joint surrounding the spine and transverse foramen. Occasionally, it is caused by herniated discs, thickened ligaments, tumors, and vertebral fractures. Usually, it occurs in patients older than 50.

Clinical Presentation
- Neck pain and stiffness
- With or without paresthesia
- Numbness
- Weakness in the neck and bilateral UEs
- If the stenosis is central, cervical myelopathy may occur and cause issues in the LEs with weakness, decreased balance, coordination, and incontinence.
- Radiographs, MRIs, and CTs are diagnostic.

Treatment
- NSAIDs, muscle relaxants, anti-depressants for chronic pain, anti-seizure drugs, opioids, and steroid injections
- PT is used for education and modalities, including traction, MH, TENS, manual techniques, and exercise for strength and flexibility.
- If conservative treatment fails, surgery is indicated, usually in the form of laminectomy.

Rheumatoid Arthritis

Rheumatoid arthritis is a chronic progressive inflammatory condition affecting the synovium and joints. Although mainly seen in the hand, wrist, and extremities, it can affect the cervical spine. Of particular concern is that it can lead to upper cervical instability and atlanto-axial subluxation, which can be a life-threatening condition and cause symptoms of cervical myelopathy, including spastic gait, balance, and bowel and bladder dysfunction.

Clinical Presentation
- Dull, achy neck pain, but can become sharp during a period of exacerbation, and limited motion.
- X-rays can be diagnostic and are used during cervical flexion to assess the integrity of the AA joint. MRI is also commonly used.

Treatment
- Cervical fusion if myelopathy is present.
- Cervical collars can provide relief, along with pain and anti-inflammatory medication/injections.
- PT can assist with education, pain-relieving modalities, gentle ROM, and strengthening.
- After the period of exacerbation passes, therapy can become more aggressive.

Concussion

Concussions fall under the category of a traumatic brain injury caused by a blow to the head. The effects are usually temporary but complications, such as postconcussion syndrome, occur and last for weeks to months after the initial injury.

Clinical Presentation
- With or without loss of consciousness
- Headaches
- Problems with concentration, memory, balance, and coordination
- Feelings of "being foggy"
- Ringing in the ears, fatigue, nausea, vomiting, slurred speech, sleep disturbance, and sensitivity to light and noise are common.
- Neurologic exam and cognitive testing should be performed; in severe cases, an MRI or CT of the brain may be necessary.

Treatment
- Medications for pain
- Vestibular therapy if balance is affected
- Optical exam if vision is impaired, including prism glasses
- PT for pain and to address any cervical spine issues that may have occurred simultaneously with the concussion.
- Once the concussion has resolved, athletes may receive additional therapy and conditioning for return to play.

Elbow

Lateral Epicondylalgia (Tennis Elbow)

Tennis Elbow causes pain in the lateral epicondyle region due to mechanical overloading and abnormal microvascular response in the extensor carpi radialis longus or brevis muscles, affecting 1 to 3 percent of the population.

Clinical Presentation
- Pain and tenderness over the lateral epicondyle, which is increased with wrist motion, gripping, and resisted finger extension of the second or third digits
- Decreased grip strength

- Injury often caused by overuse, training error for athletes, or work (manual labor or prolonged computer use and keyboarding), but some onsets are insidious.

Treatment
- Rest
- NSAIDs
- Extracorporeal shock wave therapy, ultrasound therapy, Botox injections, and corticosteroid injections
- PT provides modalities, stretching, and manual techniques, including joint mobilization and soft tissue work, strengthening (emphasis on eccentric), ergonomic recommendations and counterforce bracing.
- Recalcitrant cases may undergo surgical release. More recently, platelet-rich plasma injections have shown promise in treating lateral epicondylalgia.
- Cervical spine injury should be ruled out as contributing to symptoms.

Review Questions

1. For which of the following diagnoses are patients most likely to complain of pain on the plantar surface of the foot?
   A. Metatarsal stress fracture
   B. Pes cavus
   C. Pes planus
   D. Morton's neuroma

2. What is the most common cause of heel pain?
   A. Plantar fasciitis
   B. Achilles tendinopathy
   C. Ankle sprain
   D. Compartment syndrome

3. Pain with a standing (weight-bearing [WB]) heel raise will occur with which of the following diagnoses?
   A. Achilles tendinopathy
   B. Lateral ankle sprain
   C. Compartment syndrome
   D. Medial ankle sprain

4. The following picture shows a foot deformity that is characteristic of which of the following diagnoses?
   A. Compartment syndrome
   B. Diabetes mellitus
   C. Charcot foot
   D. Pes cavus

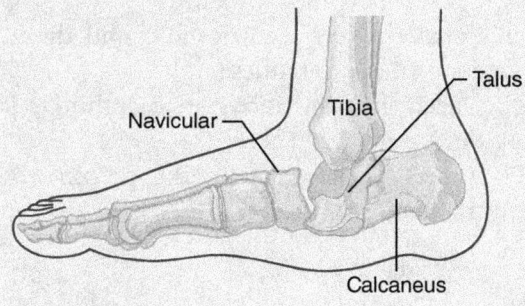

5. Which of the following is true of the Ottawa foot and ankle rules?
   A. Has a high specificity for foot and ankle fractures
   B. Has high sensitivity for foot and ankle fractures
   C. Is specific for fractures of the cuboid bone
   D. Is correlated with decreased foot and ankle range of motion (ROM)

6. Severe uncontrolled pain, swelling, and pain with a history of foot trauma is consistent with which of the following diagnoses?
   A. Pes cavus
   B. Pes planus
   C. Achilles tendinopathy
   D. Compartment syndrome

7. Limping and pain in a child's leg of insidious onset may indicate what?
   A. Intertrochanteric fracture
   B. Hip dislocation
   C. Legg-Calve-Perthes disease
   D. Hip impingement

8. Which of the following is true of intertrochanteric fractures?
   A. Affects men more than women
   B. Has a 50 to 60 percent mortality rate in the first year after the fracture
   C. Primary intervention is open reduction and internal fixation (ORIF)
   D. Carries a 30 percent chance of refracture

9. Of the following, which is the most fractured bone in the body?
   A. The femur
   B. The humerus
   C. The ulna
   D. The radius

10. A patient is being evaluated for a complaint of pain at the base of the thumb. The provider performs a Finkelstein test, and the results are positive. This is indicative of which of the following disease processes?
    A. De Quervain's tenosynovitis
    B. Carpal tunnel syndrome
    C. Ligamentous strain
    D. Trigger finger

11. The picture below depicts which deformity?
    A. Boutonniere deformity
    B. Mallet finger
    C. Swan neck deformity
    D. Subluxed distal interphalangeal joint (DIP)

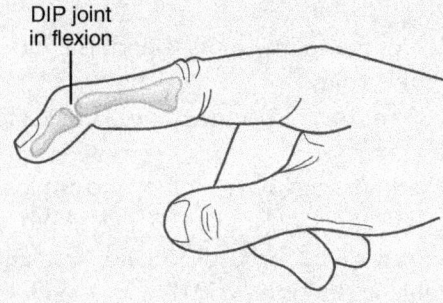

12. Thickening of the palmar skin of the hand in older adults is termed what?
    A. De Quervain's tenosynovitis
    B. Trigger finger
    C. Dupuytren's contracture
    D. Swan neck deformity

13. Raynaud's phenomenon is associated with which of the following?
    A. Men, cold climates, and a history of hypothyroid
    B. Women, scleroderma, and cold climates
    C. Men, stroke, and diabetes mellitus (DM)
    D. Women, sedentary occupation, smoking

14. What is ankylosing spondylitis?
    A. An inflammatory arthritis affecting adolescent girls
    B. An inflammatory arthritis more commonly seen in men
    C. A genetic disease affecting older men
    D. An infective arthritis affecting teenage boys

15. What is the most common type of chronic low back pain (LBP)?
    A. Degenerative lumbar disc disease
    B. Spinal stenosis
    C. Rheumatoid arthritis
    D. Osteoarthritis of the sacroiliac joint

16. Which of the following is associated with lumbar radiculopathy?
    A. Negative straight leg raise (SLR)
    B. Muscle weakness in particular distribution
    C. Dull, achy pain in the back
    D. Usually occurs bilaterally

17. The most common cause for lumbar surgery in the United States is:
    A. Spinal tumor
    B. Ankylosing spondylitis
    C. Spondylolisthesis
    D. Spinal stenosis

18. Which of the following is true of a patient with lumbar spinal stenosis?
    A. Symptoms are improved with standing.
    B. Symptoms are relieved by walking for 15 to 30 minutes.
    C. Symptoms are relieved by the patient lying on their stomach.
    D. Symptoms are improved when the patient walks bent over a shopping cart.

19. A positive Gower's sign is often found in which of the following conditions?
    A. Lumbar disc herniation
    B. Abdominal aortic aneurysm (AAA)
    C. Lumbar radiculopathy
    D. Clinical lumbar instability

20. Insidious chest wall pain can occur with which of the following?
    A. AAA
    B. C5-C6 radiculopathy
    C. Costochondritis
    D. Lumbar facet syndrome

21. Which of the following can cause thoracic pain that may radiate around to the front of the chest?
    A. Thoracic disc herniation
    B. Rib stress fracture
    C. Shingles
    D. All of the above

22. Which of the following is true of scoliosis?
    A. Associated with uneven shoulders, a leg length discrepancy, and rib hump
    B. Usually affects teenage boys and those with congenital disabilities
    C. Onset occurs in women in their third to fourth decade of life
    D. Affects approximately 20 percent of the population

23. A Milwaukee brace is a conservative treatment for which condition?
    A. Torticollis
    B. Lumbar stenosis
    C. Scoliosis
    D. Thoracic disc herniation

24. Torticollis is a shortening or spasm of which of the following muscles?
    A. Anterior scalene
    B. Subclavius
    C. Latissimus dorsi
    D. Sternocleidomastoid

25. Concentration and visual disturbances are common in which of the following conditions?
    A. Cervical disc herniation
    B. Rheumatoid arthritis (RA) affecting the cervical spine
    C. Cervical radiculopathy
    D. Concussion

Answers and Enhanced Rationales

1. Answer D is correct. Morton's neuroma is a painful condition that affects the ball of the foot, most commonly between the area of the third and fourth toe.

   Answer A is incorrect. A metatarsal stress fracture usually causes pain on the dorsal surface of the foot, which may initially be felt while playing sports but gradually progresses to pain when walking or performing daily activities.

   Answer B is incorrect. Pes cavus is a foot with an abnormally high arch that does not flatten with WB. Pes cavus presentation is variable. Patients may have increased WB on the lateral aspect of the foot and may complaint of lateral foot pain.

   Answer C is incorrect. Pes planus is commonly referred to as flat feet. Patients may present with an altered gait, such as overpronation with ambulation, or a history of ankle sprains.

2. Answer A is correct. Plantar fasciitis is one of the most common causes of heel pain. It involves pain and inflammation of a thick band of tissue, called the plantar fascia, which runs across the bottom of the foot and connects the calcaneus bone to the toes. Plantar fasciitis commonly causes stabbing pain that usually occurs with the very first steps in the morning.

   Answer B is incorrect. Achilles tendinopathy refers to tendinitis (acute) and tendinosis (chronic). The patient will complain of pain in the lower posterior area of the leg or pain directly above the heel, especially after running, sprinting, or sports activities.

   Answer C is incorrect. Ankle sprains present with pain (both at rest and with WB), bruising, and tenderness to touch. The pain typically involves the lateral ligaments or, less commonly, the medial side of the ankle.

   Answer D is incorrect. Compartment syndrome results in numbness, tingling, or pain, which may be present in the entire limb. It is assessed using the 5 Ps.

3. Answer A is correct. When performing a physical exam, most people with Achilles tendinopathy complain of pain when standing on the affected leg and raising their heel off the ground. This movement reproduces their pain.

   Answer B is incorrect. Lateral ankle sprains present with pain on the lateral aspect of the foot; swelling and bruising may be present.

   Answer C is incorrect. Compartment syndrome results in numbness, tingling, or pain, which may be present in the entire limb. It is assessed using the 5 Ps.

   Answer D is incorrect. Medial ankle sprains present with pain on the medial aspect of the foot; swelling and bruising may be present. Pain is usually continuous but worsens with WB.

4. Answer C is correct. Diabetes damages blood vessels, decreasing blood flow to the feet. Poor circulation weakens bones and can cause disintegration of the bones and joints in the foot and ankle. As a result, people with diabetes are at a high risk for developing Charcot foot. The combination of bone disintegration and trauma can warp and deform the shape of the foot.

   Answer A is incorrect. Compartment syndrome results in numbness, tingling, or pain, which may be present in the entire limb. It is assessed using the 5 Ps.

   Answer B is incorrect. DM is a common cause of Charcot foot due to the impaired vasculature to the foot. The picture shows a Charcot foot.

   Answer D is incorrect. Pes cavus (high arches) is a foot with an abnormally high arch that does not flatten with WB. Pes cavus presentation is variable. Patients may have increased WB on the lateral aspect of the foot. They do not have a visible "rocker foot," which is evident from Charcot's foot.

5. Answer B is correct. Evidence supports the Ottawa ankle rules as an accurate instrument for excluding fractures of the ankle and midfoot. The instrument has a *sensitivity* of almost 100 percent and a modest specificity, and its use should reduce the number of unnecessary radiographs by 30 to 40 percent.

   Answer A is incorrect. A systematic review of 27 studies showed the Ottawa Ankle Rules' specificity at 31 percent. Low specificity means that there is a higher likelihood of false positives.

   Answer C is incorrect. The Ottowa Ankle Rules (OARs) are used to rule out ankle and midfoot fractures and help the clinician determine if an X-ray is necessary.

   Answer D is incorrect. The OARs are used to determine areas of pain within the injured foot with palpation and if the patient can walk at least four steps. The pain with an injured ankle will likely cause decreased foot and ankle ROM.

6. Answer D is correct. Compartment syndrome causes severe pain that does not go away with analgesic medications and is not relieved when the foot is raised. More severe cases may include paresthesia, pallor, and pulselessness.

   Answer A is incorrect. Pes cavus (high arches) does not cause severe pain and is not associated with any of the "5 Ps."

   Answer B is incorrect. Pes planus does not cause severe pain and is associated with gait abnormalities.

   Answer C is incorrect. Achilles tendinopathy may be acute or chronic and presents as pain during activity. The pain of compartment syndrome occurs even if the limb is at rest.

7. Answer C is correct. Legg–Calvé–Perthes disease occurs when the blood supply is temporarily interrupted to the femoral head of the hip joint. Without sufficient blood flow, the bone begins to die and can break easily and subsequently may heal poorly.

   Answer A is incorrect. Intertrochanteric fractures are common hip fractures seen in older patients and are rarely seen in children. The patient presents with an inability to bear weight and an acute onset of hip pain.

   Answer B is incorrect. A hip dislocation causes severe pain, and the patient cannot move the affected leg. It is a medical emergency.

   Answer D is incorrect. Hip impingement syndrome presents as pain in the groin after prolonged sitting or during or after activity. There is difficulty flexing the hip beyond a right angle. It can be detected by bringing the patient's flexed knee toward the chest and rotating it inward. If this recreates the pain, then the test is positive for impingement syndrome.

8. Answer C is correct. ORIF is indicated for all intertrochanteric fractures, unless the patient's medical condition is such that any general or spinal anesthesia is contraindicated.

   Answer A is incorrect. Intertrochanteric fractures affect women three times more often than men.

   Answer B is incorrect. Hip fractures commonly occur in older people and even after surgical repair, commonly cause some functional loss. Approximately 30 percent of people with hip fracture will die within the first year; however, some studies show mortality rates to be even lower.

   Answer D is incorrect. One study revealed a 14.8 percent chance of refracture within 5 years, which is greatly influenced by age, sex, and functional status.

9. Answer D is correct. Arm fractures account for almost 50 percent of all broken bones. The radius is commonly fractured when a person tries to break their "fall on an outstretched hand" (FOOSH).

   Answer A is incorrect. The femur is the strongest bone in the body and usually requires significant force to break unless other influencing factors, such as osteoporosis, are present.

   Answer B is incorrect. A fracture of the humerus is the least common fracture of the body.

   Answer C is incorrect. Although the ulna may commonly break along with the radius, most of the force when falling on an outstretched hand is taken on the radius, and therefore, it is the most likely to fracture.

10. Answer A is correct. The Finkelstein test can help the clinician confirm De Quervain's tenosynovitis. To perform the test, the thumb is bent across the palm of the hand and then covered with the fingers. The patient then bends the wrist toward their little finger. If this causes pain, it is likely due to De Quervain's tenosynovitis.

    Answer B is incorrect. Carpal tunnel syndrome is caused by compression of the median nerve and causes numbness and tingling in the thumb, index, and middle fingers. Carpal tunnel syndrome can be tested with Tinel's sign and the Phalen's test.

Answer C is incorrect. A ligamentous strain of the hand will cause pain and stiffness. Like most strains and sprains of the limbs, there may be swelling, bruising, tenderness to palpation, and loss of function.

Answer D is incorrect. Trigger finger occurs when the affected finger or thumb locks in place when bent. The stiffness and locking tend to worsen after periods of inactivity, such as early morning.

11. Answer B is correct. Mallet finger is commonly associated with a sports or baseball injury. A flexion force on the tip of the extended finger jolts the DIP joint into flexion. Active extension power of the DIP joint is lost, and the joint rests in an abnormally flexed position.

Answer A is incorrect. The Boutonniere deformity is more commonly seen in conditions such as RA. The middle joint of the finger (proximal interphalangeal [PIP] joint) remains flexed while the DIP joint bends back and hyperextends.

Answer C is incorrect. The swan neck deformity is commonly seen with degenerative conditions, such as RA, and is characterized by hyperextension of the PIP joint and flexion of the DIP joint. It is seen in up to 50 percent of persons with RA.

Answer D is incorrect. Dislocation of the DIP is associated with fracture, tendon rupture, or forced hyperextension of the finger.

12. Answer C is correct. Dupuytren's contracture is a hand deformity that usually develops over years. Knots of tissue form under the skin, eventually creating a thick cord that pulls one or more fingers into a bent position.

Answer A is incorrect. De Quervain's tenosynovitis is a painful condition affecting the tendons on the thumb side of the wrist. Symptoms are pain and swelling near the base of the thumb and a "sticking" sensation in the thumb when moving it.

Answer B is incorrect. Trigger finger occurs when the affected finger or thumb locks in place when bent. The stiffness and locking tend to worsen after periods of inactivity, such as early morning. Typically, the trigger finger can be "popped" back into position.

Answer D is incorrect. Swan neck deformity is a degenerative condition that causes a permanent bend in the finger joints. The most common cause of swan neck deformity is rheumatoid arthritis.

13. Answer B is correct. People of all ages can have Raynaud's phenomenon. It may run in families, especially those that typically have autoimmune disorders. The primary form is the most common. It most often starts between age 15 and 25 and is most common in women and people living in cold places.

Answer A is incorrect. Raynaud's phenomenon is more common in women than men. It is often associated with other autoimmune disorders but not necessarily hypothyroidism.

Answer C is incorrect. Raynaud's phenomenon is more common in women and is not associated with stroke. Patients with DM1 (an autoimmune disorder) may develop Raynaud's phenomenon as with any other autoimmune disorder.

Answer D is incorrect. Raynaud's phenomenon is usually triggered by cold temperatures, anxiety, or stress, causing the blood vessels to spasm temporarily. Smoking can aggravate the condition by affecting the circulation to the fingers. Persons with Raynaud's should wear gloves when in cold temperatures and quit smoking.

14. Answer B is correct. Ankylosing spondylitis is an inflammatory disease that can cause some vertebrae in the spine to fuse together. This fusing makes the spine less flexible and can result in a hunched-forward posture. Ankylosing spondylitis affects men more often than women. Signs and symptoms of ankylosing spondylitis typically begin in early adulthood.

Answer A is incorrect. Ankylosing spondylitis is more common in men with approximately 80 percent experiencing symptoms by the age of 30.

Answer C is incorrect. The cause remains unknown, but there seems to be a correlation between the prevalence of AS and the presence of HLA-B27. Fewer than 5 percent are diagnosed after the age of 45.

Answer D is incorrect. AS is an inflammatory disease affecting persons in early adulthood (not teenagers). An infectious disorder does not cause it.

15. Answer A is correct. Degenerative joint disease is the most common type of low back pain. The lumbar facet joints are susceptible to wear and tear, degeneration, inflammation, and arthritic changes. This may result in pain or limited ROM.

Answer B is incorrect. Spinal stenosis is common in older adults with approximately 11 percent of adults in the United States having lumbar spinal stenosis. Although common, it is not the most common cause of chronic LBP.

Answer C is incorrect. RA is generally a genetic disorder and is more commonly seen in people with a family history of RA. It affects about 1 percent of the population worldwide.

Answer D is incorrect. Osteoarthritis can affect the sacroiliac (SI) joint, leading to bone spurs. It can cause pain, loss of function, and inflammation of the hips, pelvic region, and lower back. It is not the most common cause of LBP.

16. Answer B is correct. Radicular pain radiates into the lower extremity (thigh, calf, and occasionally the foot) directly along the course of a specific spinal nerve root. The most common symptom of radicular pain is sciatica, which is caused by spinal nerve compression in the lower back. It often will be caused by compression of the lower spinal nerve roots (L5 and S1). With this condition, leg pain and weakness may occur, depending on which nerve in the low back is affected.

Answer A is incorrect. The SLR test identifies impairment or nerve root irritation in the lower back. A negative test indicates the patient can tolerate the leg raised to 80 to 90 degrees (depending on age and overall health). A positive SLR may indicate several conditions, including lumbar disc herniation.

Answer C is incorrect. Dull, achy pain in the back is not radicular pain, as it does not radiate to a specific area along the nerve root.

Answer D is incorrect. Lumbar radiculopathy usually affects only one side of the body, depending on what nerve root is affected.

17. Answer D is correct. A lumbar laminectomy is typically performed to alleviate pain from lumbar spinal stenosis. Spinal stenosis is caused by degenerative changes that lead to enlargement of the facet joints in the back of the vertebrae.

Answer A is incorrect. A spinal tumor will cause pain at the site of the tumor due to growth. Surgery may be performed to resect the tumor. It is not the most common reason for lumbar surgery. Spinal cord tumors are typically persistent and progressive in nature.

Answer B is incorrect. Ankylosing spondylitis is an autoimmune disorder that occurs in young people, usually under the age of 40. The preferred form of treatment is PT along with NSAIDs or the use of tumor necrosis factor (TNF) blockers such as Humira, Enbrel, or Remicade. Treatment is most successful when started before the disease causes irreversible damage.

Answer C is incorrect. Spondylolisthesis occurs due to the vertebra slipping forward onto the bone below it. A back brace for support and low-impact activities, such as swimming, can treat a low-grade slippage. A higher level of slippage may require surgical intervention. It is not a common cause of lumbar surgery.

18. Answer D is correct. Standing upright and bending backward (extension) can worsen spinal stenosis symptoms. This is because lumbar flexion (bending forward) increases the diameter of the transverse foramen. Therefore, it is more comfortable for patients to sit or lean forward. Patients are frequently unable to walk long distances and often state that their symptoms are improved when bending forward while walking with the support of a walker or shopping cart (shopping cart sign).

Answer A is incorrect. Symptoms present with spinal stenosis typically get worse when standing or walking. They typically improve with sitting or leaning forward.

Answer B is incorrect. Most people with spinal stenosis cannot walk for any length of time without pain symptoms getting much worse.

Answer C is incorrect. Lying on the stomach increases pressure and strain on the back and the spine. Sleeping on the back is the best position for dealing with back pain.

19. Answer D is correct. Generally, Gower's sign is identified by how people with proximal muscle weakness stand up from the floor. A patient with lumbar instability or weakness may bend the top half of their body forward, place weight on their knees using their hands, transfer their body weight supported by their hands up their legs, and then raise to a standing position.

Answer A is incorrect. A patient with a lumbar disc herniation will not demonstrate a positive Gower's sign. Gower's sign indicates weakness of the pelvic and proximal lower limb muscles, which is not associated with disc herniation.

Answer B is incorrect. An AAA usually presents as pain in the abdomen, legs, or back. It is not associated with weakness in the lower limb muscles.

Answer C is incorrect. Lumbar radiculopathy causes sciatic pain. It is often associated with a herniated lumbar disc.

20. Answer C is correct. Costochondritis is inflammation of the junctions of the ribs with the cartilage where it attaches at the sternum. Costochondritis causes localized chest wall pain and tenderness that can be reproduced by pushing on the involved cartilage in the front of the rib cage. Costochondritis is a relatively harmless MS chest pain and usually resolves without treatment.

    Answer A is incorrect. The pain associated with an AAA is usually abdominal, low back, or leg pain. It does not involve pain in the chest wall.

    Answer B is incorrect. C5-C6 radiculopathy is associated with tingling, pain, or numbness from the neck into the shoulder and down the arm to the thumb. There may be associated weakness in the upper arm.

    Answer D is incorrect. Lumbar facet syndrome causes lower back, buttocks, or thigh pain.

21. Answer D is correct (All of the above). When considering the differential diagnoses for a patient complaining of thoracic pain, the possibility of disc herniation, rib fracture, and shingles should all be considered as potential diagnoses.

22. Answer A is correct. Scoliosis most typically occurs in those 10 to 18 years old, females more than males, and is often detected by school screenings or regular physician visits. A medical professional will look for a curvature of the spine, uneven shoulders, and protrusion of one shoulder blade, asymmetry of the waistline, or one hip higher than the other.

    Answer B is incorrect. Scoliosis is less common in teenage boys. It most often develops during growth spurts such as during puberty.

    Answer C is incorrect. Scoliosis occurs in young women during periods of rapid growth, such as during puberty. Onset in the 30s and 40s would be unusual.

    Answer D is incorrect. Scoliosis affects 2 to 3 percent of the population and tends to run in families, so there may be a genetic factor.

23. Correct answer is C. The Milwaukee brace is also known as a cervico-thoraco-lumbo-sacral orthosis. It is a back brace used to treat spinal curvatures such as scoliosis. It is a full-torso brace that extends from the pelvis to the base of the skull. This brace is normally used with growing adolescents to hold a 25° to 40° advancing curve. The brace is intended to minimize the progression to an acceptable level, not to correct the curvature.

    Answer A is incorrect. Torticollis occurs when neck muscles cause the head to twist and tilt to one side. It is also called wryneck and is most associated with newborn babies. Treatment depends on the etiology and consists of PT, heat therapy, massage therapy, and sometimes a neck collar.

    Answer B is incorrect. Lumbar stenosis is treated with anti-inflammatory medications, PT, steroid injections, and if necessary, spinal surgery. A brace does not help lumbar stenosis.

    Answer D is incorrect. Thoracic disc herniation is treated with pain medication, anti-inflammatory medications, rest, and PT.

24. Answer D is correct. Torticollis results in a fixed or dynamic posturing of the head and neck in tilt, rotation, and flexion. Spasms of the sternocleidomastoid, trapezius, and other neck muscles, usually more prominent on one side than the other, may cause turning or tipping of the head.

    Answer A is incorrect. Anterior scalene muscles allow for flexion of the cervical portion of the vertebral column. The muscles also help elevate the first rib.

    Answer B is incorrect. The subclavius muscle lies between the clavicle and the first rib. Its function is to stabilize the clavicle during shoulder and arm movement.

    Answer C is incorrect. The latissimus dorsi muscle is one of the largest muscles in the back and stretches across the lower posterior thorax. It is involved primarily in moving the shoulder and raising the trunk upward when the arms are raised above the head.

25. Answer D is correct. A concussion is a traumatic brain injury that alters the way the brain functions. Effects are usually temporary but can include headaches, visual disturbances, and problems with concentration, memory, balance, and coordination.

    Answer A is incorrect. Cervical disc herniation manifests as pain or numbness along the neck, upper arm, forearm, and fingers.

    Answer B is incorrect. The cervical spine is the third most common site of RA. It can destroy the cervical joints, including subluxation, and results in pain and neurological deficits.

    Answer C is incorrect. Cervical radiculopathy causes pain that spreads to the arm, neck, chest, and upper back. There may be paresthesia in the hand or fingers and weakness in the arm muscles.

Resources

Aldridge, T. (2004). Diagnosing heel pain in adults. *American Family Physician, 70*, 332–342.

Almond, L. M., Hamid, N. A., & Wasserberg, J. (2007). Thoracic intradural disc herniation. *British Journal of Neurosurgery, 21*(1), 32–34.

American Academy of Orthopaedic Surgeons (AAOS). (2014, September 5). American Academy of Orthopaedic Surgeons clinical practice guideline on management of anterior cruciate ligament injuries. *American Academy of Orthopaedic Surgeons,* 619.

Bare, A. A., & Guanche, C. A. (2005). Hip impingement: The role of arthroscopy. *Orthopedics, 28*(3), 266–273.

Block, J. A., & Sequeira, W. (2001). Raynaud's phenomenon. *The Lancet, 357*(9273), 2042–2048.

Bontempo, N. A., & Mazzocca, A. D. (2010). Biomechanics and treatment of acromioclavicular and sternoclavicular joint injuries. *British Journal of Sports Medicine, 44*(5), 361–369.

Bozkurt, M., Unlu, S., Cay, N., Apaydin, N., & Dogan, M. (2014). The potential effect of anatomic relationship between the femur and the tibia on medial meniscus tears. *Surgical and Radiologic Anatomy, 36*(8), 741–746.

Çakmak, S., Tekin, L., & Akarsu, S. (2014). Long-term outcome of Osgood-Schlatter disease: Not always favorable. *Rheumatology International, 34*(1), 135–136.

Carcia, C. R., Martin, R. L., Houck, J., & Wukich, D. K. (2010). Orthopaedic section of the American Physical Therapy Association. Achilles pain, stiffness, and muscle power deficits: Achilles tendinitis. *Journal of Orthopaedic & Sports Physical Therapy, 40*(9), A1–A26.

Cheung, J. P. Y., Fung, B., & Ip, W. Y. (2012). Review on mallet finger treatment. *Hand Surgery, 17*(3), 439–447.

Cortina, J., Amat, C., Selga, J., & Corona, P. S. (2014). Isolated medial foot compartment syndrome after ankle sprain. *Foot and Ankle Surgery, 20*(1), e1–e2.

Debarge, R., Demey, G., & Roussouly, P. (2011). Sagittal balance analysis after pedicle subtraction osteotomy in ankylosing spondylitis. *European Spine Journal, 20*(5), 619–625.

de Souza, M. C., de Ávila Fernandes, E., Jones, A., Lombardi Jr., I., & Natour, J. (2011). Assessment of cervical pain and function in patients with rheumatoid arthritis. *Clinical Rheumatology, 30*(6), 831–836.

Do, T. T. (2006). Congenital muscular torticollis: Current concepts and review of treatment. *Current Opinion in Pediatrics, 18*(1), 26–29.

El-Sallakh, S., Aly, T., Amin, O., & Hegazi, M. (2012). Surgical management of chronic Boutonniere deformity. *Hand Surgery, 17*(3), 359–364.

Expert Panel on Musculoskeletal Imaging, Beaman, F. D., von Herrmann, P. F., Kransdorf, M. J., Adler, R. S., Amini, B., Appel, M., Arnold, E., Bernard, S. A., Greenspan, B. S., Lee, K. S., Tuite, M. J., Walker, E. A., Ward, R. J., Wessell, D. E., & Weissman, B. N. (2017). ACR Appropriateness Criteria® Suspected Osteomyelitis, Septic Arthritis, or Soft Tissue Infection (Excluding Spine and Diabetic Foot). *Journal of the American College of Radiology, 14*(5S), S326–S337. https://doi.org/10.1016/j.jacr.2017.02.008

Forman, T., Forman, S., & Rose N. A. (2005). A clinical approach to diagnosing wrist pain. *American Family Physician, 72*(9), 1753–1758.

Franco, A. H. (1987). Pes cavus and pes planus analyses and treatment. *Physical Therapy, 67*(5), 688–694.

Fritz, J. M., Piva, S. R., & Childs, J. D. (2005). Accuracy of the clinical examination to predict radiographic instability of the lumbar spine. *European Spine Journal, 14*(8), 743–750.

Gautam, V. K., Verma, S., Batra, S., Bhatnagar, N., & Arora, S. (2015). Platelet-rich plasma versus corticosteroid injection for recalcitrant lateral epicondylitis: Clinical and ultrasonographic evaluation. *Journal of Orthopaedic Surgery, 23*(1), 1–5.

Gervais, J., Périé, D., Parent, S., Labelle, H., & Aubin, C. E. (2012). MRI signal distribution within the intervertebral disc as a biomarker of adolescent idiopathic scoliosis and spondylolisthesis. *BMC Musculoskeletal Disorders, 13*(1), 239.

Gilden, D., Mahalingam, R., Nagel, M. A., Pugazhenthi, S., & Cohrs, R. J. (2011). Review: The neurobiology of varicella zoster virus infection. *Neuropathology and Applied Neurobiology, 37*(5), 441–463.

Gude, W., & Morelli, V. (2008). Ganglion cysts of the wrist: Pathophysiology, clinical picture, and management. *Current Reviews in Musculoskeletal Medicine, 1*(3–4), 205–211.

Guly, H. R. (2002). Injuries initially misdiagnosed as sprained wrist (Beware the sprained wrist). *Emergency Medicine Journal, 19*, 41–42.

Hailer, Y. D., Montgomery, S., Ekbom, A., Nilsson, O., & Bahmanyar, S. (2012). Legg-Calve-Perthes disease and the risk of injuries requiring hospitalization: A register study involving 2579 patients. *Acta Orthopaedica, 83*(6), 572–576.

Hardy, P., & Sanghavi, S. (2009). Rotator cuff injury: Still a clinical controversy? *Knee Surgery, Sports Traumatology, Arthroscopy, 17*(4), 325–327.

Herman, A. M., & Marzo, J. M. (2014). Popliteal cysts: A current review. *Orthopedics (Online), 37*(8), e678.

Honda, H., & McDonald, J. R. (2009). Current recommendations in the management of osteomyelitis of the hand and wrist. *The Journal of Hand Surgery, 34*(6), 1135–1136.

Huisstede, B. M., Fridén, J., Coert, J. H., Hoogvliet, P., & European HANDGUIDE Group. (2014). Carpal tunnel syndrome: Hand surgeons, hand therapists, and physical medicine and rehabilitation physicians agree on a multidisciplinary treatment guideline—results from the European HANDGUIDE Study. *Archives of Physical Medicine and Rehabilitation, 95*(12), 2253–2263.

Huisstede, B. M., Hoogvliet, P., Coert, J. H., & Fridén, J. (2014). Multidisciplinary consensus guideline for managing trigger finger: Results from the European HANDGUIDE Study. *Physical Therapy, 94*(10), 1421–1433.

Ilahi, O. A., Cosculluela, P. E., & Ho, D. M. (2008). Classification of anterosuperior glenoid labrum variants and their association with shoulder pathology. *Orthopedics, 31*(3), 226.

Iversen, T., Solberg, T. K., Romner, B., Wilsgaard, T., Nygaard, Ø., Waterloo, K., . . . & Ingebrigtsen, T. (2013). Accuracy of physical examination for chronic lumbar radiculopathy. *BMC Musculoskeletal Disorders, 14*(1), 206.

Kasai, Y., Akeda, K., & Uchida, A. (2007). Physical characteristics of patients with developmental cervical spinal canal stenosis. *European Spine Journal, 16*(7), 901–903.

Kontopodis, N., Metaxa, E., Papaharilaou, Y., Tavlas, E., Tsetis, D., & Ioannou, C. (2014). Advancements in identifying biomechanical determinants for abdominal aortic aneurysm rupture. *Vascular, 23*(1), 65–77.

Kosashvili, Y., Drexler, M., Backstein, D., Safir, O., Lakstein, D., Safir, A., . . . & Gross, A. (2014). Dislocation after the first and multiple revision total hip arthroplasty: Comparison between acetabulum-only, femur-only and both component revision hip arthroplasty. *Canadian Journal of Surgery, 57*(2), E15.

Lamba, D., Pant, V. S., Joshi, M., Sah, H., & Mahara, M. (2011). A comparison study of the effects of massage therapy with and without ultrasonic therapy in medial epicondylitis. *Journal of Physiotherapy & Occupational Therapy, 5*(2), 54–57.

Lau, L. H., Kerr, D., Law, I., & Ritchie, P. (2013). Nurse practitioners treating ankle and foot injuries using the Ottawa Ankle Rules: A comparative study in the emergency department. *Australasian Emergency Nursing Journal, 16*(3), 110–115.

Liporace, F. A., Adams, M. R., Capo, J. T., & Koval, K. J. (2009). Distal radius fractures. *Journal of Orthopaedic Trauma, 23*(10), 739–748.

Maffey, L., & Emery, C. (2007). What are the risk factors for groin strain injury in sport? *Sports Medicine, 37*(10), 881–894.

Martin, R. L., Davenport, T. E., Paulseth, S., Wukich, D. K., & Godges, J. J. (2013). Orthopaedic Section American Physical Therapy Association. Ankle stability and movement coordination impairments: Ankle ligament sprains. *Journal of Orthopaedic & Sports Physical Therapy, 43*(9), A1–A40.

Melvin, J. S., & Mehta, S. (2011). Patellar fractures in adults. *Journal of the American Academy of Orthopaedic Surgeons, 19*(4), 198–207.

McKeon, K. E., & Lee, D. H. (2015). Posttraumatic Boutonnière and swan neck deformities. *Journal of the American Academy of Orthopaedic Surgeons, 23*(10), 623–632.

Miao, J., Wang, S., Wan, Z., Park, W. M., Xia, Q., Wood, K., & Li, G. (2013). Motion characteristics of the vertebral segments with lumbar degenerative spondylolisthesis in elderly patients. *European Spine Journal, 22*(2), 425–431.

Moore, J. S. (1997). De Quervain's tenosynovitis: Stenosing tenosynovitis of the first dorsal compartment. *Journal of Occupational and Environmental Medicine, 39*(10), 990–1002.

Moen, M. H., Bongers, T., Bakker, E. W., Zimmermann, W. O., Weir, A., Tol, J. L., & Backx, F. J. G. (2012). Risk factors and prognostic indicators for medial tibial stress syndrome. *Scandinavian Journal of Medicine & Science in Sports, 22*(1), 34–39.

Mulligan, J., & Amblum, J. (2014). Diagnosis and treatment of scaphoid fracture. *Emergency Nurse, 22*(3), 18–23.

Non-Surgical Management of Hip and Knee Osteoarthritis Working Group. (2014). *VA/DoD clinical practice guideline for the non-surgical management of hip and knee osteoarthritis*. Department of Veterans Affairs, Department of Defense. p. 126

Pearce, J. M. S. (2008). Observations on concussion. *European Neurology, 59*(3–4), 113–119.

Proulx, A. M., & Zryd, T. W. (2009). Costochondritis: Diagnosis and treatment. *Am Fam Physician, 80*(6), 617–620.

Rambani, R. & Hackney, R. (2015). Loss of range of motion of the hip joint: A hypothesis for etiology of sports hernia. *Muscles, Ligaments and Tendons Journal, 5*(1), 29.

Ramonda, R., Frallonardo, P., Musacchio, E., Vio, S., & Punzi, L. (2014). Joint and bone assessment in hand osteoarthritis. *Clinical Rheumatology, 33*(1), 11–19.

Roddy, E., Zwierska, I., Hay, E. M., Jowett, S., Lewis, M., Stevenson, K., . . . & Foster, N. E. (2014). Subacromial impingement syndrome and pain: Protocol for a randomised controlled trial of exercise and corticosteroid injection (the SUPPORT trial). *BMC Musculoskeletal Disorders, 15*(1), 81.

Rogers, L. C., Frykberg, R. G., Armstrong, D. G., Boulton, A. J., Edmonds, M., Van, G. H., . . . & Uccioli, L. (2011). The Charcot foot. *Diabetes Care*, 34(9), 2123–2129.

Rosenthal, M. D., Rainey, C. E., Tognoni, A., & Worms, R. (2012). Evaluation and management of posterior cruciate ligament injuries. *Physical Therapy in Sport, 13*, 196–208.

Schwartz, E. N., & Su, J. (2014). Plantar fasciitis: A concise review. *The Permanente Journal, 18*(1), e105.

Shakil, H., Iqbal, Z. A., & Al-Ghadir, A. H. (2013). Scoliosis: Review of types of curves, etiological theories and conservative treatment. *Journal of Back and Musculoskeletal Rehabilitation, 27*(2), 111–115.

Sinha, I., Lee, M., & Cobiella, C. (2008). Management of osteoarthritis of the glenohumeral joint. *British Journal of Hospital Medicine (London, England: 2005), 69*(5), 264–268.

Stein, G., Koebke, J., Faymonville, C., Dargel, J., Müller, L. P., & Schiffer, G. (2011). The relationship between the medial collateral ligament and the medial meniscus: A topographical and biomechanical study. *Surgical and Radiologic Anatomy, 33*(9), 763–766.

Szucs, P. A., Richman, P. B., & Mandell, M. (2001). Triage nurse application of the Ottawa knee rule. *Academic Emergency Medicine, 8*(2), 112–116.

Takao, T., Morishita, Y., Okada, S., Maeda, T., Katoh, F., Ueta, T., . . . & Shiba, K. (2013). Clinical relationship between cervical spinal canal stenosis and traumatic cervical spinal cord injury without major fracture or dislocation. *European Spine Journal, 22*(10), 2228–2231.

Tamburrelli, F. C., Genitiempo, M., Bochicchio, M., Donisi, L., & Ratto, C. (2014). Cauda equina syndrome: Evaluation of the clinical outcome. *European Review for Medical and Pharmacological Sciences, 18*(7), 1098–1105.

Townley, W. A., Baker, R., Sheppard, N., & Grobbelaar, A. O. (2006). Dupuytren's contracture unfolded. *BMJ: British Medical Journal, 332*(7538), 397.

Urrutia, J., & Fadic, R. (2012). Cervical disc herniation producing acute Brown–Sequard syndrome: Dynamic changes documented by intraoperative neuromonitoring. *European Spine Journal, 21*, 418–421.

Van Demark, Jr., R., Van Demark, III, R., & Helsper, E. (2015). Stress fracture of the hook of the hamate: A case report. *South Dakota Medicine, 68*(4), 157–9, 161.

Vinther, A., Kanstrup, I. L., Christiansen, E., Alkjær, T., Larsson, B., Magnusson, S. P., & Aagaard, P. (2005). Exercise-induced rib stress fractures: Influence of reduced bone mineral density. *Scandinavian Journal of Medicine & Science in Sports, 15*(2), 95–99.

Walmsley, S., Osmotherly, P. G., & Rivett, D. A. (2014). Clinical identifiers for early-stage primary/idiopathic adhesive capsulitis: Are we seeing the real picture? *Physical Therapy, 94*(7), 968–976.

Weinstein, J. N., Tosteson, T. D., Lurie, J. D., Tosteson, A. N., Blood, E., Hanscom, B., . . . & An, H. (2008). Surgical versus nonsurgical therapy for lumbar spinal stenosis. *New England Journal of Medicine, 358*(8), 794–810.

Werner, B. C., Fashandi, A. H., Gwathmey, F. W., & Yarboro, S. R. (2015). Trends in the management of intertrochanteric femur fractures in the United States 2005–2011. *Hip International, 25*(3), 270–276.

Yan, J., Sasaki, W., & Hitomi, J. (2010). Anatomical study of the lateral collateral ligament and its circumference structures in the human knee joint. *Surgical and Radiologic Anatomy, 32*(2), 99–106.

CHAPTER 11

Nervous System

Nancy L. Dennert, MS, MSN, FNP-BC, CDCES, BC-ADM

Overview of Neurological Assessment

- Exam findings can be deduced from a careful history
- Initial MINIMAL screening exams should include the following:
  - Mental status—Oriented to person, place, and time; ability to follow commands and respond appropriately
  - Cranial nerves—Visual fields, pupillary light reflex (Pupils are Equal, Round, and Reactive to Light and Accommodation [PERRLA]), extraocular muscles (EOMs), facial strength, and hearing to whisper test or finger rub
  - Motor system—Strength in upper and lower extremities, pronator drift, tandem gait walking on heels; coordination: rapid alternating movements (RAMs), finger-to-nose, heel-knee-shin
  - Reflexes—Deep tendon reflexes (DTRs); plantar, biceps, triceps, patellar, and ankle bilaterally (Graded 0 = absent, 1 = hypoactive, 2 = normal, 3 = hyperactive, 4 = clonus)
  - Sensation—Light touch, two-point discrimination, all four distal extremities, vibration on great toe bilaterally

Romberg Test

The Romberg test measures a person's sense of balance. Specifically, it measures proprioception. When a person is standing with their eyes open, they receive visual, proprioceptive, and vestibular information. With their eyes closed, they must rely on proprioception and vestibular function.

The test: The patient is asked to stand with feet together, arms at their sides, and then close their eyes for 60 seconds. A positive Romberg test occurs if the patient cannot maintain their balance (some swaying if acceptable). If the patient must move their feet or put one foot in front of the other to prevent falling or starts to fall (the examiner should stand close to prevent falling), this is considered a positive Romberg test. Further evaluation is needed.

Deficits in any area, or neurologic complaints or findings, require an expanded exam. **Figure 11-1** illustrates the functional areas of the cerebral cortex.

Cranial Nerves

To remember the cranial nerves (**Figure 11-2**), use a mnemonic "On Old Olympus's Towering Top, A Finn and German Viewed Some Hops":

- CN I: Olfactory
- CN II: Optic
- CN III: Oculomotor
- CN IV: Trochlear
- CN V: Trigeminal
- CN VI: Abducens
- CN VII: Facial
- CN VIII: Acoustic
- CN IX: Glossopharyngeal
- CN X: Vagus
- CN XI: Spinal Accessory
- CN XII: Hypoglossal

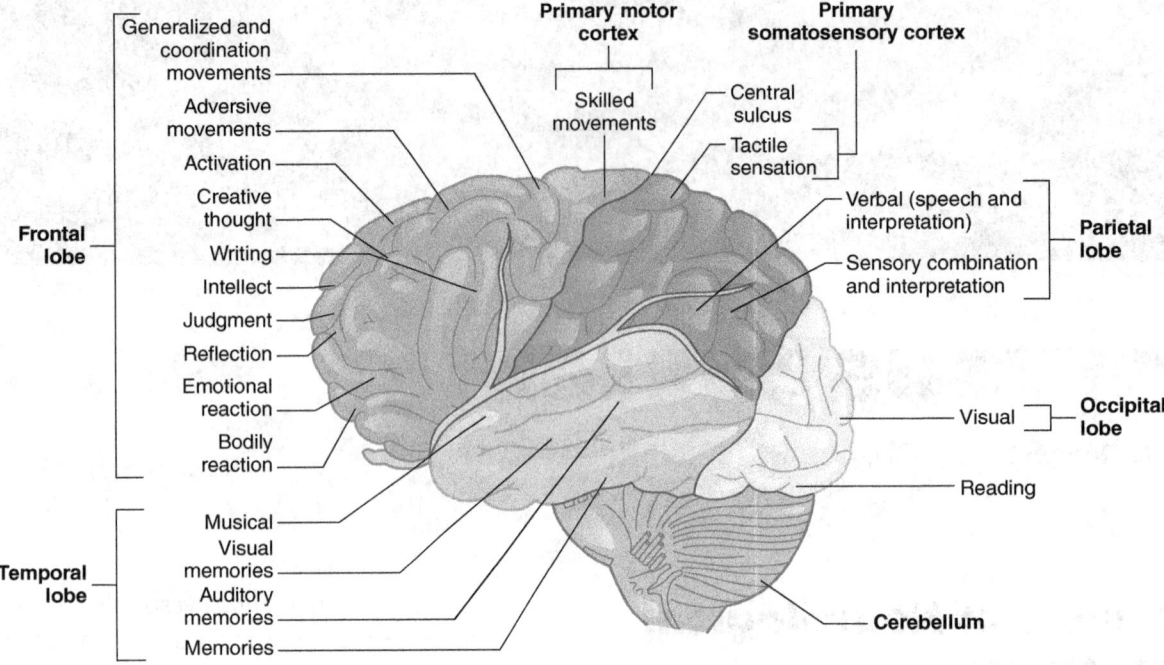

Figure 11-1 Functional Areas of Cerebral Cortex.

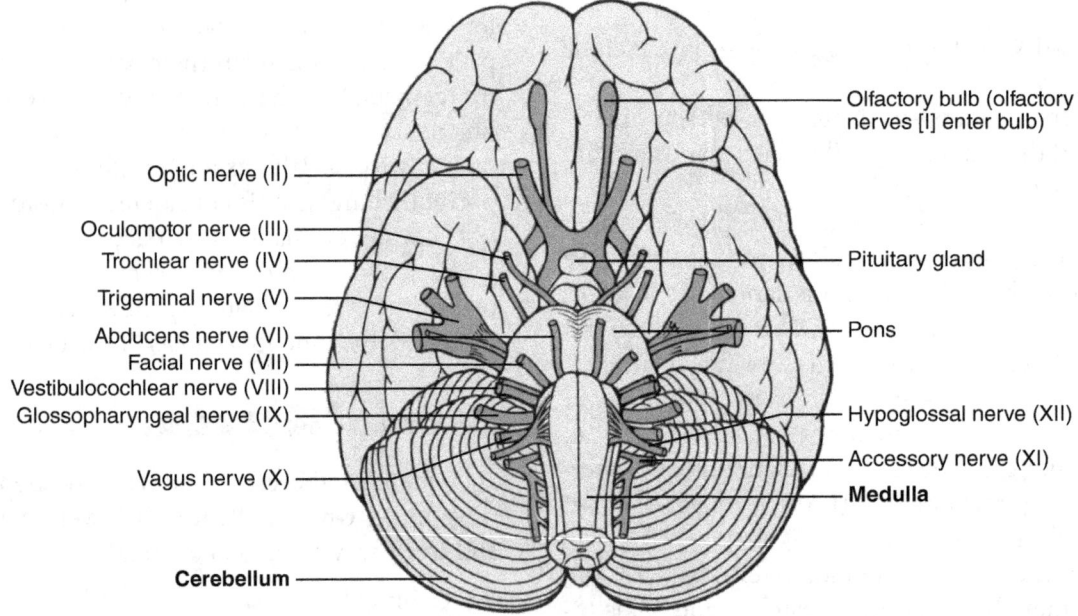

Figure 11-2 Cranial nerves.

Red Flags for Referral for Adults

- No response to treatment or improvement from standard therapy
- Focal findings suggestive of space-occupying lesion of the brain or spinal cord (unequal pupil size, papilledema with headache)
- Peripheral nerve compression
- Acute or sudden onset of symptoms—headache, change in level of consciousness (LOC), aphasia, visual change = IMMEDIATE consult/hospital
- Headaches requiring emergency care:
  - "Worst headache of my life"
  - Thunderclap headache (abrupt onset of severe pain)
  - Sudden onset of exertional headache (after sex, coughing, straining)

Brain Tumors

Brain tumors may be associated with signs of increased intracranial pressure (ICP):

- Vomiting without nausea and neuro deficits
- Headache may be in the morning, usually dull aching and increasing over time

New-onset seizures are considered mass lesions. Symptoms and deficits will be dependent on the location of the tumor.

*A classic triad that may be observed when there is increased intracranial pressure is papilledema, morning headache, and vomiting.

Stroke and Transient Ischemic Attack

Strokes are the leading cause of adult long-term disability in the United States. There is a higher incidence in men; people older than 60; Asian, Hispanic, and Black people; persons with a family history; and lower socioeconomic status (nonmodifiable risk factors).

- Modifiable risk factors include:
  - Hypertension
  - Hyperlipidemia
  - Carotid stenosis or dissection
  - Cardiac disease
  - Atherosclerosis
  - Previous stroke or transient ischemic attack (TIA)
  - Diabetes
  - Obesity and a sedentary lifestyle
  - Poor nutrition
  - Cigarette smoking
  - Alcohol consumption
  - Obstructive sleep apnea (OSA)
  - Stress
- Women: Oral contraceptive use is linked to a small increase in risk of thrombosis. Risk increased significantly with women who smoke. Estrogen should also not be used with vascular disease (preeclampsia).
- Pregnant and postpartum have higher associations (coagulopathy and preeclampsia).
- Migraine with aura is associated with a 2-fold risk of stroke.
- Illicit drug use of cocaine, heroin, and amphetamine abuse is linked to stroke.

"Time is brain"—onset of symptoms is important to assess (thrombolytic therapy window of 4.5 hours).

Sensitive Test for Stroke

- Pronator drift—Observe: Facial droop, arm weakness, and speech abnormalities—probability of stroke = 72 percent
  - Patient stands with arms outstretched and fully extended, palms up, and eyes closed. Watch 5 to 10 seconds for pronation and downward drift (+ test).

Transient Ischemic Attack

TIA is a transient episode of neurological dysfunction caused by focal brain, spinal cord, or retinal ischemia without acute infarction.

- Episode lasts less than 10 minutes and not longer than 24 hours
- Increased risk of stroke (5%) within 48 hours

Stroke

Strokes cause a reduction in cerebral blood flow to a region of the brain, resulting in vascular injury.

- Types:
  - Ischemic—(most common—85 percent) occlusion or stenosis caused by the following:
    - Atherosclerosis of large vessels extra- or intracranial (ICA, MCA)
    - Small vessel disease—lacunar stroke
    - Cardioembolic (atrial fibrillation [aFib])
    - hypercoagulable states, vasculitis or dissection, and infarcts of unknown origin (cryptogenic)

  Figure 11-3 illustrates an ischemic stroke.
  - Hemorrhagic—(15%) subarachnoid, intracerebral

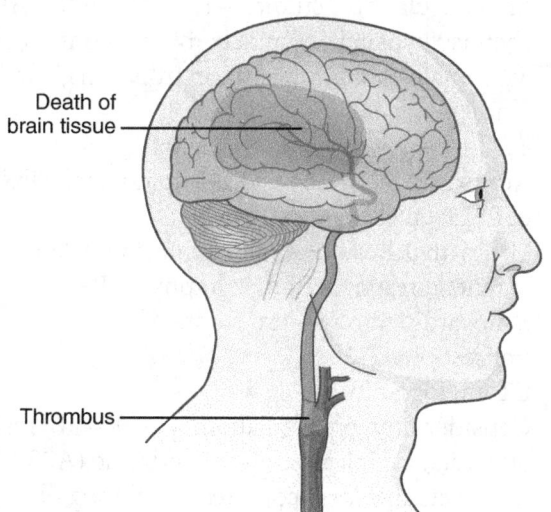

Figure 11-3 Ischemic Stroke.

Neurologic deficits represent the decreased blood flow in the affected region of the brain. Sickle cell disease is the most common cause of ischemic stroke in African American children. The treatment for a suspected stroke is **immediate referral to the ER**. Brain imaging should be taken within 24 hours of symptom onset for TIA.

> **Red Flags for Stroke**
>
> - Sudden severe headache/nausea/vomiting
> - Sudden dizziness or inability to walk
> - Sudden confusion
> - Sudden difficulty seeing in one/both eyes
> - Sudden difficulty speaking or understanding
> - Sudden numbness/weakness of one side of the body or face
> - Sudden altered level of consciousness

*Look for red flags—arm drift (pronator drift), weakness, facial droop, or abnormal speech.

Management

- Pulse oximetry
- Blood pressure
- Antiplatelet Drugs: recommended for reduction of vascular events in patients with a history of ischemic stroke.
- Aspirin (50 to 325 mg)
- Combination aspirin/dipyridamole (25 and 200 mg BID ER dipyridamole)
- Ticlopidine
- Clopidogrel 7 mg

Testing

- Immediate noncontrast CT to exclude intracerebral hemorrhage (ICH) (stroke)
- Anticoagulation studies—PT < INR, APTT, chemistry panel, complete blood count (CBC) with platelet count, cardiac troponins, creatine kinase
- ECG
- Nonurgent labs to consider—lipid panel, HbA1C, ESR, LFTs, CRP
- MRI with diffusion weighted imaging (DWI) (TIA)
- Magnetic resonance angiography (MRA)
- Echocardiography—transthoracic and/or transesophageal
- CT angiography
- Consider hypercoagulation panel—(if history warrants) antiphospholipid syndrome (APS), Factor V Leiden, B2 glycoprotein immunoglobulin M (IgM), immunoglobulin g (IgG), Protein C, Protein S, Antithrombin III

Anticoagulants

- Warfarin—an inexpensive means to prevent stroke in aFib, coagulopathies, and cardiomyopathy. Requires regular INRs with goals typically being 2.0 to 3.0. Diet issues related to vitamin K content of foods.
- Direct oral anticoagulants (DOACs)—relatively low bleeding risk with good safety profiles. In 2015, the Food and Drug Administration (FDA) approved idarucizumab (Praxbind) to reverse Pradaxa. In 2018, the FDA approved andexanet alfa (AndexXa) to reverse apixaban (Eliquis) and rivaroxaban (Xarelto).
  - NO INR needed. Check renal clearance/creatinine.
- Dabigatran (Pradaxa): 150 mg PO (by mouth) twice daily
- Rivaroxaban (Xarelto): 20 mg PO daily
- Apixaban (Eliquis)—5 mg PO twice daily

CHADS2 VAS score is used to assess the risk of stroke in nonvalvular AFib patients to determine the level of anticoagulation needed.

Concussion

A concussion is a direct, impulsive force delivered to the head, face, or body, resulting in rapid acceleration, deceleration, or rotation of the brain.

- Mild traumatic brain injury (TBI) or concussion used interchangeably—accounts for 75 percent of TBI with 3 million cases annually.
- Fewer than 10 percent of patients with sports-related concussions have LOC.
- Sports with the greatest risk—males: football and rugby, hockey, and soccer; females: soccer and basketball
- Loss of consciousness is not a reliable indicator of dysfunction or recovery.

Symptoms may present in a delayed fashion. There are three categories of signs and symptoms:

- Somatic—headaches, sleep disturbance, tinnitus, nausea/vomiting, visual disturbance, imbalance
- Cognitive—poor concentration, memory impairment, complaints of mental fog, confusion about recent events, repeating or answering questions slowly
- Neuropsychiatric—anxiety, increased fatigue, depressed mood, irritability

Clinical Management
- CT imaging is used for LOC with more serious TBIs to rule out subarachnoid hemorrhage, post-traumatic amnesia, focal neurologic deficits, skull fracture, or an alteration in mental status that persists.
- Encourage "cocooning" after injury—physical and cognitive rest, no video, schoolwork, TV, or texting for the first 48 hours.
- For athletes: no return to play until complete resolution of symptoms during exercise and rest
- Risk factors for prolonged recovery: younger age, previous concussions, headaches, and "fogginess"
- Postconcussive syndrome can develop (headache, dizziness, concentration/processing disturbance)
- Patients who experience repetitive concussions are at risk for permanent impairment, which may lead to psychiatric illnesses, dementia, and chronic traumatic encephalopathy (CTE).

Inquire as to whether the patient is on any anticoagulant therapy (NSAIDs, Aspirin [ASA]) because this would indicate a higher risk of brain hemorrhage.

Meningitis

Meningitis is the inflammation of the meninges caused by a bacterial infection. People at the extremes of age (e.g., newborns and older people) are most at risk.

Etiology
- Bacterial—*Streptococcus pneumoniae*. *Haemophilus influenzae* type B, and *Neisseria meningitidis*. Hib vaccine is now given and has decreased the incidence of H. flu and Listeria monocytogenes
- Viral—coxsackie, echo, herpes, West Nile, Epstein-Barr virus (EBV), cytomegalovirus (CMV)
- Other—Lyme, syphilis, fungal, protozoal
- Bacterial is fatal in 5 to 40 percent of cases.

Risk
- HIV
- Alcoholism
- Malignancy
- Head trauma
- Asplenia
- Complement deficiency
- College students living in dormitories
- Tuberculosis (TB)
- Infective endocarditis

Clinical Presentation
- Rapid development of fever and chills (85%)
- Headache
- Photophobia
- Nuchal rigidity
- Seizures
- Somnolence
- Rashes or petechiae
- Nausea
- Vomiting

May see findings consistent with viral presentation (e.g., tonsillar exudates, vesicular rashes, cervical adenopathy)

Signs of Meningeal Irritation
- Kernig's sign—resistance or discomfort is felt in the back and posterior thigh with passive knee extension when the patient is supine with the hip flexed at 90 degrees.
- Brudzinski's sign—passive neck flexion causes knee or hip flexion.

Prevention
- Hib vaccine
- Conjugate meningitis
- Pneumococcal vaccine

Management
This is a medical emergency.
- Lumbar puncture—cerebrospinal fluid (CSF) culture and gram stain—the only way to differentiate between viral and bacterial
- Elevated white blood cell (WBC) count is seen with more than 1,000 cells/ul—predomination of neutrophils (neutrophilic pleocytosis) bacterial
- WBC less than 1,000 in aseptic or viral meningitis, negative gram stain, no bacteria
- Polymerase chain reaction (PCR for rapid identification
- Labs: CBC, blood cultures, serum electrolytes, glucose, liver function tests (LFTs), HIV—specific tests per history

Treatment
Empiric therapy with antibiotics based on susceptibilities in specific populations and guidelines, **then** targeted therapy dictated by organism and patient population

- Age > 50 years: Vancomycin + ampicillin plus third-generation cephalosporin

- Age 18 to 50 years: Vancomycin + third-generation cephalosporin
- Age 1 to 18: Vancomycin + third-generation cephalosporin
- Age < 1 month—Ampicillin, + gentamicin or cephalosporin
- Treatment of close contacts: meningococcal meningitis (roommates, crowded environments: prisons, military)
- Ciprofloxacin, Rifampin
- Risk of neurologic sequelae, follow-up for hearing and neuropsychological testing required

Progressive Degenerative Disorders

Dementia

Dementia is the chronic deterioration in cognitive function, resulting in impairment in activities of daily living (ADLs), behavior, and deficits in intellectual functioning. **Table 11-1** (Reisberg et al., 1982) describes the variations and global deterioration scales.

Alzheimer's Disease

AD is the most common form of dementia in people ages 65 and over. Prevalence doubles every 5 years after age 65 with genetic and environmental influence. ApoE e4 gene, Down syndrome, and family history increase risk. AD is more common in women. Early onset between ages 30 and 60 is rare (10 percent). Familial, inherited cases account for 50 percent. Other causes that increase risk include:

- hypertension,
- diabetes,
- hyperlipidemia,
- Lower education level, and
- depression.

Advancing age is the greatest risk.

AD is due to amyloid neuritic plaques and neurofibrillary tangles in the brain.

- Insidious onset and gradual progression (continuing cognitive decline)
- Impairment in memory plus aphasia, apraxia, or agnosia (impairment in two cognitive domains): attention, executive function, language, social cognition
- Deficits are a significant decline in the previous level of functioning. Patients are often unaware of deficits. Forgetfulness, disorientation, poor short-term memory, and losing items are common.
- Deficits do not occur exclusively during a course of delirium.

Table 11-1 Global Deterioration Scale

- Used with primary degenerative dementia. Reisberg Stages describe the seven different stages of dementia.
  - Stages 1–3 are the predementia stages.
  - Stages 4–7 are the dementia stages.
  - Beginning in stage 5, an individual can no longer survive without assistance

Each stage lasts 3–4 years and progression is very different among patients.

1. No impairment
2. Very mild cognitive decline. Age-associated memory impairment (e.g., forgets names, misplaces things). Symptoms are not evident to loved ones.
3. Mild cognitive decline. Slight difficulty concentrating, difficulty finding the right words, increased forgetfulness. Loved ones notice.
4. Moderate cognitive decline (clear but early Alzheimer's disease [AD]), moderate dementia. Forgets recent events, can't handle finances, difficulty concentrating, in denial about symptoms. May withdraw from friends or family. Evident to medical personnel.
5. Moderately severe decline (clear functional impairment). Needs assistance with ADLs, forgets address or phone number, doesn't know where they are.
6. Severe decline (can no longer care for self). Forgets major events and recent events. Difficulty speaking.
7. Very severe decline (around-the-clock care or institutional care). Unable to speak or communicate, unable to walk, loss of motor skills.

Data from Reisberg, B., Ferris, S. H., de Leon, M. J., and Crook, T. (1982). Global deterioration scale. *American Journal of Psychiatry, 139*, 1136–1139.

- Experience behavioral problems with sleep disturbance, wandering, agitation, "sundowning," and may have hallucinations and delusions.
- Exam may appear normal; abnormal coordination and motor exam occur in advanced disease.
- Brief assessments to help determine the extent of the dementia can be done with the mini mental state examination (MMSE), neuropsychological testing, and a clock draw test.
- Labs: metabolic panel, CBC, ESR, serum thyroid stimulating hormone (TSH), Vit B12 and folic acid, LFTs, rapid plasma regain (RPR). Urine drug screen (genetic testing for familial type)
- CT/MRI—hippocampal volume loss, temporal lobe, or posterior cortical atrophy
- Positron emission tomography (PET)/single-photon emission computed tomography (SPECT) scanning
- EEG (if seizures suspected)
- Elevations in tau protein on CSF (not done routinely)

Treatment of AD
- Cholinesterase inhibitors—mild to moderate
  - Side effects
    - GI, caution with cardiac conduction abnormalities
    - Syncopal/bradycardic episodes
    - Caution with asthma
    - COPD
    - Seizure
    - GI history
- Donepizil
- Rivastigmine
- Galantamine
  - Lecanemab
  - In 2023, the FDA approved an IV infusion given every 2 weeks, which slowed the decline in people with early AD and mild symptoms.

Treatment of Moderate AD
- Memantine—slows the progression of symptoms of moderate AD. Often used in combination with a cholinesterase inhibitor.
- Antipsychotics used to treat agitation/hallucinations, delusions (Black Box Warning—increases morbidity and cardiovascular events)
  - Haloperidol—risk of tardive dyskinesia
  - Risperidone—extrapyramidal symptoms
  - Olanzapine—metabolic effects, diabetes
  - Quetiapine—orthostasis, sedating
  - Other—antidepressants: Sertraline; Anticonvulsants: valproic acid
- Nonpharmacologic
  - Psychosocial intervention
  - Physical exercise
  - Cognitive exercise
  - ADL training
  - Reality orientation
  - Socialization in familiar surroundings with routine

There is no cure.

Frontotemporal Dementia
- Frontotemporal dementia tends to occur at a younger age than other forms of dementia. Sixty percent of patients are 45 to 65 years old.
- Atrophy of the frontal lobe
- Changes in behavior, disinhibition, and language deficits (both expressive and receptive)

Dementia With Lewy Body
- The second most common form of dementia after AD.
- Typically progresses faster than AD, with a life expectancy of 5 to 8 years after diagnosis.
- Similar to Parkinson's disease dementia, cognitive decline appears first in Lewy body dementia. In Parkinson's disease dementia, the physical symptoms appear long before cognitive decline.
- Fluctuating cognition and visual hallucinations are common. Presence of Lewy bodies in subcortical and cortical structures (absence of neurofibrillary tangles).

Vascular Dementia
- Due to multiple infarcts, often comorbid with AD
- Stepwise progression of decrease in cognition with memory loss occurring later than AD
- History of hypertension, stroke, TIA, hyperlipidemia, vascular disease, and diabetes
- May see abnormal neuro exam (weakness, gait disturbance, exaggerated deep tendon reflexes [DTR])
- Lesions on CT/MRI appear in white and gray matter

Acute Neurological Disorders

Delirium
Delirium is an acute disturbance in mental functioning characterized by confusion, impaired thinking, cognition, and attention deficit with a fluctuating course.

- Patient may be hypo- or hyperalert and demonstrate incoherent or illogical speech
- Risk—advanced age, hospitalized patients

Causes
- Metabolic—electrolyte imbalance, dehydration, hypoxia, vitamin deficiency
- Medications—anticholinergics, antihistamines, lithium, sedatives, narcotics
- Withdrawal—alcohol, benzodiazepines, narcotics
- Infections—UTI, pneumonia, sepsis, influenza
- Neurologic—intracranial hemorrhage, stroke, subdural hematoma, seizure
- Endocrine—hypo/hyperthyroid
- Cardiovascular—congestive heart failure (CHF), myocardial infarction (MI), arrhythmia

Diagnostics
MMSE, CBC, chemistry profile, thyroid panel, LFTs, urinalysis, toxicology screen, CXR. Additional tests as indicated (CT, MRI, LP, EEG)

Treatment

Treat underlying illness (restore electrolyte imbalance or discontinue medication)
   Haldol for agitation—0.25 mg q 4 hour/max 2 mg/d

Headache

Diagnosis is established based on clinical findings. Patient history is the most important tool in evaluation and physical examination (PE). Special attention should be paid to gait, motor, sensory, and fundoscopic exams.

Primary

- Migraine (with and without aura)—aura occurs in 20 percent
- Tension type—most common
- Cluster

Secondary

- Result of abnormal anatomical pathology
- Abnormal neurologic exam, change in pattern of headache, systemic disease
- Increased intracranial pressure
- Intracerebral hemorrhage
- Concussion
- Tumor
- Infection
- Psychiatric

Immediate referral/treatment is needed for subarachnoid hemorrhage, giant cell arteritis, brain tumor, meningitis, ischemic stroke, and Chiari I malformation.

Red Flags (Don't miss possible diagnoses.)

- SA hemorrhage
- Meningitis/encephalitis
- Temporal arteritis
- Acute strokes
- Trigeminal neuralgia
- Hypertensive emergencies
- Mass lesions

Identify Red Flags (These headaches should prompt a CT.)

- Change in basic headache pattern
- Sudden onset, worst headache ever
- Headache accompanied by neurological signs and symptoms
- Sudden onset, especially after age 50
- Physical illness (i.e., fever, chills, nuchal rigidity, rash)
- Headache followed by physical exertion: trauma, exercise, sexual activity
- Or use a common mnemonic device developed to help diagnose secondary headaches.

SNOOP:

Systemic symptoms (fever, weight loss) or secondary headache risk factors (HIV, systemic cancer)

Neurologic symptoms or abnormal signs (confusion, impaired alertness, or consciousness)

Onset: Sudden, abrupt, or split-second

Older: New onset and progressive headache, especially in middle-aged patients under 50 (giant cell arteritis)

Previous headache history or headache progression: first headache or different (change in attack frequency, severity, or clinical features)

Migraine

- Usually unilateral with or without aura associated with nausea, with or without vomiting; photophobia; phonophobia; osmophobia, persisting 4 to 72 hours.
- Aura may precede 20 min to 1 hour before the onset of migraine; visual impairments: scotoma (blindspots), zigzag, flashing lights, paresthesia/weakness, hemianopsia.
- More common in women, strong familial patterns and menstrual patterns are triggers in 50 percent of cases.
- Triggers include fatigue, environment, weather, food, alcohol, caffeine, changes in meals, menstruation, and changes in sleep.

Management

- Diagnostics: NONE required except for neurologic findings, history, or secondary headache
- Laboratory testing: metabolic profile, thyroid function, ESR, rheumatoid arthritis (RA), Lyme, coagulation workup
- **Medical management aims to decrease the number/severity and duration of attacks and reduce impairment.**

Management of Episodic Migraines

- Nonspecific: Acetaminophen, aspirin, and caffeine can effectively treat mild or infrequent

headaches. Other medications that can be used include NSAIDs, combination analgesics, narcotics, steroids, and antinausea medications.
- Triptans—GOLD STANDARD
  - Sumatriptan, eletriptan, rizatriptan, naratriptan, almotriptan: first-line treatment of migraine headache; administration via injection, intranasal, or oral
  - Contraindications: cardiovascular disease, cerebrovascular disease, breastfeeding
  - Side effects: flushing, tingling, chest/neck/sinus/jaw discomfort.
- Ergots—acute treatment—usually migraines lasting less than 72 hours
  - Contraindications: Cardiovascular disease, cerebrovascular disease
  - Side effects: powerful vasoconstrictor; nausea; don't mix with triptan/decongestant
- NSAIDs—naproxen, ketoprofen
  - Contraindications: coronary artery bypass graft (CABG), renal impairment, gastric or peptic ulcer
- Antiemetics: metoclopramide, prochlorperazine, and diphenhydramine for acute nausea and vomiting

Prophylaxis
- When migraine attacks are severe and frequent enough to interfere with a patient's daily activities despite appropriate medical management
- Two or more headaches each week
- Medication overuse during attacks
- Severe adverse effects from medications to treat migraines or unresponsive to abortive treatment
- Contraindications to acute treatment

Miscellaneous Treatment
- Beta blockers—propranolol, timolol
  - Preferred for patients with hypertension, angina
  - Side effects: fatigue, drowsiness
  - Contraindication: asthma, COPD, CHF, type 1 diabetes
- Anticonvulsants—topiramate, gabapentin, divalproex sodium, sodium valproate
- Antidepressant—amitriptyline—preferred for anxiety, mood disorder
- Anticholinergics
  - Contraindications: advanced age, urinary retention, or heart block
  - Side effects: increased appetite and weight gain, watch for rashes, dry mouth
- Antidepressant—fluoxetine-SSRI—dose every other day (off label)

- Acetaminophen—Used in pediatric population and pregnancy
  - Contraindications: liver disease/cirrhosis

Cluster
- Men are affected by cluster headaches more than women. The headaches typically begin around age 30. Symptoms are severe, boring to the eye. It lasts 20 to 30 minutes, often several times/night, every other day up to 8/day. Often referred to as "ice pick" or "suicide" headaches.
- May demonstrate ipsilateral Horner's syndrome with conjunctival injection, lacrimation, nasal congestion, rhinorrhea, miosis, ptosis, eyelid edema, and facial sweating.
- Cluster periods may last 2 to 16 weeks, then remit for 1 year or more. Chronic patients have no remission period.
- No specific testing; rule out secondary causes; can be confused with trigeminal neuralgia or giant cell arteritis.

Treatment
- Acute therapy: the severity of the pain requires acute abortive therapy that responds quickly
- Oxygen: via facemask (FM) at 7 to 12 liters/min for 10 to 20 minutes per attack
- Triptans: Sumatriptan shot, nasal spray 1 shot or spray with headache, repeat in 2 hours as needed. Zomig can also be used for the relief of cluster headaches.
- Lidocaine intranasally
- Ergots: Dihydroergotamine (DHE) shot or spray—1 shot every 8 hours, 1 to 2 sprays in each nostril can repeat in 8 hours, up to 6 sprays per day.
- Prophylaxis: Usual Verapamil. Can use Depakote, Lithium, Topamax all titrated up.
- Steroid tapers and Medrol dose pack until preventative is effective.

Tension
- Bilateral band-like with steady, mild to moderate pain lasting 30 minutes to 2 days
- Does not interfere with activities and is not aggravated by physical activity
- Episodic tension-type headache: the most common headache disorder—aggravated by stress
- Seen in adolescents and adults
- Treat with simple analgesia, ASA, NSAIDs, and Tylenol; combine analgesics with caution, biofeedback, physical therapy, stress reduction, relaxation

> **Red Flags for Headache—Pediatric**
>
> - Unequal pupils
> - Cannot awaken
> - Worsening headache (HA)
> - Repeated vomiting
> - Seizure
> - Slurred speech
> - Increased confusion, LOC
> - Don't forget to check for hyphemas (pooling of blood in the anterior chamber between cornea and iris)

Temporal Arteritis

Giant cell arteritis (GCA) vasculitis involves the ophthalmic, temporal, and carotid systems.

- Medical emergency in the older people
- Age of onset 50 to 70, affecting women more than men
- Concerns of vision loss—visual disturbances in 50 percent of patients
- Headache localized over eye and scalp tenderness
- Associated with polymyalgia rheumatic (PMR) with joints and muscle aches
- ESR elevation 100, elevated CRP
- Associated symptoms: fever, jaw, or tongue claudication, weight loss, fatigue
- Labs: ESR, CBC, LFTs, CRP
- Surgical referral: for unclear diagnosis—temporal artery biopsy
- Imaging: duplex ultrasonography of temporal and axillary arteries

Prompt Treatment

- Oral corticosteroids—40 to 60 mg/d for 4 weeks until symptom resolution/ESR normal. Then slow taper over 1 to 2 years.
- Follow-up/referral: rheumatologist, ophthalmologist; risk of recurrence is followed every 4 to 6 weeks.

Trigeminal Neuralgia

Onset in patients under 50 years old, mostly idiopathic

- Lasts seconds to minutes, shock-like severe lancinating unilateral pain in sensory distribution of trigeminal nerve (CN V)
- Increase in frequency, arises spontaneously, triggered by sensory stimulus, chewing, talking, and touching.
- No neurologic deficit was noted.
- Exclude temporal arteritis, postherpetic neuropathy (PHN), and multiple sclerosis if bilateral.

Treatment

- First-line—carbamazepine initially 100 mg/d, gradually titrated up. 400 to 800 mg/d
- Monitor CBC and platelets for bone marrow suppression.
- Other—oxcarbamazapine, lamotrigene

Bell's Palsy

- Unilateral paralysis of CN VII, acute onset, idiopathic etiology
- Cause: HSV 1 or 2, EBV, Lyme, MS, neoplasm, aneurysm of the basilar artery
- Risk—pregnancy (3-fold increase), diabetes, trauma, syphilis
- Recovery in 65 percent at 3 months, 85 percent at 9 months
  - Steroids and Valtrex in 72 hours
- Bilateral paralysis excludes Bell's Palsy
- Forehead sparing of motor function indicates upper motor lesion (stroke, infarction)
- Symptoms: Pain near the ear, hyperacusis, distortion of taste, weakness on one side of the face, weakness of eye closure
- No sensory loss on the affected side
- Asymmetry of the mouth
- Increased tear flow, dry eye, corneal reflex intact
- Rash or vesicles around the ear—herpes zoster; Ramsay Hunt syndrome
- Tests: CBC, ESR, Lyme, HIV, glucose, CT dependent on history
- Treatment: Antivirals: Valtrex 1,000 mg TID × days—not given routinely
- Prednisone 1 mg/kg/d 6 mg/kg × 7 days without taper
- Eye protection: patch at night, artificial tears

Motor Neuron Disorders

Multiple Sclerosis

Multiple sclerosis is an autoimmune progressive neurodegenerative disease characterized by demyelination and inflammation with axonal loss in the spinal cord and brain.

- Deficits vary in time and location (CNS location and episodes)
- More common in northern latitudes, 15 percent have family history
- Clinical features: CN dysfunction—VI, palsy, nystagmus, vision loss, optic neuritis
- Impaired motor—weakness, increased tone, + Babinski, action tremor
- Sensory—changes in sensation, proprioception, vibration, numbness, tingling, paresthesias
- Cerebellar—positive Romberg test, gait imbalance, gait ataxia
- Bowel or bladder—urgency or incontinence
- Fatigue
- Lhermitte's sign: electrical sensation down the back of legs produced with flexion of the neck

There are three types of multiple sclerosis:

- Relapsing remitting—acute onset, self-limiting, recovery, some residual deficit
- Secondary progressive—develops after relapsing, remitting with slow deterioration in function, may still have some acute attacks
- Primary progressive—steady functional decline without acute onset

Diagnosis

- MRI—90 percent multifocal T2 abnormalities brain and spinal cord
- LP—CSF—oligoclonal bands (neurologist)
- Bloodwork: Screening—CBC, chem panel, HIV, ANA, B12, ESR

Treatment

- Acute exacerbations: IV methylprednisone × 5 days
- Interferon B, glatiramir acetate, natalizumab, fingolimod. Reduce the frequency of reoccurrence and long-term disability.
- Treat depression and symptoms (spasticity, bladder dysfunction) with disease progression.

Parkinson's Disease

- Clinical symptom of tremor at rest (usually one hand) due to loss of dopaminergic cells in substantia nigra
- Gradual onset asymmetry is the most common presentation (insidious).
- Decreased arm swing, bradykinesia, and rigidity detected on the symptomatic side (cogwheel)
- Clinical diagnosis and routine labs are not helpful
- Balance and gait affected with progression—risk of falls
- Rigidity and freezing
- Autonomic disturbance: constipation, urinary urgency, sweating, orthostatic hypotension
- Decreased blink rate, masked facies, anosmia
- Seborrhea

Treatment

- Neuroimaging is used to exclude other conditions.
- Treatment with dopamine agonists, levodopa-carbidopa, and MAO-B inhibitors, anticholinergics
- Physical and occupational therapy

(Benign) Essential Tremor

An essential tremor is a rhythmic oscillation of a body part—present on movement, absent at rest

- Most common movement disorder
- Affects men more than women, with a median age of onset of 15
- 2/3 of patients have a family history, first-degree relatives

Clinical Diagnosis

- Action tremor of upper distal arms and hands, partial tremor of the head
- Symmetrical presentation
- Voice may be affected
- Does not appear in sleep
- Alcohol often suppresses the symptoms
- Nicotine, caffeine, stress, anxiety, hypoglycemia, fatigue, some medications worsen symptoms
- Handwriting demonstrates the problem
- Exclude hyperthyroidism, neurologic causes, and deficits

Treatment

- Beta-adrenergic blocker
- Primidone
- Patients self-treat with premeal cocktails
- Evaluate treatment and progression by asking the patient to draw a pinwheel

CASE STUDY

An 18-year-old male college student presents to the health center on campus with an acute onset of high fever, chills, nausea, slight confusion, and headache. The exam reveals a positive Kernig's sign. He does not recall if he received the meningococcal vaccine, and his vaccination records are incomplete. He lives on campus with three other roommates who share a kitchen. He recently attended a party on campus and was playing drinking games.

Considerations for the clinician:
1. First-year college students living in dormitories have a six-fold increased risk for meningitis.
2. It is spread primarily through saliva or oral secretions. Oral contact with shared items, such as drinking glasses, increases the risk of contracting the disease.
3. The disease must be recognized promptly since symptoms may progress rapidly.
4. Estimates of 100 to 125 cases occur annually on college campuses, with 5 to 15 deaths.
5. Emergency medical services (EMS) should be initiated, and the patient should be sent to the ED immediately.
6. If positive for meningococcal meningitis, the clinician should report the positive findings to the local and state health departments.
7. Students attending the college should be notified that there is a case of bacterial meningitis and should be alerted to signs/symptoms of the disease.

Review Questions

1. A 76-year-old patient arrives at the office with his spouse with complaints of episodes of slurred speech, word-finding difficulties, and numbness in his arm. The priority in management is:
   A. tell him to take an aspirin right away.
   B. order a CT scan.
   C. send him to the ER.
   D. perform an EKG.

2. Which one of these patients is most at risk for ischemic stroke?
   A. A patient with atrial fibrillation (AFib) on Coumadin with an INR of 1.2
   B. A patient with a two-pack per day (PPD) tobacco history × 40 years who quit 5 years ago
   C. A patient on anticoagulation therapy with an INR of 4.0
   D. A hypertensive patient currently being treated with losartan

3. What is the first symptom seen in most Parkinson's patients?
   A. Intention tremor
   B. Bradykinesia
   C. Rest tremor
   D. Rigidity

4. An 82-year-old patient presents with a history of transient ischemic attack (TIA) and confusion. A sensitive neurologic test for stroke would be what?
   A. The pronator drift
   B. Epley maneuver
   C. Visual field exam
   D. Get-up-and-go test

5. The CHA2DS2 VASc Index categorizes patients with nonvalvular atrial fibrillation (AF) for stroke risk. The main purpose of using the CHA2DS2 VASc score is to help the clinician determine:
   A. which anticoagulant therapy would be most beneficial for the patient.
   B. if the patient is having a hemorrhagic stroke or an ischemic stroke.
   C. the patient's risk for a thromboembolic event in a nonanticoagulated patient.
   D. if the patient is experiencing a TIA or a stroke.

6. A patient with multiple sclerosis presents with concerns of exacerbation. The nurse practitioner (NP) knows the patient will likely present with complaints of:
   A. tremors at rest, especially in the upper extremities.
   B. fatigue, weakness, and ataxic gait.
   C. headache, nuchal rigidity, and fever.
   D. sensory deficit that follows a single dermatomal distribution.

7. A primary headache differs from a secondary headache in what way?
   A. A primary headache is the first headache of someone's life.
   B. A secondary headache presents with an aura.
   C. A secondary headache is a result of abnormal anatomic pathology.
   D. A primary headache is due to systemic disease.

8. Which of the following is the first-line treatment for essential tremor?
   A. Propranolol (Inderal)
   B. Alprazalam (Xanax)
   C. Amitryptylline (Elavil)
   D. Alcohol

9. A 62-year-old woman complains of severe lancinating pain in her right cheek that worsens with cold drinks or teeth brushing. She is afraid to chew or eat because it seems to initiate the attack. The most likely diagnosis is which of the following?
   A. Sinus infection
   B. Abscessed tooth
   C. Trigeminal neuralgia
   D. Bell's palsy

10. A 35-year-old male complains of the abrupt onset of recurrent "ice pick" headaches behind one eye. He presents to the NP's office with an acute episode. During the physical exam, the patient was noted to have tearing in one eye, ptosis, and nasal discharge/congestion. The NP's plan for therapeutic management would be which of the following?
    A. High-dose NSAIDs
    B. 7 to 10 L of high-dose oxygen for 20 minutes in the office
    C. Send to the ER for a CT scan
    D. Verapamil

11. A 72-year-old patient presents with complaints of a headache with unilateral marked scalp tenderness. You note the induration of the temporal artery. Upon checking his labs, the family nurse practitioner (FNP) expects to find which of the following?
    A. Normal CRP
    B. Erythrocyte sedimentation rate (ESR) > 100 mm/hr
    C. Thrombocytopenia
    D. Positive Western blot

12. Which of the following medications is the best choice for acute treatment of the patient who presents with unilateral headache accompanied by nausea, vomiting, photophobia, or phonophobia?
    A. Triptans
    B. Beta blockers
    C. NSAIDs
    D. Acetaminophen ES

13. Which cranial nerve (CN) is responsible for shoulder shrugging?
    A. CN X
    B. CN XI
    C. CN IX
    D. CN XII

14. Which CNs are being tested with extraocular muscles (EOM)?
    A. CN III, IV, VI
    B. CN III, IV, V
    C. CN II, III, IV
    D. CN II, IV, V

15. A patient seen by the FNP is a 16-year-old high school soccer player who suffered a Grade 1 concussion. The best advice at this time would be which of the following?
    A. Pupillary checks every hour, monitor vital signs
    B. May return to play when all symptoms have resolved
    C. Physical rest × 2 weeks, no contact sports with medical follow-up
    D. Physical and cognitive rest monitored by medical personnel × 72 hours. Monitor for emotional symptoms, headaches, difficulty remembering, feeling foggy, trouble concentrating

16. A patient had a positive Romberg test during the neurologic exam. This highlights an issue in what part of the neurologic system?
    A. The sensory system and balance
    B. Mental status
    C. The motor system
    D. The reflex system

17. Which statement below best describes a positive Romberg test?
    A. The patient is unable to walk on their heels or their toes.
    B. The patient holds their arms up and out to the side with their eyes closed and touches their nose with their index finger and alternating hands. The patient misses the tip of the nose more than 50 percent of the time.
    C. The patient stands with feet together, eyes closed, arms at side with excessive swaying—begins to fall and keeps feet far apart to maintain balance.
    D. Patient places outstretched arms with palms facing up and closed eyes. One arm goes down after 5 to 10 seconds.

18. The FNP is evaluating an 18-year-old male college student at the student health center. He has had a fever > 102°F for approximately 24 hours and complains of a severe headache. During the examination, the patient is directed to lay supine

and passively bend his neck toward his chest; he flexes his knees and hips. What is the name of this test result?
   A. Brudzinski's sign
   B. Kernig's sign
   C. Cullen's sign
   D. Lachman test

19. Bell's palsy presents as acute weakness or paralysis of the muscles supplied by which cranial nerve(s)?
    A. VI
    B. V
    C. VII
    D. VII and VIII

20. A 32-year-old patient with migraines is complaining of two migraine headaches per week despite treatment with triptans. The next consideration for treatment is which of the following?
    A. Discontinue triptans and offer butalbital/caffeine/acetaminophen (Fioricet)
    B. Order high-dose O_2 therapy to be used during migraine attacks
    C. Order an MRI to rule out a brain tumor
    D. Start propranolol as preventative therapy

21. A 32-year-old female has a history of migraines with aura. Counseling should include which of the following?
    A. Headaches resulting from aura may last much longer and be more serious than those without.
    B. The use of combined hormonal contraceptives may increase the risk of stroke.
    C. A visual scotoma (circumscribed vision loss) is caused by cerebral ischemia in the middle or posterior cerebral artery.
    D. The aura can be a jabbing "ice pick" feeling in the head or over one eye that lasts seconds.

22. An 80-year-old patient was admitted to the hospital with confusion this week. Her daughter tells the hospitalist her memory may be slipping a bit, but she was oriented and independent last week, driving herself to the market. Upon admission to the hospital, she is found to have pneumonia. Currently, she is difficult to arouse and has incoherent speech. Last night, she was up all night and seemed to know her daughter but was confused regarding place and time. Her CT was normal. The most appropriate diagnosis of consideration at this time is which of the following?
    A. Dementia
    B. Parkinson's disease
    C. Stroke
    D. Delirium

23. A 70-year-old patient has complaints of gradual memory loss without neurologic deficits. The first-line method of evaluation would be which of the following?
    A. Administering a MMSE
    B. CT of the brain
    C. Neuropsychological testing
    D. Meeting with the family to obtain a history

24. Which of the following medications should be considered as first-line therapy for patients with mild to moderate Alzheimer's disease?
    A. Anticholinergics
    B. ACE inhibitors
    C. Cholinesterase inhibitors
    D. Antidepressants

25. A 28-year-old female presents with weakness, complaints of fatigue, recent problems with diplopia, numbness of her left arm, and some bladder changes. She remembers something similar happening last year. What would be in the differential?
    A. Migraine with aura
    B. Multiple sclerosis
    C. Meningitis
    D. Pituitary tumor

Answers and Rationales

1. Answer C is correct. The patient is showing signs of a developing stroke and needs immediate intervention in the ER.

   Answer A is incorrect. Aspirin could make it worse if the concern is a stroke; it is not known if it is hemorrhagic or ischemic in origin.

   Answer B is incorrect. A CT is reasonable but should be done emergently upon admission to the ER.

   Answer D is incorrect. An EKG would be applicable for chest pain or hospital admission.

2. Answer A is correct. The patient is out of his therapeutic window and at risk for a thromboembolic event (desirable INR range is 2–3).

   Answer B is incorrect. Smokers who quit are indeed at greater risk than nonsmokers, but at 5 years, their risk drops to half that of smokers.

   Answer C is incorrect. An INR of 4.0 signifies that the patient is overly anticoagulated. The person would be at risk for a hemorrhagic stroke rather than an ischemic stroke.

Answer D is incorrect. Hypertension may increase the risk of stroke; however, this patient is treated with losartan and may have well-controlled blood pressure. Therefore, A is the best answer.

3. Answer C is correct. Asymmetric tremor at rest is usually seen in one hand as a presenting symptom of Parkinson's disease (PD).

   Answer A is incorrect. Intention tremor is also known as an essential tremor and presents symmetrically in a different population.

   Answer B is incorrect. Bradykinesia (slowness of movement, progressive hesitation, or halting in movement) is seen later in the disease.

   Answer D is incorrect. Rigidity is when the muscles become stiff and inflexible. It is seen much later in the disease.

4. Answer A is correct. The pronator drift will reveal upper motor neuron weakness if the patient's arm drifts and confusion if they cannot follow directions to perform the exam.

   Answer B is incorrect. The Epley maneuver is done to help with vertigo.

   Answer C is incorrect. An ophthalmologist usually performs the visual field exam but may be part of a regular neurologic exam to assess for vision loss. Although vision loss may occur with a stroke, this is not a sensitive test for stroke.

   Answer D is incorrect. The Get-up-and-go test is used in older people to assess for problems with mobility and/or concerns with balance.

5. Answer A is correct. CHA2DS2 VASc score is used to assess the risk of stroke in nonvalvular atrial fibrillation (AFib) patients to determine the level of anticoagulation needed.

   Answer B is incorrect. The CHA2DS2 VASc score is a risk score tool not used to differentiate hemorrhagic and ischemic strokes.

   Answer C is incorrect. There are many risk factors for stroke. AFib increases the risk of stroke fivefold. Therefore, the CHA2DS2 VASc score is used for patients with nonvalvular AFib.

   Answer D is incorrect. The CHA2DS2 VASc score is not used to differentiate a stroke from a TIA.

6. Answer B is correct. Patients experiencing a reoccurrence (exacerbation) of MS might complain of ataxia, fatigue, weakness in arms or legs, visual changes, numbness, tingling, or a feeling of pins and needles.

   Answer A is incorrect. A resting tremor is associated with Parkinson's disease.

   Answer C is incorrect. These are all symptoms of meningitis.

   Answer D is incorrect. In MS, the symptomology does not follow a single dermatomal distribution.

7. Answer C is correct. A secondary headache is associated with abnormal anatomic pathology.

   Answer A is incorrect. A primary headache is a tension, migraine, or cluster headache.

   Answer B is incorrect. A headache with aura is noted in 20 percent of migraine headaches and is a primary headache.

   Answer D is incorrect. A secondary headache (not a primary headache) may be due to systemic disease.

8. Answer A is correct. Beta blockers are the first line of treatment for essential tremors.

   Answer B is incorrect. Benzodiazepines may reduce essential tremors; however, they are not first line due to their risk of dependency.

   Answer C is incorrect. Amitriptyline is a tricyclic antidepressant primarily used to treat major depressive disorder.

   Answer D is incorrect. Some patients may try to self-medicate with alcohol, but this is not the first-line treatment. Heavy alcohol use may worsen ET.

9. Answer C is correct. Classic symptoms of trigeminal neuralgia are severe lancinating unilateral pain in the sensory distribution of the trigeminal nerve (CN-5). Often initiated by cold, chewing, or a sensory stimulus.

   Answer A is incorrect. A sinus infection causes pain or pressure in the face over the area of the sinuses.

   Answer B is incorrect. An abscessed tooth may cause severe, constant throbbing pain around the affected tooth, which may radiate to the jaw, neck, or ear.

   Answer D is incorrect. Bell's palsy causes weakness or paralysis of one side of the face.

10. Answer B is correct. The patient is exhibiting cluster headache symptoms, especially since the patient has experienced these before (recurrent). High-dose oxygen therapy is the treatment of choice.

    Answer A is incorrect. NSAIDs are not the treatment of choice to treat a cluster headache.

    Answer C is incorrect. The patient does not need to go to the ER since his presentation is characteristic of a cluster headache, which has occurred previously.

Answer D is incorrect. Although the patient may be given Verapamil as a prophylactic treatment, it is not effective in treating an acute episode.

11. Answer B is correct. The ESR would be expected to be markedly elevated with temporal arteritis (also known as Giant Cell Arteritis [GCA])

    Answer A is incorrect. The CRP would also be elevated, as it is also an inflammatory marker.

    Answer C is incorrect. The patient would likely have thrombocytosis.

    Answer D is incorrect. The Western blot is not a test used for this diagnosis.

12. Answer A is correct. Triptans are the first-line treatment for migraine headaches if the patient does not have a cardiac history.

    Answer B is incorrect. Beta blockers are used as a preventative therapy for migraine headaches, not for acute treatment.

    Answer C is incorrect. NSAIDs are beneficial for tension or episodic headaches.

    Answer D is incorrect. Extra-strength acetaminophen is also used for tension or episodic headaches.

13. Answer B is correct. CN XI (spinal accessory) allows for shoulder shrugging.

    Answer A is incorrect. CN X is the vagus nerve. The vagus nerve is the longest in the autonomic nervous system. Some of the anatomic activities of the vagus nerve are controlling heart rate, intestinal peristalsis, swallowing, and mouth movements.

    Answer C is incorrect. CN IX is the glossopharyngeal nerve. It is involved in the person's ability to swallow.

    Answer D is incorrect. CN XII is the hypoglossal nerve. It is involved in controlling speech, swallowing, and tongue movement.

14. Answer A is correct. CN III (the oculomotor nerve) innervates medial deviation and eye movement in all directions. CN IV (trochlear nerve) is involved in the downward gaze. CN VI (the abducens nerve) innervates the superior oblique muscle of the eye and allows for downward and lateral movement.

    Answer B is incorrect. CN V is the trigeminal nerve, which provides sensory innervation to the face.

    Answer C is incorrect. CN II is the optic nerve that transmits visual information.

    Answer D is incorrect. Neither CN II nor CN V is involved in EOMs.

15. Answer B is correct. A grade 1 concussion is a low-grade or mild concussion. The patient can return to normal activity once all symptoms have completely passed.

    Answer A is incorrect. Regular neurologic assessments may be needed for a severe (grade 3) concussion.

    Answer C is incorrect. Physical rest may be needed for a grade 2 or grade 3 concussion, both of which are higher-level concussions that involve a loss of consciousness. Grade 2 is less than 5 minutes of LOC. Grade 3 is more than 5 minutes of LOC.

    Answer D is incorrect. Close monitoring by medical personnel and physical and cognitive rest (cocooning) may be needed for grade 2 and certainly for grade 3 concussions. It is not necessary for a grade 1 concussion.

16. Answer A is correct. The Romberg test assesses proprioception and balance.

    Answer B is incorrect. The Romberg test does not assess mental status. This can be done with the MMSE.

    Answer C is incorrect. The Romberg test does not assess the motor system; it is a test of balance and proprioception.

    Answer D is incorrect. Reflexes are tested using a reflex hammer, and DTRs are checked.

17. Answer C is correct. If the patient begins to fall or must move their feet to prevent falling, that is a positive Romberg test.

    Answer A is incorrect. This is a heel walk test, which can assess for weakness in L5, or the toe walk test, which can assess for weakness in S1.

    Answer B is incorrect. This is known as the finger-to-nose test, which assesses cerebellar function.

    Answer D is incorrect. This is the pronator drift test and is used to assess for stroke.

18. Answer A is correct. If a patient has meningitis, flexion of the neck will elicit flexion of the knees and hips. This is called Brudzinski's sign.

    Answer B is incorrect. This test is also used to assess for meningeal irritation; however, with a positive Kernig's sign, the patient will experience resistance or pain when the knees are extended after being flexed slowly by the examiner.

    Answer C is incorrect. Cullen's sign is not related to meningitis. It is the development of ecchymosis and edema around the umbilicus. This may be associated with acute pancreatitis or ruptured ectopic pregnancy.

    Answer D is incorrect. The Lachman test is done to assess for an anterior cruciate ligament (ACL) injury or tear.

19. Answer C is correct. The CN VII (facial nerve) is the only affected nerve in Bell's palsy. CN VII innervates the muscles used in facial movement and expression.

    Answer A is incorrect. CN VI is the abducens nerve and is responsible for eye movement.

    Answer B is incorrect. CN V is the trigeminal nerve, which is divided into three branches (the ophthalmic, maxillary, and mandibular nerves) and provides sensory innervation to the face.

    Answer D is incorrect. CN VII is correct, but CN VIII (the acoustic nerve) is not affected in Bell's palsy.

20. Answer D is correct. Propranolol or other beta blockers are effective in preventing migraine headaches. Beta blockers should be initiated when the patient has two or more migraines per week.

    Answer A is incorrect. Butalbital/acetaminophen/caffeine (Fioricet) may be prescribed for tension headaches and rarely for migraine headaches. However, it is habit-forming and not considered to be an effective treatment option.

    Answer B is incorrect. High-dose O_2 therapy is considered abortive therapy for cluster headaches.

    Answer C is incorrect. The patient has migraine headaches. An MRI is not warranted.

21. Answer B is correct. The use of combined hormonal contraceptives may increase the risk of a stroke.

    Answer A is incorrect. Migraine headaches with aura are not more serious or longer lasting than those that occur without aura.

    Answer C is incorrect. A migraine headache with aura is not related to ischemia of a cerebral artery.

    Answer D is incorrect. "The "ice pick" feeling is a classic sign of a cluster headache, not a migraine headache.

22. Answer D is correct. This meets the criteria for acute mental disturbance characterized by confusion, impaired thinking, cognition, and attention deficits with a fluctuating course.

    Answer A is incorrect. The patient is demonstrating an acute episode of change in cognition. This is not consistent with a diagnosis of dementia.

    Answer B is incorrect. The patient does not demonstrate any signs or symptoms of Parkinson's disease.

    Answer C is incorrect. Although a stroke is a possible consideration, the patient has a normal CT scan and a recent diagnosis of pneumonia. Pneumonia in older people often can cause confusion.

23. Answer A is correct. The MMSE is a validated screening tool that can be used as a first-line method to evaluate concerns of memory loss.

    Answer B is incorrect. A brain CT is not considered a first-line evaluation method and is not warranted for this patient, who has gradual memory loss and no neurologic deficits.

    Answer C is incorrect. Neuropsychological testing may be necessary in the future, but it would depend on the findings of the MMSE.

    Answer D is incorrect. Meeting with the family is important, but the clinician should first identify any issues after gathering initial data.

24. Answer C is correct. Cholinesterase inhibitors are first-line treatments for patients diagnosed with mild to moderate AD. Cholinesterase inhibitors prevent the breakdown of acetylcholine and may help mitigate the symptoms of memory loss and impaired judgment.

    Answer A is incorrect. Anticholinergics block acetylcholine and inhibit nerve impulses that cause involuntary movement. They treat a variety of disorders, such as COPD or an overactive bladder.

    Answer B is incorrect. ACE inhibitors block the production of angiotensin II, and they treat hypertension, certain heart conditions, and renal disease.

    Answer D is incorrect. Antidepressants may be used for patients who have dementia, but it is not first-line therapy and will not mitigate symptoms associated with AD.

25. Answer B is correct. Multiple sclerosis presents with varying deficits at different times due to the multifocal demyelination and inflammation. Common symptoms include gait ataxia, visual loss, diplopia, paresthesia, weakness, and fatigue.

    Answer A is incorrect. The patient does not verbalize any symptoms consistent with migraine with aura.

    Answer C is incorrect. Meningitis would present with acute symptoms and typically have an accompanying headache, fever, malaise, and nuchal rigidity.

    Answer D is incorrect. Patients who have a pituitary tumor exhibit symptoms corresponding to endocrine dysfunction and may experience symptoms such as headaches, inappropriate breast milk production, irregular menstruation, weight loss or weight gain, hypotension, and rapid or irregular heart rate.

Resources

Bushnell, C., McCullough, L. D., Issam, A., Awad, M. V., Chireau, W. N., Fedder, K. L., . . . & Walterson, M. R. on behalf of American Heart Association Stroke Council, Council on Cardiovascular and Stroke Nursing, Council on Clinical Cardiology, Council on Epidemiology and Prevention, and Council for High Blood Pressure Research. (2014). Guidelines for the prevention of stroke in women: A statement for healthcare professionals from the American Heart Association /American Stroke Association. *Stroke, 45*(5), 1545–1588. https://doi.org/10.1161/01.str.0000442009.06663.48

Chia-Chun, C., Vanderpluym, J. (2020, May) Secondary headaches. *Journal of Practical Neurology. 19*(4). https://practicalneurology.com/

Centers for Disease Control and Prevention. (2014). Traumatic brain injury & concussion. https://www.cdc.gov/traumaticbraininjury/

Dodick, D. W. (2003). Clinical clues and clinical rules primary vs. secondary headache. *Advance Studies in Medicine, 3*(6C), S550–S555.

Kernan, W. N., Oybiagele, B., Black, H. R., Bravata, D. M., Chimowitz, M. I., Ezekowitz, M.D., . . .& Wilson, J. A. (2014). Guidelines for the prevention of stroke in patients with stroke and transient ischemic attack: A guideline for healthcare professionals from the American Heart Association/American Stroke Association. *Stroke, 45*(7), 2160–2236. https://doi.org/10.1161/STR.0000000000000046

Halstead, M. E., McAvoy, K., Devore, C. D., Carl, R., & Lee, M. (2013). Returning to learning following a concussion. *Pediatrics, 132*(5), 948–957. https://doi.org/10.1542/peds.2013-2867

Harmon, K. G., Drezner, J. A., Gammons, M., et al. (2013). American Medical Society for Sports Medicine position statement: Concussion in sport. *British Journal of Sports Medicine, 47*(1), 15–26.

Reisberg, B., Ferris, S. H., de Leon, M. J., and Crook, T. (1982). The global deterioration scale for assessment of primary degenerative dementia. *American Journal of Psychiatry, 139*, 1136–1139.

Rowland, L., & Pedley, T. (Eds.). (2009). *Merritt's neurology* (12th ed.). Lippincott Williams & Wilkins.

Silberstein, S. D., Holland, S., Freitag, F., Dodick, D. W., Argoff, C., & Ashman, E. (2012, April). Evidence-based guideline update: Pharmacologic treatment for episodic migraine prevention in adults. Report of the Quality Standards Subcommittee of the American Academy of Neurology and the American Headache Society. *Neurology, 78*(17), 1337–1345. https://dx.doi.org/10.1212/WNL.0b013e3182535d20

Silberstein, S. D., Lipton, R. B., & Dalessio, D. J. (2001). Overview, diagnosis, and classification. In S. D. Silberstein, R. B. Lipton, & D. J. Dalessio (Eds.), *Wolff's headache and other head pain* (7th ed.). Oxford University Press.

Suchowersky, O., Reich, S., Perlmutter, J., et al. (2006). Practice parameter: Diagnosis and prognosis of new onset Parkinson's disease (an evidence-based review): Report of the Quality Standards Subcommittee of the American Academy of Neurology. *Neurology, 66*, 968–975.

Tunkel, A., Hartman, B. J., Kaplan, S. L., Kaufman, B. A., Roos, K. L., Scheld, W. M., & Whitley, R. J. (2004). IDSA guideline: practice guidelines for the management of bacterial meningitis. *Clinical Infectious Diseases. 39*(9), 1267–1284. https://doi.org/10.1086/425368

Zesiewicz, T. A., Elble, R., Louis, E. D., et al. (2005). Practice parameter: Therapies for essential tremor: Report of the Quality Standards Subcommittee of the American Academy of Neurology. *Neurology, 64*, 2008–2020.

CHAPTER 12

Endocrine System

Nancy L. Dennert, MS, MSN, FNP-BC, CDCES, BC-ADM

Diabetes Mellitus

Etiology

Diabetes mellitus (DM) is a chronic illness requiring continuous medical care. The nurse practitioner must work with the patient and the patient's healthcare team to identify a therapeutic treatment plan that optimizes risk-reduction strategies. The plan should be patient-centered, tailored to the individual, and support diabetes self-management.

Diabetes Facts

- 10.5 percent of the entire global adult population has diabetes.
- By 2045, it is projected that 1 in every 8 adults will have diabetes.
- More than 90 percent have type 2 diabetes.
- Driving factors are obesity, decreased physical activity, an aging population, and socioeconomic factors.
- Racial disparities in diagnosed diabetes in the United States:
  - 12.6 percent of African Americans
  - 11.8 percent of Hispanics
  - 8.4 percent of Asian American people
  - 7.1 percent of non-Hispanic White people
  - 24.1 percent of Native Americans in southern Arizona

Diagnosis of Prediabetes

- Prediabetes is the term used for an individual who has one or more of the following characteristics (should have at least one confirmatory test):
  - Fasting plasma glucose (FPG) 100 to 125 mg/dL (impaired fasting glucose)
  - 2-hour post 75 g oral glucose tolerance test (OGTT) 140 to 199 mg/dL (impaired glucose tolerance)
  - Hemoglobin A1C (HbA1C) 5.7 to 6.4 percent (those with HbA1C higher than 6 percent should be considered very high risk for development of DM)

The majority of individuals with prediabetes will develop type 2 diabetes within 10 years.

Clinical Presentation/Assessment Findings

Diagnosis of DM occurs if the individual has one of the following characteristics. (The individual should have at least one confirmatory test if there is only one positive test result.) Confirmatory testing is unnecessary if the individual presents with a positive result for more than one of these tests.

- Hemoglobin HbA1C ≥ 6.5 percent
- FPG ≥ 126 mg/dL (No caloric intake × 8 hours)
- 2-hour post 75 g OGTT ≥ 200 mg/dL
- Patients may present with symptoms such as polyuria, polydipsia, polyphagia, fatigue, and a random (in-office) glucose of ≥ 200.

Screening Recommendations for Both Prediabetes and Diabetes

Adults

- Asymptomatic adults of any age who have a BMI greater than 25 (or if Asian American, a BMI greater than 23), with one or more additional risk factors for diabetes, which may include high-risk ethnicity, family history, central obesity, dyslipidemia (particularly those with high triglycerides and low HDLs), hypertension (HTN).

- All individuals over the age of 45 who are overweight or obese.
- Screening can be done with the HbA1C, FPG, or a 2-hour 75-g OGTT. Diagnosis of asymptomatic individuals should only occur with repeat confirmatory testing.
- Normal tests of individuals meeting the criteria should be repeated at least every 3 years.

Children

Screen asymptomatic children who are overweight (> 85th percentile) and who have two or more of the following risk factors:

- Family history of type 2 DM in first- or second-degree relative
- High-risk ethnicity
- Have a condition associated with insulin resistance: HTN, dyslipidemia, polycystic ovarian syndrome (PCOS), acanthosis nigricans, large for gestational age (LGA), or small for gestational age (SGA).
- Maternal history of gestational diabetes during the child's gestation
- Screening should occur every 3 years.

Differential Diagnosis

There are four recognized types of diabetes mellitus.

1. Type 1 diabetes (formerly known as juvenile diabetes): To more closely identify the pathology of the disease, type 1 diabetes is now known as "immune-mediated diabetes." There are approximately 1 million immune-mediated type 1 diabetics in the United States. The etiology of immune-mediated diabetes is pancreatic beta cell destruction, which usually leads to absolute insulin deficiency.
2. Type 2 diabetes: Results from a progressive loss of insulin secretion on the background of insulin resistance. There is a strong association between genetic predisposition (inherited) and obesity. This is the fastest-growing population of all types of DM. There are approximately 30 million type 2 diabetics in the United States.
3. Gestational diabetes (GDM): Diabetes that develops in the second or third trimester of pregnancy.

> **Clinical Pearl**
>
> Diabetes that occurs in the first trimester is considered overt diabetes, not gestational diabetes.

4. Diabetes due to other causes (e.g., diseases or disorders that affect the pancreas, such as cystic fibrosis, partial pancreatectomy, or pancreatic cancer). Additionally, diabetes that develops as a result of exposure to certain medications, such as glucocorticoids, HIV medications, and some psychiatric and immunosuppressive medications.

Clinical Management (A, B, C)

A = HbA1C

B = Blood Pressure

C = Cholesterol

Hemoglobin A1C

The hemoglobin A1C reflects the approximate average of blood glucose levels over the last 3 months. The ADA goal for **most** diabetics is an HbA1C lower than 7 percent (equates to an average blood glucose of 154). The American Association of Clinical Endocrinologists (AACE) set this goal at less than 6.5 percent. However, both the ADA and the AACE recognize that there are times when a less stringent HbA1C goal is appropriate. Although an HbA1C of less than 7 percent is ideal, other factors to consider are disease duration, life expectancy, significant comorbidities, patient attitude, available resources, and support systems.

In theory, an individual can achieve an HbA1C lower than 7% if they meet the following criteria:

1. Fasting (8-hour minimum fasting period) blood glucose level between 80 and 130 mg/dL
2. A 2-hour postmeal (postprandial) blood glucose of less than 180. Additionally, the patient should maintain a blood glucose level of less than 180 mg/dL.

Blood Pressure/Renal Function Assessment

Clinical trials have demonstrated that keeping the blood pressure less than 130/80 for most individuals with diabetes can help reduce the risk of developing kidney damage.

- Most diabetics with HTN or the presence of microalbumin in the urine will be placed on an angiotensin-converting enzyme (ACE) inhibitor or

an angiotensin receptor blocker (ARB) to maintain blood pressure at a goal of less than 130/80 and to prevent or reduce the presence of microalbuminuria.
- The clinician should measure for microalbuminuria annually. If positive, a confirmatory test should be repeated within 3 months. If the patient continues to have a positive result with a microalbumin level greater than 30 mcg/ml, the patient and clinician should institute measures to reduce microalbuminuria and improve renal function.
- The microalbumin test can be performed as a random spot collection of urine. When positive with confirmatory testing, it should be checked by the clinician every 3 months to assess for progression or improvement in renal function.
- Individuals with diabetes should be referred to a nephrologist in the presence of persistent microalbuminuria, a glomerular filtration rate of less than 30, and/or hematologic evidence of a decline in renal function.

Cholesterol

The 2023 ADA Standards of Medical Care have been revised to recommend when to initiate and intensify statin therapy:

- Obtain lipid profile at diagnosis and every 5 years if under age 40 with no cardiovascular disease (CVD) or lifestyle factors. No statin therapy.
  - With CVD factors: Moderate-high dose statin therapy and lifestyle therapy
  - With overt CVD: High-dose statin therapy
- Ages 40 to 75 without CVD risk factors: Moderate statin therapy.
- Ages 40 to 75 with CVD risk factors: High-dose statin therapy.
- For those older than 75, the same recommendation applies to those ages 40 to 75, except that the risk/benefit profile should be considered and titrated downward if needed.

Clinical Pearl

All patients with diabetes over the age of 40 are recommended to be on statin therapy.

Complication of Diabetes

Diabetic Ketoacidosis

Diabetic ketoacidosis (DKA) is severe and potentially life-threatening.

- DKA is more commonly seen in Type I DM but can occur with Type II DM, especially in the case of illness.
- DKA is more likely to occur when patients have physiologic stress, such as infections (e.g., urinary tract infections [UTIs], pneumonia), myocardial ischemia, or other medical or surgical-related illnesses.
- DKA may develop rapidly, sometimes developing in less than 24 hours. Clinical features of DKA may include Kussmaul's respirations, nausea, vomiting, abdominal pain, anorexia, dehydration, and fatigue.
- Patients with advanced DKA may become comatose. Treatment of DKA requires hospitalization with fluid and electrolyte repletion and insulin therapy.

DKA: Laboratory Findings
- PH < 7.3
- Bicarbonate < 18
- Anion gap > 10
- Osmolality < 320
- Hyperglycemia > 250 mg/dL
- Ketones: present

Clinical Pearl

Not all patients who develop DKA have an elevated glucose level over 250. There have been cases of euglycemic DKA. This may occur in patients on SGLT-2 inhibitors. The clinician should always be alert for DKA in any patient with diabetes, even in a euglycemic state.

Hyperglycemic Hyperosmolar State

Hyperglycemic hyperosmolar state (HHS) is a severe and potentially life-threatening diabetic complication. It is more commonly seen in patients with Type 2 DM.

- Hyperglycemia may be severe and occurs when a patient has a blood glucose level greater than 600 mg/dL and sometimes as high as 1,000 mg/dL. HHS develops more slowly and more subtly than DKA. It may take days to weeks to develop, and the hyperosmolar state results in severe fluid loss and dehydration.
- Most patients with HHS will have some degree of neurologic disturbance, which may manifest as irritability, stupor, spasticity, hyperreflexia, seizures, and coma. HHS requires hospitalization to provide fluid and electrolyte repletion, along with insulin administration.

HHS Laboratory Findings
- PH > 7.3
- Bicarbonate > 18
- Anion gap: Variable

- Osmolality > 320
- Hyperglycemia > 600 mg/dL
- Ketones: Rare

Pharmacologic Agents for Type 2 Diabetes Mellitus

Biguanides: Metformin

- Typically, the first agent used for Type 2 diabetics is a biguanide (metformin).
- Reduces hepatic glucose production, enhances insulin sensitivity in muscle and fat cells, and lowers HbA1C by 1 to 1.5 percent. The usual dose is 1,000 mg twice daily; needs to be titrated to that dose. Adverse effects include GI distress in up to 50 percent of patients. It may promote weight loss.
- May increase the risk of lactic acidosis in patients with renal disease, alcohol abuse, or advanced age people.
- With radiological studies: discontinue (d/c) metformin 24 hours before the procedure until 48 hours afterward (until hydration is reestablished).
- Can improve ovulatory function (think pregnancy).
- Approved for use in children over the age of 10.

Dipeptidyl Peptidase Inhibitors

- Dipeptidyl peptidase inhibitors (DPP-4) inhibits the enzyme that breaks down glucagon-like-peptide-1 (GLP-1) and glucose-dependent insulinotropic polypeptide (GIP)
- Januvia (sitagliptin) 100 mg daily (adjust dosage downward for renal impairment)
- Onglyza (saxagliptin) 5 mg daily (adjust dosage downward for renal impairment)
- Tradjenta (linagliptin) 5 mg daily (no adjustment needed for renal impairment)
- Nesina (alogliptin) 6.25, 12.5, 25 mg (adjust dosage downward for renal impairment)
- Can be monotherapy. Often used in combination with metformin.
- No hypoglycemia and weight neutral.
- Can be expensive.
- Additional lowering of HbA1C by 0.5 to 1.0 percent.

Clinical Pearl

All DPP-4 inhibitors end in "gliptin" generically.

GLP-1 RAs (Glucagon-Like Peptide Receptor Agonists)

- Daily: Byetta (exenatide), Victoza (liraglutide), Rybelsus (semaglutide—oral)
- Weekly: Bydureon (long-acting exenatide), Tanzeum (albiglutide), Trulicity (dulaglutide), Ozempic (semaglutide), Mounjaro (tirzepatide—both a GLP1-RA combined with GIP)
- Increases insulin secretion in response to carbohydrates.
- Prevents excessive hepatic glucose production by suppressing glucagon release.
- Slows gastric emptying and signals the brain to recognize increased satiety. This results in reduced food intake.
- Promotes weight loss.
- Decreases HbA1C by 0.5 to 1.5 percent.
- GI adverse events: Nausea and diarrhea or constipation (usually self-limiting of approximately 8 to 10 weeks)
- May increase the risk of pancreatitis.
- If the patient is taking a DPP-4 inhibitor, stop the drug when initiating GLP-1 (both together will increase the risk of pancreatitis).
- Rats in clinical trials developed medullary thyroid carcinoma. Do not use in patients with personal or family history of medullary thyroid cancer. Do not use in patients with a history of multiple endocrine neoplasia type 2 (MEN 2).

Clinical Pearl

All GLP1-RA's have generic names ending in "tide"

SGLT-2 Inhibitors (Sodium-Glucose Co-Transporter 2 Inhibitors)

Examples of the SGLT-2 co-transport inhibitors are:

- Invokana (canagliflozin) 100 mg or 300 mg QD
- Farxiga (dapagliflozin) 5 mg or 10 mg QD
- Jardiance (empagliflozin) 10 mg or 25 mg QD

SGLT-2 advantages:

- Blocks glucose reabsorption by the kidney, increasing glucosuria.
- No hypoglycemia
- Decrease in blood pressure
- Weight loss occurs because of the loss of glucose (calories) in the urine.
- Approximate HbA1C reduction of 1 percent

SGLT-2 disadvantages:
- May cause genitourinary infections.
- May cause Fournier's gangrene.
- May cause volume depletion/hypotension/dizziness.
- Transient increase in potassium or creatinine
- May cause an increase in low density lipoproteins (LDL).

> **Clinical Pearl**
>
> All SGLT-2 inhibitors have generic names ending in "flozin"

Thiazolidinediones
- Actos (pioglitazone) 15 to 45 mg/daily. Avandia (rosiglitazone)
- Decrease insulin resistance in peripheral tissue/decrease hepatic glucose production
- May also decrease triglycerides (TG) and increase high density lipoproteins (HDL).
- Side Effects: weight gain, edema (contraindicated for patients with congestive heart failure [CHF])
- Decreases HbA1C by 1 to 1.5 percent

Alpha-Glucosidase Inhibitors
- Precose (acarbose) and Glyset (miglitol)
- Delays carbohydrate (CHO) digestion and decreases postprandial glucose.
- Useful in patients with mild glucose intolerance associated with postprandial hyperglycemia
- Can cause bloating and flatulence due to the increased transit time of food through the digestive system.
- Decreases HbA1C by 0.5 percent.

> **Clinical Pearl**
>
> The thiazolidinediones (TZDs) (only two) both have generic names ending in "glitazone"

Sulfonylureas
- Glyburide, Glipizide, Glimepiride
- Stimulates insulin secretion
- Risk of hypoglycemia
- Weight gain
- Caution in patients with sulfa allergies and renal or liver impairments
- Cost effective
- Improve HbA1C by 1 to 2 percent

Meglitinides
- Repaglinide (Prandin) and nateglinide (Starlix)
- Similar to sulfonylureas, they stimulate the pancreas to produce more insulin. More rapid onset/shorter duration
- Side Effects: hypoglycemia and weight gain
- Frequent dose scheduling (with each meal)
- Useful for those with sulfa allergy
- Monotherapy or use with metformin
- Decreases HbA1C by 1 by 1.5 percent.

Insulin
Start insulin when the following conditions are present:
- Any newly diagnosed type 1
- Severe hyperglycemia (> 300 mg/dL) or HbA1c > 10 percent
- Signs of dehydration
- Signs of acidosis or ketosis

> **Clinical Pearl**
>
> If the patient has an HbA1C greater than 10 percent or blood sugar greater than 300, the patient is considered glucose toxic and should have insulin therapy. Once the glucose toxicity resolves and the patient's condition improves, insulin can be discontinued from the regimen of the patient with type 2 diabetes. It is important to remember that insulin can be added to the regimen at any time. It can be added to oral therapy whenever necessary. Usually, initiation for a type 2 diabetic is done with basal insulin.

Basal insulins (glargine, detemir, degludec) are typically taken before bed and provide background insulin (no peak) for approximately 24 hours. When initiating basal insulin, it is usually started at 0.1 to 0.2 units/kg/day. Consider discontinuing the sulfonylurea when initiating short-acting insulin (given before meals). **The greatest risk of insulin therapy is hypoglycemia.**

Short-acting insulins: lispro (Humalog), aspart (Novolog), glulisine (Apidra).

Hypoglycemia
The Rule of "15"

If an individual has symptoms of low blood sugar, they should check their blood sugar. If low (below 70), follow the "rule of 15."

- Eat or drink 15 grams of fast-acting sugar (4 glucose tablets, 4 ounces of fruit juice, ½ can of regular soda).
- Recheck blood sugar after 15 minutes. If it is still low, repeat with 15 grams of fast-acting sugar.
- Once blood sugar is over 100, the individual should have a small snack with protein and carbohydrates, such as half a sandwich and milk, to sustain the blood glucose level.

Clinical Pearl

Sometimes, a patient will feel symptomatic even when their blood sugar is not low (below 70). This commonly occurs in individuals who have chronically high blood sugars. In that case, the individual with diabetes can initiate the same treatment as is done for "true" hypoglycemia. However, the clinician should reinforce to the individual with diabetes that this is not a normal physiologic response, and they should work together to bring the patient to a more normal state of hypoglycemic awareness.

Diabetic Self-Management Education and Support Services (DSMES):

- Uses a team approach.
- Assists the patient with decision-making necessary for diabetes self-management.
- Considers the needs and goals of the patient. It is always patient-centered.
- Supports informed decision-making and self-care.

Medical Nutrition Therapy (MNT)

- Individualized eating patterns with meal planning
- Provided by a registered dietitian or nutritionist skilled in providing diabetes-specific MNT.
- The treatment plan for MNT should take a collaborative approach and include all providers caring for the patient with diabetes.

Brief Case Study and Considerations for the Clinician

A 28-year-old Asian American male presents to his primary care physician's (PCP) office with complaints of fatigue, thirst, and frequent urination. He has no other symptoms. He is known to the clinician and has no significant past medical history (PMH). His BMI is 27, and he reports 5 pounds of unintentional weight loss. His vital signs are BP 90/60, apical HR=100, Respirations-16 unlabored, and afebrile. The rest of his physical exam is unremarkable except for dry mucous membranes. He reports no recent illnesses. There is no history of use of toxic substances. He takes no medications. Family history includes a father with type 2 DM and a mother with Hashimoto's hypothyroidism. The clinician obtains a random blood glucose (BG) and HbA1C in the office.

Results: Random BG = 224. Hgb A1C = 10%

Considerations for the Clinician

- The etiology or type of DM the patient has is not known. Further testing is required.
- Father has Type 2 DM (strong genetic risk with a first-degree relative).
- Mother has an autoimmune disorder (increases patient risk of autoimmune disorders).
- The patient falls into a high-risk ethnicity.
- A BMI of 27 is overweight for this patient. Asian American people are considered overweight when their BMI exceeds 23.
- The patient is considered glucose toxic and must begin insulin at this time.
- Inform the patient that, depending on the test results, he may not need insulin therapy later when his BG is under control.
- No symptoms of DKA or HHS at this time. Discuss with the patient the symptoms of both DKA and HHS and to go to ED if symptoms occur.
- Unintentional weight loss is likely due to dehydration.
- The patient should start on basal insulin (0.1 to 0.2 units/kg/day). Have the patient self-administer in the office today.
- Encourage an increased intake of noncarbohydrate fluids such as water.
- Patient should be given a glucometer with written and verbal instructions for use.
- Patient needs to be instructed on "the rule of 15" regarding the risk of hypoglycemia.
- The patient needs a nutrition referral.
- The patient needs an endocrine referral.

Thyroid Disorders

Etiology

- Bilobar structure located in the neck
- 2 lobes connected by isthmus at the level of the cricoid cartilage
- The thyroid gland produces and stores thyroid hormone.
- Production of thyroid hormone is dependent on ingestion of iodine.
- Triiodothyronine (T3) and thyroxine (T4) are bound to plasma proteins.

- The majority of T4 is bound to plasma proteins; a small amount of free T4 circulating in serum reflects thyroid activity.
- Eighty percent of T3 is formed in the liver, kidneys, and muscles as a breakdown of T4; the remaining 20 percent is secreted directly by the thyroid.
- The anterior pituitary releases thyroid-stimulating hormone (TSH) in response to thyrotropin-releasing hormone (TRH).
- TSH is inhibited by circulation of T3 and T4 (negative feedback system).
- TSH level is a good indicator of thyroid function; sensitive and specific.
- TSH normal range varies between 0.40 to 4.5u/ml (normal levels may vary slightly depending on the assay used by the laboratory).
- Hyperthyroid (TSH < 0.40)
- Hypothyroid (TSH > 4.5)
- Euthyroid (TSH = 0.40–4.5)
- The American Thyroid Association recommends screening men and women every 5 years beginning at age 35. Screen women over 50 years of age or with any symptoms.
- The United States Preventative Services Task Force (USPTSF) does not recommend routine screening.

Clinical Presentation

Hypothyroidism
- Fatigue
- Weight gain
- Constipation
- Dry skin
- Dry, coarse, or brittle hair, thinning hair
- Cold sensitivity
- Depression
- Slow movements, "foggy" thoughts
- Muscle aches or joint pains.

Hyperthyroidism
- Weight loss
- Tachycardia or arrhythmia
- Nervousness, anxiety, irritability
- Hand tremors
- Sweating
- Heat insensitivity
- Frequent bowel movements
- Hunger
- Fatigue
- Thinning skin
- Sleep disturbances
- Warm, moist skin
- Muscle weakness

Clinical Pearl

A goiter is not diagnostic for hyper- or hypothyroidism. It is an indicator that the thyroid is overworked. Further testing is necessary.

Clinical Management

Laboratory and Diagnostic Tests: Initial Testing

1. Free T4 and TSH
   - Free T4 (thyroxine) normal range is 4.5 to 12.0.
   - Low T4 with elevated TSH confirms hypothyroidism.
   - High T4 with low TSH confirms hyperthyroidism.
   - TSH may rise before the drop in T4 is observed (subclinical hypothyroidism).
2. Radioactive Iodine (RAI) Uptake Test
   - Useful for diagnosing hyperthyroidism
   - Measures the amount of iodine taken up by the thyroid gland
   - Increased uptake of iodine in hyperthyroid, goiter
   - Decreased uptake of iodine in subacute thyroiditis, hypothyroidism
   - Check for allergy to shellfish
   - Not useful if patients are already on thyroid replacement
3. Thyroid Ultrasound
   - Measures size and shape of the gland, homogenous, solid, or cystic nodule
   - If suspicious for cancer, can obtain a sample of cells with ultrasound-guided fine-needle aspiration (FNA)
4. Radionucleotide Thyroid Scan (if suspecting nodule, cancer)
   - "Hot area" hyperfunctioning nodule is present—90 percent benign
   - "Cold area" hypofunctioning nodule is present—5 to 10 percent malignant

Hypothyroidism
- Most common form of thyroid disorders
- Symptoms can mimic normal aging
- 10 × more common in women

- 1 out of every 50 people, age 60 and older
- Low levels of circulating thyroid hormone cause clinical manifestations
- High TSH and low free T4
- Ninety-five percent of all cases are primary hypothyroidism caused by underfunctioning of the thyroid gland.
- Autoimmune (Hashimoto's thyroiditis) is the most common cause.
- Goiter may or may not be present.
- Check antithyroid antibody titer (thyroid peroxidase [TPO] autoantibody). A positive result indicates Hashimoto's disease (autoimmune type).

Other less common causes of primary hypothyroidism include:

- Ablative therapy
- Thyroidectomy (for goiter or cancer)
- Iodine deficiency
- Pharmacologic agents such as lithium or amiodarone
- Transient postpartum thyroiditis. It may occur in 5 to 10 percent of postpartum women.

Secondary Hypothyroidism

- Rare: 5 percent of all cases
- Neoplasm of the pituitary gland or hypothalamus
- Hypopituitarism (pituitary adenoma)
- Congenital (cretinism)

Physical exam findings may include:

- Pale/cool/coarse/dry skin
- Dry, coarse hair
- Eyelid and facial edema (lid lag or ptosis)
- Slow speech
- Neurologic signs such as delayed reflexes (patellar "hang-up" reflex)
- Bradycardia
- Cardiomyopathy
- Anemia
- Dyslipidemia
- Hyponatremia (if edema present)

Treatment

- Replace thyroid hormone with levothyroxine (T-4), the gold standard.
- Some patients will ask for liothyronine (T-3) or a combination of both T-3 and T4.

Hyperthyroidism

- Excess secretion of thyroid hormones (T4 and T3)
- Also known as thyrotoxicosis
- Common causes:
  - Graves' disease in 60 to 80 percent of all cases (autoimmune)
  - 15 percent of cases are older than 60
  - May be related to a hyperfunctioning thyroid nodule
  - Toxic nodular goiters account for 5 percent of cases
  - More common in patients older than 40 with a long-standing history of multinodular goiters
  - Thyroid inflammatory diseases: leakage of thyroid hormone from damaged or inflamed gland (postviral illness, postpartum thyroiditis)

Clinical Pearl

Both endogenous and exogenous hyperthyroidism (caused by overreplacement of thyroid hormone) can cause tachyarrhythmia and/or atrial fibrillation. Include a cardiac assessment when performing the workup of a patient who has hyperthyroidism.

Physical exam findings:

- Skin smooth, soft, palmar erythema, diaphoresis
- Nails clubbing, onycholysis
- Eye exam may show exophthalmos, lid lag, palpebral fissures
- Neck: thyroid enlargement—may have goiter
- Respiratory: dyspnea
- Cardiac: tachycardia, arrhythmias
- Musculoskeletal (MS): proximal weakness, tremors, hyperreflexia
- Neuro/MS: restless, labile, irritable, decreased concentration, memory loss

Treatment options for hyperthyroidism:

- There is no treatment to reverse the underlying autoimmune cause of Graves' disease.
- Treatment options to control the production of thyroid hormone and/or symptom control include:
  - Beta blockers to control sympathomimetic symptoms (usually propranolol unless contraindicated); may also use calcium channel blockers (CCBs)
  - Antithyroid drugs (thioamides)
  - Ablative therapy with radioactive iodine (RAI-131)
  - Surgical thyroidectomy (may be partial or total)

Ablative Therapy with RAI-131
- First-line treatment option
- Concentrates in the thyroid gland, causing atrophy of thyroid tissue
- Adverse side effect: development of permanent hypothyroidism. Patients need to be informed of this since they will likely need life-long replacement therapy with levothyroxine.
- Not to be used in pregnancy or nursing. Patients should wait at least 6 months post-RAI ablative therapy before attempting pregnancy.

Thioamides
Thioamides inhibit the formation of T3 and T4. Examples of thioamides include:
- MMI (methimazole) 10 to 20 mg q 8 hours (daily, every 8 hours)
- PTU (propylthiouracil) 50 to 100 mg q 6 to 8 hours (daily, every 6 to 8 hours)
- The patient typically will obtain a euthyroid state in 4 to 6 weeks.
- Generally, thioamides are not the first-line choice of treatment due to the risk of agranulocytosis and hepatitis.

Thyroidectomy (Partial or Total)
- Occasionally used in patients with large goiters and thyroid nodules resistant to radioiodine therapy.
- Pregnant women, children
- Complications:
  - Laryngeal nerve damage
  - Hypoparathyroidism (hypocalcemia)

Disorders of the Parathyroid Glands

Etiology
- Parathyroid glands are four small glands located within or behind the thyroid gland
- Controls serum calcium and phosphorous levels
- Produces parathyroid hormone (PTH)
- Hyperparathyroidism (HPT) is far more common than hypoparathyroidism.
- Primary hyperparathyroidism is due to enlargement and overproduction of PTH. Usually due to a parathyroid adenoma. Almost always benign tumors.
- Secondary hyperparathyroidism is generally related to other diseases (often renal disease) or status post intestinal surgery.

Clinical Presentation
- Asymptomatic or vague symptoms may be discovered through routine lab work or a workup for osteoporosis or renal calculi.
- Weakness/fatigue
- Muscle cramps
- Headaches
- Osteoporosis/osteopenia
- Renal calculi
- Nonspecific abdominal pain
- Mood disturbances
- Severe hypercalcemia; the patient may develop coma or death.

Clinical Pearl
Hypercalcemia is also observed in patients with metastatic cancer. It is essential that the NP immediately follows up with lab work and diagnostic imaging to help differentiate HPT from metastatic cancer.

Clinical Management
Laboratory Workup
- PTH, calcium, phosphorous, vitamin D, metabolic panel
- DEXA scan to measure bone mineral density
- 24-hour urine for calcium
- Imaging of kidneys to assess for renal calculi or renal disorder
- Sestamibi parathyroid scan
- Thyroid ultrasound
- Referral: Patients with HPT should be followed by endocrinology.

Treatment
- Watchful waiting (if calcium levels are only moderately elevated and there are no other symptoms). This will require regular monitoring of calcium levels and bone density.
- Surgical removal of affected parathyroid gland(s) is the preferred treatment.
- Cinacalcet (Sensipar), a calcimimetic drug, may trick the parathyroid glands into not producing as much PTH.
- Hormone replacement therapy (HRT) for postmenopausal women may help maintain bone density but does not address the underlying problem.
- Bisphosphonates prevent bone calcium loss but do not address the underlying problem.

Patient Education

- Drink plenty of fluids to lessen the incidence of renal calculi.
- Regular exercise with strength training for bone health
- 600 iu of vitamin D daily
- 1,200 mg of calcium daily for women over age 51 or men over age 71. Preferably, at least half of this should come from dietary calcium.

Evaluation and Follow-Up

- Patients who have had a parathyroidectomy need close monitoring of calcium, vitamin D, and PTH levels. Teach the patient to monitor for signs and symptoms of low calcium (tetany) following surgery.

> **Red Flag**
>
> A patient whose lab results reveal an elevated calcium level with a normal PTH level (inappropriately normal), a normal vitamin D level, and normal renal function who is not taking excessive amounts of calcium should be considered suspicious for malignancy and needs to follow up as soon as possible.

Hypoparathyroidism

Etiology

- A rare condition usually caused by accidental damage to the parathyroid glands from head or neck surgery. It may also be caused by radiation therapy to the neck.
- A rare genetic condition in children is called DiGeorge syndrome.
- Hypomagnesemia—parathyroid glands need magnesium to function properly.

Signs and Symptoms

Related to low calcium levels in the blood—muscle cramps, tetany, abdominal pain, confusion, cardiac arrhythmias.

Clinical Management

- Laboratory testing: PTH, calcium, magnesium, phosphorous, 24-hour urine for calcium
- ECG

Pharmacologic Management

- Calcium and vitamin D supplementation
- May need PTH injections (although this increases the risk for osteosarcoma, so only used when absolutely necessary)

Nonpharmacologic Management

- Diet high in calcium and low in phosphorous
- Refer to endocrinology

Adrenal Disorders

Addison's Disease: Chronic Adrenal Insufficiency

- A deficiency of the adrenal hormones cortisol and aldosterone.
- Addison's disease usually develops slowly and most commonly during a person's middle age.
- Often undiagnosed until it has progressed beyond the early stages. However, during a stressful period, the symptoms can worsen very quickly and cause an Addisonian crisis, which may be life-threatening.
- Primary adrenal insufficiency is caused by damage to the adrenal gland from autoimmune disease, infection, tuberculosis, or cancer.
- Secondary adrenal insufficiency is caused by the failure of the pituitary gland to produce ACTH or by a reduction of CRH (corticotropin-releasing hormone) in the hypothalamus.

Symptoms

- Fatigue
- Muscle weakness
- Hypotension
- Hypoglycemia
- Nausea/vomiting
- Salt cravings
- Weight loss
- Hyperpigmentation

Diagnosis

- The most unique symptom is hyperpigmentation, often in non–sun-exposed areas.
- ACTH stimulation test: a patient is given ACTH, and subsequent cortisol levels are measured in the serum and the urine. People with Addison's disease do not respond to the ACTH hormone.
- If ACTH is positive, the patient may require a CRH stimulation test. The patient is given IV CRH, and serial measurements of both cortisol and ACTH are taken. Patients with Addison's disease have low cortisol levels and high ACTH levels if the secondary cause is related to the hypothalamus.

- Additional tests for primary adrenal insufficiency are:
  - ultrasound of the abdomen, kidneys, and adrenal glands;
  - TB skin testing;
  - antibody testing to assess for autoimmune origin; and
  - MRIs and CT scans, which can help assess for secondary causes, such as abnormalities within the pituitary gland or the hypothalamus.

Treatment
- Patients are typically referred to an endocrinologist for care, treatment, and follow-up.
- Patients are treated with cortisol replacement, such as hydrocortisone, prednisone, or dexamethasone.
- With primary adrenal insufficiency, there is a greater chance of aldosterone deficiency, and the patient is maintained with fludrocortisone (Florinef) daily.
- Dosages are adjusted during increased stress, illness, surgery, or trauma. Patients should carry injectable hydrocortisone to use in case of emergency.

Cushing Syndrome
- Cushing syndrome (CS) is a rare condition in people aged 20 to 50 caused by excessive production of cortisol and ACTH.
- CS is uncommon and affects women three times more often than men. It is a type of Cushing disease caused by a pituitary adenoma, which causes an overproduction of ACTH. The adenoma is almost always benign.
- ACTH independent: Exogenous—occurs when excess steroids are taken into the body. Drug-induced Cushing syndrome is the most common reason for ACTH-independent CS.
- ACTH independent: Endogenous—caused by adrenal adenomas or carcinomas. Excess cortisol is rarely due to excess production by the adrenal gland itself.

Diagnostic Tests
- First-line tests: Establish diagnosis
  - 24-hour urinary test for free cortisol (urine for free cortisol [UFC]: Three samples are taken. Normal levels are less than 100 mcg/24 hours).
  - Dexamethasone suppression test (DST): Patient is given 1 mg of dexamethasone between 11:00 p.m. and 12:00 midnight. In the morning, serum cortisol measurements above 5 mcg/dL indicate CS.
- Second-line tests: Differentiate the cause
  - ACTH measurements
  - High-dose DST testing
  - CRH stimulation test
  - Pituitary MRI

Treatment
- Discontinue the causative medication
- Inhibit steroid synthesis with pharmacologic treatments, such as ketoconazole, mitotane (Lysodren), metyrapone (Metopirone), and etomidate (Amidate).
- Transphenoidal surgery for pituitary tumors or radiation therapy.

Review Questions

1. The nurse practitioner (NP) reviews the laboratory values of a 28-year-old male patient who presents to the office to establish care with a primary care provider. The lab results from the previous week indicate an HbA1C of 7.2 percent. The NP obtains a fasting blood sugar in the office of 142. The patient denies any significant past medical history and states he "feels fine." The nurse practitioner recognizes that the patient has:
   A. developed type 1 diabetes.
   B. developed type 2 diabetes.
   C. diabetes and further testing is required.
   D. prediabetes.

2. The NP has been working with a 40-year-old single mother who has diabetes and who has two teenage children. The patient has an HbA1C of 8.0 percent. The patient and provider agree upon a plan designed to achieve glycemic control and set a target date of 6 months. When the patient returns six months later, her HbA1C is 7.8 percent. The NP would then:
   A. encourage the patient to take greater responsibility for her health, reinforcing the concept that she is a role model for her children.
   B. reassess the plan and consider barriers such as income, health literacy, and family dynamics.

C. encourage the patient to design a plan to meet her and her family's needs.
D. explain to the patient that if there is improvement in her HbA1C, the plan is a success.

3. The NP reviews the laboratory values of a patient during a follow-up office visit. The NP observes the following results in the chart:
September: HbA1C = 6.6 Fasting glucose = 118
December: HbA1C = 6.8 Fasting glucose = 122
The NP is correct in noting:
A. the patient does not meet the criteria to establish a diagnosis of diabetes mellitus (DM).
B. the patient partially meets the criteria for establishing a diagnosis of DM, but further confirmatory testing is required.
C. the patient has DM.
D. the HbA1C and fasting tests should be repeated in 3 months to confirm a diagnosis of DM.

4. The American Diabetes Association (ADA) recommends using laboratory testing to screen for prediabetes in asymptomatic people. The recommendation is to perform this screening on:
A. all children who are overweight or obese.
B. all adults with a BMI greater than 25 with one or more risk factors for DM.
C. all adults and children as part of their complete routine physical exams.
D. all children who were born to mothers who have had gestational diabetes.

5. Impaired fasting glucose (IFG) and impaired glucose tolerance (IGT) are both markers for prediabetes. Both IFG and IGT are closely associated with:
A. autoimmune disorders such as hypothyroidism, rheumatoid arthritis, and Sjögren's syndrome.
B. elevations in liver enzymes and inflammatory markers such as C-reactive protein.
C. obesity, coronary artery disease, and peripheral vascular disease.
D. central obesity, high triglycerides, low high density lipoproteins (HDLs), and hypertension (HTN).

6. Which of the following laboratory results would strongly indicate that the patient has prediabetes?
A. An HbA1C between 5.5 and 5.7
B. A 2-hour postprandial glucose between 110 and 140, after a 75-g oral glucose tolerance test
C. A fasting glucose between 100 and 125 after an 8-hour fasting interval
D. An HbA1C of greater than or equal to 6.5 percent.

7. Immune-mediated diabetes accounts for 5 to 10 percent of all DM and is caused by autoimmune destruction of the pancreatic beta cells. Which of the following statements is true regarding immune-mediated diabetes?
A. It will develop during early childhood or adolescence.
B. Patients with immune-mediated diabetes have a BMI less than 25.
C. The rate of beta cell destruction is more rapid in some individuals and slower in others.
D. Initial treatment with oral hypoglycemic agents is appropriate until there is a complete loss of beta cell function.

8. Type 2 diabetes mellitus is associated with insulin resistance. Which of the following statements about insulin resistance is true?
A. Patients with insulin resistance have decreased insulin production.
B. Insulin resistance may improve with weight loss and exercise.
C. Insulin resistance and type 2 DM are progressive diseases that eventually lead to absolute insulin deficiency.
D. Insulin resistance is a genetic trait and thus cannot be altered or improved.

9. Diabetes self-management education and support (DSMES) encourages patients to make informed decisions. This approach is most successful when:
A. patients with diabetes are provided with enough education and information to make an informed decision.
B. it is patient-centered and responsive to the patient's educational, psychosocial, and behavioral needs.
C. the patients are given written directions that outline a specific medication regimen and goal.
D. a consensus model is used, which considers multiple disciplines involved in caring for individuals with diabetes.

10. Medical nutrition therapy (MNT) is integral to DSMES. Which of the following aspects of MNT would most support the patient?
A. All patients with type 2 diabetes should be encouraged to lose between 2 and 8 kilograms of their body weight.
B. All healthcare team members involved with the individual with diabetes should be knowledgeable about MNT and support its implementation.

C. All patients with DM need to know how to count carbohydrates and limit the amount of carbohydrates in each meal.
D. Menus and easy recipes for the patient to create at home should be provided.

11. A patient asks how they could help themselves if they feel like their blood glucose is low. The NP teaches the patient about the "Rule of 15." This is used when the diabetic experiences hypoglycemia but is still capable of helping themselves. The "Rule of 15" instructs the patient to:
   A. take 15 units of insulin for every 15 grams of carbohydrate ingested.
   B. have 15 grams of protein, 15 grams of fat, and 15 grams of carbohydrate in equal portions for each meal.
   C. ingest 15 grams of carbohydrates, wait 15 minutes, and recheck their blood glucose level. Repeat as necessary until symptoms abate or blood glucose is less than 100.
   D. Immediately inject 15 milligrams of a glucagon hypoglycemic emergency kit into their midthigh muscle.

12. An overweight patient with diabetes verbalizes that he is interested in beginning therapy with a GLP-1 RA to improve his diabetic control and assist with weight loss. The nurse practitioner must first assess the patient for a personal or family history of:
   A. medullary thyroid cancer.
   B. papillary thyroid cancer.
   C. familial hereditary polyposis.
   D. polycystic kidney disease.

13. A patient presents to the primary care office for an initial evaluation. The patient is complaining of polyuria and polydipsia and exhibits symptoms of dehydration. An HbA1C is obtained that reveals an HbA1C of 12.7 percent. The NP should initiate therapy with:
   A. metformin.
   B. a GLP-1 RA.
   C. insulin.
   D. a sulfonylurea.

14. The patient is reviewing her labs with the NP. She inquires about the significance of the HbA1C test. The NP explains:
   A. "It represents the serum glucose level."
   B. "It reflects the postprandial (after-meal) increase of the serum glucose."
   C. "It represents the percentage of red blood cells that contain hemoglobin."
   D. "It correlates with the average serum glucose level of the previous 90 days."

15. A type 2 diabetic patient is started on pharmacologic therapy that is expected to assist with weight loss. Which pharmacologic therapy may assist with weight loss?
   A. A dipeptidyl peptidase inhibitor (DPP-4 inhibitor)
   B. A thiazolinedione (TZD)
   C. A sodium-glucose co-transporter 2 inhibitor (SGLT-2 inhibitor)
   D. A sulfonylurea

16. Diabetic retinopathy is the most common cause of new cases of blindness among adults aged 20 to 74 years. It is associated with the duration of the disease, as well as microvascular damage. When present, which of the following conditions would alert the nurse practitioner to recommend an immediate ophthalmic evaluation?
   A. Orthostatic hypotension
   B. Nephropathy
   C. Coronary artery disease
   D. Gastroparesis

17. A 38-year-old female patient with type 1 diabetes has developed persistent microalbuminuria, as evidenced by two specimens collected over a 6-month period. The patient is normotensive. The NP would be correct in recommending that the patient:
   A. continue with watchful waiting and repeat urine microalbumin annually.
   B. restrict the protein in their diet to no more than 60 kilograms of protein per day.
   C. Obtain a serum pregnancy test, and if negative, initiate ACE-inhibitor therapy.
   D. Repeat the test using a first-morning urine sample obtained with a clean-catch, midstream collection method.

18. The most sensitive laboratory indicator of overall thyroid function is to evaluate the level of circulating:
   A. free T4.
   B. free T3.
   C. Thyroid stimulating hormone (TSH).
   D. thyroid peroxidase antibody (TPO).

19. Thioamides may cause severe side effects. Before initiating treatment with a thioamide, the NP should obtain a baseline:
   A. coagulation study.
   B. renal function test.
   C. complete blood count (CBC) with differential.
   D. dexa scan.

20. The NP is evaluating the lab results of a 52-year-old female patient with a history of Hashimoto's hypothyroidism. The NP observes that the patient's TSH indicates overtreatment with her thyroid replacement medication. She instructs the patient to reduce her dosage by taking her levothyroxine 6 days per week instead of 7. The patient responds, "I don't want to do that since it will make me gain weight. Why can't I just stay at this dose?" What is an appropriate response from the NP?
    A. "Thyroid replacement medication is not to be used for weight loss."
    B. "Decreasing the medication dosage one day a week will not affect your weight."
    C. "You may continue at the same dosage for now. If you should start to feel jittery or have symptoms consistent with hyperthyroidism, we will need to reduce your dosage at that time."
    D. "Over-replacement with thyroid hormone puts you at risk for developing cardiac arrhythmias."

21. A patient with primary adrenal insufficiency will often have which of the following classic presenting symptoms?
    A. Hypertension
    B. Weight gain
    C. Hyperpigmentation
    D. Increased appetite

22. A patient with primary adrenal insufficiency might be expected to have which of the following lab results?
    A. Hypokalemia
    B. Hyponatremia
    C. Hyperglycemia
    D. Hypocalcemia

23. A patient has hypercalcemia and an elevated PTH level. Additional laboratory findings are normal renal function and vitamin D levels. What is the most likely diagnosis for this patient?
    A. Cushing's syndrome
    B. Primary hyperparathyroidism
    C. Metastatic disease of unknown origin
    D. Hyperthyroidism

24. A patient with an elevated 24-hour urine for cortisol can be diagnosed as having which of the following?
    A. Cushing's disease
    B. Cushing's syndrome
    C. Hypercortisolemia of undetermined origin
    D. Primary adrenal hyperplasia

25. A 60-year-old female patient who has been lost to follow-up presents to her PCP's office after a 5-year interval. She reports feeling fatigue, weakness, and a recent fall at home with a hairline fracture of her right ulnar bone. Her right forearm is immobilized in a cast. The NP reviews her labs from the hospital and finds her most recent serum calcium level is 10.8 mg/dl, and her PTH level is 88 pg/ml. Vitamin D level is 36, and renal function is normal. Her ECG reveals normal sinus rhythm (NSR). Which would be most appropriate for the NP to do first?
    A. Obtain stat DEXA scan
    B. Obtain stat endocrine referral
    C. Obtain stat cardiology referral
    D. Begin Cinacalcet (Sensipar) to lower her calcium levels

Answers and Rationales

1. Answer C is correct. The patient meets the criteria to be diagnosed with diabetes. The clinician would be unable to determine what type of diabetes the patient has without further testing.

   Answer A is incorrect. The patient has diabetes. To be diagnosed with Type 1 diabetes, the patient would need confirmatory testing for autoantibodies and the presence or absence of C-peptide. (C-peptide is often present in early DM 1 but is typically lower than normal as the beta cell destruction occurs.)

   Answer B is incorrect. The patient needs further testing. If autoantibodies are negative and C-peptide is present (or may be elevated), then a diagnosis of type 2 DM may be made.

   Answer D is incorrect. The patient has an HbA1C of 7.2 percent and a fasting BG of 142. Both meet the criteria for diagnosing DM.

2. Answer B is correct. The NP needs to reassess the plan and work with the patient to identify barriers to achieving the goal.

   Answer A is incorrect. The NP and patient are collectively responsible for the patient's health and goal setting. Telling the patient that she needs to do better as a role model for her children is both demoralizing and guilt inducing.

   Answer C is incorrect. The patient cannot be expected to design a plan without input from her healthcare professional.

Answer D is incorrect. Although the patient's HbA1c slightly improved, her current result of 7.8 percent does not indicate glycemic control.

3. Answer C is correct. The patient meets the criteria for establishing DM. An HBA1c at or greater than 6.5 percent is diagnostic for diabetes. The 3-month interval then indicates confirmatory testing is completed.

Answer A is incorrect. The patient meets the criteria for diagnosis with an HbA1c greater than 6.5 percent. The fact that the patient has impaired fasting glucose (IFG), which is greater than 126, is not significant since the HbA1c is already diagnostic in this case.

Answer B is incorrect. The patient meets the criteria for DM and has had repeat labs that reveal the same result of an HbA1C greater than 6.5 percent.

Answer D is incorrect. The HbA1c test indicates the average blood glucose value over a 3-month period. The patient has already had two tests that are 3 months apart, and both are positive indicators for DM.

4. Answer B is correct. The ADA recommends screening for prediabetes and diabetes in all adults with a BMI > 25 and at least one other risk factor.

Answer A is incorrect. Although obesity is a known risk factor for developing diabetes, there is no current recommendation to screen all overweight children.

Answer C is incorrect. According to the ADA and the USPSTF, screening for diabetes is not part of a routine complete physical exam. The clinician should screen for DM if known risk factors or other health indicators warrant screening.

Answer D is incorrect. Children who are born to mothers who had gestational diabetes do have a slightly higher risk of developing DM themselves. However, screening all children with mothers who had gestational diabetes is not the recommended standard of care.

5. Answer D is correct. Central obesity, high triglycerides, and low HDLs are consistent with metabolic syndrome, which is closely associated with prediabetes and diabetes.

Answer A is incorrect. DM type 1 is an autoimmune disorder and may be associated with a first-degree relative who has an autoimmune disorder. However, DM 2, which is the vast majority of patients with DM, is not an autoimmune disorder.

Answer B is incorrect. Elevations in liver enzymes and inflammatory markers would need further evaluation and are not necessarily associated with DM.

Answer C is incorrect. Obesity, coronary artery disease, and peripheral vascular disease are all associated with diabetes. However, these are more closely associated with long-standing DM and not necessarily prediabetes. Answer D is the best answer to this question.

6. Answer C is correct. An individual with a fasting blood glucose of 100 to 125 mg/dl after an 8-hour fast is diagnostic for prediabetes.

Answer A is incorrect. An A1c of 5.7 to 6.4 percent is diagnostic of prediabetes, but 5.5 to 5.7 percent is considered normal.

Answer B is incorrect. A 2-hour postprandial blood glucose between 110 to 140 mg/dl is an expected result.

Answer D is incorrect. An HbA1C greater than or equal to 6.5 percent is diagnostic for diabetes, not prediabetes.

7. Answer C is correct. The rate of beta cell destruction with immune-mediated diabetes is highly individualized. It may take months or sometimes years until enough beta cell destruction has occurred to cause symptoms.

Answer A is incorrect. A common misconception is that autoimmune (type 1) diabetes always develops in early childhood or adolescence. Although autoimmune diabetes commonly develops during youth (ages 0 to 19), it can develop at any age. Recent studies from the United Kingdom have shown that half of all new cases are identified in adults over the age of 20.

Answer B is incorrect. There is no association between BMI and the development of type 1 diabetes.

Answer D is incorrect. Although there may be some response to oral hypoglycemic agents until complete beta cell destruction, insulin is the treatment of choice for all persons diagnosed with immune-mediated diabetes, even when there is some beta cell function.

8. Answer B is correct. Weight loss and exercise is an effective nonpharmacologic intervention that may reduce insulin resistance.

Answer A is incorrect. Patients with insulin resistance produce adequate insulin. Often, they overproduce insulin and have an elevated C-peptide level.

Answer C is incorrect. Insulin resistance and type 2 DM may be progressive but do not necessarily lead to absolute insulin deficiency. Type 2 diabetes is not an autoimmune disease, and beta cell function may continue throughout a patient's lifetime.

Answer D is incorrect. Although there is a genetic component to both type 2 DM and insulin resistance, many nonpharmacologic and pharmacologic factors can improve and reduce insulin resistance.

9. Answer B is correct. DSMES must be patient centered and responsive to the patient's educational, psychosocial, and behavioral needs. Otherwise, it is unlikely to be successful.

Answer A is incorrect. The patient is provided with enough education to assist in decision-making, but this should be shared decision-making with the clinician. Education and information alone do not ensure that self-management will be successful.

Answer C is incorrect. A written plan is useful when it is patient-centered and responsive to the patient's needs. It may help the patient to remember the complexities associated with DSMES. However, a written plan is not the nature of DSMES.

Answer D is incorrect. While a consensus model is an important component of care for the patient with diabetes, collaboration and coordination with other disciplines will provide the patient with the optimum medical treatment. DSMES is a specific concept related to self-management through education and self-recognition of the individual's needs.

10. Answer B is correct. All healthcare team members involved with the patient with diabetes should be knowledgeable about MNT and support its implementation. There should be consistent recommendations by all healthcare team members to promote these life-long behavioral modifications.

Answer A is incorrect. The need for weight loss is specific and individualized to the patient. There are some patients with type 2 DM who do not benefit from weight loss as they may already be thin or have a normal weight (BMI of 20 to 25).

Answer C is incorrect. The patient should understand carbohydrate management in their diet, but it is not essential that all persons with diabetes count carbohydrates.

Answer D is incorrect. While providing the patient with menus and recipes may be helpful, it is not integral to the concept of MNT. MNT is a nutrition-based treatment generally provided by a registered dietitian or nutritionist.

11. Answer C is correct. The purpose of the "rule of 15" is to provide a patient with easy-to-remember instructions during periods of hypoglycemia.

Answer A is incorrect. The "rule of 15" is used for patients experiencing low blood glucose. If the patient were to take insulin, this could cause unresponsiveness, coma, or even death.

Answer B is incorrect. Ingesting protein or fat to correct hypoglycemia is of no benefit to the patient. The patient must ingest a quick-acting carbohydrate.

Answer D is incorrect. Glucagon emergency kits contain 1 mg of glucagon and are used when the patient's hypoglycemia causes confusion or unresponsiveness, and the patient is unable to help themselves.

12. Answer A is correct. GLP-1 RA therapy should not be used by patients with a personal or family history of medullary thyroid cancer, as this drug could cause medullary thyroid cancer to develop.

Answer B is incorrect. There is no known association between GLP-1 RA therapy and the development of papillary thyroid cancer.

Answer C is incorrect. There is no known association between GLP-1 RA therapy and the development of hereditary polyposis.

Answer D is incorrect. There is no known association between GLP-1 RA therapy and the development of polycystic kidney disease.

13. Answer C is correct. The patient is symptomatic, and an A1C of 12.7 percent indicates glucose toxicity. The patient should be assessed further for HHS or DKA. Insulin initiation is the only appropriate therapy at this time.

Answer A is incorrect. Starting metformin is inappropriate for this patient and would likely be harmful in the setting of severe dehydration.

Answer B is incorrect. A GLP-1 RA would only be appropriate later when the patient is no longer glucose toxic and only if the patient has type 2 DM.

Answer D is incorrect. A sulfonylurea is not appropriate if it is determined that the patient has autoimmune diabetes (Type 1) and is not appropriate for this patient who is glucose toxic and needs insulin.

14. Answer D is correct. The HbA1C test reflects the average glucose detected on the hemoglobin molecule. Since red blood cells (RBCs) have a typical lifespan of 90 days, this is an extrapolated number given as a percentage based on the glycated hemoglobin.

    Answer A is incorrect. Stating that it represents the serum glucose level is misleading as the patient needs to understand that this number is based on an average of their serum glucose levels over 90 days.

    Answer B is incorrect. It does not reflect the after-meal increase but rather the average glucose of the previous 90 days.

    Answer C is incorrect. RBCs contain hemoglobin. This answer does not explain how their average blood glucose is determined.

15. Answer C is correct. SGLT-2 inhibitors promote weight loss by removing glucose from the bloodstream at the level of the kidneys, and the excess glucose is subsequently excreted in the urine.

    Answer A is incorrect. A DPP-4 inhibitor is weight neutral.

    Answer B is incorrect. A TZD will typically cause some weight gain, most commonly associated with fluid retention.

    Answer D is incorrect. A sulfonylurea may cause weight gain due to increasing insulin production.

16. Answer B is correct. The microvascular complications associated with DM are those that cause damage to tiny vessels, such as those found in the retina and the nephrons of the kidneys, due to chronically elevated glucose. Retinopathy, nephropathy, and neuropathy are all considered to be the microvascular complications of DM and often develop simultaneously.

    Answer A is incorrect. Orthostatic hypotension is not associated with microvascular complications.

    Answer C is incorrect. Coronary artery disease is associated with DM. However, it is a **macro**vascular complication, not a **micro**vascular complication.

    Answer D is incorrect. Gastroparesis is associated with prolonged uncontrolled DM due to damage to the nerves innervating the stomach. Although this could be considered a type of microvascular complication due to its association with neuropathy, answer B is the best answer.

17. Answer C is correct. Initiating an ACE inhibitor may help delay the further progression of microalbuminuria. Since the patient is normotensive, the patient should start on a low dose and monitor for hypotension.

    Answer A is incorrect. The patient already has had confirmatory testing with two specimens collected at 6-month intervals.

    Answer B is incorrect. Restricting protein in the diet is not an appropriate recommendation unless the patient has evidence of severe renal impairment. A nephrologist, in association with a nutritionist, decides to restrict protein.

    Answer D is incorrect. Two spot urine specimens for microalbuminuria 6 months apart are considered confirmatory testing in the patient with DM. It is not necessary to obtain a clean catch midstream morning urine.

18. Answer C is correct. The TSH is used to evaluate thyroid function. The negative feedback system produces TSH in the pituitary gland and reflects thyroid function. Generally, no further testing is needed if the TSH level is normal.

    Answer A is incorrect. Free T4 reflects the amount of thyroxine that is unbound to protein (thyroglobulin). It is one test that helps to determine thyroid function but is not the best indicator for overall thyroid function.

    Answer B is incorrect. T3 (triiodothyronine) is one hormone produced by the thyroid gland. Other tissues in the body also produce it.

    Answer D is incorrect. TPO is an antibody that indicates an autoimmune disease. The presence of TPO is most seen with Hashimoto's hypothyroidism but may also be seen with Graves' disease.

19. Answer C is correct. Thioamides are associated with agranulocytosis. Patients on thioamides should have their CBC monitored at regular intervals.

    Answer A is incorrect. Patients on thioamides do not need to have coagulation studies.

    Answer B is incorrect. Thioamides may cause agranulocytosis or hepatotoxicity. The liver metabolizes thioamides. CBC and liver function tests (LFTs) should be obtained at baseline.

    Answer D is incorrect. Thioamides are not associated with osteoporosis.

20. Answer D is correct. If a patient is overtreated with thyroid replacement hormone, this may cause cardiac arrhythmias or atrial fibrillation. This response will answer the patient's question and provide the rationale for avoiding overreplacement with thyroid hormone.

Answer A is incorrect. It is important to tell the patient that thyroid medication is not a weight loss medication.

Answer B is incorrect. It is unlikely that the patient would gain weight related to being in a euthyroid state. The NP should reinforce that thyroid medication is not a weight loss drug.

Answer C is incorrect. It would not be appropriate to have the patient continue at the same dose and continue in a hyperthyroid state due to the risks of cardiac arrhythmias. The patient needs to understand that thyroid medication is titrated to achieve a euthyroid state, which may need periodic dose adjustments.

21. Answer C is correct. Hyperpigmentation due to ACTH-induced melanogenesis is a classic finding of primary adrenal insufficiency. It typically affects mucocutaneous surfaces and pressure areas such as elbows and palmar creases.

    Answer A is incorrect. A patient with primary adrenal insufficiency (Addison's disease) will typically experience hypotension, not HTN.

    Answer B is incorrect. Weight loss and loss of appetite, along with nausea or vomiting, are symptoms associated with Addison's disease.

    Answer D is incorrect. Loss of appetite accompanied by nausea and/or vomiting are typical presenting symptoms.

22. Answer B is correct. A patient with primary adrenal insufficiency may have low aldosterone levels. Therefore, they would excrete sodium and likely have hyponatremia.

    Answer A is incorrect. A low aldosterone level would cause the patient to retain potassium and, therefore, experience hyperkalemia, not hypokalemia.

    Answer C is incorrect. Patients with Addison's disease do not have adequate circulating cortisol and subsequently experience hypoglycemia and fatigue.

    Answer D is incorrect. Primary adrenal insufficiency causes decreased cortisol levels and often decreased aldosterone levels. Neither of these hormones is involved in the production or secretion of calcium. Calcium levels are controlled by parathormone from the parathyroid glands.

23. Answer B is correct. The patient's lab values are consistent with primary hyperparathyroidism. The elevated calcium level is a result of the elevated PTH level. The fact that renal function and vitamin D levels are normal makes this the most likely diagnosis.

    Answer A is incorrect. Cushing's syndrome is associated with elevated cortisol and glucose levels. The calcium levels are not affected.

    Answer C is incorrect. Although the clinician should always consider the possibility of metastatic disease with an elevated calcium level, the high PTH level is indicative of primary hyperparathyroidism. If the patient had a low or normal PTH level and an elevated calcium level, metastatic disease would be part of the differential diagnoses.

    Answer D is incorrect. Hyperthyroidism does not affect PTH levels.

24. Answer C is correct. The patient has hypercortisolemia, but the origin cannot be determined without further testing.

    Answer A is incorrect. Cushing's disease is a type of Cushing's syndrome that occurs when a pituitary adenoma makes too much ACTH. An elevated cortisol level may be Cushing's disease, but the patient would need to have further testing, such as an MRI of the brain, to assess for a pituitary adenoma.

    Answer B is incorrect. Elevated 24-hour urine indicates elevated cortisol; however, it is not enough to confirm a specific diagnosis.

    Answer D is incorrect. Primary adrenal hyperplasia causes low cortisol levels and is treated with steroids.

25. Answer B is correct. The patient needs immediate referral to an endocrinologist to determine the source of the elevated PTH level. The most common cause of hyperparathyroidism is a parathyroid adenoma. This may be seen with a thyroid ultrasound.

    Answer A is incorrect. A DEXA scan can help diagnose osteoporosis/osteopenia, but it is not diagnostic for determining the cause of hyperthyroidism.

    Answer C is incorrect. Elevated calcium levels can lead to arrhythmias. This patient had an ECG with NSR. A cardiology referral may be needed, but this would not be the first intervention.

    Answer D is incorrect. Although the patient may use cinacalcet to lower calcium levels, nephrologists use it more often in patients with renal failure. Surgical removal of the parathyroid adenoma is the gold standard for treating hyperparathyroidism.

Resources

American Diabetes Association (2022). *Standards of Medical Care in Diabetes-2022* Abridged for Primary Care Providers. *Clinical diabetes: a publication of the American Diabetes Association, 40*(1), 10–38. https://doi.org/10.2337/cd22-as01

Bancos, I., Hahner, S., Tomlinson, J., & Arlt, W. (2015). Diagnosis and management of adrenal insufficiency. *The Lancet Diabetes & Endocrinology, 3*(3), 216–226. https://doi.org/10.1016/S2213-8587(14)70142-1

Barthel, A., Benker, G., Berens, K., Diederich, S., Manfras, B., Gruber, M., Kanczkowski, W., Kline, G., Kamvissi-Lorenz, V., Hahner, S., Beuschlein, F., Brennand, A., Boehm, B. O., Torpy, D. J., & Bornstein, S. R. (2019). An update on Addison's disease. *Experimental and Clinical Endocrinology & Diabetes: Official journal, German Society of Endocrinology [and] German Diabetes Association, 127*(2-03), 165–175. https://doi.org/10.1055/a-0804-2715.

Black, C., Donnelly, P., McIntyre, L., Royle, P., Shepherd, J. J., & Thomas, S. (2007). Meglitinide analogues for type 2 diabetes mellitus. *Cochrane Database of Systematic Reviews, 2*(CD004654). https://doi.org/10.1002/14651858.CD004654.pub2

Cunningham, A. M., & Freeman, A. M. (2022). Glargine Insulin. In *StatPearls*. StatPearls Publishing.

Dicker, D. (2011). DPP-4 Inhibitors: Impact on glycemic control and cardiovascular risk factors. *Diabetes Care, 34*(2). https://doi.org/10.2337/dc11-s229

El Sayed, N. A., Aleppo, G., Aroda, V. R., Bannuru, R. R., Brown, F. M., Bruemmer, D., Collins, B. S., Gaglia, J. L., Hilliard, M. E., Isaacs, D., Johnson, E. L., Kahan, S., Khunti, K., Leon, J., Lyons, S. K., Perry, M. L., Prahalad, P., Pratley, R. E., Seley, J. J., Stanton, R. C., & Gabbay, R. A. (2022). Standards of care in diabetes. *Diabetes Care, 46*, S41–S48.

Garber, J. R., Cobin, R. H., Gharib, H., Hennessey, J. V., Klein, I., Mechanick, J. I., Pessah-Pollack, R., Singer, P. A., Woeber, K. A., & American Association of Clinical Endocrinologists and American Thyroid Association Taskforce on Hypothyroidism in Adults (2012). Clinical practice guidelines for hypothyroidism in adults: Cosponsored by the American Association of Clinical Endocrinologists and the American Thyroid Association. *Endocrine practice: Official journal of the American College of Endocrinology and the American Association of Clinical Endocrinologists, 18*(6), 988–1028. https://doi.org/10.4158/EP12280.GL

Heidelbaugh, Joel. J. (2014). *Type II diabetes mellitus, a multidisciplinary approach*. Elsevier.

Henske, J. A., Griffith, M. L., & Fowler, M. J. (2009). Initiating and titrating insulin in patients with type 2 diabetes. *Clinical Diabetes, 27*(2), 72–76. https://doi.org/10.2337/diaclin.27.2.72

Inzucchi, S. E., Berganstat, R. M., Buse. J. B., Diamant, M., Ferranini, E., Nauck, M., & Matthews, D. (2015). Management of hyperglycemia in type 2 diabetes: A patient-centered approach. *Diabetes Care, 38*(140), 140–149. https://doi.org/10.2337/dc14-2441

Korytkowski. M. T. (2004). Sulfonylurea treatment of type 2 diabetes mellitus: Focus on glimeperide. *Pharmacotherapy, 24*(5), 606–620.

Ladenson, P. W., Singer, P. A., Ain, K. B., Bagchi, N., Bigos, S. T., Levy, E. G., Smith, S. A., Daniels, G. H., & Cohen, H. D. (2000). American Thyroid Association guidelines for detection of thyroid dysfunction. *Archives of Internal Medicine, 160*(11), 1573–1575. https://doi.org/10.1001/archinte.160.11.1573

National Institute of Diabetes and Digestive and Kidney Diseases (NIDDK), NIH. *Cushing's Syndrome*. Available at: https://www.niddk.nih.gov/health-information/endocrine-diseases/cushings-syndrome. Last reviewed May 2018.

Reid, T. S. (2013). Practical use of glucagon-like peptide-1 receptor agonist therapy in primary care. *Clinical Diabetes, 31*(4), 148–157.

Rugge, J. B., Bougatsos, C., & Chou, R. (2015). Screening and treatment of thyroid dysfunction: An evidence review for the U.S. Preventative Services Task Force. *Annals of Internal Medicine, 162*(1), 35–45. https://doi.org/10.7326/M14-1456

Standards of Medical Care in Diabetes. (2023). *Diabetes Care, 46* (S1), S1–S93.

Toft, D. J., & Spinasanta, S. (2014). *Addison's disease and adrenal insufficiency*. http://www.endocrineweb.com/conditions/addisons-disease/addison-disease-adrenal-insufficiency-overview

Vijayaraghavan, K. (2010). Treatment of dyslipidemia in patients with type 2 diabetes. *Lipids in Health and Disease, 9*, 144. https://doi.org/10.1186/1476-511X-9-144

CHAPTER 13

Hematology

Susan M. DeNisco, DNP, APRN, FNP-BC, FAANP

The nurse practitioner (NP) needs to be proficient in ordering labs and interpreting the results as part of the patient encounter in the primary care setting. These clinical tools provide essential information that can be used to screen for common problems or as part of the decision-making process when confirming a suspected diagnosis. Although the development of the presumed diagnosis depends upon obtaining a detailed history and physical examination, the NP must rely on knowledge of the underlying etiology and developing a systematic approach to evaluating the complete blood count (CBC).

Laboratory Testing

Anemia

- One of the most common hematological conditions encountered in primary care is anemia.
- Anemia is a decrease in red blood cells (RBCs) as measured by the red cell count, the hematocrit, or the red cell hemoglobin content.
- Anemia is associated with several International Classification of Diseases (ICD-10) diagnostic codes.
- Anemia is not a disease but a manifestation of an underlying pathology that alters hematological homeostatic mechanisms.

Laboratory Testing and Normal Ranges

- Decreased hemoglobin (Hgb), hematocrit (HCT), and/or the RBC count indicates anemia.
- Normally, the Hgb to HCT ratio is 1 to 3 (i.e., 14 grams of Hgb correlates with an HCT of 42 percent).
- This ratio is relatively constant, even in most anemic states, but may be altered in cases of severe dehydration or overhydration.
- When evaluating Hgb, HCT, and RBCs in the individual with anemia, it is important to remember that anemias are commonly classified according to **cell size:**
  - Microcytic
  - Macrocytic
  - Normocytic

  and cell color:
  - Hypochromic
  - Normochromic

This knowledge leads to a systematic approach to evaluating anemia; consistency is key.

Mean Corpuscular Volume Is Key!

- **The first RBC index that should be evaluated in the individual with anemia is the mean corpuscular volume (MCV).**
- MCV measurement, reported in femtoliters, measures an RBC's average volume (or size) and helps determine the type of anemia.
- The MCV allows the anemia to be classified as follows:
  - normocytic [800 to 100 fL] [normal]
  - microcytic [< 80 fL] [small]
  - macrocytic [100 fL] [large]

Mean Corpuscular Hemoglobin Concentration

- The mean corpuscular Hgb concentration (MCHC), the average concentration of Hgb in RBCs, is commonly evaluated next.
- The MCHC provides information regarding the color of the cells as follows:
  - 32 to 37 g/dl = normochromic [normal color]
  - < 32 g/dl = hypochromic [pale]
  - The MCHC is diminished in microcytic anemias and is normal in macrocytic anemias.
- **Table 13-1** identifies the common indices used to evaluate anemia patients.

Peripheral Smear

- A peripheral blood smear is often triggered to be performed on an automated CBC if abnormal cells are detected.
- Should be ordered when there is a particular concern for a specific diagnosis.
- The peripheral smear allows for the evaluation of the health of the bone marrow.
- It evaluates the shape of RBCs and the presence of abnormal circulating cells (**Table 13-2**).

Red Cell Distribution Width

- Red cell distribution width (RDW) is a component of the CBC that indicates the degree of variation in size (homogeneity or heterogeneity) among the circulating RBCs.
- Cells developed in a healthy environment should be similar in size.
- A variation of less than 15 percent is considered normal.

Table 13-1 Hematological Indices Evaluated in Patients With Anemia

Index	Normal Value
RBC	4.5–6.0 million/mm³
Hgb	Male 14–18 g/100 mL; Female 12–16 g/100 mL
HCT	Male 40–54%; Female 37–48%
Platelets	150,000–450,000
MCV	80–100 fL
MCHC	32–37 g/dL
Reticulocyte Count	1–2%

Table 13-2 Clues to Causes of Anemia Found Within the Peripheral Smear

RBC Morphology	Common Causes or Associated Conditions
Spherocytes	Hereditary Spherocytosis Autoimmune Hemolytic Anemia
Schistocytes	Hemolysis Microangiopathic Hemolytic Anemias
Elliptocyte/Ovalocyte	Iron Deficiency Anemia Folic Acid Anemia
Teardrop Cells	Iron Deficiency Anemia
Sickle Cells	Sickle Cell Disease
Target Cells	Alpha Thalassemia
Bite Cells	G6PD Deficiency
Basophilic Stippling	Thalassemia Lead Toxicity

- In *acute* states, RDW is often increased (reported as anisocytosis; RDW greater than 15 percent).
- In *chronic* anemia, RDW may normalize as more circulating RBCs are produced of abnormal size.

Clinical Pearl

The lab index that has demonstrated reliability as an *early* marker of microcytic and macrocytic anemias is the RDW.

Reticulocyte Count

- A reticulocyte count (normal = 0.5 to 2 percent) measures the proportion of immature (i.e., "young red blood cells") RBCs in the blood.
- The reticulocyte count helps to determine if the bone marrow is functioning properly and responding adequately to the need for additional RBCs.
- The reticulocyte count will rise in response to therapy for iron deficiency anemia (IDA), B12 and folate deficiency, resolution of acute bleeding, hemolysis, and leukemia and erythropoietin (EPO) treatment.
- Reticulocytosis is less than 2.5 percent of the total RBC count.

- If there is no reticulocytosis following the above treatments and conditions, then the NP needs to consider bone marrow failure (aplastic anemia).

Microcytic Anemia

- Microcytic anemias are characterized by the presence of smaller-sized RBCs (microcytes) that are represented on the hemogram as a decreased MCV.
- **IDA is the most common cause of microcytic anemia in children and adults and the number one cause of anemia worldwide.**
- **Common reasons for IDA include:**
  - chronic blood loss: GI bleed, menorrhagia;
  - nutritional deficiency;
  - increased need for iron during pregnancy; and
  - lead toxicity in children.
- RBCs are microcytic (small) and hypochromic (pale).
- Decreased MCV less than 80 fL.
- Decreased serum iron.
- Increased iron-binding capacity.
- Decreased serum ferritin.
- **Anemia of chronic disease is most often normocytic anemia but can be microcytic in 20 percent of cases.**
- Thalassemia is a less likely cause of microcytic anemia.

Common Signs and Symptoms

- Pallor of skin, conjunctiva, and nail beds
- Fatigue
- Shortness of breath on exertion
- Pica
- Severe IDA
  - Spoon-shaped nails (koilonychia)
  - Systolic murmur
  - Tachycardia
  - Heart failure

Treatment of Iron Deficiency Anemia

- Treat the underlying cause.
- Oral replacement with up to 300 mg of elemental iron daily in divided doses for adolescents and adults.
- Ferrous sulfate, which contains 65 mg of elemental iron in each 325 mg tablet, is better absorbed than other preparations.
- Take iron supplements with vitamin C or orange juice for better absorption.
- Increase fiber and fluids to prevent constipation.
- Stools may turn black and cause gastritis.
- Eat iron-rich foods (e.g., red meat, legumes, tofu, dark green vegetables, shellfish, etc.).
- Avoid taking iron with antacids, dairy products, quinolones, and tetracycline.
- Iron stores (serum ferritin) may take 4 to 6 months to return to normal levels with supplementation.
- Serum iron levels rise earlier in the treatment process and reflect recent intake. A noticeable increase in Hgb may not occur until after 2 to 4 weeks of supplementation.
- Reticulocytosis should be noted within 3 to 10 days.

Clinical Pearl

Iron deficiency typically manifests as microcytic, hypochromic anemia.

Thalassemia

- A group of autosomal recessive hematologic disorders caused by defects in the synthesis of one or more of the hemoglobin alpha or beta chains.
- Malformation of RBCs, increasing hemolysis.
- Found incidentally on a CBC that shows mild microcytic, hypochromic anemia.
- **The gold standard test for diagnosis is hemoglobin electrophoresis.**
- *Alpha thalassemia* occurs more commonly in people originating from Southeast Asia, China, and occasionally Africa.
- The alpha thalassemia trait is a mild form of anemia, not requiring therapy.
- Alpha thalassemia trait hemoglobin electrophoresis will be normal.
  - On CBC with peripheral smear, look for microcytosis [low MCV]
  - Target cells
  - An MCH always below 27 pg
  - RBC counts are usually higher than normal.
- Alpha thalassemia major, however, requires frequent RBC transfusions and, in some instances, iron chelation therapy.
- *Beta thalassemia* occurs in those originating from Mediterranean countries. Those with the beta thalassemia trait are asymptomatic and usually do not require treatment.
  - On Hgb electrophoresis, look for elevated HgB A2 =/- HgB F.

- On CBC with peripheral smear, look for microcytic cells (low MCV), hypochromic cells, and variations in size and shape (anisocytosis and poikilocytosis).
- **Thalassemia major**, also known as **Cooley's anemia**, is detected during infancy and requires lifelong treatment with frequent RBC transfusions.
- Beta thalassemia major causes hemolytic anemia, poor growth, and skeletal abnormalities during development.
- Persons with the thalassemia trait have a normal life expectancy, but those with beta thalassemia major often die from cardiac complications of iron overload by 30 years of age.
- Parents with any combination of alpha or beta thalassemia syndromes place a child at risk for the disorder.
- Each child of two carrier parents is at a 25 percent risk of the disease (1 in 4 children).
- Preconception genetic counseling and screening of parents is recommended.
- If a parent is positive for the trait, a prenatal diagnosis can be made with fetal blood sampling or chorionic villi sampling.

Clinical Pearl

Ferritin level and serum iron levels are normal in thalassemia trait.

Macrocytic Anemia

- Macrocytic anemia represents a group of pathological conditions associated with RBCs of insufficient numbers in which the cells are larger than normal.
- Although many specific etiologies are known to cause macrocytic anemias, the two **most common are vitamin B12 and folic acid deficiency.**
- Other causes include postgastrectomy patients, bariatric surgery patients, strict vegans, and patients with celiac disease and small bowel disease.
- Drug-induced causes include heavy alcohol consumption and anti-epileptic drugs (carbamazepine [Tegretol], phenytoin [Dilantin], and methotrexate).
- Prolonged use of the following:
  - Histamine H2 blocker use for more than 12 months
  - Metformin use for more than 4 months
  - Proton pump inhibitor use for more than 12 months

Vitamin B12 Deficiency Anemia

- Most common cause of macrocytic anemia.
- **Vitamin B12 deficiency, especially pernicious anemia (lack of intrinsic factor to absorb B12)**, is the most prevalent underlying etiology, especially in those between 60 and 75 years old.
- Pernicious anemia is an autoimmune disorder caused by the destruction of parietal cells in the fundus, resulting in the cessation of intrinsic factor production.
- Intrinsic factors are needed to absorb B12 from the small intestine.
- Symptoms of vitamin B12 deficiency include:
  - a smooth, sore, beefy red tongue (aka glossitis), and
  - neurological symptoms (e.g., paresthesia in hands and feet, peripheral neuropathy, hyporeflexia, extremity weakness, incoordination, difficulty with gait).

Lab Testing for Macrocytic Anemias

- When macrocytic anemia is suspected, the next step is to obtain a vitamin B12 level and folic acid level.
- To determine if macrocytic anemia is related to vitamin B12 or folic acid deficiency, homocysteine (Hcy) and methylmalonic acid (MMA) levels should be drawn.
- Both MMA and Hcy will be elevated in vitamin B12 deficiency.
- Only Hcy will be elevated in folate deficiency.
- Other lab tests for pernicious anemia include:
  - Antiparietal cell antibodies (APCAs) and
  - Anti-intrinsic factor (IF) antibodies.

Treatment for B12 Deficiency

- The traditional approach is to give Cobalamin 1,000 mcg IM weekly for four weeks and then monthly for life.
- Cobalamin 1,000 mcg of oral replacement daily may be an acceptable alternative for those with sufficient absorption in the small intestine.
- The response time to appropriate vitamin B12 replacement is usually rapid, with reticulocytosis occurring within 2 to 5 days and peaking within 5 to 7 days.
- Hct normalization occurs within weeks, but full hematological recovery may take up to 2 months.

Folic Acid Deficiency Anemia
Etiology
- **Folic acid deficiency anemia** (FADA) is a macrocytic anemia caused by folate (folic acid) deficiency due to increased requirements, impaired absorption in the proximal jejunum, and drug antagonism or inadequate intake.
- FADA can lead to an accumulation of Hcy, which can contribute to cognitive decline, stroke, and heart disease.
- Causes of decreased absorption
  - Bariatric surgery
  - Celiac disease
  - Chronic alcohol intake
  - Crohn's disease
  - Gastric and small bowel resection
  - Zinc deficiency
  - Medications that reduce folic acid absorption
- Decreased dietary intake
  - Restrictions related to chronic disease
  - Overcooking vegetables
  - Low citrus intake
  - Older people, infants, alcoholics
- Increased requirements for folic acid
  - Chronic hemolytic anemia
  - Infection and malignancy
  - Pregnancy and breastfeeding

Signs and Symptoms
- The common picture is an older patient and a male with an alcohol disorder.
- Fatigue, pallor, decreased appetite, smooth sore tongue, diarrhea
- Memory loss, decreased concentration, confusion, irritability, and depression
- As with other anemias, shortness of breath, tachycardia, palpitations, and heart failure if severe

Treatment Plan
Labs
- CBC with peripheral smear: decreased Hgb and Hct, increased MCV greater than 100, macro-ovalocytes, and hyper-segmented neutrophils
- A serum folic acid less than 2.5 ng/mL
- MMA and Hcy levels to rule out a coexisting vitamin B12 deficiency
- Urine human chorionic gonadotropin (HCG) if considering pregnancy

Dietary Measures
- Leafy green vegetables
- Grains
- Legumes
- Liver

Medications
- Folic acid replacement for adults is 1 mg/day.
- The CDC (1992) recommends that all women between 15 and 45 years consume 0.4 mg of folic acid daily to minimize the risk of neural tube defects.
- Women with a previous history of birthing a child with a neural tube defect should increase their folic acid intake to 4 mg daily beginning 1 month before planned conception and continue this dose through the first 3 months of pregnancy.

Evaluation
- In response to supplementation, reticulocytosis occurs rapidly and peaks within 7 to 10 days.
- Hct levels usually return to normal within 1 month.
- If levels are not rising as expected and coexisting vitamin B12 anemia has been ruled out, keep in mind that IDA coexists in one-third of patients with vitamin B12 or folate deficiency.

Medications that lower folic acid levels include anti-epileptic drugs such as carbamazepine (Tegretol), phenytoin (Dilantin), methotrexate, sulfasalazine, and Bactrim.

> **Test Taking Tip**
>
> Folate deficiency will show a decrease in folate level, an increase in Hcy level, and an MCV greater than 100.

Normocytic Anemias

Normocytic anemias can be divided into two major etiologies:

1. Decreased RBC production
2. Increased RBC loss or destruction

Anemia of chronic disease (ACD), the most common form of normocytic anemia and the second most common cause of anemia worldwide, is associated with decreased RBC production.

Anemia of Chronic Disease
Etiology
- Normocytic (MCV=80 to 96 fL) and normochromic anemia with normal RDW.

- Underlying pathophysiology includes decreased activity of the bone marrow, inadequate production of EPO or decreased response to EPO, and decreased RBC lifespan.
- ACD is associated with a variety of chronic disorders: infection, inflammation, malignancy, and other systemic diseases (i.e., chronic renal disease, advanced liver disease, rheumatic arthritis, and/or endocrine disorders).

Signs and Symptoms
- Fatigue, pallor, weakness, cold intolerance
- Palpitations, dyspnea on exertion, activity intolerance
- Systolic murmur
- Hepatosplenomegaly (HSM)

Common Lab Findings
- Low circulating serum iron and transferrin levels.
- Total iron binding capacity (TIBC) in ACD is low.
- Serum ferritin will be normal or increased.
- Rare for the Hct to drop below 25 percent.
- Hgb usually is maintained at 8 to 12 g/dL.

Treatment
- Timely identification and management of the underlying etiology.
- Since ACD is caused by underproduction of EPO, recombinant human EPO supplementation is common: 50 to 150 IU/kg three times a week.
- Target goal for correction of Hgb with EPO is 11 to 12 g/dL.
- Hgb levels greater than this have demonstrated no additional health benefits but are associated with an increased risk of cardiovascular events.
- Coexisting IDA and ACD iron supplements may be necessary for proper erythropoiesis.

Clinical Pearl
The kidneys are responsible for most of the body's EPO production.

Normocytic Hemolytic Anemias
Etiology
- Hemolytic anemia represents approximately 5 percent of all anemias and can be categorized as follows:
  - Congenital/inherited (e.g., sickle cell disease [SCD], hereditary spherocytosis or elliptocytosis, thalassemia, or G6PD deficiency)
  - Acquired (e.g., microangiopathic hemolytic anemias [disseminated intravascular coagulation [DIC], hemolytic uremic syndrome [HUS], or thrombotic thrombocytopenic purpura [TTP], transfusion of ABO-incompatible blood, use of toxic chemicals or drugs, presence of prosthetic heart valves, or hemodialysis)
- Consider hemolysis if there is a precipitous fall in Hgb, significant reticulocytosis, and/or spherocytes (small, dense RBCs with a loss of biconcave shape) or RBC fragments on the peripheral smear.
- Most sensitive measure of hemolysis is lactate dehydrogenase (LDH).
- LDH is released into circulation when RBCs are destroyed and Hgb is released from damaged erythrocytes, leading to an increase in indirect bilirubin (typically not exceeding 3 mg/dl) and urobilinogen levels.
- Serum haptoglobin (which binds to free Hgb) is also sensitive to hemolytic anemia.
- With intravascular hemolysis, Hgb is released from cells and is bound by haptoglobin.
- Circulating free haptoglobin levels decline.
- Direct Coombs' test can evaluate autoimmune hemolytic anemia; it evaluates for immunoglobulin G (IgG) alloantibodies or autoantibodies and their complement proteins, which bind to and destroy erythrocytes.
- Persistent hemolysis may result in the development of jaundice, bilirubin gallstones, or skin staining from hemosiderosis.
- Iron overload may occur in patients who have received multiple transfusions.

Glucose-6-Phosphate Dehydrogenase Deficiency Anemia
Etiology
- Glucose-6-phosphate dehydrogenase (G6PD) deficiency is the most common enzyme deficiency worldwide, impacting 400 million people.
- The X-linked inherited disorder has multiple variants, with different gene mutations resulting in varying levels of enzyme deficiency and symptom manifestation, including neonatal hyperbilirubinemia and acute or chronic hemolysis.
- G6PD most commonly affects persons of African, Mediterranean, Asian, or Middle-Eastern descent.
- The conversion of nicotinamide adenine dinucleotide phosphate to its reduced form in erythrocytes is the basis of diagnostic testing for the deficiency, which is confirmed by fluorescent spot tests.

- Acute hemolysis is typically self-limiting but can be severe enough to warrant a transfusion and is caused by exposure to an oxidative stressor (i.e., infection, oxidative drugs, and/or fava beans).
- Treatment is geared toward avoidance of these and other stressors.
- Medications to avoid include quinolones, sulfonamides, nitrofurans, antimalarials, and anthelmintics.

Sickle Cell Anemia
Etiology
- SCD describes a group of blood cell disorders in which individuals inherit abnormal Hgb and Hgb S.
- Approximately 100,000 Americans have SCD, and while the majority of these are Black people, some individuals are of Hispanic, southern European, Middle Eastern, and Asian Indian descent.
- The most severe form of the disease occurs when individuals inherit Hgb SS, one Hgb S gene from each parent.
- Individuals who have inherited normal Hgb (Hgb A) from one parent and Hgb S from the other are known to have sickle cell trait and may transmit the defective gene to offspring.
- Approximately 1 in 13 Black infants are born with sickle cell trait, while 1 in every 365 is born with SCD.
- All 50 states and the District of Columbia require newborn screening for SCD.

Signs and Symptoms
- Sickle cells lack the flexibility of normal RBCs and adhere to vessel walls, impeding flow and limiting oxygenation to tissues, which results in the symptomatology associated with SCD:
  - Acute pain/vaso-occlusive crises
  - Acute chest syndrome
  - Stroke (up to 24 percent of those with Hgb SS will suffer a stroke by age 45)
  - Retinal detachment, heart failure, pulmonary hypertension, leg ulcers, and kidney or liver damage.
  - SCD patients are also prone to hemolytic anemia.
  - Normal RBCs live 90 to 120 days; however, sickle cells last only 10 to 20 days.
  - Individuals with SCD live with mild to moderate anemia.
  - Severe, life-threatening anemia in children can occur with a splenic sequestration crisis (trapping of RBCs in the spleen) or an aplastic crisis (acute bone marrow suppression usually caused by parvovirus B19 infection).

Treatment
- CBC is a screening test.
- Gold standard testing is hemoglobin electrophoresis.
- Sickle cell is an autosomal recessive pattern genetic disease.
- Genetic counseling if both partners are at risk.
- If each parent has the sickle cell trait, 1 out of 4 children will have the disease.
- Adhere to the vaccine schedule to prevent infection.
- Needs to be managed by hematologist.

Clinical Pearl
Hemoglobin electrophoresis will show an increase in HbS and HbF, reticulocytosis, and hemolytic anemia

Abnormalities of the White Blood Cells

In addition to evaluating RBCs and their indices, the NP should have foundational knowledge of conditions associated with abnormalities of white blood cells (WBCs).

WBCs can be categorized into two groups:
- Granulocytes (basophils, eosinophils, and neutrophils)
- Agranulocytes (lymphocytes and monocytes)

WBC counts in adults range from 4,500 to 10,500/mm^3, and differential components help determine the body's response to acute and chronic infections, inflammatory conditions, allergic reactions, immunodeficiencies, and hematologic malignancies (**Table 13-3**).

Leukocytosis (Elevated WBC Count)
Etiology
- Usually indicative of benign conditions, including infections and inflammatory processes.
- May be a manifestation of a more serious etiology, such as leukemia or a myeloproliferative disorder.
- Other causes may be stress, anemia, immune system disorders, severe allergic reactions, trauma, bronchogenic carcinomas, uremia, medications

Table 13-3 Common Conditions Resulting in Elevations of Circulating WBCs

WBC Component	Function	Normal Range	Conditions Resulting in Elevated Levels
Neutrophils (Polys or Segs)	First responders to bacterial infections	30–70%	Acute bacterial infections
Lymphocytes	Immune responses against antigens	15–40%	Viral infections Leukemia
Monocytes	Assists with phagocytosis and regulates immunity	2–8%	Autoimmune disorders Severe bacterial infections Chronic infections
Eosinophils	Targets antigen antibodies for destruction; regulates inflammation	0–5%	Allergic disorders Parasitic infections
Basophils	Hypersensitivity reactions; allergic responses	0–3%	Parasitic infections Some allergic disorders Inflammation
Bands	Triggered to target bacterial infections with neutrophils	0–4%	Severe bacterial infections

(quinine, corticosteroids, and epinephrine), acute hemolysis, hemorrhage, splenectomy, polycythemia vera, and pregnancy.
- Leukocytosis is most associated with an increase in the absolute number of mature neutrophils but can also reflect an increase in lymphocytes, eosinophils, monocytes, or basophils.

Leukopenia (Decreased WBC Count)

- Also known as" neutropenia," leukopenia is observed when the WBC supply is depleted by infection or treatments, such as chemotherapy or radiation, or when stem cell abnormalities disrupt bone marrow function.
- Other causes of leukopenia may be viral infections, congenital disorders characterized by diminished bone marrow function, cancer, other diseases that damage bone marrow, or autoimmune disorders.
- Symptoms may include anemia, fatigue, fever, headache, stomatitis, pneumonia, menorrhagia, and thrombocytopenia.
- Treatment is aimed at managing the underlying condition and minimizing the risks of infection.

Neutrophils

- Neutrophils (polys or segs) are the body's most numerous and important leukocytes.
- Through phagocytosis, they constitute the body's preliminary defense against infection.
- In a healthy adult, most neutrophils circulating in the bloodstream are mature (segmented); however, the term "left shift" refers to an increase in the proportion (0.1 percent) of bands (stabs), immature neutrophils with a banded-appearing nucleus.
- The left shift typically indicates bacterial infection but may also occur when there is inflammation or necrosis.
- *Bacterial infections typically cause neutrophilia,* which is the most common form of leukocytosis.
    - Trauma, inflammatory disorders, burns, acute hemorrhage, sepsis, cigarette smoking, malignancy, uremia, and metabolic processes may also cause the condition.
- *Neutropenia* can be caused by insufficient or injured bone marrow stem cells, increased destruction of neutrophils in circulation, shifts in neutrophils from circulating blood to the tissues, infections (e.g., tuberculosis and viral infections), or nutritional deficiencies.

Eosinophils

- Eosinophils play two major roles in the body: destroying foreign substances and regulating inflammation.
- Eosinophils are (a) phagocytic, (b) target antigen-antibodies for destruction, and (c) become

increasingly active during allergic reactions and parasitic infections.
- *Eosinophilia* can occur in the blood or body tissues and may be due to asthma, autoimmune disorders, infections, dermatologic conditions, allergic events, eczema, hay fever, or leukemia.
- *Eosinopenia* can occur with Cushing's syndrome, stress, or corticosteroid therapy.
- Treatment is generally unnecessary because the immune system can compensate adequately for other WBC components.

Basophils
- Basophils are the least numerous of the WBCs and are responsible for hypersensitivity reactions and allergic responses with receptors for immunoglobin E (IgE).
- Basophils contain a multilobed nucleus and granules comprised of histamine, heparin, and serotonin.
- The cells can be stained with a base dye (methylene blue); hence the name basophil, meaning "base-loving."
- *Basophilia* may indicate asthma, allergic reactions to food, drugs or parasites, anaphylaxis, infections, inflammatory conditions (e.g., IBD dermatitis), or myeloproliferative disorders.
- *Basopenia* may stem from thyroid disorders, urticaria, ovulation, pregnancy, radiation, chemotherapy, or infections.

Lymphocytes
- Lymphocytes are the primary components of the body's immune system and are the second most common WBCs.
- Lymphocytes circulate in blood, lymph fluid, and body tissues, such as the spleen, thymus, bone marrow, lymph nodes, tonsils, and liver.
- The three main types are T cells, B cells, and natural killer cells, which are critical for immune responses against antigens.
- *Lymphocytosis* (increased number) may indicate acute or chronic infections (viral or bacterial), including mononucleosis or tuberculosis, cancer of the blood (leukemias) or lymphatic system, or an autoimmune disorder causing chronic inflammation. A common reason for lymphocytosis is lymphocytic leukemia.
- *Lymphocytopenia* (decreased number) may be caused by acquired diseases, such as infectious diseases, autoimmune disorders, steroid therapy, aplastic anemia, Hodgkin's disease, radiation, and chemotherapy.

Monocytes
- Monocytes are structurally the largest of the WBCs.
- Monocytes migrate from blood to tissue within a few hours after bone marrow production and develop into macrophages and dendritic cells.
- Once converted, monocytes assist other WBCs in removing dead or damaged tissues, destroying cancer cells, and regulating immunity against foreign substances.
- *Monocytosis* (increased number) occurs in response to chronic infections, autoimmune disorders, blood disorders, and cancers.
- *Monocytopenia* (decreased number) can occur in response to toxins bacteria release into the bloodstream and in those receiving chemotherapy.

Abnormalities of Platelets
- The final factor of the CBC that NPs are commonly required to evaluate is the platelet count.
- Platelets are components of blood cells developed from megakaryocytes in the bone marrow that are essential for coagulation.
- Most platelets circulate in the blood; however, approximately one-third are stored in the spleen.
- The typical life cycle of a platelet is 7 to 10 days.
- The normal range of platelets, also referred to as thrombocytes, is 150,000 to 450,000/µL.

Thrombocytosis
- **Thrombocytosis** is defined as a platelet count of more than 450,000/µL.
  - *An overproduction of platelets in the bone marrow causes primary thrombocytosis.*
  - Most patients with primary thrombocytosis are asymptomatic, and treatment entails the lifelong use of hydroxyurea to suppress platelet production.
  - Low-dose aspirin may be needed to reduce the risk of thrombus formation.
  - Complications of primary thrombocytosis include thrombosis, gastrointestinal (GI) bleeding, and, in rare instances, progression to acute myeloid leukemia.
  - **Secondary thrombocytosis** is caused by an underlying disease, such as anemia, cancer, inflammation, infection, surgery (splenectomy), or certain medications.
  - Symptoms of secondary thrombocytosis may include headaches, weakness, dizziness,

bruising, bleeding, chest pain, and loss of consciousness.
- A diagnosis is made while interpreting a routine CBC; however, bone marrow aspiration may be needed.
- Treatment is aimed at resolving the underlying cause.

Thrombocytopenia

- Thrombocytopenia is defined as a platelet count of less than 150,000/μL and is often found incidentally when obtaining a CBC.
- If present, symptoms may include easy bruising (ecchymosis and petechiae), bleeding from mucous membranes, spontaneous epistaxis, excessive bleeding from wounds, and hematuria.
- Causes of thrombocytopenia are multifactorial:
  - Impaired production of platelets (i.e., viral infections, aplastic anemia, chemotherapeutic drugs, cancers, alcohol, myelodysplastic syndrome)
  - Increased destruction of platelets (i.e., transfusion reactions, medications such as digoxin, quinine, quinidine, acetaminophen, and rheumatologic conditions)
  - Autoimmune conditions, thrombotic thrombocytopenia purpura (TTP), immune thrombocytopenic purpura (ITP), heparin-induced thrombocytopenia (HIT)
  - Severe infections, hemolysis, elevated liver enzymes and low platelets (HELLP) syndrome
  - Splenic sequestration (i.e., chronic alcohol misuse, liver disease, gestational thrombocytopenia).
- Treatment depends on the severity and underlying cause.
- Most patients do not require regular transfusions of platelets.
- In severe thrombocytopenia, steroids are used to suppress the autoimmune attack on platelets.
- IV antibodies or IVIG can be used in patients who are not responsive to steroids.

Review Questions

1. A 20-year-old college student presents with complaints of excessive fatigue, fever, and exudative pharyngitis, which is accompanied by anterior and posterior cervical lymphadenopathy. What white blood count (WBC) findings would support the suspected diagnosis?
   A. Increased neutrophils with more than 10 percent bands
   B. Increased lymphocytes with more than 10 percent atypical lymphocytes
   C. Increased total leukocytes, with an increased proportion of basophils
   D. Increased total leukocytes, with an increased proportion of eosinophils

2. Which of the following laboratory findings are most consistent with anemia related to folic acid deficiency?
   A. Decreased mean corpuscular volume (MCV) and decreased mean corpuscular Hgb concentration (MCHC)
   B. Decreased MCV and normal MCHC
   C. Increased MCV and normal MCHC
   D. Normal MCV and normal MCHC

3. The family nurse practitioner (FNP) evaluates a complete blood count (CBC) that reveals an abnormally low hemoglobin (Hgb), hematocrit (Hct), and red blood cell (RBC) count. Which of the following lab values would assist the FNP in determining if the anemia was microcytic or macrocytic?
   A. Ferritin level
   B. MCV
   C. MCHC
   D. Total iron binding capacity (TIBC)

4. Which of the following conditions is associated with normocytic anemia?
   A. A deficiency in vitamin B12 intake or absorption
   B. Chronic blood loss
   C. Concurrent chronic illness (i.e., chronic kidney disease)
   D. Inadequate globin synthesis

5. The FNP is following up with a patient previously diagnosed with anemia who complains of a sore tongue, numbness, and tingling of the hands and feet. The FNP recognizes that she needs to address the patient's response to:
   A. the administration of erythropoietin (EPO).
   B. ferrous sulfate supplementation.
   C. folic acid supplementation.
   D. vitamin B12 supplementation.

6. The FNP is following up with a young adult woman previously diagnosed with microcytic, hypochromic anemia. The FNP recognizes that it is most important to rule out:
   A. abnormal uterine bleeding.
   B. gastrointestinal bleeding.
   C. inadequate intake of folic acid.
   D. low carbohydrate diet fads.

7. When interpreting findings in an individual with leukocytosis, the FNP recognizes that a "left shift" is represented by an increase in the proportion of:
   A. eosinophils.
   B. lymphocytes.
   C. monocytes.
   D. neutrophils.

8. Hemolytic anemia may be an inherited condition. Which of the following is not an inherited condition related to hemolytic anemia?
   A. Hereditary spherocytosis
   B. Pernicious anemia
   C. Glucose-6-phosphate dehydrogenase deficiency (G6PD)
   D. Sickle cell anemia

9. Women of childbearing age should have an adequate intake of what micronutrient to decrease the risk of fetal neural tube defects?
   A. Folic acid
   B. Iron
   C. Vitamin B6
   D. Vitamin B12

10. What is the most likely diagnosis for a 66-year-old patient with the following CBC findings?
    WBC: $7.1 \times 10^3/\mu l$
    RBC: $3.32 \times 10^3/\mu l$
    Hgb: 11.3 g/dL
    Hct: 34.4%
    MCV: 91 fL
    MCHC: 32 g/dL
    Plt: $364 \times 10^3/\mu l$
    RDW: 13.4%
    Reticulocytes: 0.9%
    A. Anemia of chronic disease
    B. Folate deficiency anemia
    C. Iron deficiency anemia (IDA)
    D. Vitamin B12 deficiency anemia

11. What is the most likely diagnosis for a patient with the following CBC findings?
    WBC: $8.8 \times 10^3/\mu l$
    RBC: $3.01 \times 10^3/\mu l$
    Hgb: 10.3 g/dL
    Hct: 32.2%
    MCV: 74 fL
    MCHC: 28.3 g/dL
    Plt: $400 \times 10^3/\mu l$
    RDW: 18.4%
    Reticulocytes: 2.1%
    A. Anemia of chronic disease
    B. Folate deficiency anemia
    C. IDA
    D. Vitamin B12 deficiency anemia

12. The FNP is seeing a patient taking ferrous sulfate. Which statement by the patient demonstrates a need for additional education?
    A. "I should take my medication with orange juice to increase absorption."
    B. "I should take one tablet twice a day."
    C. "It is best to take the iron on an empty stomach."
    D. "It is recommended that I take enteric-coated iron with meals."

13. The nurse practitioner (NP) knows that the differential diagnosis list for a full-term newborn who has jaundice in the first 24 hours of life and an elevated bilirubin level should include the following (select all that apply):
    A. Sickle cell anemia
    B. Thalassemia
    C. G6PD deficiency
    D. Physiologic neonatal hyperbilirubinemia

14. When evaluating the patient with megaloblastic anemia who does not have neurological symptoms, the FNP recognizes that the most likely diagnosis is:
    A. an underlying hemolytic process.
    B. folic acid deficiency.
    C. iron deficiency.
    D. suppression of the bone marrow.

15. The gold standard for diagnosing sickle cell disease (SCD) is a(n):
    A. bone marrow aspiration.
    B. direct antiglobulin test (DAT).
    C. hemoglobin electrophoresis.
    D. indirect Coombs' test.

16. A 20-year-old black male was recently treated for a minor skin infection with sulfamethoxazole/trimethoprim DS twice daily for 10 days. He returns to the clinic complaining of fatigue, yellowing

of his skin and eyes, and dark urine. These symptoms lead the NP to suspect which of the following?
A. G6PD deficiency
B. Pernicious anemia
C. SCD
D. Thalassemia

17. A 16-year-old female is experiencing an asthma exacerbation following exposure to cats at her neighbor's home. Which leukocyte will likely be elevated?
A. Basophils
B. Eosinophils
C. Monocytes
D. Neutrophils

18. A 33-year-old pregnant female with a history of beta thalassemia trait consults with the NP about her child's risk of inheriting the disorder. The father of the child is uninvolved in the prenatal planning, and it is unknown whether he is a carrier. The most appropriate action by the NP is to:
A. counsel the mother about pregnancy termination options.
B. discuss that a prenatal diagnosis cannot be made.
C. explain that the chances of the child inheriting the disease are 50 percent.
D. refer the patient for genetic counseling.

19. Which of the following lab tests confirms a diagnosis of iron deficiency when evaluating microcytic anemia?
A. Hgb electrophoresis
B. Platelet count
C. Serum ferritin
D. Vitamin B12 level

20. A 30-year-old female recently began treatment with ferrous sulfate 325 mg by mouth three times daily between meals. She presents to the NP for a repeat CBC after one month of iron therapy. Lab values are as follows: Hgb 12.0 g/dL, HCT 36%, MCV 82, and MCHC 32 g/dL. What is the most appropriate follow-up course of action by the NP?
A. Continue the current treatment regimen
B. Decrease oral iron supplementation
C. Increase oral iron supplementation
D. Switch to IV iron therapy

21. A 60-year-old female is following up with the NP for a recent diagnosis of pernicious anemia, and she would like to know how long she will need to continue treatment with vitamin B12. The most appropriate response by the NP is:
A. 1 to 3 months.
B. 3 to 6 months.
C. 6 to 12 months.
D. lifelong.

22. An 80-year-old White male with alcohol use disorder complains of fatigue, decreased appetite, and occasional palpitations. He denies neurological complaints. His CBC reveals the following: Hgb 8.0 g/dL, HCT 24%, and MCV 110. Which would be the most likely diagnosis?
A. Anemia of chronic disease
B. Folic acid deficiency anemia
C. IDA
D. Vitamin B12 deficiency anemia

23. The NP is following up with a patient who was recently diagnosed with vitamin B12 deficiency. To assess the effectiveness of dietary education, the FNP should focus on the patient's intake of which food source?
A. Broccoli
B. Chicken
C. Legumes
D. Lettuce

24. Following an upper respiratory infection, a 5-year-old boy presents to the clinic with his mother with complaints of unexplained purple discolorations to his upper and lower extremities, frequent nosebleeds, and petechiae. The CBC reveals a normal white blood cell count, normal hemoglobin and hematocrit levels, and a decreased platelet count. Which diagnosis is most likely?
A. Aplastic anemia
B. Idiopathic thrombocytopenia purpura (ITP)
C. Sickle cell disease
D. Reactive thrombocytosis

25. A 12-year-old boy with fatigue, dyspnea, pallor, and easy bruising presents for evaluation by the NP. The CBC reveals pancytopenia. Which test should be used to confirm the suspected diagnosis?
A. ANA screen
B. Bone marrow biopsy
C. Folate level
D. Hgb electrophoresis

Answers and Rationales

1. Answer B is correct. The scenario is consistent with the classic triad seen with infectious mononucleosis: fever, exudative pharyngitis, and adenopathy. Within mono, the characteristic CBC findings include absolute lymphocytosis in which more than 10 percent of the cells are atypical.

   Answer A is incorrect. A normal band cell count is 10 percent or less, but a count of more than 10 percent can be a clinical indicator of sepsis.

   Answer C is incorrect. It is called basophilia when there is an increase in total leukocytes, or white blood cells, and an increase in the proportion of basophils. Basophilia is the rarest form of leukocytosis and can be a sign of infection, leukemia, or autoimmune disease.

   Answer D is incorrect. Eosinophilia describes abnormally high levels of a type of WBC called an eosinophil. Several conditions, including parasitic infection, drug reactions, allergies, and cancer, can cause it.

2. Answer C is correct. Folic acid deficiency results in impaired RNA and DNA synthesis within the developing erythrocyte and the development of immature and dysfunctional enlarged RBCs (megaloblasts). Because hemoglobin synthesis is not impaired, RBCs formed in the presence of folic acid deficiency retain their normal MCHC and color.

   Answer A is incorrect. Low MCV and MCHC may indicate iron-deficiency anemia, microcytosis, and thalassemia.

   Answer B is incorrect. In normochromic microcytic anemias, the RBCs are small (MCV) but the appropriate color (MCHC). This can indicate a normal amount of iron and hemoglobin. This type of anemia may indicate chronic inflammation, infection, or diseases that prevent RBCs from developing properly.

   Answer D is incorrect. Normocytic normochromic anemia is the type of anemia in which the circulating RBCs are the same size (normocytic, MCV) and have a normal red color (normochromic, MCHC). Most of the normochromic, normocytic anemias are a consequence of other diseases. Anemia of chronic disease may be secondary to infections, malignancies, autoimmune disorders, or chronic renal failure.

3. Answer B is correct. The MCV is the lab value that reflects RBC size or average volume. Based on MCV, cells are classified as normocytic (80 to 100 femtoliters [fL]), microcytic (< 80 fL), or macrocytic (> 100 fL). The first RBC index that should be evaluated in the individual with anemia is the MCV.

   Answer A is incorrect. Ferritin is a protein that stores iron in cells; ferritin level measures the amount of iron stored in the body. Normal ferritin levels vary by age and sex. The ferritin level should be ordered after determining the results of your CBC.

   Answer C is incorrect. MCHC is a measurement of the amount of hemoglobin present in RBCs. It is most useful when used in conjunction with other CBC results.

   Answer D is incorrect. The TIBC blood test measures transferrin's capacity to bind with iron and transport it throughout the body. Iron studies, which typically include total serum iron level, TIBC, transferrin, and transferrin saturation, are essential for diagnosing patients suspected of iron deficiency, overload, inflammatory conditions, or poisoning.

4. Answer C is correct. Normocytic anemia, with an MCV of 80 to 100 fL, correlates with anemia of chronic disease.

   Answer A is incorrect. A deficiency in vitamin B12 results in the development of macrocytic anemia.

   Answer B is incorrect. Chronic blood loss is associated with IDA and microcytic anemia.

   Answer D is incorrect. Inadequate globin synthesis occurs in beta thalassemia, a microcytic anemia.

5. Answer D is correct. The case presentation is that of vitamin B12 deficiency.

   Answer A is incorrect. EPO is indicated for patients with chronic kidney disease (CKD), which causes low EPO levels; signs and symptoms include fatigue, weakness, and shortness of breath.

   Answer B is incorrect. Ferrous sulfate supplementation is commonly used to treat IDA. Symptoms of iron deficiency can present as fatigue, weakness, shortness of breath, pica and pagophagia, tachycardia, altered mental status, hypothermia, and increased risk of infection.

   Answer C is incorrect. Although glossitis may occur with folic acid deficiency, paresthesias of the hands and feet in a stocking/glove distribution are characteristic of pernicious anemia; thus, evaluating the patient's response to vitamin B12 supplementation is important.

6. Answer A is correct. In young adult women, abnormal uterine bleeding is a common cause of IDA, a microcytic, hypochromic anemia.

   Answer B is incorrect. Bleeding from the GI tract is a more common cause of IDA in older adults.

   Answer C is incorrect. Inadequate intake of folic acid would result in macrocytic anemia.

   Answer D is incorrect. Low carbohydrate diets still allow adequate iron intake from meat and green leafy vegetables.

7. Answer D is correct. The term "left shift" is almost always associated with neutrophils. The left shift means that the population of cells is shifted toward most immature cells, with an increased percentage of immature neutrophils (i.e., bands, metamyelocytes, and myelocytes) being present to fight infection. Neutrophils account for between 55 percent and 70 percent of total WBCs.

   Answer A is incorrect. Eosinophils account for between 1 percent and 4 percent of total WBCs.

   Answer B is incorrect. Lymphocytes account for between 20 percent and 40 percent of total WBCs.

   Answer C is incorrect. Monocytes account for between 2 percent and 8 percent of total WBCs.

8. Answer B is correct. Inadequate absorption of vitamin B12 causes pernicious anemia. The symptoms of pernicious anemia develop slowly and subtly and may not be recognized right away.

   Answer A is incorrect. In contrast, hemolytic anemias (hereditary spherocytosis) caused by the premature destruction of RBCs, or hemolysis, occur when the bone marrow cannot produce RBCs fast enough to compensate for those being destroyed. These anemias can be acquired or congenital.

   Answers C and D are incorrect. Other inherited conditions include G6PD deficiency, sickle cell anemia, and thalassemia.

9. Answer A is correct. Folic acid deficiency in early pregnancy has been linked to the teratogenic effect of neural tube defects.

   Answer B is incorrect. Iron deficiency is the most common nutritional deficiency in pregnant women. It is associated with poor pregnancy outcomes and preterm delivery but not neural tube defects.

   Answers C and D are incorrect. Vitamin B6 and B12 are important nutrients during pregnancy and can be safely taken together. Vitamin B12 may be especially beneficial to patients who consume a plant-based-only diet.

10. Answer A is correct. The MCV of this patient with anemia reveals normocytic anemia.

    Answer C is incorrect. IDA is a microcytic anemia (low MCV).

    Answers B and D are incorrect. Folic acid and vitamin B12 deficiencies produce RBCs larger than normal cells (elevated MCV), consistent with macrocytic anemia.

11. Answer C is correct. The low MCV of this patient with anemia reveals microcytic anemia.

    Answer A is incorrect. Anemia of chronic disease is most commonly a normocytic anemia.

    Answers B and D are incorrect. Folic acid and vitamin B12 deficiencies produce larger RBCs than normal cells, which is called macrocytic anemia.

12. Answer D is correct. Iron is best absorbed when taken on an empty stomach but does have GI effects that limit tolerability (i.e., nausea and epigastric discomfort); taking iron supplementation with food can decrease absorption by two-thirds. The use of enteric-coated preparations limits the absorption in the duodenum.

    Answers A, B and C indicate the patient is already informed about the proper use of iron supplementation and needs no further education.

13. Answers A, B, C, and D are correct. Sickle cell anemia, thalassemia, and G6PD deficiency are all inherited hematologic disorders that should be considered. When neonatal jaundice is clinically identified, the underlying etiology of neonatal hyperbilirubinemia must be determined. In most neonates, unconjugated hyperbilirubinemia is the cause of clinical jaundice. However, some infants have conjugated hyperbilirubinemia, which is always pathologic and signifies an underlying medical or surgical etiology.

14. Answer B is correct. Megaloblastic anemia correlates with macrocytic anemia. Of the macrocytic anemias, vitamin B12 commonly produces a variety of neurological symptoms because of its relationship with methylmalonic acid and methionine. In contrast, folic acid deficiency does not manifest with neurological symptoms. Vitamin B12 and folic acid deficiencies are the leading causes of megaloblastic anemia.

Answer A is incorrect. An underlying hemolytic process correlates with normocytic anemia when RBCs are destroyed, which can be caused by intrinsic or genetic (i.e., sickle cell anemia, hereditary spherocytosis, G6PD deficiency, thalassemia, etc.) or extrinsic factors (acquired hemolytic anemia related to autoimmune disorders, HIV, certain cancers, etc.).

Answer C is incorrect. Iron deficiency is the most common cause of microcytic anemia.

Answer D is incorrect. Suppression of the bone marrow can cause normocytic, normochromic anemia, in which RBCs are a normal size and color. Aplastic anemia is a rare and serious condition that prevents the body from producing enough new blood cells.

15. Answer C is correct. Hemoglobin electrophoresis identifies variant and abnormal hemoglobins, including hemoglobin S (HbS) or sickle hemoglobin. It can be used to differentiate those who have SCD (in which at least one of the two abnormal inherited genes will result in the production of hemoglobin S) and sickle cell anemia (in which the individual has inherited two hemoglobin S genes, hemoglobin SS [HbSS], the most common and severe type of the disease).

Answer A is incorrect. Bone marrow aspiration is considered one of the most valuable diagnostic tools for evaluating hematologic disorders. Indications include, but are not limited to, lymphoproliferative disorders such as chronic lymphocytic leukemia (CLL), Hodgkin and non-Hodgkin lymphoma, hairy cell leukemia, myeloproliferative disorders, myelodysplastic syndrome, and multiple myeloma.

Answer B is incorrect. A DAT, a direct Coombs' test, indicates which antibodies are attached to RBCs. The test can be used to diagnose a variety of conditions, including, but not limited to, the following: autoimmune hemolytic anemia, drug-induced immune hemolysis, lupus, lymphoma, or other malignant disease.

Answer D is incorrect. Indirect Coombs' tests, also known as an antibody screen or indirect antiglobulin test (IAT), are blood tests that look for antibodies in the blood that could react with RBCs. The test can be used for various reasons, including prenatal screening for Rh compatibility, screening for blood product compatibility, etc.

16. Answer A is correct. G6PD deficiency is a genetic disorder in which the body doesn't have enough of the G6PD enzyme to help protect the RBCs from oxidative insult. The most common presentation is hemolytic anemia, leading to symptoms of jaundice, pallor, fatigue, dark urine, tachycardia, and dyspnea. G6PD is on the X chromosome and tends to affect more men than women. The hemolytic anemia is most often triggered by an oxidative stressor such as bacterial or viral infections and certain medications (sulfonamides, analgesics, antimalarials, antihelminths). Hemolytic anemia can also occur after eating fava beans, inhaling pollen from fava plants (a reaction called favism), or exposure to mothballs.

Answer B is incorrect. Pernicious anemia is a complex disease with a clear autoimmune basis. Megaloblastic anemia is caused by vitamin B12 deficiency secondary to intrinsic factor (IF) deficiency in the ileum. Anti-IF antibodies inhibit B12 from binding to IF, preventing B12/IF complex formation and intestinal absorption. It usually occurs in patients over 60 years old, and the physical examination may be notable for pallor, dry skin, jaundice, glossitis (tender, smooth, red tongue), and tachycardia.

Answer C is incorrect. SCD is an inherited hemolytic anemia with abnormal Hgb and Hgb S. Sickle cell anemia is characterized by hemolysis, vaso-occlusive crises (VOC), and organ damage.

Answer D is incorrect. Thalassemia is a chronic inherited autosomal recessive hematologic disorder caused by defects in synthesizing one or more hemoglobin alpha or beta chains. These defects cause malformation of RBCs and increase hemolysis. Depending on the type of thalassemia, symptoms vary from mild to severe.

17. Answer B is correct. The leukocytes that increase during an allergic reaction are the eosinophils. Eosinophils regulate inflammation and destroy foreign substances. The normal percentage of eosinophils on a CBC differential is 0 to 5 percent. Eosinophilia occurs when a large number of eosinophils are recruited to a particular site in the body and are most commonly triggered by allergic disorders and parasitic infections.

Answers A, C, and D are incorrect. Basophils, monocytes, and neutrophils play a role in the immune response to allergens, but to a lesser degree than eosinophils. Current research is aimed at studying the role these leukocytes have in allergic inflammation, protective immunity against parasitic infections, and regulation of innate and acquired immunity.

18. **Answer D is correct.** Parents with any combination of alpha or beta thalassemia syndromes place a child at risk for the disorder. Each child of two carrier parents is at a 25 percent risk of the disease. If a parent is positive for the trait, a prenatal diagnosis can be made with fetal blood sampling or chorionic villi sampling. Genetic counseling is an integral and necessary component of comprehensive care for patients and parents affected by all forms of thalassemia disease and traits. Genetic counseling is the process of providing information and support to individuals and families with a diagnosis and/or risk of occurrence of an inherited disorder. A licensed genetic counselor should provide services.

    Answers A, B, and C are incorrect. Review the section on Thalassemia.

19. **Answer C is correct.** Ferritin is a protein found within cells that stores iron for later use. Serum ferritin reflects the body's iron storage capacity and is the most useful test for diagnosing IDA. Serum ferritin levels are often ordered with other iron tests, such as the TIBC. Ferritin levels are low in IDA and elevated in iron overload, inflammation, or infection. A normal ferritin level is 12 to 300 ng/mL in males and 12 to 150 ng/mL in females.

    Answer A is incorrect. Hgb electrophoresis is most used to screen for SCD and thalassemia.

    Answer B is incorrect. A normal platelet count is 150,000 to 450,000 per microliter (mcL) of blood. This range is generally applicable to all adults. A low platelet count, also known as thrombocytopenia, can have many causes, including immune thrombocytopenia (ITP), bone marrow issues, heavy alcohol use, liver disease, infections, and so on. A high platelet count, or thrombocytosis, can be caused by the overproduction of thrombopoietin, interleukin-6, other cytokines, or catecholamines in inflammatory, infectious, or neoplastic conditions or secondary to stress.

    Answer D is incorrect. Vitamin B12 level is used to evaluate low levels of serum B12 secondary to pernicious anemia, low B12 vitamin intake, digestive disorders, and so on.

20. **Answer A is correct.** An increase in hemoglobin by 1 g/dL within 1 month of iron supplementation demonstrates an adequate response to treatment and confirms the diagnosis of IDA. In adults, therapy should be continued for 3 months after hemoglobin is corrected to restore ferritin stores.

    Answer B is incorrect. Decreasing the iron supplementation would be wrong as the patient needs to maximize their treatment.

    Answer C is incorrect. The partient is showing adequate response to the current treatment regimen.

    Answer D is incorrect. A patient with an HgB of 12.0 g/dL is not a candidate for IV iron therapy. Candidates for IV iron therapy would include: patients with IDA refractory to oral iron therapy and patients with chronic gastrointestinal bleeding, and inflammatory bowel disease (IBD), and heart failure.

21. **Answer D is correct.** Pernicious anemia is an autoimmune disorder caused by the destruction of parietal cells in the gastric fundus, resulting in the cessation of IF production. The intrinsic factor is important for absorbing vitamin B12 from the small intestine. Since pernicious anemia is irreversible, lifetime supplementation of B12 (injections, nasal, or high-dose oral route) is necessary.

    Answers A, B, and C are incorrect. One to 3 months, 3 to 6 months, and 6 to 12 months are short-term treatment regimens that may be appropriate for vitamin B12 deficiency resulting from inadequate dietary intake and by adding foods containing B12.

22. **Answer B is correct.** A folate deficiency typically causes macrocytosis without neurological manifestations. The most common causes are inadequate dietary intake, malnutrition, and excessive alcohol intake. Folate food sources include green leafy vegetables, grains, beans, and liver. The classic presentation is an older patient and/or older male with alcoholic use disorder with signs and symptoms of anemia such as weakness, fatigue, difficulty concentrating, irritability, headache, palpitations, or shortness of breath.

    Answer A is incorrect. Chronic disease anemia presents as normocytic (MCV = 80 to 96 fL) and normochromic anemia with normal red cell distribution width (RDW).

    Answer C is incorrect. IDA presents as a microcytic anemia (MCV < 80) and decreased ferritin level.

    Answer D is incorrect. While vitamin B12 deficiency anemia is a macrocytic anemia (MCV >

100 fL), patients usually present with a smooth, sore, beefy red tongue and significant neurological symptoms, such as paresthesia in hands and feet, peripheral neuropathy, hyporeflexia, extremity weakness, incoordination, and difficulty with gait.

23. Answer B is correct. Vitamin B12 is naturally found in animal products, including fish, meat, poultry, eggs, milk, and milk products.

    Answers A, C, and D are incorrect. Vitamin B12 is generally absent in plant-based foods, such as broccoli, legumes, and lettuce. However, fortified breakfast cereals are an option for strict vegetarians.

24. Answer B is correct. ITP is a syndrome characterized by a decrease in platelets, which causes a reduced ability for primary clotting and leads to purpura and petechiae. The cause is unknown, but most cases are acute in children and tend to follow a viral illness. The condition is diagnosed with a CBC; isolated thrombocytopenia is the hallmark finding.

    Answer A is incorrect. Aplastic anemia has similar symptoms, including a low platelet count; however, the patient will also have a decrease in hemoglobin, hematocrit, and WBCs secondary to bone marrow failure.

    Answer C is incorrect. SCD lab work typically shows low hemoglobin levels, reduced RBC count, increased WBC count, elevated reticulocytes, and sickle-shaped cells. Platelets are often increased.

    Answer D is incorrect. Reactive thrombocytosis is an abnormally high platelet count in the absence of chronic myeloproliferative disease secondary to an infection, inflammation, and hemorrhage.

25. Answer B is correct. Aplastic anemia is a serious blood disorder caused by bone marrow failure characterized by pancytopenia and marrow hypoplasia. Therefore, the first tests to order when evaluating a patient for suspected aplastic anemia include a CBC with differential reticulocyte count, peripheral blood smear, and a bone marrow biopsy with cytogenic evaluation. A bone marrow biopsy typically demonstrates hypocellular marrow without abnormal cells.

    Answers A, C, and D are incorrect. An ANA screen, folate level, and Hgb electrophoresis will not provide the necessary information to assist in this diagnosis.

Resources

Ankara, A., & Kumar, A. (2022, October 22). Vitamin B12 deficiency. In: *StatPearls* [Internet]. StatPearls Publishing. https://www.ncbi.nlm.nih.gov/books/NBK441923/

Baird, D. C., Batten, S. H., Carl, W., & Sparks, S. K. (2022). Alpha- and beta-thalassemia: Rapid evidence review. *American Family Physician. 105*(3), 272–280. https://www.aafp.org/pubs/afp/issues/2022/0300/p272.html

Bajwa, H., & Basit, H. (2023, August 8). Thalassemia. In: *StatPearls* [Internet]. StatPearls Publishing. https://www.ncbi.nlm.nih.gov/books/NBK545151/

Cash, J. C. (2024). *Family practice guidelines* (6th ed.). Springer Publishing.

Centers for Disease Control. (1992). Recommendations for the use of folic acid to reduce the number of cases of spina bifida and other neural tube defects. *MMWR, 41*(RR-14). https://www.cdc.gov/mmwr/preview/mmwrhtml/00019479.htm

Fischbach, F. T., Fischbach, M., & Stout, K. (2021). *Fischbach's manual of laboratory and diagnostic tests with access* (11th ed.). Lippincott Williams & Wilkins.

Onimoe, G., & Rotz, S. (2020). Sickle cell disease: A primary care update. *Cleveland Clinic Journal of Medicine, 87* (1): 19–27. https://doi.org/10.3949/ccjm.87a.18051. https://www.ccjm.org/content/ccjom/87/1/19.full.pdf

Richardson, S. R., & O'Malley, G. F. (2022, September 26). Glucose-6-phosphate dehydrogenase deficiency. In: *StatPearls* [Internet]. StatPearls Publishing. https://www.ncbi.nlm.nih.gov/books/NBK470315/

Turner, J., Parsi, M., & Badireddy, M. Anemia. (2023, August 8). In: *StatPearls* [Internet]. StatPearls Publishing. https://www.ncbi.nlm.nih.gov/books/NBK499994/

CHAPTER 14

Renal and Genitourinary Urinary System

Susan M. DeNisco, DNP, APRN, FNP-BC, FAANP

Review of Normal Kidneys Findings

- The kidneys are found in the retroperitoneal space.
- The right kidney is slightly displaced by the liver and is lower than the left.
- Nephrons, containing the glomeruli, are the kidney's functional units.
- The kidneys produce approximately 1,500 mL of urine daily.

Renal Function

- The kidneys are involved in the regulation of fluids and electrolytes.
- The antidiuretic hormone (ADH) and aldosterone produced by the kidneys help promote water reabsorption in the body and excrete waste products.
- Waste products include creatinine, urea, and uric acid.
- Kidneys are involved in the production of red blood cells through the production of erythropoietin, which stimulates the production of bone marrow.
- Kidneys secrete the following hormones: renin and bradykinin (blood pressure [BP]), prostaglandins (renal perfusion), calcitriol, and vitamin D3 production (bone).

Laboratory Findings

- Serum creatinine
  - Male: 0.7 to 1.3 mg/dL
  - Female: 0.6 to 1.1 mg/dL
- Normal: eGFR > 90 ml/min
- Renal failure: eGFR (glomerular filtration rate) < 15 ml/min [stage V kidney disease]
- Oliguria: urine output < 400 ml daily in adults
- Blood urea nitrogen (BUN) not as sensitive as creatinine and eGFR
  - High BUN can be seen in acute renal failure, high protein diet, hemolysis, heart failure, and medications.

Urinary Tract Infections

Acute Cystitis

- A urinary tract infection (UTI) can also be called acute cystitis.
- Acute cystitis is a urinary bladder inflammation most often caused by fecal flora.
- Bacteria usually ascend via the urethra into the bladder.
- The most common pathogen responsible for outpatient UTIs is **Escherichia coli.**
- Other pathogens to consider are Staphylococcus, Proteus, Klebsiella, Pseudomonas, Enterobacter, and Enterococci.

- Most common signs and symptoms:
  - Dysuria
  - Frequency, urgency
  - Suprapubic tenderness
  - Hematuria

Acute Pyelonephritis

- When bacteria migrate to the kidneys, pyelonephritis can ensue.
- Pyelonephritis results when one or both upper urinary tracts are involved.
- Signs and symptoms include those involved in acute cystitis:
  - Fever, chills
  - One-sided flank or groin pain
  - Nausea and vomiting
- Causes of pyelonephritis include nephrolithiasis/urolithiasis, pregnancy, neurogenic bladder, and vesicoureteral reflux.

> **Clinical Pearl**
> White blood cell (WBC) casts, proteinuria, and hematuria are associated with pyelonephritis.

Risk Factors for Urinary Tract Infection

- UTIs can be uncomplicated, complicated, or recurrent.
- Female gender; pregnancy
- Use of spermicide in female patients
- History of UTI or recurrent infections
- Recurrent UTIs: three or more in 1 year or three infections in 6 months
- Diabetes mellitus or immunocompromised
- Failure to void after intercourse or frequent intercourse
- Constipation in children
- Other risks: low fluid intake, poor hygiene, infected renal calculi, and instrumentation

Diagnosis

- Acute cystitis made primarily by history (dysuria and frequency and suprapubic tenderness on physical exam)
- Urinalysis (microscopic or dipstick):
  - Positive nitrites. Sensitivity 80 to 90 percent; specificity 94 to 98 percent.
  - Leukocyte positive > 10/mcL
  - Hematuria may be present.
- Urine culture is often unnecessary in acute cystitis.
- Obtain a urine culture to see if pyelonephritis is suspected, if complicating factors are present, and for recurrent UTI.
- Urine Culture and Sensitivity:
  - positive for infection with bacteria ≥ 100,000 CFU/ml with pyuria
  - Sensitivity > 90 percent
  - Urine culture with multiple bacteria: a contaminated sample
- Imaging studies should be obtained in infants or children with an initial febrile UTI or women with recurrent UTIs.
- No imaging studies are needed for patients with uncomplicated UTIs.

> **Clinical Pearl**
> Large numbers of squamous epithelial cells in the urine sample can indicate a contaminated sample.

Differential Diagnosis

- Vaginitis
- Urethritis
- Structural urethral abnormalities
- Painful bladder syndrome
- Pelvic inflammatory disease
- Nephrolithiasis/urolithiasis
- Prostatitis

Treatment

Resolution of symptoms should occur approximately 48 hours after initiation of therapy. A urinary analgesic (Pyridium) can be given, in addition to the antibiotic regimen, to help alleviate symptoms.

Uncomplicated UTI

First line:
- 3-day course of Bactrim (trimethoprim/sulfa)
- Sulfa allergy: 5- to 7-day course of Macrobid (nitrofurantoin)
- Phenazopyridine (Pyridium) BID x 2 days
  - Orange color to urine
  - Stain contact lenses
  - Avoid in patients with liver or renal disease

Second line:
- 3-day course of quinolone (contraindicated in pregnancy)
- 7-day course of amoxicillin or first-generation cephalosporin

Complicated UTI

- Initial empiric treatment should be initiated and modified per urine culture and sensitivity results.
- Treat for 7 days or longer:
  - Males
  - Diabetics
  - Pregnant women
  - Children or older people
  - Immunocompromised
  - Recurrent UTIs
  - Anatomic abnormalities of kidneys or ureters

Follow-Up

- No test of cure is necessary for uncomplicated UTI.
- Urine culture and sensitivity should be obtained for persistent symptoms.
- Rule out bacterial prostatitis in men.
- Refer to urologist if persistent bacteriuria or recurrent UTI.
- May consider antibiotic prophylaxis for recurrent UTI (>3/year).
- Consider postcoital UTI prophylaxis following intercourse.
- In pregnancy, refer to an obstetrician if pyelonephritis is suspected or develops.

Prevention

- Encourage patients to remain well hydrated. The recommended daily allowance (RDA) for fluids in healthy adults is 30 mL/kg/day.
- Instruct female patients on proper hygiene.
- Avoid constipation.
- Use of spermicide/diaphragm increases the risk of UTI.
- Encourage micturition after intercourse.
- No sufficient evidence to promote the use of cranberry products.
- Educate patients that Pyridium may cause an orange-red discoloration of bodily fluids (urine, sweat, tears).

Clinical Pearl

Indications for hospitalization in patients with acute pyelonephritis include inability to maintain oral hydration, persistently high fever > 101°F, toxic appearance, immunocompromised, concern for sepsis, or issues with medication adherence.

Test Tip

Be able to interpret urinalysis results and distinguish between acute cystitis and acute pyelonephritis.

Nephrolithiasis/Urolithiasis

- Urinary lithiasis (kidney stones) occurs when protein, crystals, or other substances accumulate and obstruct the urinary flow.
- Stones can be in the kidney, bladder, ureters, or urethra.
- The most common types of kidney stones:
  - Calcium oxalate (70 to 80 percent)
  - Struvite (magnesium, ammonium, or phosphate) (15 percent)
  - Uric acid (7 percent)
  - Cysteine (<1 percent).
- The most common manifestation of kidney stones is renal colic.
- Presents as sudden onset of moderate to severe pain at the costovertebral angle junction or flank area, often radiating to the groin area.
- Dysuria, frequency, urgency, pink-tinged urine, nausea, and vomiting can also be present. Fever and chills may indicate infection.
- Complications of untreated nephrolithiasis can lead to kidney damage and/or renal failure.

Incidence and Risk Factors

- Kidney stones are more prevalent in Caucasians.
- Male: 15 percent; female: 6 percent
- Typically, in patients younger than 50 years old.
- Recurrence rate is 30 to 50 percent over 5 years.
- Family history of nephrolithiasis increases risk.

Evaluation

- Often made with a good history and focused physical examination.
- Renal ultrasonography if pregnant or suspect hydronephrosis.
- Noncontrast spiral CT scan (sensitivity 94 to 97 percent).
- Complete blood count (CBC) to evaluate for infection.
- Metabolic panel to assess levels of calcium, uric acid levels, renal function, and hydration status.
- Urinalysis:

- microscopic and/or gross hematuria
- pH > 7 suspect struvite
- pH < 5 suspect uric acid
- Consider kidney, ureter, and bladder [KUB] X-ray to evaluate radiopaque stones
- Consider 24-hour urine collection which will be obtained to assess for:
  - calcium citrate,
  - oxalate, or
  - other sedimentation.

Differential Diagnosis
- Hydronephrosis
- Glomerular nephritis
- UTI
- Pyelonephritis
- Ectopic pregnancy
- Dysmenorrhea
- Acute intestinal obstruction
- Acute mesenteric ischemia
- Herpes zoster

Treatment
- Initial treatment usually focuses on pain management:
  - Both opioids and nonsteroidal anti-inflammatory drugs (NSAIDs) may be appropriate.
- Promote stone passage by prescribing:
  - Terazosin (alpha blocker)
  - Nifedipine (calcium channel blocker)
  - Tamsulosin (alpha blocker)
- Urine straining to identify the stone type.
- Urology referral for urosepsis, acute renal failure, anuria, unremitting pain, nausea, or vomiting.
- Stone removal via lithotripsy, ureteroscopy, and percutaneous nephrolithotomy.
- Calcium stones: a thiazide diuretic or potassium citrate may be ordered.
- Uric acid stones: Allopurinol may be prescribed to decrease uric acid levels.
- Cystine stones: Increase fluid intake and urinary alkalinization.

Follow-Up and Prevention
- Increase fluid intake up to 2 to 3 L/daily
- Calcium oxalate stone formation can be minimized by decreasing the intake of oxalate-rich foods, such as rhubarb, beets, okra, nuts, spinach, and chocolate.
- Increase intake of calcium-rich foods but caution patients about calcium supplements.
- A low-sodium and low-animal-protein diet has been shown to decrease the incidence of nephrolithiasis.
- Maintain optimal body weight to reduce risk.
- Referral to a urologist for stones larger than 10 mm and stones larger than 5 mm in patients who failed to pass the stone within 4 weeks of starting an alpha blocker

Clinical Pearl
The urinalysis will show hematuria in most patients.

Kidney Disease
Classification
- Renal Insufficiency:
  - Defined as a GFR of 25 to 30 mL/minute or a reduction in renal function of 25 percent.
  - There is a mild elevation of urea and serum creatinine.
- Acute Kidney Injury (AKI):
  - Diagnosed with sudden onset of increased BUN, serum creatinine, and an elevation of other kidney waste products.
  - Progression to complications such as fluid overload, hyperkalemia, metabolic acidosis, hypocalcemia, hyperphosphatemia, and uremia.
- Chronic Kidney Disease:
  - End-stage kidney disease
  - Significant loss of kidney function (< 10 percent functioning).
- Uremia:
  - Sequala of renal failure manifested by elevations of blood urea and serum creatinine levels, as well as symptoms of fatigue, anorexia, nausea, vomiting, pruritus, and neurological changes.
- Azotemia:
  - Elevations in blood urea levels with/without elevated serum creatinine levels.

Acute Kidney Injury
- Characterized by a sudden decline in renal function.
- Decreased GFR
- Elevated serum creatinine and blood nitrogen levels.
- Associated with a 50 to 80 percent mortality rate and is a result of hypovolemia, decreased kidney perfusion, and/or toxic/inflammation of renal cells, leading to decreased kidney function.

- Risk factors:
  - Hypertension, heart failure, diabetes mellitus, sepsis, and hypovolemia
  - Use of nephrotoxic medication, contrast materials, and hospitalization
  - Medications that limit GFR: angiotensin-converting enzyme inhibitors (ACE-I), angiotensin II receptor blockers (ARB), nonsteroidal anti-inflammatory drug (NSAID), protease inhibitors, and aminoglycosides

Signs/Symptoms of AKI

- Sudden onset of edema, weight gain, oliguria, or anuria
- Anorexia, apathy, fatigue, arrhythmia, nausea and vomiting, change in mental status, seizures
- Dyspnea on exertion (DOE), jugular venous distension (JVD), hypertension +/or hypotension
- Bilateral edema and cool extremities

Treatment Goals

- Identify at-risk patients in the primary care setting, intervene quickly, and refer patients to specialists and/or the ED.
- Minimize progression to chronic kidney disease (CKD) and maintain eGFR > 60.
- Maintain HbA1C less than 7 percent.
- Maintain normotensive BP.

Chronic Kidney Disease

CKD is defined as:

- Persistent and progressive reduction in glomerular filtration rate (GFR) < 60 ml/min/1.73m^2; and/or
- Albuminuria > 30 mg of urinary albumin per gram of urinary creatinine

The five stages of chronic kidney diseases are described in **Table 14-1**.

Incidence

- Most common in patients older than 65.
- More common in non-Hispanic Black adults.
- Prevalence is greatest in patients with poorly controlled diabetes and hypertension.

Other Predisposing Risk Factors

- Cardiovascular (CV) disease
- Chronic use of NSAIDs
- Autoimmune disorders
- Polycystic kidney disease
- Urinary tract obstruction (i.e., benign prostatic hyperplasia [BPH] or kidney stones)
- Recurrent UTIs
- Smoking and exposure to other toxins
- Family history of kidney disease

Evaluation

- A thorough history is conducted, including a review of medications and physical examination.
- The patient may be asymptomatic in stages I and II.
- Patients may present with vague symptoms of fatigue, anorexia, nausea, and pruritus.
- Physical exam findings may include the following:
  - Signs of volume overload (i.e., weight gain, edema, and shortness of breath)
  - Signs of volume depletion (i.e., fatigue, postural dizziness, tachycardia, and decreased skin turgor)
  - Rashes and skin lesions
  - Abnormal bruit in renal artery stenosis
  - Palpable enlarged kidneys in polycystic kidney disease
  - Peripheral neuropathy

Initial Laboratory Testing

- Basic metabolic panel for increased serum urea and creatinine levels
- Urinalysis for evaluation of proteinuria or albuminuria and the presence of WBCs and red blood cells (RBCs)
- Albumin-specific urine dipstick to assess for albumin-to-creatinine ratio (ACR)
- CBC to assess anemia and/or infection
- May also evaluate the patient for hypocalcemia, elevated parathyroid hormone (PTH)
- Other common lab findings may include hyperkalemia, hyperphosphatemia, and metabolic acidosis, depending on the severity and stage

Imaging Studies

- Renal ultrasound to rule out obstructions, cysts, or masses
- Vascular duplex ultrasound to assess for renal artery stenosis

Treatment

The purpose of treatment is to preserve kidney function and prevent future deterioration:

- Manage hypertension and control diabetes
- Prevent CV complications by lowering cholesterol and BP
- Correct fluid/electrolyte abnormalities

Table 14-1 Stages of Chronic Kidney Diseases

Stage	GFR*	Description	Treatment
1	> 90	Normal kidney function but urine findings or structural abnormalities or genetic trait point to kidney disease	Observation, control of BP. Annual test for microalbuminuria.
2	60–89	Mildly reduced kidney function, and other findings (as for stage 1) point to kidney disease	Observation and control of BP and risk factors. Medication that may help slow progression of kidney disease (i.e., ACE inhibitors, ARBs, SGLT2 inhibitors, or non-steroid mineralocorticoid receptor blockers).
3A 3B	45–59 30–44	Moderately reduced kidney function	Observation, control of BP and risk factors. Nutritional and dietary counseling to help support kidney function.
4	15–29	Severely reduced kidney function	Planning for end-stage renal failure. Referral to nephrologist.
5	< 15 or on dialysis	Very severe, or end-stage kidney failure (sometimes call "established renal failure")	Treatment choices. Evaluate for renal transplant.

*All GFR values are normalized to an average surface area (size) of 1.73m^2
Data from The National Kidney Foundation. (2022). *Estimated glomerular filtration rate (eGFR)*. Retrieved from https://www.kidney.org/atoz/content/gfr#download-nkf-fact-sheet-egfr

- Treat/prevent infections
- Ensure adequate nutrition
- Drug regimen review and discontinuation of nephrotoxic medications
- Smoking cessation to prevent worsening of kidney function
- Referral to nephrology for patients with Stage III CKD and comorbid systemic autoimmune disorders, pregnancy, and multiple myeloma

Follow-Up and Prevention

- Educate patient regarding the importance of controlling their hypertension and diabetes.
- Maintain dietary changes (low sodium, potassium, and protein as prescribed).
- Avoid nephrotoxic drugs such as NSAIDs and contrast imaging drugs.
- Maintain proper hydration.
- Promptly report any urgent symptoms of decreased urination, hematuria, edema, nausea, vomiting, fatigue, chest pain, and changes in mental status, as these can indicate worsening kidney function.

Clinical Pearl

Patients with preexisting kidney disease and/or diabetes are at increased risk of kidney damage from contrast media; a rise in creatinine will be seen within 24 to 48 hours after administration.

Urinary Incontinence

Urinary incontinence (UI) is defined as a lack of bladder control resulting in involuntary urine leakage. It can majorly impact quality of life, leading to depression, anxiety, and social isolation. **Table 14-2** classifies the types of urinary incontinence.

Epidemiology

- The prevalence of UI increases with advanced age and in long-term care residents.
- Stress incontinence is mostly seen in younger females; the highest incidence is seen between the ages of 45 and 49, while urgency incontinence is more prevalent in older females.
- Male patients with prostate problems are also common.

Risk Factors for UI

- Obesity
- Parity, including mode of delivery: higher rates in vaginal delivery
- Age
- Ethnicity/race—more prevalent in Caucasians than African Americans

Table 14-2 Types of Urinary Incontinence

Type	Definition	Patient Scenario
Urge incontinence	Involuntary urine leakage with strong symptoms of urgency "overactive bladder."	45-year-old female with history of cystitis reports sudden strong need to urinate when there is no bathroom facility nearby
Stress incontinence	Involuntary urine loss with the increase of intra-abdominal pressure occurring with coughing, sneezing, and laughing in the absence of bladder contraction.	50-year-old female who had three vaginal deliveries reports loss of urine when coughing and sneezing
Overflow incontinence	Urine leakage occurs with an overdistended bladder, often seen with incomplete emptying of the bladder. It is caused by detrusor underactivity of bladder outlet obstruction.	40-year-old female with schizoaffective disorder who has been taking an antipsychotic agent for her mood over the past year
Mixed incontinence	Stress and urge incontinence	65-year-old postmenopausal female who is overweight urgently needs to use the bathroom, especially when taking ballroom dance classes
Functional incontinence	Involves a fully functional urinary system but occurs with the inability to toilet oneself in a timely manner.	85-year-old male patient who uses a wheelchair, has dementia, and lives in an extended care facility
Transient Incontinence	Transient incontinence is urinary leaking that spontaneously reverses after the underlying cause is resolved.	60-year-old female who had several episodes of urinary leakage during a recent UTI who was treated with an antibiotic and symptoms resolved

- Tobacco use and caffeine intake
- Vaginal atrophy
- Medical history of hypertension, diabetes, benign prostatic hyperplasia (BPH), stroke, depression, hormone replacement therapy, neurologic disorders, cognitive impairment, cancer, genitourinary radiation, or surgery, such as hysterectomy
- Medications (reversible) (i.e., antihypertensive agents, analgesics, psychotropics, alcohol, and antihistamines)

Evaluation

- Initial evaluation will attempt to distinguish the type of UI and identify potential reversible causes.
- Diagnosed with a thorough history and physical examination, including a pelvic exam to rule out vaginal atrophy.
- A urinalysis is obtained to rule out infection.
- Kidney function testing is not routinely done except in cases of urinary retention to rule out hydronephrosis.
- Further testing may be undertaken, such as a bladder stress test, postvoid residual test, urodynamic testing, and urethral mobility evaluation.
- Refer to urology in cases of hematuria, abdominal/pelvic pain associated with incontinence, abnormal physical exams, such as prolapsed bladder, and incontinence associated with new neurologic symptomatology.

Treatment

- Anticholinergic medications, such as oxybutynin (Ditropan, Oxytrol), tolterodine (Detrol), darifenacin (Enablex), solifenacin (Vesicare), trospium (Sanctura), fesoterodine (Toviaz), are utilized.
- Serotonin and norepinephrine reuptake inhibitors (SNRIs) like Cymbalta may be effective for stress incontinence.
- Use of beta-3 adrenergic agonists like mirabegron (Myrbetriq) or vibegron (Gemtesa) for overactive bladder
- Exercises, such as pelvic floor muscle training (Kegel) with or without biofeedback, and bladder training
- Medical devices such as electric or magnetic electrostimulation
- Treatment of underlying reversible causes, such as infection, or obstructions, such as those caused by prostate enlargement or pelvic organ prolapse

Follow-Up and Prevention

- Discuss weight loss if the patient has obesity.
- Discuss the importance of glycemic control in patients with diabetes.
- Keep a bladder diary.
- Avoid intake of potential triggers, such as caffeine, alcohol, and spicy or acidic foods, that can irritate the bladder.
- Decrease fluid intake before bed.
- Patient to seek medical care if symptoms, such as dysuria, hematuria, pelvic/abdominal pain, fever, and chills, develop.

Clinical Pearl

First-line treatment for incontinence should be aimed at lifestyle modifications such as weight reduction, weight loss, dietary changes, fluid restriction, caffeine reduction, and smoking cessation.

Test Tip

Anticholinergic agents can cause urinary retention; severe, decreased gastric motility; and uncontrolled narrow-angle glaucoma.

Review Questions

1. The most common bacteria involved in acute uncomplicated urinary tract infection (UTI) is:
   A. *Klebsiella*.
   B. *Escherichia coli*.
   C. *Clostridium difficile*.
   D. *Staphylococcus*.

2. A young female visits your clinic and complains of burning with urination. She states that she had these same symptoms about six months ago and was diagnosed with a UTI. She reports that a 3-day course of antibiotics was effective. Upon further questioning, it is uncovered that she has just become sexually active. Patient education should include the following (select all that apply):
   A. Voiding after intercourse may prevent recurrent UTIs.
   B. Using a spermicide may increase the risk of UTI.
   C. Drinking 6 ounces of cranberry juice daily may prevent future UTIs.
   D. Using prophylactic antibiotics if she develops recurrent UTIs.

3. The most common stone composition of nephrolithiasis is:
   A. struvite (magnesium, ammonium, and phosphate).
   B. calcium oxalate.
   C. cysteine.
   D. uric acid.

4. A 25-year-old female comes to the office complaining of right-sided abdominal pain that has radiated to the groin area for the last 2 days. She has felt nauseated and has had a decreased appetite. The differential diagnosis will include the following (select all that apply):
   A. Ectopic pregnancy
   B. Pyelonephritis
   C. Constipation
   D. Acute intestinal obstruction

5. In educating a female patient with nephrolithiasis, the family nurse practitioner (FNP) reviews with the patient the following (select all that apply):
   A. Adequate hydration may decrease her risk of reoccurrence.
   B. Decreasing the intake of oxalate-rich foods may prevent reoccurrence.
   C. Advising her to increase her intake of cranberry juice or take cranberry supplements.
   D. Explaining that she has a 50 percent increased risk of reoccurrence over the next 5 years.

6. The FNP diagnoses a UTI in a 33-year-old female who provides a history of dysuria, frequency × 48 hours, and a urine dipstick that was positive for nitrites. She admits to having had two UTIs in the last 6 months. The FNP initiates antibiotic therapy with ciprofloxacin. The patient calls the FNP two days later to state that she has developed a fever. What is the next step?
   A. Change her antibiotic.
   B. Have her return and obtain a urinalysis, urine culture, and sensitivity.
   C. Refer to urology.
   D. Tell her to increase hydration and take Tylenol (acetaminophen) for fever.

7. While reviewing the laboratory results of a 32-year-old man who came to the office for a complete physical exam 2 days earlier, it is noted that his blood urea nitrogen (BUN) and creatinine levels are as follows: 19 mg/dL (normal 7 to 18 mg/dL) and 1.4 mg/dL (normal 0.6 to 1.2 mg/dL). Previous results from 6 months prior were within normal limits. What's the next step?
   A. Tell the patient to increase his consumption of fluids.
   B. Check a urinalysis.
   C. Repeat the bloodwork and assess medication intake.
   D. Tell the patient, "Not to worry." These elevations are minimal, and you will recheck them in 6 months at the next follow-up visit.

8. A 44-year-old African American female comes to the office to discuss symptoms of stress incontinence that she has been having for the last 3 months. The FNP tells her that:
   A. her symptoms may resolve if she loses some weight.
   B. her race is associated with a higher prevalence of incontinence.
   C. stress incontinence is usually seen in older females, while urge incontinence is more prevalent in younger-aged females.
   D. fluid intake has no impact on her symptoms.

9. A 26-year-old female is being treated for cystitis. She informs the FNP that this is the third reoccurrence in almost a year. The FNP proceeds to ask her about her fluid intake. Which of the following would the FNP encourage her to stop drinking?
   A. Fruit juice
   B. Coffee
   C. Water
   D. Lemonade

10. A 52-year-old male patient presents to the office after a brief pyelonephritis hospitalization. He is currently on the second day of a 7-day course of antibiotics. Patient education includes which of the following?
    A. If you develop dysuria, increase oral fluids for 2 days.
    B. Continue your antibiotic until you are asymptomatic.
    C. Return to the office in 7 to 10 days for a repeat urinalysis, a urine culture, and sensitivity.
    D. If you develop urinary frequency, decrease PO fluid intake.

11. Stage V chronic kidney disease (CKD) is diagnosed when the estimated glomerular filtration rate (eGFR) is below which of the following?
    A. 15 ml/min
    B. 20 ml/min
    C. 25 ml/min
    D. 30 ml/min

12. What is the leading cause of CKD?
    A. Hypotension
    B. Anemia
    C. Prostate cancer
    D. Diabetes mellitus

13. Kidney disease is associated with which of the most dangerous electrolyte imbalances?
    A. Hypermagnesemia
    B. Hyponatremia
    C. Hyperkalemia
    D. Hypercalcemia

14. A 66-year-old man with a medical history that includes CKD comes to the clinic. When discussing nutrition, which of the following diets should he eat?
    A. High carbohydrate, high protein diet
    B. High calcium, high potassium, low protein diet
    C. Low protein, low sodium, low potassium diet
    D. Low protein, high potassium

15. The FNP is seeing a 32-year-old male who states, "I think I'm having kidney stones again." The FNP expects the patient to describe his pain as:
    A. dull and aching pain in the costovertebral area.
    B. diffused abdominal aching and cramp-like pain.
    C. sharp pain radiating to the spine.
    D. excruciating pain that comes and goes and radiates to the groin.

16. A 44-year-old male with a history of kidney stones is being seen in the primary care clinic. In reviewing his chart, it is noted that the patient's kidney stones are made up of uric acid crystals. He should be told to avoid which of the following (select all that apply)?
    A. Tuna fish
    B. Liver
    C. Apples
    D. Carrots

17. A 59-year-old man comes to the office for a hypertension follow-up. His blood pressure (BP) today is 128/82. While reviewing his recent laboratory value, it is noted that his creatinine is 1.9 mg/dL. Which of his following medications should be discontinued at this time?
    A. Beta blockers
    B. Calcium-channel blockers
    C. Direct-acting vasodilators
    D. Angiotensin-converting enzyme (ACE) inhibitors

18. Which of the following are normal kidney changes resulting from aging (select all that apply)?
    A. Decreased bladder capacity
    B. Nocturnal polyuria
    C. Kidney enlargement
    D. Decreased glomerular filtration rate

19. A 28-year-old female is diagnosed with an uncomplicated UTI. She is currently on an oral contraceptive, has not missed any of her pills, and her last menstrual period (LMP) was 2 weeks ago. She is allergic to sulfa drugs that caused hives in the past. Which first-line antibiotic treatment should the NP prescribe?
    A. Amoxicillin
    B. TMP-SMX
    C. Nitrofurantoin
    D. Ciprofloxacin

20. A 74-year-old female complains of urinary incontinence. She feels urgency, but osteoarthritis in her hip prevents her from making it to the bathroom in time. For the past 12 years, she has been experiencing urinary leakage when she coughs or sneezes. She has a history of hypertension. Which of the following is the first best-choice therapy for this patient?
    A. A trial of oxybutynin (Ditropan)
    B. Referral to a urologist for a cystoscopy
    C. Kegel exercises and timed voiding
    D. Topical vaginal estrogen

21. Which type of incontinence is caused by weak bladder muscles?
    A. Overflow incontinence
    B. Urge incontinence
    C. Stress incontinence
    D. Transient incontinence

22. An older adult patient is diagnosed with an acute UTI. Which drug class may put the patient at risk for an Achilles tendon rupture?
    A. Sulfonamides
    B. Quinolones
    C. Cephalosporins
    D. Penicillin

23. Which of the following is considered the best overall measure of kidney function and is used to stage CKD?
    A. Creatinine clearance
    B. Glomerular filtration rate (GFR)
    C. BUN
    D. Serum Creatinine

24. A patient presents with acute renal colic pain, hematuria, nausea and vomiting. Based on these presenting symptoms, which of the following diagnostic tests should the NP order to confirm the suspected diagnosis?
    A. Abdominal X-ray
    B. Ultrasound of the kidneys and bladder
    C. Intravenous pyelography
    D. CT of the abdomen and pelvis without contrast

25. A 35-year-old is being evaluated for microscopic hematuria. Which of the following diagnoses can easily be ruled out?
    A. Kidney stones
    B. Bladder cancer
    C. Acute pyelonephritis
    D. Renal artery stenosis

Answers and Rationales

1. Answer B is correct. The most common bacteria involved in UTIs is the gut bacteria *Escherichia coli*. It accounts for 85 percent of all infections.

    Answers A, C, and D are incorrect. For uncomplicated UTIs, other causative agents are (in order of prevalence): Answer A: *Klebsiella pneumoniae*, Answer D: *Staphylococcus saprophyticus*, *Enterococcus faecalis*, group B Streptococcus (GBS), *Proteus mirabilis*, *Pseudomonas aeruginosa*, *Staphylococcus aureus*, and *Candida* spp. Answer C: *Clostridioides difficile*, formerly known as *Clostridium difficile* and often called C. difficile or C. diff., is a germ (bacterium) that causes diarrhea and colitis.

2. Answers A, B, and D are correct. Recommended treatments for recurrent UTIs include maximizing personal hygiene factors, avoiding spermicides, wiping correctly, increasing fluid intake and hydration, using vaginal estrogens if appropriate, and use of postcoital antibiotic prophylaxis is appropriate for women with frequent episodes of cystitis that are associated with sexual activity.

Answer C is incorrect. There is no current evidence supporting the use of cranberry products.

3. Answer B is correct. Calcium oxalate makes up about 70 to 80 percent of kidney stones.

   Answers A, C, and D are incorrect. Struvite accounts for 15 percent of kidney stones, uric acid for 7 percent, and cysteine for only 1 percent.

4. Answers A, B, and D are correct. In the case presentation, the following conditions need to be ruled out: hydronephrosis, glomerular nephritis, UTI/pyelonephritis, dysmenorrhea, acute intestinal obstruction, acute mesenteric ischemia, herpes zoster, and ectopic pregnancy in females.

   Answer C is incorrect. Common signs of constipation are difficult and painful bowel movements, bowel movements fewer than three times a week, and bloated or uncomfortable feeling in the lower abdomen.

5. Correct Answers A, B, and D. Recommend increasing fluid intake to 2 to 3 L/day. Calcium oxalate stone formation can be minimized by decreasing the intake of oxalate-rich foods, such as rhubarb, beets, okra, nuts, spinach, and chocolate. A low-sodium and low-animal-protein diet has been shown to decrease the incidence of nephrolithiasis.

   Answer C is incorrect. The evidence for recommending cranberry juice/supplement is inconclusive. Increased water intake is advised to minimize stone formation.

6. Answer C is correct. The patient can rapidly deteriorate during this time. It is best to have her seen by a urologist immediately.

   Answer A is incorrect. The patient has already been on antibiotics several times during the past 6 months and may have developed antibiotic resistance.

   Answer B is incorrect. The results of a urine culture and sensitivity will take approximately 48 hours to return.

   Answer D is incorrect. While Tylenol may reduce her fever, she needs to be evaluated for pyelonephritis.

7. Answer C is correct. Repeat the test to ensure that a laboratory error did not occur. Intake of NSAIDs needs to be ruled out in the acute onset of kidney disease.

   Answer A is incorrect. Increasing water intake can help prevent kidney stones and may slow the progression of CKD.

   Answer B is incorrect. While a urinalysis can help detect kidney disease by measuring the amount of albumin in the urine, in this case, rechecking the bloodwork would be the first step.

   Answer D is incorrect. If an unexpected result and stable clinical context occur, consider repeating the creatinine level within 48 to 72 hours to determine whether any creatinine changes are truly dynamic acute kidney injury (AKI) or relatively stable/false positive.

8. Answer A is correct. Stress incontinence is more prevalent in people with obesity.

   Answer B is incorrect. White females have a higher incidence of stress incontinence than African Americans.

   Answer C is incorrect. Stress incontinence is more prevalent in younger females, while urge incontinence is more frequently seen in older females.

   Answer D is incorrect. Adequate hydration is important; however, fluids should be limited at bedtime. Caffeine and alcohol may worsen symptoms.

9. Answer B is correct. Caffeine and alcohol are known bladder irritants; therefore, they should be avoided to decrease the risk of cystitis.

   Answer A is incorrect. Fruit juices are acceptable.

   Answer C is incorrect. Drinking six to eight 8-oz glasses of water daily is recommended.

   Answer D is incorrect. Lemonade may be acceptable if it is not too acidic.

10. Answer C is correct. Once the antibiotic treatment is complete, return to the office in 7 to 10 days for repeat urinalysis, culture, and sensitivity.

    Answer B is incorrect. The patient should complete the entire course of the prescribed antibiotic.

    Answers A and D are incorrect. If symptoms of cystitis develop, he should contact his healthcare provider immediately. Increasing PO fluid intake is also encouraged.

11. Answer A is correct. Stage V CKD, or "end-stage renal disease," occurs when the eGFR is less than 15 ml/min.

    Answer B is incorrect. eGFR of 20ml/minute indicates Stage 4 CKD.

    Answer C is incorrect. eGFR of 25ml/minute indicates Stage 4 CKD.

    Answer D is incorrect. eGFR of 30ml/minute indicates Stage 3B CKD. Review Table 14-1: Stages of CKDs.

12. Answer D is correct. Uncontrolled diabetes mellitus and hypertension are the most common causes of kidney disease.

    Answer A is incorrect. Hypotension can affect many organs in the body, including the brain, heart, and other vital organs, but it is not a cause of CKD.

    Answer B is incorrect. Anemia of chronic renal disease, also known as anemia of CKD, is a form of normocytic, normochromic, and hypoproliferative anemia caused by CKD.

    Answer C is incorrect. Prostate cancer does not cause CKD.

13. Answer C is correct. Kidney disease often causes hyperkalemia, which can lead to dangerous cardiac arrhythmias.

    Answer A is incorrect. Hypermagnesemia is an uncommon electrolyte disorder. It occurs in approximately 10 to 15 percent of hospitalized patients with renal failure.

    Answer B is incorrect. Hyponatremia is common in patients with kidney disease; however, symptoms may be absent in mild hyponatremia and non-life-threatening in moderate hyponatremia (i.e., nausea and vomiting, headache, confusion, loss of energy, drowsiness, fatigue, etc.).

    Answer D is incorrect. Hypercalcemia is most often associated with primary hyperparathyroidism and malignancies.

14. Answer C is correct. Patients with CKD need to consume a low-protein, sodium, and potassium diet. The subfunctioning kidney cannot adequately excrete the by-products of protein metabolism. A low-sodium diet will help control hypertension.

    Answer A is incorrect. A high-protein diet (HPD) can be harmful to people with CKD. HPDs can cause glomerular hyperfiltration, leading to glomerulosclerosis, tubulointerstitial inflammation, and fibrosis.

    Answer B is incorrect. Patients with CKD are at risk for hyperkalemia and should consume foods lower in potassium.

    Answer D is incorrect. While a low-protein diet will reduce the workload on the kidneys, a high-potassium diet is typically contraindicated.

15. Answer D is correct. Acute renal colic is generally caused by acute obstruction of the urinary tract by calculus. It is frequently associated with nausea, vomiting, and excruciating pain that comes and goes and radiates to the groin.

    Answer A is incorrect. Dull and aching pain in the costovertebral is a common presentation in patients with pyelonephritis.

    Answer B is incorrect. Diffuse abdominal aching and cramp-like pain are commonly associated with constipation, irritable bowel syndrome, food allergies, lactose intolerance, food poisoning, stomach virus, indigestion, gas, diarrhea, menstrual cramps, and ovulation pain.

    Answer C is incorrect. Sharp pain radiating to the spine can have many causes, including injuries, disc problems, sciatica, and other underlying conditions, such as pancreatitis.

16. Answers A and B are correct. Uric acid can be decreased by consuming a low-purine diet and avoiding red meats and shellfish. Alcoholic beverages should be avoided.

    Answers C and D are incorrect. Fruits and vegetables and dairy products, such as milk, cheese, and yogurt, are low in purine. They are a good fit for a diet to manage uric acid or prevent gout.

17. Answer D is correct. ACE inhibitors are contraindicated in kidney disease. Because they are metabolized through the kidneys, they can cause kidney injury.

    Answer A is incorrect. Beta blockers are often recommended for patients with CKD because they can help slow kidney damage by lowering BP and reducing strain on blood vessels.

    Answer B is incorrect. Calcium-channel blockers are extensively hepatically metabolized and can be continued in patients with CKD.

    Answer C is incorrect. Direct-acting vasodilators (hydralazine, minoxidil, nitrates, nitroprusside) are not contraindicated in kidney disease.

18. Answers A, B, and D are correct. Decreased bladder capacity, nocturnal polyuria, and decreased glomerular filtration rate are all common renal changes as the body ages.

    Answer C is incorrect. Aging causes the kidneys to shrink, resulting in the loss of cortical kidney tissue due to decreased renal blood flow.

19. Answer C is correct. Nitrofurantoin (Macrobid) is a first-line treatment for acute uncomplicated UTIs, cystitis, and urethritis in nonpregnant women allergic to sulfa.

    Answer A is incorrect. Amoxicillin, or first-line generation cephalosporin, is a second-line treatment for an acute uncomplicated UTI.

Answer B is incorrect. TMP-SMX is a sulfa drug.

Answer D is incorrect. Ciprofloxacin (quinolone) is a second-line treatment for an acute uncomplicated UTI. While this patient is not pregnant she is of child bearing age and the NP needs to consider that quinolones are contraindicated in pregnancy.

20. Answer C is correct. Kegel exercises are the first-line treatment for patients with urge and stress incontinence.

    Answer A is incorrect. While anticholinergic agents like Oxybutynin and Fesoterodine fumarate are useful, they are contraindicated in patients with hypertension.

    Answer B is incorrect. Referral to a urologist for a cystoscopy may be an option following the trial of Kegel exercises and bladder training.

    Answer D is incorrect. Topical vaginal estrogen is a common treatment for atrophic vaginitis (i.e., vaginal dryness, itching, and burning) and painful urination in women who have experienced menopause.

21. Answer C is correct. Weak bladder muscles cause stress incontinence.

    Answer A is incorrect. Overflow incontinence occurs with an overdistended bladder, often seen with incomplete emptying of the bladder.

    Answer B is incorrect. Urge incontinence is involuntary urine leakage with strong symptoms of urgency and "overactive bladder."

    Answer D is incorrect. Transient incontinence is urinary leaking that spontaneously reverses after the underlying cause is resolved.

22. Answer B is correct. All patients who are prescribed quinolones are at risk of rupturing their Achilles tendon.

    Answers A, C, and D are incorrect. Sulfonamides, cephalosporins, and penicillin do not cause this potential risk.

23. Answer B is correct. GFR is the best index of overall kidney function; a decreasing GFR is characteristic of progressive kidney disease.

    Answers A, C, and D are incorrect. Creatinine clearance, BUN, and serum creatinine are all tests that can help evaluate kidney function; however, the best overall indicator of glomerular function is the GFR.

24. Answer D is correct. CT scan of the abdomen and pelvis without contrast is the preferred diagnostic test for nephrolithiasis. It can also detect hydronephrosis with a sensitivity of 94 to 97 percent and a specificity of 96 to 100 percent.

    Answer A is incorrect. An abdominal X-ray, also known as a kidney, ureter, and bladder (KUB) X-ray, can help show the location and size of kidney stones in the urinary tract. However, X-rays aren't always the best choice for diagnosing kidney stones because they can miss smaller ones like uric acid.

    Answer B is incorrect. Ultrasound is less accurate and has greater variability than a CT scan but is an acceptable alternative in pregnant patients or where ionizing radiation is to be avoided.

    Answer C is incorrect. Intravenous pyelography (IVP) is a tool for assessing flank and lower back pain and hematuria. It is useful in diagnosing congenital anomalies of the urinary tract, urinary calculi, enlarged prostate, neoplasms of the kidney, ureter, bladder, and scars and strictures of the urinary tract. However, it has a sensitivity of 52 to 85 percent and a specificity of 97 to 100 percent for detecting ureteral calculi.

25. Answer D is correct. Renal artery stenosis is the narrowing of the renal arteries. It is commonly seen in patients over the age of 50 with comorbid hypertension and hyperlipidemia.

    Answers A, B, and C are incorrect. Hematuria is not associated with renal artery stenosis but can be present in patients.

Resources

American Urologic Association. (2024). *Non-oncology guidelines*. https://www.auanet.org/guidelines-and-quality/guidelines/non-oncology-guidelines

Cash, J. C. (2024). *Family practice guidelines* (6th ed.). Springer Publishing.

Fischbach, F. T., Fischbach, M., & Stout, K. (2021). *Fischbach's manual of laboratory and diagnostic tests with access* (11th ed.). Lippincott Williams & Wilkins.

Goyal, A., Daneshpajouhnejad, P., Hashmi, M. F., et al. (2023, November 25). Acute kidney injury. In: *StatPearls* [Internet]. StatPearls Publishing. https://www.ncbi.nlm.nih.gov/books/NBK441896/

Gupta, K. (2023). *Acute complicated urinary tract infection (including pyelonephritis) in adults and adolescents*. UpToDate. https://www.uptodate.com/contents/acute-complicated-urinary-tract-infection-including-pyelonephritis-in-adults-and-adolescents

McKinney, J. L., Keyser, L. E., Pulliam, S. J., & Ferzandi, T. R. (2022, March). Female urinary incontinence evidence-based treatment pathway: An infographic for shared decision-making.

Journal of Women's Health, 31(3), 341–346. https://doi.org/10.1089/jwh.2021.0266

Mottl, A. K., & Nicholas, S. B. (2023). *KDOQI commentary on the KDIGO 2022 update to the clinical practice guideline for diabetes management in CKD.* https://www.ajkd.org/article/S0272-6386(23)00883-1/fulltext#articleInformation

National Kidney Foundation. (2022). *Estimated glomerular filtration rate (eGFR).* https://www.kidney.org/atoz/content/gfr#download-nkf-fact-sheet-egfr

Nojaba, L., & Guzman, N. (2023, August 8). Nephrolithiasis. In: *StatPearls* [Internet]. StatPearls Publishing. https://www.ncbi.nlm.nih.gov/books/NBK559227/

Pearle, M. S., Goldfarb, D. S., Assimos, D. G., Curhan, G., Denu-Ciocca, C. J., Matlaga, B. R., Monga, M., Penniston, K. L., Preminger, G. M., Turk, T. M., White, J. R., & American Urological Association. (2014). Medical management of kidney stones: AUA guideline. *The Journal of Urology, 192*(2), 316–324. https://doi.org/10.1016/j.juro.2014.05.006

Stanford Antimicrobial Safety and Sustainability Program. (2024). *SHC clinical pathway: Management of urinary tract infections—adult patients.* https://med.stanford.edu/content/dam/sm/bugsanddrugs/documents/clinicalpathways/SHC-UTI-Guideline.pdf

CHAPTER 15

Sexually Transmitted Infections

Shirley Kuan, MSN, APRN, AGNP-C

Nurse practitioners (NPs) should review the *Sexually Transmitted Infection Treatment Guidelines* recommended by the Centers for Disease Control and Prevention (2021a) for the most up to date and relevant information regarding screening, testing, and treatment.

This information is broken down into sexually transmitted infection (STI) risk factors, screening, testing, physical exam, complications, and treatment recommendations. Special attention is given to specific populations (i.e., adolescents, **men** who **have sex** with **men** [MSM], and pregnant patients). The following review of the most common STIs was guided by the Centers for Disease Control and Prevention.

Chlamydial Infections

Etiology

In the United States, *Chlamydia trachomatis* is the most common bacterial sexually transmitted infection (STI), with the highest prevalence among individuals older than 24 years. All people are typically asymptomatic when infected. Thus, it is important to utilize screening tests to detect chlamydia infection. Annual screening of all sexually active women younger than 25 years is recommended, as is screening of older women at increased risk for infection (e.g., women aged 25 years or older who have a new sex partner, more than one sex partner, a sex partner with concurrent partners, or a sex partner who has an STI) (CDC, 2021).

Clinical Presentation/ Assessment Findings

- History of Present Illness
  - Chlamydia can be spread through vaginal, anal, or oral sex with someone that is infected.
  - Transmission does not require penetration or ejaculation.
  - Pregnant individuals may transmit the infection to their baby during childbirth and cause ophthalmia neonatorum (conjunctivitis) or pneumonia in some infants.
  - Symptom presentation
    - Females may report mucopurulent vaginal discharge, dysuria, dyspareunia, and lower abdominal discomfort.
    - Males may report dysuria and/or urethral discharge.
    - Inguinal lymphadenopathy may present in all genders.

Clinical Management

- Laboratory and Diagnostic Studies (Both Gonorrhea and Chlamydia)
  - Nucleic acid amplification tests (NAAT) are highly sensitive tests used to detect both *C. trachomatis* and *N. gonorrhoeae*.
  - Vaginal, penile-meatal, oral, and rectal swabs can be collected by a provider or self-collected in a clinical setting.

- Urine specimens may be collected for all patients.
- Individuals positive for chlamydia should also be tested for HIV, gonorrhea, and syphilis.
- **Pharmacologic**
  - Doxycycline 100 mg orally 2 times/day for 7 days, azithromycin 1 g in a single dose, *or* levofloxacin 500 mg orally once daily for 7 days.
    - Doxycycline is efficacious for *C. trachomatis* infections of urogenital, rectal, and oropharyngeal sites.
    - Azithromycin is highly efficacious for urogenital *C. trachomatis* infections.
    - Levofloxacin is an effective alternative but is more expensive.
    - Side effects: nausea, GI upset, photosensitivity (avoid sun or use sunscreen)
  - During pregnancy, treatment includes azithromycin 1 g orally in a single dose or amoxicillin 500 mg orally 3 times a day for 7 days.
  - If there is suspicion of possible *pelvic inflammatory disease* (PID) infection, treat with either:
    - Ceftriaxone 500 mg* IM once *plus* doxycycline 100 mg 2 times a day for 14 days with metronidazole 500 mg orally 2 times a day for 14 days
    - Cefoxitin 2 g IM once and probenecid 1 g orally once concurrently *plus* doxycycline 100 mg 2 times a day for 14 days with metronidazole 500 mg orally 2 times a day for 14 days
    - Other parenteral third-generation cephalosporins (i.e., ceftizoxime or cefotaxime) *plus* doxycycline 100 mg 2 times a day for 14 days with metronidazole 500 mg orally 2 times a day for 14 days

  * For persons weighing greater than 150 kg, 1 g of ceftriaxone should be administered.
  - Expedited partner therapy (EPT) is the clinical practice of treating the sex partners of a person diagnosed with an STI without the sexual partner needing to be seen or evaluated by a healthcare provider (HCP). It is recommended to offer treatment to all sexual partners the infected person had sexual encounters with for the past 60 days. If they had not had sex during the 60 days before diagnosis, then the HCP should offer EPT to the most recent sexual partner.
    - EPT is permissible in 46 states and potentially allowable in 4 states (CDC, 2024).
    - Use the *CDC* (2024) website to see if EPT is legal in your state.

- **Patient Education**
  - Patient education should include abstaining from sexual intercourse for 7 days posttreatment.
  - Limit the number of sex partners.
  - Avoid douching.
  - Get regular screenings.
  - Use contraception.

Evaluation and Follow-Up
- **Follow-Up**
  - All patients treated for chlamydia and/or gonorrhea should be retested about 3 months after treatment for a test of cure. Earlier testing is not recommended unless there is suspicion of failure in therapeutic adherence, persistent symptoms, or possible reinfection.
  - Pregnant individuals should have a test of cure 4 weeks after completion of treatment.
- **Complications**
  - **Pelvic inflammatory disease (PID)**
    - An acute ascending multiorganism bacterial infection of the upper genital tract in females
    - If left untreated, it can lead to infertility.
    - Ceftriaxone (Rocephin) 500 mg* IM in a single dose *plus* doxycycline 100 mg orally 2 times a day for 14 days with metronidazole 500 mg orally 2 times a day for 14 days

  *Individuals weighing more than 150 kg will require 1 g of ceftriaxone to be administered IM.
    - Cefoxitin 2 g IM in a single dose and probenecid 1 g orally administered concurrently in a single dose *plus* doxycycline 100 mg orally 2 times a day for 14 days with metronidazole 500 mg orally 2 times a day for 14 days
    - Other parenteral third-generation cephalosporins (i.e., ceftizoxime or cefotaxime) *plus* doxycycline 100 mg 2 times a day for 14 days with metronidazole 500 mg 2 times a day for 14 days

Risk Factors
- History of PID
- Multiple sex partners and/or one with STI
- Young, age 15 to 25
- Inconsistent use of condoms
- Recent IUD placement

> **Exam Tip**
>
> Adnexal tenderness is a sensitive physical exam finding for PID. Cervical wall motion tenderness or the "chandelier sign" is also a criteria for diagnosing PID.

Gonococcal Infection

Etiology

In the United States, *Neisseria gonorrhoeae* is the second most reported bacterial STI. Annual screening of all sexually active women aged younger than 25 years is recommended, as is screening of older women at increased risk for infection (e.g., women age 25 years or older who have a new sex partner, more than one sex partner, a sex partner with concurrent partners, or a sex partner who has an STI) (CDC, 2021a). Annual screening is recommended for MSM.

- Risk Factors
  - Inconsistent and incorrect use of condoms
  - Individuals with multiple partners or nonmonogamous relationships
  - Previous or coexisting STIs
  - Sex workers

Clinical Presentation/Assessment Findings

- **History of Present Illness**
  - Clinical presentations include symptoms from localized inflammatory reactions, including urethritis, cervicitis, pharyngitis, epididymitis, prostatitis, and PID. In addition, complaints of dysuria, frequency, pelvic or testicular pain, and purulent discharge may be present. Disseminated infection can cause meningitis, endocarditis, and/or arthritis-dermatitis. **Many patients may be asymptomatic; therefore, screening patients at risk is indicated.**
- **Physical Assessment Findings**
  - Mucopurulent urethral, cervical or anal discharge, typically thick, yellowish or greenish
  - Unilateral epididymitis
  - Cervical friability
  - Cervical wall motion tenderness
  - Pharyngeal exudates
  - Cervical lymphadenopathy
  - Disseminated gonococcal infection with fever, skin lesions, arthritis, and tenosynovitis
  - Ophthalmia neonatorum in infants can present with purulent eye drainage and orbital edema

Clinical Management

- Laboratory and Diagnostic Studies
  - Refer to the previous chlamydia section.
  - Test of cure should be done for anyone with pharyngeal gonorrhea 7 to 14 days after initial treatment through a culture or NAAT.
  - Test of cure is unnecessary for those with uncomplicated urogenital or rectal gonorrhea.
- Pharmacologic

Uncomplicated gonococcal infection of cervix, urethra, rectum, and pharynx *There is no alternative for treating pharyngeal gonorrhea	Ceftriaxone 500 mg* IM in a single dose for individual's weighing < 150 kg If chlamydial infection has not been excluded, treat for chlamydia with doxycycline 100 mg orally 2 times/day for 7 days *Individuals weighing > 150 kg, 1 g ceftriaxone should be given
Alternative if ceftriaxone is unavailable	Gentamicin 240 mg IM in a single dose Plus Azithromycin 2 g orally in a single dose Or Cefixime* 800 mg orally in a single dose *If chlamydial infection has not been excluded, treat for chlamydia with doxycycline 100 mg orally 2 times/day for 7 days

Evaluation and Follow-Up

> **Clinical Pearls**
>
> - If the gonorrhea test is positive, it is recommended to co-treat for chlamydia if the infection has not been excluded with doxycycline 100 mg orally 2 times a day for 7 days.

- Refer to the previous chlamydia section.

Trichomoniasis

Etiology

Trichomonas vaginalis is a protozoan parasite with a flagellum that affects approximately 2.6 million individuals in the United States. It is one of the most prevalent nonviral STIs worldwide. It infects genitourinary tissue and can cause inflammation. Symptoms may include pruritis, dysuria, and irritation.

Clinical Presentation/Assessment Findings

- History of Present Illness
  - Most individuals with trichomoniasis may have minimal or no genital symptoms. Untreated infections can persist for months to years. Transmission of the infection can occur through penile–vaginal sex, infected vaginal fluids, or fomites among women who have sex with women.
  - **Males** may experience symptoms of dysuria, penile pruritis or irritation, pain with ejaculations, and/or penile discharge.
  - **Females** may experience dysuria, vaginal discharge that may be malodorous, diffuse, or yellow-greenish with or without vulvar irritation.
- Physical Assessment Findings
  - A "strawberry cervix" can be found on colposcopy. It is the result of small points of bleeding on the cervical surface.

Clinical Management

- Laboratory and Diagnostic Studies
  - NAATs are more sensitive than traditional wet-mount microscopy among women for detecting *T. vaginalis*. For females, vaginal swabs (self-collected or clinician collected), endocervical swabs, and urine samples may be used to be tested for *T. vaginalis*.
  - Testing for males is done through urinary samples.
  - Due to the high rate of reinfection in females treated for *T. vaginalis*, retesting is recommended for all sexually active women 3 months after treatment, regardless of the treatment status of sexual partners. There is insufficient data to support retesting of men after treatment.
- Pharmacologic

Treatment for Women	Treatment for Men
Metronidazole 500 mg 2 times a day for 7 days Alternative: Tinidazole 2 g orally in a single dose	Metronidazole 2 g orally in a single dose Alternative: Tinidazole 2 g orally in a single dose

- Patient Education
  - Infected individuals should abstain from sex until they and their sexual partner have completed their treatment course and all symptoms resolved.
  - Douching is not recommended as it may disrupt the vaginal pH and increase the risk of vaginal infections.

Evaluation and Follow-Up

Clinical Pearls

- Individuals affected with *T. vaginalis* should be tested for other STIs, such as HIV, syphilis, gonorrhea, and chlamydia.

Herpes Simplex Virus (HSV-1 and HSV-2)

Etiology

HSV is a very common infection that is lifelong. It affects 1 out of 6 individuals in the United States between the ages of 14 and 49. Infections may be asymptomatic or may show up as outbreaks of blisters and sores. It is primarily transmitted through skin-to-skin contact with the infected areas, often through kissing, oral sex, vaginal sex, or anal sex. Herpes is most infectious when the sores are wet and open. However, herpes can also shed and get passed to others when the skin appears normal and there are no sores.

Herpes is treatable but not curable. Most individuals who are infected may never have any symptoms as the virus stays dormant in the body. Active infections may cause painful blisters or ulcers that can recur over time.

Clinical Presentation/Assessment Findings

- History of Present Illness
  - HSV-1: Typically causes oral infections but can still appear in the genitals.
  - HSV-2: Typically causes genital infections but can still appear in the oral region.
  - An infected person may experience prodromal symptoms (e.g., burning, itching, and tingling) on-site before the eruption of a cluster or small vesicles sitting on an erythematous base.

- Clinical symptoms may include painful, recurrent, and vesicular or ulcerative lesions in the oral or anogenital region.
- Initial herpes outbreak may last from 2 to 4 weeks.

Clinical Management

- **Laboratory and Diagnostic Studies**
  - Lesions can be swabbed for HSV through type-specific virologic testing of the lesion by NAAT or culture.
    - Type-specific serologic assays should be requested to distinguish HSV-1 versus HSV-2 infection.
    - If samples were taken from older lesions or in the absence of lesions, they may fail to detect HSV but not rule out the absence of HSV as viral shedding is only intermittent.
    - Random or blind genital swabs are discouraged as they will have a low sensitivity for diagnosing genital HSV infection.
  - Individuals with HSV-2 infections have a two-to-threefold increased risk of acquiring HIV and thus should be co-tested for HIV.
- **Pharmacologic**
  - The goal of antiviral medication is either:
    - treat genital herpes infections.
      - Episodic treatments are best started within 1 day of lesion onset or during the prodrome that precedes the outbreak.
    - prevent symptomatic recurrences (suppressive treatment), improve quality of life, and suppress the virus to prevent transmission to sexual partners.
      - Since HSV-2 recurrence diminishes over time, an annual discussion should be had with the patient regarding their desire to continue suppressive therapy.
      - Lab monitoring is unnecessary as adverse events and the development of HSV antiviral resistance related to long-term use are uncommon.
  - Systemic antiviral drugs can neither eradicate latent viruses nor affect the risk, frequency, or severity of recurrences once the drugs are stopped.

First Episode (Primary Genital Herpes)	Episodic Treatment (Flare-up)	Suppressive Therapy
Acyclovir+ 400 mg orally 3 times/day for 7–10 days OR **Famciclovir** 250 mg orally 3 times/day for 7–10 days OR **Valacyclovir** 1 g orally 2 times/day for 7–10 days *All treatments may be extended if healing is incomplete after 10 days of therapy +Acyclovir 200 mg 5 times/day can also be used but not recommended due to frequency of dosing	**Acyclovir** 800 mg orally 2 times/day for 5 days OR **Acyclovir** 800 mg orally 3 times/day for 2 days OR **Famciclovir** 1 g orally 2 times/day for 1 day OR **Famciclovir** 500 mg once, followed by 250 mg 2 times/day for 2 days OR **Famciclovir** 125 mg 2 times/day for 5 days OR **Valacyclovir** 500 mg orally 2 times/day for 3 days OR **Valacyclovir** 1 g orally once daily for 5 days *Acyclovir 400 mg orally 3 times/day is also effective but is not recommended because of frequency of dosing.	**Acyclovir** 400 mg orally 2 times/day OR **Valacyclovir** 500 mg orally once a day * OR **Valacyclovir** 1 g orally once a day OR **Famciclovir** 250 mg orally 2 times/day *Valacyclovir 500 mg once a day may be less effective than other Valacyclovir or acyclovir dosing regimen for individuals with frequent episodes (i.e., >10 episodes/year).

- **Patient Education**
  - Herpes cannot live outside the body, so transmission is not possible through hugging, holding hands, coughing, sneezing, or sitting on toilet seats.
  - Individuals with symptoms of oral herpes should avoid sharing objects that have touched saliva and oral contact with others, such as kissing or oral sex.
  - Individuals with symptoms of genital herpes should abstain from sexual activity.
  - Consistent and correct use of condoms is the best way to reduce the risk of transmission of genital herpes and other STIs.

Evaluation and Follow-Up

Clinical Pearls

- In rare instances, herpes can be transmitted from mother to child during delivery, causing neonatal herpes.
- For all genital ulcers, rule out syphilis and HSV infections.
- Severe and recurrent outbreaks should alert the provider to test for HIV infection.

Human Papillomavirus

Etiology

About 150 types of human papillomavirus (HPV) have been identified, and at least 40 types infect the genital area. Most sexually active individuals may contract HPV at some point in their lifetime and be unaware.

High-risk oncogenic types include HPV types 16 and 18 and cause most cervical, vulvar, vaginal, penile, anal, and oropharyngeal cancers.

Clinical Presentation/ Assessment Findings

- **History of Present Illness**
  - HPV typically does not cause any symptoms and is self-limiting. It typically infects the anogenital area but can infect other areas, such as the mouth and throat. It is typically transmitted through vaginal and anal sex. It may be transmitted through oral and genital-to-genital contact without penetration.
  - HPV types that cause genital warts (Condyloma acuminata) are different from types that can cause cancer.

- **Physical Assessment Findings**
  - Anogenital warts may be tender and pruritic depending on location and size.
    - Warts typically appear as a flat, papular, or pedunculated growth.
    - It can be found around the vaginal introitus, under the foreskin of an uncircumcised penis, the shaft of a circumcised penis, the cervix, the vagina, urethra, perianal skin, anus, or scrotum.

Clinical Management

- **Laboratory and Diagnostic Studies**
  - Diagnosis can be made by visual inspection and confirmed by biopsy.
- **Prevention Through Vaccination**
  - Three HPV vaccines, Cervarix, Gardasil, and Gardasil 9, are licensed in the United States.
    - Only Gardasil 9, a 9-valent vaccine that targets HPV 6, 11, 16, 18, 31, 33, 45, 52, and 58, is available in the United States.
    - Vaccination is routinely recommended for all adolescents aged 11 or 12 years; it can be started at age 9. Catch-up vaccination can be given to all people through age 26.
      - If initiated before their 15th birthday, two doses of the HPV vaccine are recommended. The second dose would be 6 to 12 months after the initial dose (0, 6 to 12 months).
      - Three doses of the HPV vaccine are recommended if initiated on or after the 15th birthday. The second dose would be administered 1 to 2 months after the first, and the third dose would be 6 months after the first dose (0-1-2, 6 months).
      - The three-dose regimen is also recommended for those with primary or secondary immunocompromising conditions that may reduce cells.
    - Shared clinical decision-making regarding the HPV vaccine should be discussed with adults between the ages of 26 and 45 who are not adequately vaccinated.
- **Treatment**
  - Treatment of external anogenital warts/genital warts/Condyloma acuminata

Patient Applied	Provider Administered
Imiquimod 3.75% or 5% cream*+ Or Podofilox 0.5% solution or gel+ Or Sinecatechins 15% ointment*	Cryotherapy with liquid nitrogen or cryoprobe Or Surgical removal via scissor excision, shave excision, curettage, laser, or electrosurgery Or Trichloroacetic acid (TCA) or bicloroacetic acid (BCA) 80%–90% solution

*May weaken condoms and vaginal diaphragms
+Contraindicated in pregnancy

- **Patient Education**
  - Consistent and correct use of condoms can reduce the chances of acquiring and transmitting HPV and developing HPV-related diseases (i.e., genital warts or cervical cancer).
  - Limiting the number of sexual partners can reduce the rate of transmission and acquisition.
  - The timing of HPV acquisition cannot be definitively determined as genital warts may appear months or years after initial acquisition.
  - Females with genital warts do not need more frequent pap testing compared with other females.

Evaluation and Follow-Up

Clinical Pearls

- Even after treatment, genital warts may recur, especially during the first 3 months.

Exam Success Tip

- HPV strains 16 and 18 are oncogenic/carcinogenic.
- Treatments that are contraindicated in pregnancy include podofilox and imiquimod.

Syphilis

Etiology

Syphilis is a systemic disease caused by *T. pallidum*. Transmission typically occurs during the primary and secondary stages, where sores, ulcers, or a rash are present. It can spread through vaginal, anal, or oral sex. The bacteria can enter through the anus, vagina, penis, mouth, or broken skin. During pregnancy, the infected mother can transmit the infection to their baby through vertical transmission. Syphilis is not transmitted through fomites. Without treatment, syphilis can lead to life-threatening complications such as blindness, deafness, paralysis, and damage to other organs.

Prevalence is highest among men, especially MSM.

Clinical Presentation/Assessment Findings

- **History of Present Illness**
  - Signs and symptoms are dependent on the stage of infection.
  - **Primary syphilis (2 to 12 weeks after exposure)**
    - A single or multiple painless ulcer/chancres can appear in the individual's oral or anogenital region and last for a few weeks or months. During this stage, syphilis can easily be passed through vaginal, anal, or oral sex.
    - It can also present with multiple, atypical, or painful lesions.
  - **Secondary syphilis (1 to 6 months after resolution of sores)**
    - Nonpruritic maculopapular rash may appear and cover the entire body, including the palms and soles of the feet.
    - Mucocutaneous lesions
    - Flu-like symptoms and lymphadenopathy may appear.
    - These symptoms may come and go for months or years.
  - **Latent infections (asymptomatic and can last up to 20 years)**
    - Occurs after symptoms of secondary syphilis resolve.
    - Individuals are not infectious during the late latent stage.
    - Detected with serologic testing.
    - Early latent syphilis: acquired within the preceding year.
    - Late latent syphilis or latent syphilis of unknown duration: all other cases detected with a positive serologic testing.

- **Tertiary syphilis**
  - It can involve gummatous lesions, cardiac disease, and neurological symptoms such as cognitive impairment, movement disorder, tabes, dorsalis, and general paresis.
- Syphilis can affect the central nervous system (CNS) and lead to neurosyphilis, otosyphilis, and ocular syphilis. These complications can occur at any stage of syphilis. Ocular syphilis can result in permanent vision loss. Otosyphilis can result in permanent hearing loss.

Clinical Management

- **Laboratory and Diagnostic Studies**
  - Two types of syphilis serological tests (treponemal and nontreponemal tests) are used to diagnose syphilis.
    - Traditional algorithm
      - First step: Screening test (nontreponemal tests): venereal disease research laboratory (VDRL) or rapid plasma reagin (RPR). If reactive, a confirmatory test is necessary.
        - Nontreponemal test antibody titers may correlate with disease activity and are important for monitoring treatment response.
      - Second step: Confirmatory test (treponemal tests): T. pallidum passive particle agglutination (TP-PA) assay, T. pallidum haemagglutination (TPHA) test, enzyme immunoassays (EIAs), chemiluminescence immunoassays (CIAs), or fluorescent treponemal antibody absorbed (FTA-ABS) tests.
    - If both RPR (or VDRL) and FTA-ABS (or other treponemal test) are reactive, this is indicative of a syphilis infection.
    - When monitoring labs, ensure the use of the same labs remains consistent. For example, if RPR is used before treatment, it will be used for posttreatment titer comparison.
    - When monitoring pretreatment RPR or VDRL and posttreatment RPR or VDRL, a positive response is true if titers decrease fourfold or more.
      - For example: pretreatment (0 months) RPR 1:64, 6 months posttreatment RPR 1:32, 12 months posttreatment RPR 1:16, 18 months posttreatment.
- **Pharmacologic**
- **Indication for Referral**
  - If there is suspicion of CNS involvement, the patient should be referred to the appropriate specialties, including infectious disease, ophthalmology, and otolaryngology.
  - Consider referral to infectious disease if there is a poor response to treatment, penicillin allergy, or if the primary care provider is not familiar with syphilis management.

Primary and Secondary Syphilis in Adults	Latent Syphilis in Adults	Tertiary Syphilis Among Adults
Benzathine penicillin G 2.4 million units IM in a single dose	**Early Latent Syphilis: Benzathine penicillin G** 2.4 million units IM in a single dose **Late Latent Syphilis: Benzathine penicillin G** 7.2 million units total, administered as 3 doses of 2.4 million units IM each at 1-week intervals **If penicillin allergy, treatment for late latent or syphilis of unknown duration** Doxycycline 100 mg 2 times a day for 28 days Or Tetracycline 500 mg orally 4 times/day for 28 days	**Tertiary Syphilis with normal cerebrospinal fluid (CSF) examination: Benzathine penicillin G** 7.2 million units total, administered as 3 doses of 2.4 million units IM each at 1-week intervals

Evaluation and Follow-Up

- Clinical and serologic evaluation should be performed at 6 and 12 months for primary and secondary syphilis.
  - More frequent evaluation may be necessary if there are concerns about repeat infection or if follow-up is uncertain.
  - Treatment success will show a serological response (titers) of at least a fourfold decrease from pretreatment to posttreatment titers.
- Clinical and serologic evaluation should be performed at 6, 12, and 24 months for latent syphilis.
- Management of sex partners
  - Sexual transmission of *T. pallidum* mainly occurs only when mucocutaneous lesions are present. It is uncommon to erupt after the first year of infection.
  - Individuals who come into sexual contact with those who have been identified to have primary, secondary, or early latent syphilis should be evaluated clinically and serologically and treated accordingly:
    - Sexual partner(s) from the previous 90 days before the patient's diagnosis should be treated for early syphilis, even if RPR or VDRL are negative.
    - The treatment plan for sexual partner(s) from more than 90 days before the patient's diagnosis:
      - If RPR or VDRL is either not immediately available or follow-up is uncertain, treat presumptively for early syphilis.
      - If RPR or VDRL is negative, there is no treatment.
      - If RPR or VDRL is positive with a confirmatory treponemal test being positive, then treat based on clinical and syphilis stage.

Clinical Pearls

- False-positive nontreponemal tests can result from other medical conditions such as autoimmune conditions, vaccinations, injection drug use, pregnancy, and older adulthood.
- When receiving treatment for syphilis, typically early syphilis, a patient may have a Jarisch-Herxheimer reaction. This is a reaction to the treatment of penicillin and not an allergy.

The patient may experience an acute febrile reaction along with headaches, myalgia, and fever within the first 24 hours of initial syphilis treatment.
- Antipyretics can be used to help with symptom management.
- In pregnant patients, it may induce early labor or lead to fetal distress, but this risk should not delay therapy.

Human Immunodeficiency Virus

Etiology

- Prevalence
  - By the end of 2021,
    - about 1.2 million people aged 13 years and older in the United States were found to be living with human immunodeficiency virus (HIV).
      - Of all those individuals, only about 87 percent knew they had HIV.
    - MSM accounted for 67 percent of all new HIV diagnoses in the United States and dependent areas. Individuals who identify as heterosexual accounted for 22 percent, injection drug use accounted for about 7 percent of all HIV diagnoses, and 5 percent were individuals who were both MSM and endorsed injection drug use.
    - Black individuals accounted for 40 percent of all HIV diagnoses, while it was 29 percent for White and 25 percent for Latino/Hispanic individuals.
      - The disproportionate rate of prevalence in Black/African American people is likely related to health disparities, racism, stigma, and inequities in access to HIV care and prevention.
    - The highest age group with HIV was individuals 55 years of age and older, and the next highest were those between 45 and 54 years of age.
    - HIV prevalence was the highest in the southern regions of the United States, accounting for about 47 percent, and the northeast accounted for 20 percent.
- HIV is a retrovirus. Once it enters the host (CD4) cell, it converts its RNA (ribonucleic acid) to DNA (deoxyribonucleic acid) via its enzyme reverse transcriptase.

- There are two types, HIV-1 and HIV-2. HIV-2 has the highest prevalence in West Africa and accounts for fewer than 1 percent of all HIV infections in the United States. The dominant type in the United States is HIV-1.
- **Risk Factors**
  - Sexual intercourse with an HIV-infected individual
  - History of other STIs
  - Multiple sexual partners
  - Homelessness
  - Incarceration
  - Gay, bisexual, or other MSM
  - Sharing needles, syringes, or other drug injection equipment

Clinical Presentation/Assessment Findings

- **History of Present Illness**
  - In the absence of treatment, HIV infection advances in three stages, getting worse over time. It gradually destroys the immune system and leads to acquired immunodeficiency syndrome (AIDS). There is no cure, but treatment with antiretroviral therapy (ART) can prevent progression and help people live longer and healthier lives.
- **Stage 1: Acute HIV infection**
  - During this stage, the virus attacks the infection-fighting cells (CD4 T lymphocytes) of the immune system.
  - The viral load is high, and individuals are highly infectious and contagious.
  - Many may experience *flu-like symptoms*, such as fever, night sweats, oral ulcers, chills, malaise, lymphadenopathy, pharyngitis, myalgia, or skin rash.
    - Typically occurs 2 to 4 weeks after infection
    - Symptoms may last
  - Some may be asymptomatic
- **Stage 2: Chronic HIV infection (aka asymptomatic HIV or clinical latency)**
  - If left untreated, it can last >10 years and progress to the next stage.
  - HIV viral load continues to increase and can still be transmitted.
  - Individuals may not have any symptoms during this phase.
- **Stage 3: AIDS**
  - The most severe stage of HIV infection is when it has damaged the immune system, leading to a weakened immune system.
  - Increased risk of *opportunistic infections* and other severe infections.
    - Opportunistic infections recommended for prophylaxis include pneumonia (*Pneumocystis*) and *toxoplasma* encephalitis.
    - Prophylaxis for disseminated *Mycobacterium avium*, cryptococcal meningitis, cytomegalovirus infection, or coccidioidomycosis is not recommended.
  - AIDS state is considered when the CD4 lymphocyte count is less than 200 cells/mm^3.

Clinical Management

- **Laboratory and Diagnostic Studies**
  - HIV testing is recommended at least once for all persons aged 15 to 65.
  - More frequent testing is recommended for those with higher risk:
    - Sexually active gay, bisexual, and other MSM may benefit from more frequent screening (every 3 to 6 months)
  - HIV can be diagnosed with HIV ½ Ag/Ab combination immunoassays. These are both highly sensitive and specific.
    - If repeatedly reactive, a supplemental HIV-1/HIV-2 antibody differentiation assay is done ("reflex").
      - This will confirm the results of the initial combination assay and determine whether the infection is from HIV-1, HIV-2, or both.
    - If reactive immunoassay is noted, but a negative supplemental antibody test is found, then an HIV RNA test is warranted to determine whether the discordance represents an acute HIV infection.
- **HIV RNA PCR**
  - Detects HIV-1 RNA (viral presence/viral load)
  - Can detect HIV as early as 10 to 33 days after exposure
- **Rapid POC HIV** test can be used to make a preliminary diagnosis of HIV infection in less than 20 minutes.
  - NOTE: a rapid test cannot detect someone who has an acute infection.
- Everyone should be tested for HIV infection as part of routine screening, with CDC guidelines recommending this for those ages 13 to 64, all prenatal patients, and more frequent screening for those at high risk (every 3 to 6 months).

Opportunistic infections	Organism	Indication for primary prophylaxis	Treatment
Pneumocystis Pneumonia (PCP)	Pneumoncystis jirovecii previously called Pneumocystis carnii, a fungus	CD4 count less than 200 cells/mm^3	**Preferred Therapy** ■ Trimethoprim-sulfamethoxazole (Bactrim DS) once daily **Alternative Therapy** ■ Dapsone$^+$ ■ Atovaquone ■ Pentamidine
Toxoplasma Encephalitis	Toxoplasma gondii, a protozoan	CD4 count less than 100 cells/mm^3	**Preferred Therapy** ■ Trimethoprim-sulfamethoxazole (Bactrim) **Alternative Therapy** ■ Dapsone$^+$ ■ Atovaquone ■ Pentamidine

+Before starting dapsone, it is necessary to check the glucose-6-phosphate dehydrogenase (G6PD) level because dapsone may trigger hemolytic anemia in patients with G6PD deficiency.

- **Pharmacologic**
  - **Prophylaxis for Opportunistic Infections (Primary Prevention)**
  - **Antiretroviral Therapy (ART)**
    - Initiated as soon as possible for all individuals with HIV infection regardless of CD4$^+$ T-cell count to preserve individual health and prevent HIV transmission.
    - Typically, it includes the use of a combination of antiretroviral (ARV) regimens that have three active drugs from two or more drug classes.
    - The best sign of treatment success is an undetectable viral load (< 50 copies/mL)
      - HIV RNA PCR is used to monitor the progression of the disease and the response to ARV treatment.
      - CD4 count will typically increase as viral load decreases, a sign that the individual's immune system is improving.
- **Recommended Vaccines**
  - COVID-19
  - HPV (until age 26)
  - Pneumococcal (pneumonia)
  - Tetanus, diphtheria, and pertussis (whooping cough).
    - Every 10 years
  - Hepatitis A
  - Hepatitis B
  - Influenza (flu)
  - Zoster (Shingles) (for those ages 18 or older)
  - Meningococcus
  - Measles/mumps/rubella (MMR) is contraindicated unless the patient's CD4 count is over 200 cells/mm^3.
- **Indication for referral**
  - Individuals with a diagnosis of HIV should be managed by someone knowledgeable about infectious diseases such as HIV.
  - Referral for mental health disorders or substance use may be needed.

Evaluation and Follow-Up

Clinical Pearls

- HIV antibody tests can detect HIV 23 to 90 days after exposure. Most rapid tests and self-tests are antibody tests.
- HIV Ag/Ab test can detect HIV between 18 and 45 days after exposure.
- NAT test can detect HIV 10 to 33 days after exposure.

- **Patient Education**
  - Do not handle cat litter or eat uncooked or undercooked meat (risk of toxoplasmosis).
  - Avoid bird stool due to the risk of histoplasmosis.
  - Turtles, snakes, and other amphibians may be infected with salmonella.
  - Use gloves when cleaning animal cages or when handling stool.
- **Education to Prevent Transmission of HIV**
  - Consistent and appropriate use of condoms
  - Do not share needles or syringes if you inject drugs.
  - Do not share toothbrushes, razors, or other items with blood on them.

- For mothers with HIV, do not breastfeed the baby.
- Limit your number of sexual partners.

Preexposure Prophylaxis

- Numerous studies have documented the very low risk of transmission of HIV in a patient who has the undetectable virus. If the sexual partner is using preexposure prophylaxis (PrEP), the risk of transmission is extremely low.
- Daily oral PrEP is recommended as a prevention option for sexually active individuals at an increased risk of HIV infection, such as:
  - anyone with an ongoing sexual relationship with an HIV-infected partner, and
  - anyone who does not use condoms and engages in high-risk sexual behaviors, including multiple partners.

- Check for HIV infection before starting medications and check for HIV every 3 months thereafter.

Postexposure Prophylaxis: Healthcare Workers

- Postexposure prophylaxis (PEP) is given after a possible exposure to HIV.
  - If there is suspicion of possible exposure to HIV at work, during sex, sharing needles, or through sexual violence, individuals should be recommended to go to the healthcare provider or ED right away.
- A minimum of three ARV drugs are used.
- If prescribed PEP, it will be taken for 28 days.
- The best time to start PEP is as soon as possible, no later than 72 hours postexposure.

Review Questions

1. Due to drug resistance in gonococcal infections, which drug is no longer recommended for use in the United States?
   A. Ciprofloxacin
   B. Ceftriaxone
   C. Azithromycin
   D. Doxycycline

2. A 23-year-old male patient presents with complaints of "bumps" on his penis. Upon examination, raised lesions, which appear to be genital warts, are noted, and a sample is sent for testing that returns positive for HPV. Treatment options include which of the following?
   A. Valacyclovir 500 mg bid for 5 days
   B. Imiquimod 3.75% to the affected area once a day at bedtime for 8 weeks
   C. Corticosteroid cream 1% bid after showers for 2 weeks
   D. Azithromycin 1 g orally once

3. Treatment for a positive chlamydial infection in a pregnant person is:
   A. Valacyclovir 500 mg bid for 5 days.
   B. Imiquimod 3.75% to the affected area once a day at bedtime for 8 weeks.
   C. Corticosteroid cream 1% bid after showers for 2 weeks.
   D. Azithromycin 1 g orally once.

4. Upon visualizing a wet mount for a patient reporting greenish-colored vaginal discharge, trichomonads with 3 to 6 flagella are noted. Treatment for this patient will include:
   A. Valacyclovir 500 mg orally bid for 5 days.
   B. Imiquimod 3.75% to the affected area once a day at bedtime for 8 weeks.
   C. Metronidazole 2 g orally once.
   D. Doxycycline 100 mg orally bid for 7 days.

5. Which patient should be started on opportunistic infection *Pneumocystis jirovecii* pneumonia prophylaxis?
   A. A 52-year-old male with an HIV viral load of 60,000 copies and a CD4 absolute count of 364
   B. A 22-year-old female with an HIV viral load of 325,000 copies and a CD4 absolute count of 325
   C. A 44-year-old female with an HIV viral load of 1,230 copies and a CD4 absolute count of 185
   D. An 18-year-old male with an HIV viral load that is undetectable and a CD4 absolute count of 255

6. A 24-year-old female patient asks the nurse practitioner (NP) about herpes infections since her new partner told her he might have been exposed to it in a previous relationship. Which of the following statements is *inaccurate* and should *not* be the NP's response?
   A. "As long as your partner wears a condom, you do not have to worry about getting genital herpes."
   B. "You and your partner can be tested for herpes type 1 and type 2 to check if you have been infected, since it could be asymptomatic."
   C. "There is no cure for herpes infections."
   D. "Genital herpes can be type 1 and/or type 2."

7. A patient with a penicillin allergy who needs antibiotics for an infection may safely be given any of the following EXCEPT:
   A. TMP-SMX.
   B. doxycycline.
   C. cephalexin.
   D. azithromycin.

8. A new patient is candid during her history interview and admits her sexual partner is HIV+. She states they usually use condoms, but on occasion, they take the risk and have unprotected intercourse. She also states they have talked about having a baby together at some point in the future since her partner is well-controlled on his antiretroviral (ARV) therapy. The nurse practitioner counsels the patient about preexposure prophylaxis (PrEP). Choose the most appropriate response from the following choices:
   A. "It is never advisable to have unprotected intercourse with someone who is HIV infected."
   B. "We need to get you HIV-tested today."
   C. "There are some options we can discuss."
   D. "I can write you a prescription for antiretroviral therapy today so you don't get infected."

9. Postexposure prophylaxis to HIV should commence within which timeframe?
   A. Less than 74 hours postexposure
   B. Less than 4 days postexposure
   C. Only if it has been less than 72 hours postexposure
   D. Postexposure treatment can begin within a week postexposure

10. Complications of tertiary syphilis may include:
    A. seizures and psychosis.
    B. rashes and fevers.
    C. shingles and pneumonia.
    D. respiratory and renal failure.

11. Treatment of syphilis in pregnancy must be with:
    A. doxycycline.
    B. metronidazole.
    C. keflex.
    D. penicillin.

12. Vaccinations for HPV are:
    A. the same for males and females.
    B. only indicated for females.
    C. different in age ranges for MSM.
    D. not indicated once the patient is 18 years of age.

13. What is the most reported STI in the teenage and early adulthood years?
    A. HSV
    B. Syphilis
    C. Chlamydia
    D. Babesiosis

14. A 17-year-old female comes into the clinic with a chief complaint of vaginal discharge. Upon questioning, she says she has a new sexual partner, and they often do not use condoms. The discharge is yellowish, and the patient complains of dysuria. The nucleic acid amplification test (NAAT) is positive for chlamydia. The nurse practitioner writes a prescription for which of the following medications?
    A. Flagyl 2 g orally once
    B. Keflex 500 mg orally once
    C. Zithromax 1 g orally once
    D. Levaquin 500 mg orally once

15. The NP knows that patient education is important in treating STIs. When treating a patient who has a positive chlamydia test, which of the following statements should be discussed in addition to telling the patient that the sexual partner(s) should be treated as well? Choose the best answer.
    A. "It is important that you abstain from sexual intercourse for 7 days and until your partner has gotten treated."
    B. "It is not risky to have intercourse as long as your partner wears a condom."
    C. "Once you have had chlamydia, it is not possible to get reinfected."
    D. "Getting tested for other STIs is not necessary once the medication has been taken."

16. For females, it is imperative to get tested and treated for STIs. Patient education should include which of the following? Choose the best answer.
    A. Sexually transmitted infections in adolescents indicate a need for more parental supervision.
    B. Having chlamydia or gonorrhea will cause difficulty when the patient is trying to conceive.

C. Having an STI can cause pelvic inflammatory disease (PID), which can cause infertility.
D. Using sex "toys" will prevent the spread of STIs.

17. An HIV-infected patient gets a diagnosis of AIDS when the CD4 cell count is below which of the following?
    A. 250 cells/mm^3
    B. 350 cells/mm^3
    C. 500 cells/mm^3
    D. 200 cells/mm^3

18. A 23-year-old man presents for evaluation of a new nontender penile lesion that has slowly developed over several weeks. He is sexually active with male partners and inconsistently uses condoms. He denies other symptoms, has no chronic medical problems, and has no antibiotic allergies. Physical examination reveals a 1-cm, nontender ulcer on the dorsal surface of his penis and no other significant findings. Laboratory studies reveal a positive syphilis enzyme immunoassay (EIA) and a positive rapid plasma reagin (RPR) at a titer of 1:32. He has never been diagnosed with or treated for syphilis in the past. An HIV-1/2 antigen-antibody test is negative.

    Which one of the following options is the most appropriate therapy for this man?
    A. Amoxicillin 500 mg orally three times a day for 7 days
    B. Azithromycin 2 g orally once
    C. Benzathine penicillin G 2.4 million units intramuscular in a single dose
    D. Benzathine penicillin G 7.2 million units total, administered as three doses of 2.4 million units intramuscular, each given at 1-week intervals

19. HPV infection is:
    A. a virus or germ called HPV or human papillomavirus.
    B. the cause of genital warts.
    C. commonly found in people regardless of gender.
    D. passed from one person to another during sexual contact.

20. "Chandelier's sign" is associated with which condition?
    A. Inflammatory knee pain due to Lyme disease
    B. Cervical motion tenderness due to PID
    C. A meningeal inflammation sign apparent during neurological examinations of arthritis
    D. Optic nerve damage found upon assessment of cranial nerve II

21. PID is rare before menarche, during pregnancy, or after menopause. Which of the following is NOT a risk factor for PID?
    A. Older age (>35 years)
    B. Low socioeconomic status
    C. Presence of bacterial vaginosis
    D. Previous PID

22. After initiating treatment for a patient with syphilis, the NP suspects a Jarisch-Herxheimer reaction. Which of the following clinical manifestations support the NP's suspicions (select all that apply)?
    A. Hives
    B. Fever and shaking chills
    C. Myalgias
    D. Abdominal pain

23. Which one of the following statements is TRUE regarding recommendations for routine screening for chlamydial infection in the United States for women who have sex with men?
    A. Annual screening is recommended for all sexually active women between 35 and 44 years of age.
    B. Annual screening is recommended for all sexually active women between 25 and 34 years of age.
    C. Annual screening is recommended for all sexually active women younger than 25 years of age.
    D. Routine screening for chlamydial infection is not recommended for women, regardless of age.

24. A 24-year-old woman is diagnosed with cervical chlamydia at a health department clinic. She has no symptoms, and a test obtained for gonorrhea at the same time is negative. She had her menstrual period about 10 days ago and has not had any sexual contact in the past 3 weeks. Which of the following is the recommended regimen for treating the cervical chlamydial infection in this woman?
    A. Levofloxacin 500 mg orally as a single dose
    B. Doxycycline 100 mg orally twice daily for 7 days
    C. Amoxicillin 500 mg orally three times daily for 7 days
    D. Ceftriaxone 250 mg as a single intramuscular dose

25. A 25-year-old woman is evaluated in the emergency department with a report of having experienced sexual violence approximately 8 hours prior. She denies dysuria, vaginal discharge, or genital lesions. Pelvic examination is negative for cervical motion tenderness, discharge, lacerations, or discharge. Which of the following should routinely be included in baseline testing for cisgender women following a sexual assault evaluation?

A. Herpes simplex virus (HSV) PCR swab and serologic testing for hepatitis B virus (HBV) and hepatitis C virus (HCV)
B. Nucleic acid amplification testing (NAAT) for chlamydia, gonorrhea, and trichomoniasis
C. Herpes simplex virus (HSV) antibody and nucleic acid amplification testing (NAAT) for chlamydia and gonorrhea
D. Serologic testing for herpes simplex virus (HSV), HIV, and hepatitis C virus (HCV)

Answers and Rationales

1. Answer A is correct. Fluoroquinolones used to be prescribed for gonorrhea; however, due to resistance, the CDC now recommends cephalosporins for treating gonorrhea.

    Answer B is incorrect. Ceftriaxone given IM is the recommended treatment for uncomplicated and pharyngeal gonorrhea.

    Answer C is incorrect. Azithromycin is an acceptable alternative treatment for uncomplicated gonorrhea if ceftriaxone is not available.

    Answer D is incorrect. Doxycycline is not a recommended treatment for gonorrhea due to some strains showing antimicrobial resistance.

2. Answer B is correct. Anogenital warts can spontaneously disappear within 1 year. Other treatment options include imiquimod, podofilox, sinecatechins, cryotherapy, surgical removal, and TCA or BCA solutions. It is also important to discuss the patient's vaccination history against HPV. If he has not already received the vaccine, he should be recommended a 3-dose series for further protection.

    Answer A is incorrect. Anogenital warts are typically self-limiting. No oral antiviral medication is currently available for treatment against HPV.

    Answer C is incorrect. Topical corticosteroids are commonly used to treat many inflammatory and autoimmune dermatological conditions. They are not indicated for treating anogenital warts, and long-term use of topical corticosteroid therapy may contribute to the reactivation of anogenital warts due to immunosuppression.

    Answer D is incorrect. HPV is a viral infection, and antibiotics would be ineffective against it as they are used to destroy bacterial cell membranes.

3. Answer D is correct. Chlamydia is most common in persons 24 years of age and younger and is the most common reportable STI. Since the patient is pregnant, we have to be cautious in prescribing antibiotics to avoid toxicity and harm to the fetus. The CDC recommends 1 g of azithromycin or, alternatively, 500 mg BID for 7 days of amoxicillin. A test of cure will be necessary 4 weeks after therapy as a persistent chlamydia infection can cause severe sequelae in the mother and fetus.

    Answer A is incorrect. Valacyclovir is an antiviral medication. It will be ineffective against a bacterial infection.

    Answer B is incorrect. Imiquimod is used to spot treat anogenital warts. We will need an antibiotic to treat this infection systemically.

    Answer C is incorrect. Chlamydia is a bacterial infection that can disseminate if left untreated and lead to infertility. The patient will need to take an antibiotic to eradicate it. A topical corticosteroid will not help kill the bacteria. Individuals with chlamydia are also commonly asymptomatic.

4. Answer C is correct. Trichomoniasis is the most common nonviral STI in the United States. Metronidazole can also be given 500 mg orally twice a day for 1 week. Tinidazole 2 g orally once is another option.

    Answer A is incorrect. Valacyclovir is an antiviral medication. It cannot kill trichomoniasis, a protozoan parasite. Metronidazole is both an antibacterial and antiprotozoal agent.

    Answer B is incorrect. Imiquimod is used to spot treat anogenital warts.

    Answer D is incorrect. Nitroimidazole, such as metronidazole and tinidazole, is the treatment standard for trichomoniasis as it is both a bactericidal and antimicrobial agent. Doxycycline is ineffective against trichomoniasis.

5. Answer C is correct. HIV+ patients whose CD4 cell count falls below 200 cells/mm^3 need to start

on Bactrim (TMP-SMX) or an alternative (dapsone, Mepron) as a prophylaxis.

Answer A is incorrect.

Answer B is incorrect.

Answer D is incorrect.

6. **Answer A is correct.** Because shedding of HSV can occur outside the area that condoms cover, they may not be 100 percent effective.

    Answer B is incorrect. This is true. Appropriate counseling and treatment options should be discussed if HSV is detected in either partner.

    Answer C is incorrect. This is true. There is currently no cure for HSV available.

    Answer D is incorrect. HSV-1 is typically most common in the oral region but can still appear in the genital region. HSV-2 is typically most common in the genital region but can also appear in the oral region.

7. **Answer C is correct.** Cross hypersensitivity can occur when using beta-lactam antibiotics. Up to 10 percent can occur, in particular, with first-generation cephalosporins.

    Answer A is incorrect. Trimethoprim-sulfamethoxazole belongs to a drug class called sulfonamides and is unrelated to penicillin.

    Answer B is incorrect. Doxycycline belongs to a drug class called tetracyclines and is unrelated to penicillin.

    Answer D is incorrect. Azithromycin belongs to a drug class called macrolides and is unrelated to penicillin.

8. **Answer C is correct.** Developing a trusting relationship is essential in this scenario. Discussing the need for her partner to have his HIV well controlled with undetectable viral load is important. The need for this patient to understand the side effects of antiretroviral (ARV) agents, as well as understand the need to take this medication every day, is vital for it to be efficacious. Encourage this patient to attend her partner's next medical visit with the HIV specialist to further discuss planning for preconception care.

    Answer A is incorrect. Many individuals living with HIV can have a healthy sexual relationship with their partners if they take the necessary precautions. Partners without HIV should be taking PrEP daily to prevent the infection of HIV. Condoms should be used for additional protection against other STIs. Routine testing is also advised to identify any infections that need to be treated.

    Answer B is incorrect. The patient is interested in talking about conceiving. Although the discussion regarding their HIV status will be discussed, it is not the only thing we should focus on.

    Answer D is incorrect. We can definitely start the patient on PrEP the same day and get labs drawn, but this needs to be part of the overall discussion with the patient.

9. **Answer C is correct.** Although postexposure prophylaxis (PEP) will not guarantee that a person will not become infected with HIV, studies have shown that if treated with the appropriate antiretrovirals initiated within 72 hours or 3 days, the risk of infection is significantly reduced. The treatment course is for 28 days.

    Answer A is incorrect.

    Answer B is incorrect.

    Answer D is incorrect.

10. **Answer A is correct.** Complications of tertiary syphilis may include seizures and psychosis. Untreated syphilis can result in multisystem diseases, including severe neurological issues.

    Answer B is incorrect. Rashes and fever typically appear in secondary syphilis.

    Answer C is incorrect. Shingles and pneumonia are not complications of tertiary syphilis.

    Answer D is incorrect. When left untreated, patients can develop tertiary syphilis, which can lead to gummatous lesions, cardiac disease, and neurological symptoms. Renal disease is rare but can occur in secondary, latent, and tertiary syphilis. Respiratory failure manifestations can be secondary to neurosyphilis, which causes muscle weakness or paralysis in the lungs.

11. **Answer D is correct.** Most states require prenatal testing for syphilis to prevent congenital syphilis. Penicillin G is the only known effective treatment against syphilis during pregnancy.

    Answer A is incorrect. Although doxycycline is an acceptable alternative treatment for syphilis, it is not the recommended choice for pregnancy. Taking it during pregnancy *may affect tooth and bone development in the unborn baby.*

    Answer B is incorrect. Metronidazole is classified as pregnancy category B, indicating that animal studies have not shown any evidence of harm to the fetus and is indicated for the treatment of trichomonas.

Answer C is incorrect. Data are insufficient to recommend cephalosporins (Keflex) for treatment of maternal infection and prevention of congenital syphilis.

12. Answer A is correct. Vaccinations are indicated for 11 to 12 years through 26 years of age.

Answer B is incorrect. The HPV vaccine is available for everyone.

Answer C is incorrect. There are no special recommendations for MSM.

Answer D is incorrect. Vaccination is recommended for up to 26 years of age. Shared clinical decision-making regarding the vaccine is done for adults between 26 and 45.

13. Answer C is correct. Chlamydia is the most reported STI in those 24 years of age and younger. Thus, it should be part of screening for sexually active young people and those 25 years and older with risk factors.

Answer A is incorrect. HSV is a common infection but is not a reportable STI.

Answer B is incorrect. Syphilis is a common STI that has been increasing in rates in the United States, but rates of chlamydia are higher. It has the highest prevalence among men and MSM.

Answer D is incorrect. Babesiosis is a parasitic infection spread through blacklegged (deer) ticks. It is not an STI.

14. Answer C is correct. The correct answer is Zithromax 1 g orally once.

Answer A is incorrect. Flagyl is also known as metronidazole and is not a recommended treatment for chlamydia.

Answer B is incorrect. Keflex, also known as cephalexin, is not a recommended treatment for chlamydia.

Answer D is incorrect. Levaquin, also known as levofloxacin, is a possible alternative for the treatment of chlamydia, but it is taken at 500 mg for 7 days.

15. Answer A is correct. Reinfection can occur if both partners are not treated appropriately. The patient should be counseled on the benefits of condom use in decreasing the risk of STI acquisition.

Answer B is incorrect. Although condoms are a great way to reduce the risk of transmission, they are not 100 percent effective.

Answer C is incorrect. It is possible to get reinfected with chlamydia again. That is why it is important to ensure that all partners are treated appropriately and abstain from sexual intercourse for 7 days posttreatment.

Answer D is incorrect. It is recommended for additional testing for other STIs, such as gonorrhea, HIV, and syphilis, to minimize other disease transmission.

16. Answer C is correct. Having an STI can cause PID, which can cause infertility. Even subclinical PID can cause infertility; therefore, it is imperative to screen those at risk for STIs.

Answer A is incorrect. It is more important to educate and counsel patients on safe sex practices so they can continue them into adulthood.

Answer B is incorrect. Untreated chlamydia and gonorrhea can increase the risk of developing PID that can cause infertility.

Answer D is incorrect. Sharing sex toys also has risks of passing STIs as they can retain bodily fluids, such as semen, vaginal secretions, saliva, and blood.

17. Answer D is correct. An AIDS diagnosis is given when a patient has a low CD4 cell count (200 or less), an AIDS-defining condition, and/or when CD4 cells are less than 14 percent of all lymphocytes.

Answer A is incorrect.

Answer B is incorrect.

Answer C is incorrect.

18. Answer C is correct. The patient is likely in the stages of primary syphilis due to the presence of a nontender ulcer on his penis. Benzathine penicillin G 2.4 million units intramuscular in a single dose is the correct treatment for syphilis.

Answer A is incorrect. Amoxicillin is not the recommended treatment for syphilis.

Answer B is incorrect. Azithromycin is not the recommended treatment for syphilis.

Answer D is incorrect. The patient is in the primary stage of syphilis, so a single dose is appropriate. This treatment is for patients who are in the latent or tertiary stage of syphilis.

19. All answers are correct. There are more than 100 types of HPV. Over 40 types affect the genitals and put the person at risk for cancer.

20. Answer B is correct. During the pelvic examination, severe discomfort causes the patient to reach toward the ceiling (where chandeliers hang).

    Answer A is incorrect. Inflammatory knee pain is not associated symptom of PID.

    Answer C is incorrect. When we are concerned about meningitis, we may try to see if the patient exhibits the Kernig's or Brudzinski's sign.

    Answer D is incorrect. Assessing for optic nerve damage in a patient is not done in patients with PID.

21. Answer A is correct. Older age is not a risk factor. Women younger than 35 years are at higher risk.

    Answer B is incorrect. Low socioeconomic status is a risk factor for PID, particularly if the patient has gonorrhea or chlamydia.

    Answer C is incorrect. If left untreated, it can increase the risk of developing PID.

    Answer D is incorrect. Individuals with previous history of PID are at increased risk for recurrence of infection.

22. Answers B and C are correct. The Jarisch-Herxheimer reaction is a febrile self-limiting reaction accompanied by headache, chills, and myalgia that occurs within the first 24 hours of being treated for a spirochetal infection.

    Answer A is incorrect. If the patient had a preexisting rash, it may worsen the rash, but it does not cause hive-like reactions.

    Answer D is incorrect.

23. Answer C is correct. Annual screening is recommended for all sexually active women younger than 25 years of age. Most chlamydial infections in women are asymptomatic and often go undiagnosed. Therefore, routine screening for chlamydial infection is extremely important in women who fall within the age groups with the highest rates for acquisition of *Chlamydia trachomatis* because untreated chlamydial infection in women has been linked to PID, chronic pelvic pain, ectopic pregnancy, and infertility. High rates of chlamydial infection in women in the United States occur among those 20 to 24 years of age, with the next highest rate in women 15 to 19 years of age.

    Answer A is incorrect.

    Answer B is incorrect.

    Answer D is incorrect.

24. Answer B is correct. The preferred treatment for uncomplicated chlamydial infections at urethral, cervical, rectal, and oropharyngeal sites is doxycycline 100 mg twice daily for 7 days. Azithromycin, which was previously a preferred regimen, is now an alternative regimen for the treatment of genital and extragenital chlamydia infections in nonpregnant persons.

    Answer A is incorrect. Levofloxacin may be used to treat both chlamydia and gonorrhea; however, the dosing is 500 mg by mouth daily for 7 days. In addition it is an expensive medication and use is currently limited due to concerns about antibiotic resistance.

    Answer C is incorrect. Amoxicillin might be a good antibiotic for treating chlamydia, but it's not the recommended first-line treatment.

    For most people, doxycycline will be given first as per the CDC guidelines, but alternative regimens such as azithromycin can also be administered.

    Answer D is incorrect. Ceftriaxone is used as first line treatment for gonorrhea and is not effective against chlamydia.

25. Answer B is correct. The most diagnosed infections among women who have been sexually targeted with violence include chlamydia, gonorrhea, BV, and trichomoniasis. However, a positive test does not necessarily mean it was acquired during the targeted violence due to its prevalence among the population. Testing is still important as a means of identifying and treating as appropriate due to the risk of possible complications from the infection, such as PID.

    Answer A is incorrect. HSV is not routinely tested. Testing for Hepatitis B can be done, but it is recommended for the patient to receive a postexposure vaccination.

    Answer C is incorrect.

    Answer D is incorrect. Testing for HIV is appropriate, and PEP may be given on a case-by-case basis according to risk.

Resources

Center for Disease Control. (2024, July 16). *Sexually transmitted infections: Legal status of expedited partner therapy (EPT)*. https://www.cdc.gov/sti/php/ept-legal-status/?CDC_AAref_Val=https://www.cdc.gov/std/ept/legal/default.htm

Center for Disease Control. (2021a). *Sexually transmitted infections treatment guidelines*. https://www.cdc.gov/std/treatment-guidelines/default.htm

Center for Disease Control (2021b). *Sexually transmitted infections: trichomoniasis*. https://www.cdc.gov/std/treatment-guidelines/trichomoniasis.htm

Center for Disease Control. (2021c). *Sexually transmitted infections: Genital herpes*. https://www.cdc.gov/std/treatment-guidelines/herpes.htm

HIV.gov. (2024). *Guidelines for the prevention and treatment of opportunistic infections in adults and adolescents with HIV*. https://clinicalinfo.hiv.gov/en/guidelines/hiv-clinical-guidelines-adult-and-adolescent-opportunistic-infections/immunizations

Meites, E., Szilagyi, P. G., Chesson, H. W., Unger, E. R., Romero, J. R., & Markowitz, L. E. (2019). Human papillomavirus vaccination for adults: Updated recommendations of the advisory committee on immunization practices. *Morbidity and Mortality Weekly Report, 68*: 698–702. http://dx.doi.org/10.15585/mmwr.mm6832a3

Meites, E., Kempe, A., & Markowitz, L. E. (2016). Use of a 2-dose schedule for human papillomavirus vaccination—updated recommendations of the advisory committee on immunization practices. *Morbidity and Mortality Weekly Report, 65*(49); 1405–1408. http://dx.doi.org/10.15585/mmwr.mm6549a5

National HIV Curriculum. (2024). *The stages of HIV infection*. https://hivinfo.nih.gov/understanding-hiv/fact-sheets/stages-hiv-infection

National STD Curriculum. (2024). *Home page*. https://www.std.uw.edu/

CHAPTER 16

Integumentary

Nancy L. Dennert, MS, MSN, FNP-BC, CDCES, BC-ADM

Approximately 49 percent of all adult outpatient/primary care visits are for skin conditions. Patients with chronic and common medical problems (obesity/diabetes) have increased the number of incidences, and these numbers are higher in the pediatric population.

The skin's primary function is to protect underlying body structures from invasion by microorganisms, control body heat, eliminate body waste through perspiration, and prevent injury to body structures.

There are three layers: epidermis, dermis, and subcutaneous fat (**Figure 16-1**).

History

Obtain a history noting duration, rate of onset, location, and symptoms, as well as family history, allergies, medications, occupation, and previous treatments. The history is a vital component of the assessment.

The patient should be examined in appropriate lighting, and the skin should be viewed from a distance to seek patterns. Close inspection aids in diagnosis. Physical examination documentation should include the following:

- Primary lesion
- Type of lesion
- Shape of individual lesion
- Arrangement of multiple lesions
- Distribution of lesions
- Color
- Consistency and feel

Terminology

- **Distribution**: localized, regional, generalized
- **Lesion morphology**: wheals, macules, papules
- **Secondary characteristics**: thick, silvery, scaly, thickening, lichenification
- **Shape/Arrangement**: round/discoid, oval, annular, linear, stellate
- **Border/Margin**: discrete, indistinct, active, irregular, advancing
- **Pigmentation**: flesh, pink, erythematous, salmon, tan-brown, black, pearly, violaceous, yellow, etc.
- **Atrophy**: thinning of skin
- **Bulla**: vesicle or large blister filled with fluid; a bleb
- **Crust**: dried serum, blood, or purulent exudate; slightly elevated, size/color may vary
- **Cyst**: closed sac or pouch with a definite wall containing fluid, semifluid, or solid material
- **Erosion**: loss of part of the epidermis, depressed
- **Excoriation**: abrasion or loss of the epidermis by trauma, chemicals, burns, or other factors
- **Fissure**: linear crack or break from the epidermis to the dermis; may be moist or dry
- **Keloid**: scar formation in the skin following trauma or surgical incision. Response out of proportion to the amount of scar tissue required for normal repair
- **Lichenification**: cutaneous thickening and hardening of epidermis, secondary to persistent rubbing, itching, skin irritation
- **Macule**: flat, circumscribed area with change in color of skin; < 1 cm diameter
- **Nodule**: elevated, firm, circumscribed, deeper in the dermis than papule, 1–2 cm diameter
- **Papule**: elevated, firm, circumscribed; < 1 cm diameter
- **Patch**: flat, nonpalpable, irregular-shaped macule > 1 cm diameter

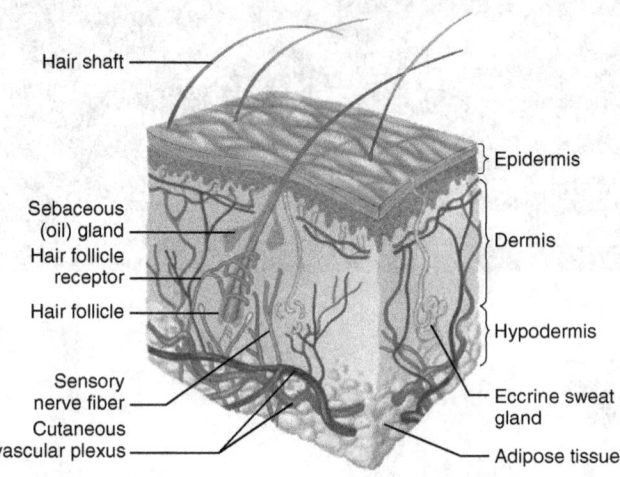

Figure 16-1 Epidermis, dermis, and subcutaneous fat.

- **Plaque**: elevated, firm, rough lesion; flat top surface; > 1 cm diameter
- **Pustule**: elevated, superficial lesion; similar to vesicle but filled w/purulent fluid
- **Scale**: heaped up keratinized cells; flaky skin, irregular, thick or thin, dry or oily, varies in size
- **Scar**: thin to thick fibrous tissue that replaces normal skin following injury to the dermis
- **Telangiectasia**: dilated, superficial blood vessel
- **Tumor**: elevated, solid, may/may not be clearly demarcated, deeper in the dermis; > 2 cm diameter
- **Ulcer**: loss of epidermis and dermis, concave, varies in size
- **Vesicle**: elevated, circumscribed, superficial, not into the dermis, filled w/fluid; < 1 cm diameter
- **Wheal**: elevated, mostly round; solid, transient; variable diameter, white in the center with a pale red periphery

Actinic Keratosis

- Most common lesions seen in dermatology
- Characterized as precancerous
- Presents on sun-damaged skin
  - Head, neck, upper trunk, arms, and legs
- Macules or patches with mild erythema and a distinctive scale you can feel
- Described as a scaly spot that won't go away or peels and comes back
- 10 to 20 percent can become squamous cell carcinoma (SCC) if not treated.
- Tenderness and bleeding are concerning.
- Treatment
  - Liquid nitrogen (LN2) is the most widely used modality
  - Topical fluorouracil (5FUs): carac, efudex
  - Topical imiquimod, also solaraze gel
- Prevention
  - Sunscreen, vitamin C, retinoids

Seborrheic Keratoses

- Benign skin lesion
- Sharply circumscribed
- Measures anywhere from 0.2 cm to 3 cm
- Colors vary from very dark brown, brown, tan
- Stuck on appearance
- Surface can be rough or smooth
- Genetic predisposition
- Treatment: usually cryosurgery, shave biopsy, electrosurgery, and curettage

Skin Cancers

- Most common cancer in all genders.
- One in five people in the United States will develop skin cancer in their lifetime.
- Forty to 50 percent of people in the United States will have at least one skin cancer by age 65.
- Treatment for nonmelanoma skin cancer (NMSCs) increased by 77 percent from 1992 to 2006.
- Ninety percent of NMSC is caused by UV radiation.
- Divided into NMSC and melanoma

Basal Cell

- Most common skin cancer
- 2.8 million diagnosed yearly
- Locally invasive, metastasis rare
- Commonly found in sun-exposed areas
- Fair skin is most at risk, but all skin types as well.
- History of sunburns, sun damage
- Arises from the basal epidermal layer
- Nodular
  - Accounts for 60 percent of basal cell carcinoma (BCC)
  - Raised, translucent papule or nodule with telangiectasias
  - Ulcers may form
  - Bleeding common
  - Can be pigmented and easily confused as a nodular melanoma
- Superficial BCC
  - Erythematous scaling patch
  - Can look like an actinic keratosis (AK)
  - Most common on the trunk and extremities but may present on the face

- Morpheaform
  - Flat, slightly atrophic lesion, infiltrative
  - Can be white or pink; may appear like a scar
- Treatment
  - Mohs surgery if on the face or morpheaform
  - Excision
  - Electrodessication and curettage (E, D, and C)
  - Aldara (imiquimod): alone or in combo with E, D, and C
  - Very rarely LN2

Squamous Cell Carcinoma

- Second most common form of skin cancer
- Arises from sun-damaged skin
- Most common on sun-exposed areas
- Flat or thickened scaly lesion with erythematous base
- Many times, tender to touch, described as bleeding or becoming larger
- Potential for metastasis is related to size, location, and depth of invasion
- Always have biopsied
- Immunocompromised patients at higher risk
- Can arise from actinic keratosis
  - Treatment
  - Always excision or Mohs
  - Radiation if lymph node involvement

Squamous Cell Carcinoma in Situ

- Also called Bowen's disease
- Slightly elevated, red, scaly plaques with surface fissures and some pigmentation
- Well-defined borders
- Can resemble psoriasis, superficial BCCs
- Slower growing and low chance of becoming invasive
- Treatment
  - Excision
  - Electrodessication and curettage (E, D, and C)
  - Topical 5FUs
  - Aldara

Melanoma

- One person dies from melanoma every 57 minutes.
- Most melanoma diagnoses are White men over the age of 50.
- Majority of mutations found are caused by UV.
- One or more blistery sunburns doubles the odds.
- Survivor has nine times the chance of another melanoma.
- Caught early = 99 percent survival rate, but falls to 15 percent when more advanced
- Originates from melanocytes, the cells that produce the pigment melanin that colors our hair, skin, and eyes.
- Usually appears as black or brown, but can also be pink, white, purple, skin-colored
- Follow the ABCDE
  - Asymmetry
  - Border
  - Color
  - Diameter
  - Elevation
- Changing lesion or new lesion that is quickly enlarging
- Risk factors
  - Immediate family member diagnosed
  - Fair skin
  - History of sunburns
  - Multiple nevi
  - UV exposure
  - Tanning booths
- High risk of distant metastasis, especially in the brain, lungs, liver, and GI tract
- The most important prognostic factor is thickness and if ulceration is present
- Treatment depends on stage:
  - Surgery
  - Immunotherapy
  - Chemo/radiation

Acne Vulgaris

- Disease of pilosebaceous unit
- Appears near puberty
- Intensity and severity varies
- Psychosocial effects can be devastating
- Divided into inflammatory and noninflammatory
- Treatment options dependent on the type of acne
  - Noninflammatory
    - Open comedones: blackhead
    - Closed comedones: whitehead
  - Treatment
    - Retinoids preferred
      - RAM, Differin, Tazorac
    - Benzoyl peroxide (BPO) as well, wash, topical
    - Exfoliation: over-the-counter (OTC) scrubs
  - Inflammatory
    - Papulopustular or cystic
    - Mild, moderate, severe
    - Watch for scarring, more aggressive

- Treatment
    - Topical BPO/clindamycin (Duac, Acanya)
    - Retinoids
    - Oral doxycycline; Accutane if scarring

Rosacea

- Inflammatory disorder affecting central face, chin, forehead
- Rarely seen in people younger than 30 years old
- More common in women
- Genetic predisposition and actinic damage
- Erythema and telangiectasis, superficial pustules
- Treatment
    - Daily sunscreen
    - Avoid triggers
    - Metrogel, Finacea, sodium sulfacetamide, and/or oral tetracycline
    - Laser for redness

Xerosis (Dry Skin)

- Most common on the back and extremities
- Generalized fine scale, no erythema
- Seen more in winter months
- Moisturization is important; stay away from fragrances
- If severe, test for hypothyroidism
- Occasionally need to use a topical steroid

Cellulitis

- Acute inflammatory condition
- Deeper infection of the skin
- Usually caused by *S. aureus* but may be caused by many different bacteria entering through a break in the skin
- Characterized by local pain, swelling, heat, erythema
- Occurs anywhere on the body
- Treatment
    - Oral antibiotics: cephalosporin, doxycycline if concerned about MRSA
    - Hibiclens
    - Topical steroid

Cysts

- Self-contained sacs of purulent material, bacteria, white blood cells (WBCs)
- Commonly seen in women in axillae, groin, and legs (areas where shaving is common)

- Treatment
    - Incision and drainage (I+D) most effective
    - Oral antibiotics: tetracycline family, cephalosporin
    - Kenalog injection

Folliculitis

- Blocked hair follicles result in small pustules
- Usually, *S. aureus*
- Can occur in any hair-bearing area
- Treatment
    - BPO washes
    - Clindamycin topical
    - Oral doxycycline

Dermatitis

- Types
    - Contact
    - Irritant
    - Allergic
- Very common (plants, acids, metals, soaps, perfumes, lotions, etc.)
- Caused by hypersensitivity response
- Erythema, vesicles, urticarial lesions
- Complaints of burning, itching, redness
- Treatment
    - Topical steroid, antihistamines, oral prednisone tapering dose
    - Remember, steroid use on the face is not recommended for long periods or with higher potency steroids

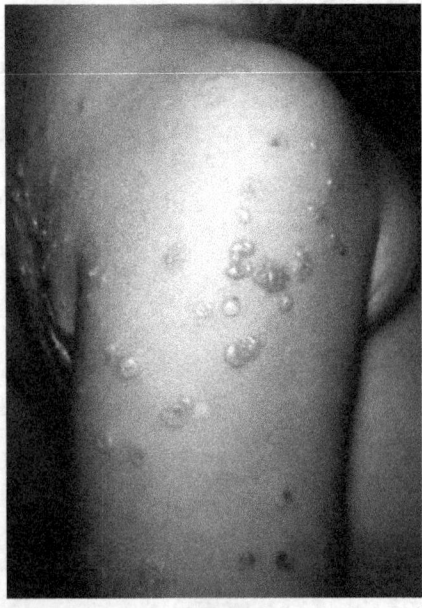

Dermatitis rash on arm
Courtesy of Centers for Disease Control and Prevention.

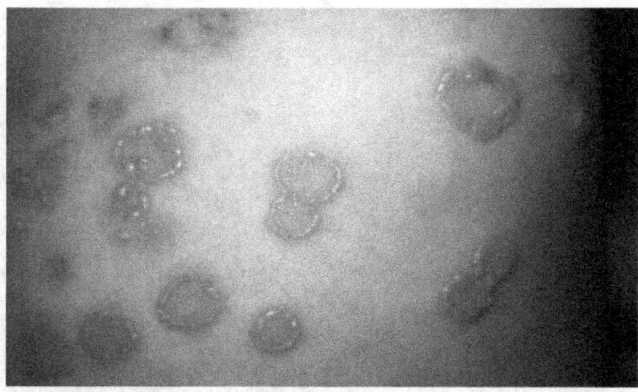

Dermatitis rash on buttock
Courtesy of Centers for Disease Control and Prevention.

Atopic Dermatitis: Eczema

- Consider personal, familial history of atopy, common in people with allergic disorders and/or asthma
- Cause: dysfunction in the epidermis
- Symptoms: intense itching, erythema, small bumps, skin flaking
- Scratching can cause skin inflammation, which worsens with itching
- Affects infants' front of arms/legs/cheeks/scalp
- Affects adults' back of neck/elbow creases/posterior knees
- "The itch that rashes"
- Cutaneous expression of atopic state
- Thought to be a problem with immunoregulatory abnormalities, including IgE, IL 4, and mast cell tryptase
- Can occur anywhere on the body
- Fragrance-free detergents, softeners, sheets
- Dove soap, Cetaphil cleanser
- Daily moisturization
- Recommend lotion face, cream body
- Decrease heat in shower, house temp
- Topical corticosteroids as needed
- Antihistamines may help

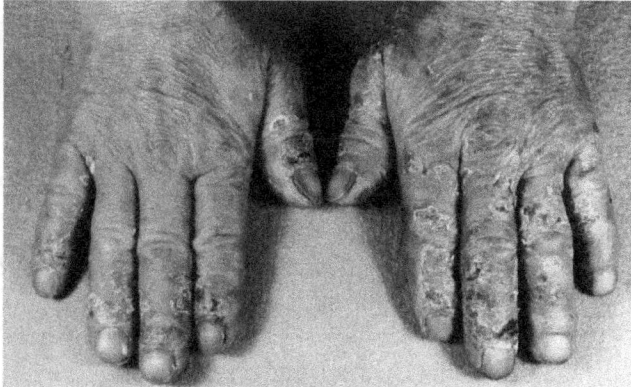

Eczema rash on hands
Courtesy of Centers for Disease Control and Prevention.

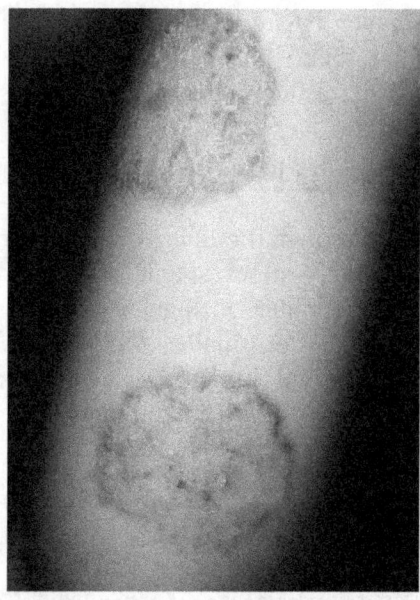

Excema rash on arm
Courtesy of Centers for Disease Control and Prevention.

Seborrheic Dermatitis

- Common chronic disorder
- Characteristic greasy scales overlying erythematous patches or plaques
- Commonly seen in Parkinson's patients, people with cerebrovascular accidents (CVAs), and HIV; the vast majority have no underlying illness. This is evident in babies as "cradle cap"; otherwise, it is rare in children.
- The most common location is the scalp (dandruff), face, eyebrows, lids, and nasolabial folds.
- Usually causes itching, burning.
- Treatment
  - Ketoconazole
  - Selenium sulfide
  - Steroid shampoos

Psoriasis

- Chronic inflammatory skin disorder
- Alteration in cell kinetics of keratinocytes; overabundance of T cells in affected cells; other immunologic factors
- Pink, sharply demarcated papules and plaques covered by silvery scale
- Lesions are variably pruritic
- Occurs equally in all people
- Tends to run in families
- The most common type is plaque.
- Most common areas are elbows, knees, and scalp. Also seen on hands, feet, and nails.
- Always ask about joint pain.
- Treatment
  - Topical steroids
  - Topical vitamin D (Dovonex)

- Coal tar (shampoos, especially)
- Phototherapy
- Methotrexate, cyclosporin, biologics

Pityriasis Rosea

- Cause unknown; thought to be a viral trigger
- Herald patch appears first: large pink scaling patch on abdomen or thigh
- Will then develop smaller oval pink scaling macules on the trunk, sometimes legs and arms
- Generally asymptomatic; mild itch at times
- Self-limiting up to 6 to 8 weeks

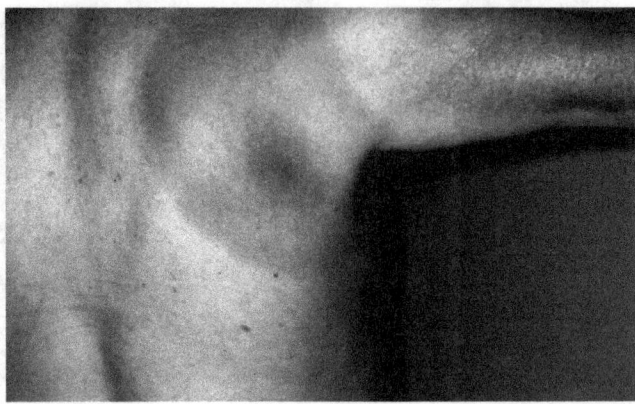

Erythema Migrans rash on shoulder
Courtesy of Centers for Disease Control and Prevention.

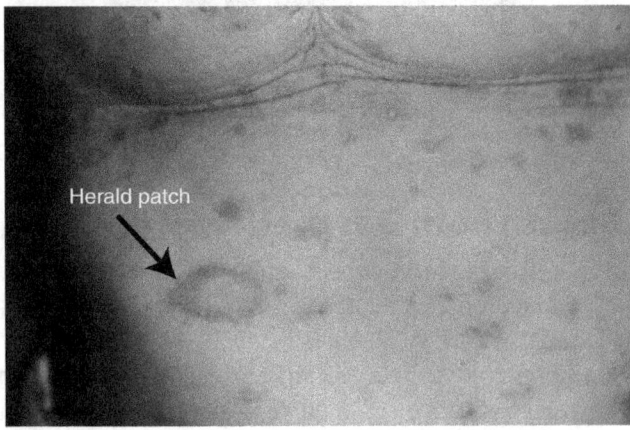

Pityriasis Rosea
Courtesy of Center for Disease Control and Prevention.

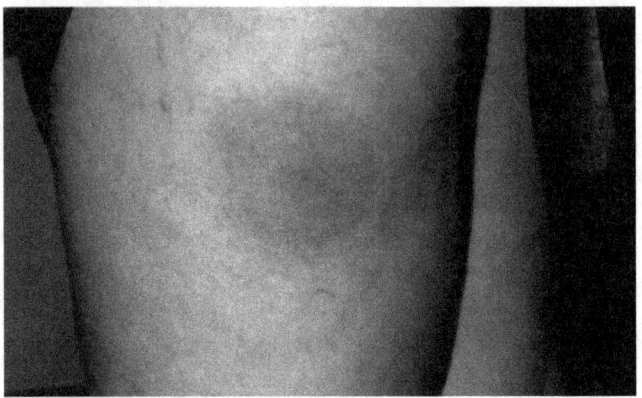

Erythema Migrans rash on thigh
Courtesy of Centers for Disease Control and Prevention.

Erythema Migrans

- A common finding in Lyme disease seen in about 70 percent of the cases.
- It is a characteristic rash that can help differentiate erythema migrans (EM) from other rashes and skin disorders.
- EM develops within 3 to 30 days after a deer tick bite and is caused by the bacterium *Borrelia burgdorferi*.

Characteristics of EM Rash

- Occurs on average 7 days after tick bite at the site of the bite.
- Rarely itchy or painful. It may feel warm to the touch.
- Expands gradually—up to 12 inches in diameter.
- Sometimes, as it enlarges, there is a central clearing, often referred to as the "bull' s-eye rash."
- It does not always appear as a classic "bull's-eye rash"; therefore, obtaining a history of possible exposure is essential to assist in diagnosis.
- If left untreated, EM rashes may occur elsewhere on the body and, in some cases, multiple areas of the body.

- Early symptoms of Lyme disease:
  - Fever
  - Headache
  - Fatigue
  - Erythema migrans at the site—develops in 70 percent of infected persons
- Untreated Lyme disease:
  - A wide range of symptoms depends on the stage of the infection and may include:
    - Facial paralysis (Bell's Palsy)
    - Arrhythmias
    - Arthritis and/or intermittent pain in muscles, joints, and tendons
    - Inflammation of the brain and spinal cord
- Diagnosis
  - Consider the signs and symptoms of the patient.
  - Consider the likelihood of exposure to the blacklegged tick (deer tick).
  - Generally, the tick must remain attached for 48 hours to transmit the disease.
  - One of every three deer ticks have the bacterium that causes Lyme disease.
  - The CDC recommends two-step testing: the enzyme immunoassay (EIA) and the Western blot (WB).

- Patients recently infected may test negative.
- Patients who receive early antibiotic treatment are less likely to seroconvert.
- Treatment
  - Treatment regimens for those patients with EM rash are adjusted depending on the patient's age, medical history, and pregnancy/breastfeeding status.
  - The most common antibiotic treatments are doxycycline (10 days), amoxicillin (14 days), or cefuroxime.
  - Azithromycin may be used if the patient is intolerant or allergic to the three most commonly used antibiotics. If azithromycin is used, the patient needs to be reassessed to resolve symptoms.

Warts: Verruca Vulgaris

- Cutaneous neoplasms caused by HPV (more than 50 types identified)
- Appear anywhere on the body
- Many resolve spontaneously in 1 to 2 years
- Spread through contact
- Treatment
  - LN2
  - Canthacur
  - Salicylic acid
  - Candida injection
  - Laser

Skin Tags

- Very common
- Benign skin lesion
- Found on face, neck, axillae
- More prevalent in Black people than White people
- 1 to 2 mm outcroppings of skin
- Caused by friction, changes in weight
- Scissor removal

Impetigo

- Common superficial bacterial infection
- Caused by group A beta-hemolytic *Streptococci* or *Staph aureus*.
- Primary lesion is a superficial pustule that ruptures and forms a characteristic honey-colored crust.
- Ecthyma is a variant of impetigo that usually occurs on lower extremities.
  - Characterized by "punched out" ulcerative lesions
- Treatment
  - Bactroban, Keflex, doxycycline

Dermatophytosis

Tineas: Capitis, Corporis, Cruris, Pedis

- Usually caused by an overgrowth of fungal organisms commonly found on the skin.
- Scaling erythematous lesions, annular on the scalp and body. Moccasin on lateral feet.
- Look for macerated skin between toes.
- Potassium hydroxide (KOH), if available; look for hyphae
- Treatment
  - Scalp: Griseofulvin since hair follicles are affected
  - Body, feet: Naftin cream/gel bid (two times a day) for 2 to 4 weeks
- Oral antifungal if severe enough

Onychomycosis

- Fungal infection in nail/bed
- More common in toes than fingers
- Yellowish, sometimes darker (brownish/bluish) discoloration of the nail; white color is candida
- Treatment
  - Topicals are a first-line treatment due to liver toxicity with oral antifungal agents.
  - Always use a gel or solution because it penetrates better.
  - Use urea gel in conjunction if the nail is thickened.
  - Loprox gel, Naftin gel
  - If oral, Diflucan; if candida, Lamisil fungal

Tinea Versicolor

- Overgrowth of yeast from sweating
- Pink velvety scaling patches on the upper body
- Sun causes hypopigmentation
- Treatment
  - Selsun 2.5% shampoo, leave on 10 minutes, rinse off: use daily for 2 weeks
  - Loprox solution daily, potentially ongoing
  - Diflucan weekly for 2 weeks for severe cases

Herpes Zoster (Shingles)

- Cutaneous viral infection involving a single dermatome, unilateral
- Reactivation of varicella virus that entered cutaneous nerves with chicken pox
- All ages inflicted
- Stress and sickness activate it.
- Contagious to pregnant persons, immunocompromised people, and nonimmunized children

Chapter 16 Integumentary

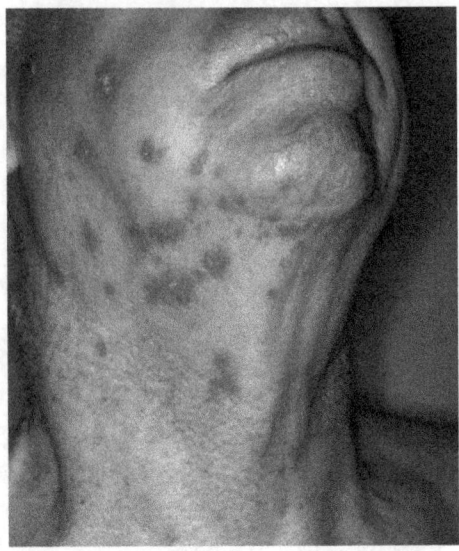

Herpes Zoster (Shingles) on neck
Courtesy of Centers for Disease Control and Prevention.

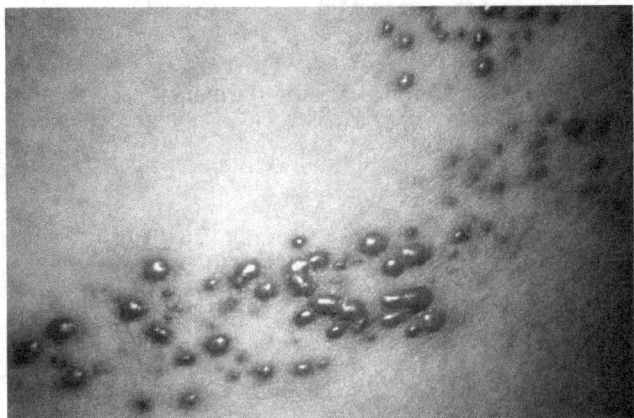

Closeup of Herpes Zoster (Shingles)
Courtesy of Centers for Disease Control and Prevention.

- Best outcome if treated within 24 to 48 hours
- Complaints of itch, pain before rash appears
- Clustered vesicles on an erythematous base
- Postherpetic neuralgia can last months
- Treatment
  - Valacyclovir 1 gm three times a day for 7 days (or acyclovir)

Vitiligo

- Hypopigmented macular lesions 5 mm to 5 cm or more
- Occurs equally in all people
- Appears in all races
- Affects 1 percent of the population
- Etiology unknown, three hypotheses: autoimmune, neurogenic, self-destruct
- Also can be related to immunotherapy treatment in cancer.

Three General Patterns of Depigmentation

- Focal: lesions in a single general area
- Segmental: lesions on one side of the body
- Generalized: widespread distribution

Treatment

- Short-burst topical steroids
- Protopic 0.1 ointment bid (two times a day), short exposure to sun after application
- Sunscreen and sun protection education

Alopecia Areata

- Skin condition that causes a sudden loss of patches of hair on the scalp and other parts of the body
- Nonscarring: no permanent damage to the hair follicle
- Most people, hair eventually grows back, with 80 percent of people recovering in 1 year
- Occurs equally in all people, all races equally, can develop at any age
- Not life threatening; no physical pain; cosmetic effect can be devastating
- Thought to be the body attacking the pigment in the hair follicle
- Stress can be a trigger
- Sometimes seen in correlation with vitiligo

Treatment

- High-potency topical steroid
- Kenalog injections

Urticaria (Hives)

- Distinct, raised areas of skin that itch intensely and are red with a pale center
- Approximately 25 percent of people will experience at least once in their lifetime
- Acute, brief, or chronic
- Also, physical urticarias: triggered by certain types of physical stimulation
- Dermatographism (skin writing)—skin welts when stroked firmly or scratched
- Angioedema can also develop with hives; occurs deeper in the skin, and causes puffiness of the face, eyelids, ears, mouth, hands, feet, and genitalia
- Triggers: Drugs, physical contact with allergens, insect stings, food allergies, infections
- Treatment: Antihistamines, avoid heat, oral steroids

CASE STUDY

A 20-year-old college student comes to the health center complaining of fever, headache, and malaise. She also complains of a sore throat lasting 2 days. Her temperature is 101.2°F, and she verbalizes having had a fever for the past 3 days. The rest of her vital signs are unremarkable. She has no significant past medical history (PMH). No recent sick contacts. Lives in off-campus housing with two roommates. She went camping with her partner at a local state park 1 week ago. Her partner is not sick. She has taken no medications except for Ibuprofen 600 mg every 8 hours for the past 3 days with some relief of symptoms. She is sexually active. No toxic habits. No known drug allergies (NKDA).

A physical exam reveals a well-nourished woman who is alert and oriented (A&O) x3. Limited neurologic exam is within normal limits with positive intraocular movements (WNL. +EOMs), no photophobia, no nuchal rigidity. Appetite is WNL—no nausea, vomiting, diarrhea, or constipation. There is an area of erythema on her right popliteal fossa that is well-circumscribed, warm to touch, nonpruritic, and flat. There is no central clearing. She states that there were a lot of "bugs" around the campsite but does not recall if she was bitten by anything other than mosquitoes.

The NP obtains a rapid strep test, influenza swab, and COVID-19 swab. All are negative. With this information, what should the NP consider next?

- Lyme disease is likely diagnosed due to recent outdoor activity and the presentation of fever, headache, malaise, and EM-type rash.
- EM rash is not always a "bull's-eye" rash with central clearing. Central clearing often appears later, but an early EM rash may just present as an erythematic patch.
- Always consider meningitis as a possible differential diagnosis for college students with headaches, fever, and malaise. Document neuro evaluation.
- Obtain pregnancy tests, as most of the standard treatments for Lyme disease are teratogenic.
- Order ELISA and Western blot tests. These tests are likely negative in the early stage of Lyme disease but may seroconvert after 4 to 6 weeks. Obtain again 4 to 6 weeks later.
- If the pregnancy test is negative, begin treatment with doxycycline 100 mg PO BID for 10 days or amoxicillin 500 mg PO TID for 14 days.

Review Questions

1. The nurse practitioner (NP) uses the correct terminology to describe the *morphology* of a lesion. Which of the following is an appropriate description?
   A. "The lesion has irregular borders."
   B. "The lesion is a macule."
   C. "The lesion is erythematous."
   D. "The lesion is scaly."

2. A patch can be differentiated from a macule by observing that a patch is:
   A. less than 1 cm in diameter.
   B. elevated, firm, circumscribed, and less than 1 cm in diameter.
   C. an elevated, firm, rough lesion with a flat top surface greater than 1 cm in diameter.
   D. a flat, nonpalpable, irregular-shaped macule greater than 1 cm in diameter.

3. Vitiligo can be described as what?
   A. Distinct raised areas of the skin that are pruritic
   B. Hypopigmented macular lesions ranging in size from 5 mm to 5 cm or greater
   C. A loss of skin pigment and hair due to injury at the base of the hair follicle
   D. A progressive thickening and hardening of the epidermis

4. A 36-year-old female patient presents to the medical office with an EM rash in her axillary region that has progressed in size over the past week. The patient removed a tick from her axilla and disposed of it. The patient has no known allergies. The NP considers treatment. What is the NP's priority consideration?
   A. Determine how long the tick may have been attached to her axilla
   B. Assess pregnancy and/or lactation status
   C. Order two-step laboratory testing with both the enzyme immunoassay (EIA) and Western blot (WB) tests before initiating treatment
   D. Begin immediate treatment with doxycycline 100 mg PO BID for 10 days

5. A patient presents to the office with concerns about the sudden loss of patches of hair from her scalp. She denies any recent changes in the use of hair products. She does not pull or tug at her hair. The

NP diagnoses the patient with alopecia areata. Which of the following statements made by the NP would provide the most reassurance to the patient?
   A. "There is no treatment, but it is always a benign condition."
   B. "If we can identify the causative agent, we may be able to prevent further hair loss."
   C. "A 1% topical naftifine cream (Naftin) applied BID for 2 to 4 weeks may help prevent further hair loss."
   D. "Eighty percent of all people with this condition will have spontaneous hair regrowth within 1 year."

6. A 35-year-old female patient is seen in the primary care office with concerns about multiple small, pink, oval scaling macules that have appeared on her trunk. There is no associated pain or pruritus. There is one significantly larger scaly patch observed on the abdomen. The NP diagnoses the patient as having what?
   A. Roseola
   B. Pityriasis rosea
   C. Contact dermatitis
   D. Rosacea

7. An 8-year-old male child is seen in the clinic with a superficial pustule along his inner forearm that started as a mosquito bite. There is a characteristic honey-colored crust covering the entire lesion. The NP diagnoses the patient with which of the following?
   A. *Staph aureus* or Group A beta-hemolytic *Streptococcus* infection
   B. Group B beta-hemolytic *Streptococcus* infection
   C. Community-acquired Methicillin-resistant *Staph aureus*
   D. Tinea corporis

8. A patient is seen in the primary care office. The patient has a maculopapular rash with distinct vesicles on the lateral left trunk that follow along a dermatome. The patient states that the rash has been there for 3 days. Which of the following is important educational information that should be provided to the patient?
   A. The patient is experiencing a reactivation of the chicken pox virus and is not contagious.
   B. The patient is contagious and must avoid pregnant persons, immunocompromised individuals, and nonimmunized children.
   C. The patient is only contagious for the first 48 to 72 hours that the rash is present.
   D. The patient is not contagious. The rash may remain for many months, and there is no treatment.

9. Which of the following is the preferred treatment for herpes zoster (shingles)?
   A. Ketoconazole 200 mg tablet PO daily for 10 to 14 days
   B. Lotrisone topical cream 0.5%; apply to the affected area for 2 weeks
   C. Diflucan 150 mg, one tablet PO daily for 14 days
   D. Valacyclovir 1 g TID for 7 days

10. The preferred therapy for onychomycosis is topical agents. If the NP uses oral agents, the NP should first obtain lab work to determine what?
    A. The patient's renal function
    B. The patient's hepatic function
    C. The patient's coagulation factors
    D. The patient's immune competency

11. A patient presents to the office with an apparent allergic reaction to an unknown antigen. The patient has pruritic hives on his arms, legs, trunk, and face. The patient has no difficulty breathing or swallowing, his lungs are clear, and there is no swelling of the lips or tongue. With this information, the NP should choose which of the following options for treatment?
    A. One-time dose of epinephrine via EpiPen stat in office
    B. Oral antihistamines, cool compresses, and oral corticosteroids
    C. Topical steroid cream to be applied to all affected areas for 1 week or until lesions disappear
    D. Second-generation antihistamines and warm compresses to the affected areas for 20 minutes TID

12. What is the most common lesion seen in dermatology?
    A. Basal cell skin cancer
    B. Squamous cell skin cancer
    C. Actinic keratosis
    D. Nonmelanoma skin cancer (NMSC)

13. An 18-year-old female patient presents to the office with complaints of papulopustular cystic acne on her forehead, chin, and upper back areas. The NP is concerned with psychosocial effects as well as physiological long-term scarring. The NP decides to initiate therapy with which of the following?
    A. Exfoliation therapy
    B. Topical clindamycin
    C. Isotretinoin (Accutane)
    D. Retinoids

14. A patient complains of a pruritic red rash that appeared on his body several days ago. The NP obtains a skin scraping, applies potassium hydroxide (KOH), and visualizes multiple hyphae under the microscope. The NP diagnoses the patient with which of the following?
    A. Herpes zoster
    B. Seborrheic dermatitis
    C. Tinea corporis
    D. Onychomycosis

15. The NP can expect to find more frequent skin conditions in which population?
    A. The adolescent population
    B. The population with diabetes
    C. People who primarily work outdoors
    D. Healthcare workers

16. A patient has been told to have Mohs surgery on a cancerous lesion. The patient asks what Mohs surgery is. The NP explains that:
    A. the cancerous lesion is removed, as well as the surrounding lymph nodes.
    B. the surface area of the lesion is excised, and the underlying area is cauterized to prevent further growth.
    C. the lesion is excised and examined under a microscope to determine if wound edges are free from cancer or if further excision is required.
    D. a wide excision is performed to avoid having to do further surgery.

17. The NP describes a patient's skin on his lower extremities as taut, shiny, and hairless. The nurse practitioner knows that this skin appearance is consistent with which of the following?
    A. Aging skin
    B. Venous insufficiency
    C. Arterial insufficiency
    D. Chronic, long-term sun exposure

18. A 45-year-old male patient presents to the clinic concerned about a mole on his upper back. The NP examines the mole and notes it is well-circumscribed, dark brown, circular, and 7 mm in diameter. The NP refers the patient to dermatology for excision and biopsy. Which of the following characteristics was most concerning to the NP?
    A. Location
    B. Size
    C. Color
    D. Border configuration

19. A patient presents to the primary care provider concerned about a distinct rash that has appeared on his lower leg. It is nonpruritic, 6 cm in diameter, with an annular homogenous erythema appearance and central clearing. The NP inquires as to whether the patient:
    A. has young children in the household with tinea corporis (ringworm).
    B. is immunocompromised.
    C. has been outdoors doing yard work, camping, or hiking in the past several weeks.
    D. has had a rash that appeared like this in the past.

20. Most cases of melanoma are seen in which of the following?
    A. White women over the age of 50
    B. White men over the age of 50
    C. White women with blue eyes and red or blond hair
    D. Any person of northern European descent

21. An important prognostic factor for a patient diagnosed with melanoma is which of the following?
    A. The number of blistering sunburns the patient has experienced over their lifetime
    B. A family history of melanoma
    C. The thickness of the lesion and if ulceration is present at the time of diagnosis
    D. The diameter of the lesion

22. A 35-year-old female patient presents to the NP for a routine physical exam. During the skin assessment, the patient comments about a lesion on the dorsal portion of her lower left leg. Which of the following statements made by the patient is the most concerning?
    A. "I think this mole is a different color than my other moles."
    B. "This mole seems like it grew overnight."
    C. "This mole is larger than the other moles on my body."
    D. "Sometimes this mole is itchy."

23. A patient's chances of developing a melanoma are closely related to which of the following?
    A. The number of melanocytes present in the dermis
    B. The number of blistering sunburns the patient has experienced in their lifetime
    C. The amount of time they have spent outdoors
    D. Chronic exposure to known carcinogens such as free radicals

24. An 18-year-old Black male travels to a tropical area for vacation. He asks the NP if he must wear sunscreen higher than SPF 8. The NP makes her recommendation to the patient based on the knowledge that:
    A. the large amount of deeply pigmented melanocytes will protect him from sun damage.
    B. the patient can sunburn and is still considered at risk for developing melanoma.
    C. the patient is not at risk for melanoma but should try to avoid sunburn to prevent skin damage.
    D. protecting his skin now will prevent premature skin aging.

25. Actinic keratosis is the most common lesion seen in dermatology. When providing education to the patient about actinic keratosis, the NP explains that it is a(n):
    A. form of skin cancer.
    B. precancerous lesion.
    C. area of increased pigmentation.
    D. area of hypopigmentation caused by sun damage.

Answers and Enhanced Rationales

1. Answer B is correct. "Morphology" is the term used to identify the shape. The terms "macule," "papule," or "patch" identify the shape of a lesion.

   Answer A is incorrect. This only gives information about the outer perimeters of the lesion.

   Answer C is incorrect. Erythema describes the appearance and color/pigmentation of a lesion.

   Answer D is incorrect. Scaly describes a heap of keratinized cells and flaky skin. Scaly lesions may be thick or thin, dry or oily, and vary in size and shape.

2. Answer D is correct. A patch is a flat, nonpalpable, irregular-shaped macule greater than 1 cm in diameter.

   Answer A is incorrect. A patch is a macule that is greater than 1 cm in size.

   Answer B is incorrect. A patch is flat, nonpalpable, and greater than 1 cm in size. This answer describes a papule.

   Answer C is incorrect. A patch is neither elevated nor palpable or less than 1 cm. Answer C describes plaque.

3. Answer B is correct. Vitiligo consists of hypopigmented lesions of varying size.

   Answer A is incorrect. This describes hives or wheals.

   Answer C is incorrect. Vitiligo is an autoimmune disorder. Loss of pigment is not related to injury at the base of the hair follicle.

   Answer D is incorrect. A progressive thickening and hardening of the epidermis describes the process of lichenification, which occurs with persistent or chronic rubbing, itching, or skin irritation.

4. Answer B is correct. The priority for this patient is to determine pregnancy status or assess if the patient is breastfeeding to determine the correct course of therapy.

   Answer A is incorrect. While it is helpful to determine if the tick was attached for longer than 48 hours, most patients will not know how long the tick has been attached, and the presence of an EM rash after tick removal is generally enough to diagnose Lyme disease.

   Answer C is incorrect. Two-step testing is recommended and should be ordered for this patient. However, it is not the priority as treatment should be started immediately for Lyme disease due to the patient's classic presentation of EM rash and history of recent tick bite.

   Answer D is incorrect. While this is the correct treatment for early-stage Lyme disease, assessing pregnancy/lactation status is a priority because doxycycline is contraindicated in pregnancy/lactation.

5. Answer D is correct. This is the only answer that provides reassurance to the patient by providing information that hair growth is likely to reoccu

   Answer A is incorrect. Some treatments that may help the patient with alopecia areata are topical steroids, Kenalog injections into the scalp, and minoxidil.

   Answer B is incorrect. Alopecia areata is an immune response in which the immune system attacks the hair follicles. It is most likely caused by a combination of genetic and environmental factors.

   Answer C is incorrect. Naftin is an antifungal agent used for tinea pedis or tinea corporis. Alopecia areata is not caused by a fungus.

6. **Answer B is correct.** The significantly larger scaly patch on the patient's abdomen is known as a "herald patch" and is a classic sign seen with pityriasis rosea.

   Answer A is incorrect. Roseola is a rash caused by the herpes virus. It generally occurs before age 3 and is commonly called the "sixth disease." The rash lasts approximately 3 days.

   Answer C is incorrect. A hypersensitivity response causes contact dermatitis. The patient generally complains of itching or burning in the affected areas.

   Answer D is incorrect. Rosacea is an inflammatory disorder affecting the nose, cheeks, forehead, and chin.

7. **Answer A is correct.** The patient is showing classic signs of impetigo, which is consistent with a history of scratching a pruritic lesion, such as a mosquito bite. This is caused by a *Staph aureus* or group A beta-hemolytic *Streptococcus* infection.

   Answer B is incorrect. Group B strep infection is commonly found in the gastrointestinal (GI) and genitourinary (GU) tracts. Newborns are susceptible to infection if the mother is positive for Group B strep in the GU tract.

   Answer C is incorrect. Any *Staph aureus* infection can be MRSA. However, there is no indication of this at the time of presentation, and the child had a mosquito bite that he was likely scratching.

   Answer D is incorrect. Tinea corporis is a fungal infection of the skin or scalp that appears as a circular patch with a raised scaly edge.

8. **Answer B is correct.** Shingles is contagious until all lesions are dried and crusted over. The patient should be instructed to avoid pregnant persons, immunocompromised individuals, and nonimmunized children who do not have a history of chicken pox.

   Answer A is incorrect. The patient is experiencing a reactivation of the varicella virus. However, the patient remains contagious while active lesions are not dried and crusted.

   Answer C is incorrect. The patient remains contagious until the vesicles are crusted over and dried, which may take 2 to 4 weeks.

   Answer D is incorrect. The rash may remain for several weeks and sometimes longer. During this time, the patient is contagious until all vesicles are crusted over. Antivirals, such as Zovirax, if started within 3 days, may decrease the symptoms and the duration of the outbreak.

9. **Answer D is correct.** Herpes zoster (shingles) is a virus and would respond best to antiviral treatment. The treatment should be started as early as possible to shorten the duration and intensity of the outbreak.

   Answer A is incorrect. Ketoconazole is an antifungal agent and is not effective for viruses.

   Answer B is incorrect. Lotrisone cream is a combination of an antifungal agent and a steroid cream. It is not an appropriate treatment for shingles.

   Answer C is incorrect. Diflucan is an antifungal agent. Herpes zoster is a virus.

10. **Answer B is correct.** Onychomycosis, by definition, is a fungal infection of the nails. Antifungal agents have the possibility of being hepatotoxic. Therapy should include complete blood count (CBC) and liver function tests (LFTs) every 4 to 6 weeks.

    Answer A is incorrect. Antifungal agents are not considered to be nephrotoxic.

    Answer C is incorrect. Coagulation factors are not needed to begin therapy if the liver function tests (LFTs) are within normal limits (WNL).

    Answer D is incorrect. The patient's immune competency should be assessed. If treatment is longer than 6 weeks, check CBC every 6 weeks.

11. **Answer B is correct.** The most appropriate treatment would be oral antihistamines, cool compresses, and oral corticosteroids.

    Answer A is incorrect. The patient is not experiencing any signs of anaphylaxis. However, it is appropriate to prescribe an EpiPen since further exposure to the antigen may cause anaphylaxis.

    Answer C is incorrect. A topical steroid would likely be ineffective since the patient is experiencing a significant histamine response.

    Answer D is incorrect. Oral antihistamines may provide some relief. However, this patient would benefit most from oral corticosteroids. Using warm compresses would increase vasodilation and make the symptoms worse.

12. **Answer C is correct.** Actinic keratosis is a precancerous lesion and the most common lesion in dermatology.

    Answer A is incorrect. Basal cell carcinoma is the most common *cancerous* lesion seen in dermatology.

    Answer B is incorrect. Squamous cell carcinoma is the second most common *cancerous* lesion seen in dermatology.

Answer D is incorrect. NMSC refers to all cancerous lesions of the skin that are not melanomas.

13. Answer C is correct. Isotretinoin is the most effective treatment of those listed.

    Answer A is incorrect. Exfoliation therapy removes the skin's most outer layer (epidermis) and is ineffective for cystic acne.

    Answer B is incorrect. Topical clindamycin is effective in treating mild acne because it slows the growth of bacteria on the skin. However, it is not the most effective treatment for cystic acne.

    Answer D is incorrect. Retinoids may be used for moderate to severe acne by reducing the amount of clogged pores or dead cells on the skin. They were first used in 1971. However, they are not the most effective treatment available.

14. Answer C is correct. The appearance of hyphae under the microscope indicates that dermatophytes are present. Also known as "ringworm," this is a common skin disorder.

    Answer A is incorrect. Herpes zoster (shingles) has an entirely different presentation due to the reemergence of the varicella virus.

    Answer B is incorrect. Seborrheic dermatitis is most common on the scalp (dandruff). It may be seen on the face, eyelids, ears, and chest and appears like patches of greasy skin covered with flaky white or yellow scales. It may disappear without treatment or with medicated shampoo.

    Answer D is incorrect. Onychomycosis is a fungal infection of the nails.

15. Answer B is correct. Persons with diabetes are more prone to skin conditions because both bacteria and fungi thrive in warm, moist environments where large amounts of glucose are present.

    Answer A is incorrect. The adolescent population has increased cases of acne vulgaris, which is commonly related to hormonal changes. Other than acne, they are not more prone to skin conditions than the general population.

    Answer C is incorrect. People who work outdoors may have an increased occurrence of skin cancers but not necessarily other skin conditions.

    Answer D is incorrect. Healthcare workers have increased exposure to organisms through contact. However, wearing PPE negates this risk.

16. Answer C is correct. Mohs surgery is designed to minimize the amount of tissue that needs to be removed while ensuring that all wound edges are clear of cancer.

    Answer A is incorrect. Mohs surgery removes the cancerous lesion, but there is no intention to remove surrounding lymph nodes.

    Answer B is incorrect. Removing only the lesion's surface area and cauterizing the underlying tissue is often used to remove noncancerous lesions.

    Answer D is incorrect. The purpose of Mohs surgery is to minimize the removal of healthy tissue.

17. Answer C is correct. Taut, shiny, hairless skin is most commonly seen in arterial insufficiency. Patients have decreased delivery of oxygen and nutrients to the area. Patients often complain of claudication, ulcers, or infections in the affected areas.

    Answer A is incorrect. Aging skin loses elasticity and subcutaneous tissue and has subsequent thinning.

    Answer B is incorrect. Venous insufficiency presents as a noticeable darkening of the skin to a dark brown, brown, yellow, or dark red. There may be skin ulceration and pain in the affected areas.

    Answer D is incorrect. Long-term sun exposure can lead to wrinkles, age spots, scaly patches (actinic keratosis), and an increased risk of skin cancer.

18. Answer B is correct. Using the ABCDE method, the NP would know that any mole larger than 6 mm in diameter should be excised and evaluated for possible melanoma.

    Answer A is incorrect. Although the location of the mole on the upper back is a concern, it is not the most concerning characteristic. In women, the melanoma lesions appear more often in their lower extremities, while in men, they seem more common on the torso, especially the back.

    Answer C is incorrect. The coloration of the mole is most significant if a mole changes color, looks different than the others present on the skin, or varies in colors within the mole itself.

    Answer D is incorrect. Melanomas commonly have an irregular, scalloped, or poorly defined border.

19. Answer C is correct. The patient presents with a classic appearance of erythema migrans, commonly called the "bull's-eye" rash. Inquiry should be made about whether the patient has been exposed to ticks recently.

Answer A is incorrect. The characteristics of this rash are not consistent with the appearance of the rash of tinea corporis (ringworm).

Answer B is incorrect. Patients who are immunocompromised are at greater risk of developing skin infections. However, this patient's presentation is inconsistent with any infection.

Answer D is incorrect. The classic presentation of this EM rash does not correlate to the appearance of a previous rash other than if the patient was undiagnosed and untreated for a previous infection with Lyme disease.

20. Answer B is correct. Men older than 50 have the highest rates of melanoma.

    Answer A is incorrect. Melanoma cases are highest in women aged 15 to 49.

    Answer C is incorrect. Although White persons with blue eyes and red or blond hair (thus more common to have lighter skin with less protective melanin) have a higher risk, the highest risk is associated with White men.

    Answer D is incorrect. White persons are commonly of northern European descent. However, age, sun exposure, and a history of blistering sunburns are the most significant risk factors.

21. Answer C is correct. Thickening or ulceration at the time of diagnosis is an important indicator of the prognosis for the patient.

    Answer A is incorrect. Although the number of blistering sunburns is a significant risk factor for the development of melanoma, it is not considered a *prognostic* indicator.

    Answer B is incorrect. A family history of melanoma is a risk factor but not a *prognostic* indicator.

    Answer D is incorrect. The diameter of the lesion is a characteristic to be considered with a melanoma. However, in and of itself, it is not a significant *prognostic* indicator.

22. Answer B is the correct answer. Any mole that has grown quickly should be immediately evaluated and biopsied, as this is a typical characteristic of a malignant melanoma.

    Answer A is incorrect. Although color is one of the considerations in the ABCDE evaluation method, a change in color or two or more colors in the same mole would have a larger significance.

    Answer C is incorrect. Any mole larger than 6 mm should be further evaluated. However, rapid growth "overnight" would be more concerning.

    This question has no information regarding the current size of the mole being assessed.

    Answer D is incorrect. Complaining of an itchy mole is not one of the characteristics assessed using the ABCDE method (asymmetry, border, color, diameter, evolving).

23. Answer B is correct. The number of blistering sunburns a person has had in their lifetime is a significant factor. A patient with one or more blistering sunburns doubles their chance of developing a melanoma.

    Answer A is incorrect. The number of melanocytes present is not the most significant factor for developing melanoma. Persons with darker skin have more melanocytes but can still burn their skin with UV rays.

    Answer C is incorrect. The amount of time a person spends outdoors is insignificant if the person is protecting the exposed skin areas with a sunscreen SPF 30 or greater.

    Answer D is incorrect. Free radicals are not a known factor in the development of malignant melanoma. Free radicals are linked to aging and oxidative stress, which theoretically will cause cell damage over time.

24. Answer B is the correct answer. Dark-skinned people have a larger number of melanocytes, but they can still sunburn and may still develop melanoma.

    Answer A is incorrect. All persons, regardless of skin color, should protect their skin from UV rays of the sun by wearing sunscreen with a SPF greater than 30.

    Answer C is incorrect. Any person, regardless of skin color, can potentially develop a melanoma. Age, sun exposure, and sunburn are all known risk factors. Dark-skinned persons are more than three times more likely to be diagnosed at later stages when it is more difficult to treat.

    Answer D is incorrect. Protecting his skin from the sun will help prevent premature skin aging later in life, but this is not the primary rationale for wearing sunscreen greater than SPF 30.

25. Answer B is correct. Actinic keratosis is the most common lesion seen in dermatology. It is important that the patient understand that these are precancerous lesions that need to be assessed and/or removed to prevent progression to skin cancer.

Answer A is incorrect. Actinic keratosis is not skin cancer, although it is a precancerous lesion.

Answer C is incorrect. Actinic keratosis is a rough, scaly skin patch that enlarges slowly. Cryosurgery is the most common treatment using liquid nitrogen.

Answer D is incorrect. It is not hypopigmented and is associated with chronic sun damage and exposure. The most valuable education is explaining to the patient that actinic keratosis is a precancerous lesion.

Resources

Kugeler, K. J., Earley, A., Mead, P. S., & Hinckley, A. F. (2022). Surveillance for Lyme disease after implementation of a revised case definition—United States. *MMWR Morbidity and Mortality Weekly, 73*, 118–123. http://dx.doi.org/10.15585/mmwr.mm7306a1

Lau, G. S. (2014). *Dermatology in primary care.* Unpublished manuscript—PowerPoint, Dermatology Associates of Glastonbury, Connecticut.

Lyons, F. (2015). *Solving skin rash in primary care.* Advance Healthcare Network for NPs and PAs. http://nurse-practitioners-and-physician-assistants.advanceweb.com/Features/Articles/Solving-Skin-Rash-in-Primary-Care.aspx

National Cancer Institute. (2018). *Common moles, dysplastic nevi, and risk of melanoma.* U.S. Department of Health and Human Services. https://www.cancer.gov/types/skin/moles-fact-sheet

Pietrangelo, A., & Potter, D. (2024). *Healthline.* Everything You Need to Know About Melanoma. https://www.healthline.com/health/skin-cancer/melanoma

Swetter, S., & Geller, A. (2014). Perspective: Catch melanoma early. *Nature, 515*(117). https://doi.org/10.1038/515S117a

PART IV

Reproductive Health, Pediatric and Adolescent Health, Gerontology, and Mental Health Review

CHAPTER 17	Women's Health and Female Reproductive System 325
CHAPTER 18	Men's Health 365
CHAPTER 19	Pediatrics 381
CHAPTER 20	Geriatrics 403
CHAPTER 21	Mental Health in Primary Care 425

CHAPTER 17

Women's Health and Female Reproductive System

Sarah E. DeNisco, MSN, APRN, FNP-BC

Normal Findings

Anatomy

Breasts

- "Tail of Spence"
  - Upper outer quadrant of the breast that extends into the axillary region
  - Common site for breast cancer development
- Simple Breast Cysts
  - Benign, fluid-filled cysts that are round or oval
  - Common in women between 35 to 50 years
- Fibroadenomas
  - Benign tumor that presents as a well-defined, mobile mass on physical examination or ultrasound
  - They persist during the reproductive years, may increase in size during pregnancy or with estrogen therapy, and usually regress after menopause due to a hormonal relationship.
  - Common in women between 15 to 35 years
  - An ultrasound is the imaging test of choice, but some women may need a needle biopsy to confirm the diagnosis.

Cervix

- Cervix: a fibrous, muscular band that holds the bottom of the uterus closed and keeps the fetus inside during pregnancy
- Cervical Ectropion
  - Benign finding. Occurs when cells from inside the cervical canal grow onto the outside surface of the cervix
  - Presents as bright-red, bumpy tissue with an irregular surface
  - Often seen with increased estrogen production (e.g., pregnancy, use of birth control pills). It can change in size/shape and will regress over time.

Uterus

- The uterus consists of two sections: the upper portion (which contains the uterine corpus and fundus) and the lower portion (which contains the cervix).
- It is the organ of menstruation. The fertilized egg implants here, maintaining and protecting the developing fetus until birth.
- Uterine Fibroids (Leiomyoma)
  - It can cause the uterus to feel firm, nontender, irregularly enlarged, and textured.
  - The patient may be asymptomatic or present with heavy menstrual bleeding, pelvic pain or cramping, and bleeding between periods (pain is most commonly present after 35 years).
  - Usually benign; it can cause urgency if the fibroid is pressing on the bladder.
  - On rare occasions, fibroids can be malignant and cause uterine cancer.

🚩 Red Flag

Dominant Breast Mass/Breast Cancer
- Painless, hard, immovable, single dominant lesion with irregular borders
- Nurse practitioner (NP) should order a mammogram and refer patient to a breast surgeon for biopsy.

Inflammatory Breast Cancer
- Acute onset of a red, swollen, and warm area in the breast that is rapidly growing
- May also present with breast tenderness or itching, axillary adenopathy, and skin thickening or dimpling ("peau d'orange")
- May mimic mastitis. Suspect in women with progressive breast inflammation that does not respond to antibiotics.

Paget's Disease
- Raw, scaly, vesicular, or ulcerated lesion that begins on the nipple and spreads to the areola of one breast
- Patient may complain of itching, pain, or burning sensation.
- Half of women will have a breast mass.

BRCA-1 and BRCA-2 Associated Hereditary Breast and Ovarian Cancer
- Patients with a personal or family history of breast, ovarian, prostate, or pancreatic cancer may benefit from genetic counseling so that they may evaluate their risk for these cancers.
- Women with BRCA1 or BRCA2 gene mutation (or both) have up to a 72 percent risk of being diagnosed with breast cancer in their lifetime.
- Breast cancer susceptibility genes are inherited in an autosomal dominant pattern. Ashkenazi Jewish people (European ethnicity Jewish) are at higher risk for BRCA 1/2 mutations.
- Women who have a high lifetime risk should undergo an annual screening mammogram, annual breast MRI, and clinical breast exam every 6 to 12 months beginning 10 years before the age of diagnosis of the youngest family member.

Ovarian Cancer
- Patients may present with vague symptoms of abdominal bloating or discomfort, low-back pain, pelvic pain, dyspareunia, changes in bowel habits, and unusual fatigue.
- Most patients are diagnosed when it has already spread beyond the ovary, which accounts for the poor survival rate.
- Assess family history of two or more first- or second-degree relatives with a history of ovarian cancer, a combination of ovarian and breast cancer, or have an Ashkenazi Jewish ethnicity. Women with high-risk family history should be referred for genetic counseling and testing.

Ovaries
- Maturation, development, and ejection of eggs. The ovaries secrete hormones, including estrogen, progesterone, and testosterone.
- Palpable Ovary
  - The ovaries become atrophied during menopause. A palpable ovary in a menopausal woman is always abnormal.
  - If palpable, order a pelvic/intravaginal ultrasound and refer to a gynecologist to rule out ovarian cancer.

Menstrual Cycle

Phases
- Normal bleeding with menses occurs every 26 to 40 days. No two women are alike, and each has a unique cycle. The following is based on a 28-day menstrual cycle:
- Follicular (Days 1 to 14)
  - The hypothalamus signals the anterior pituitary gland to release follicle-stimulating hormone (FSH) → FSH stimulates the ovaries to produce follicles, which each contain an immature egg → the healthiest egg will eventually mature, while the rest of the follicles are reabsorbed into the body → the maturing follicle creates a surge in estrogen, which thickens the lining of the uterus to prepare a nutrient-rich environment for a potential embryo
- Ovulatory (Day 14)
  - Rising estrogen levels during the follicular phase trigger the anterior pituitary gland to release luteinizing hormone (LH) → the

ovary releases the mature egg, which migrates down the fallopian tube toward the uterus to be fertilized by sperm
- Luteal (Days 14 to 28)
  - After the follicle releases the egg, it transforms into the corpus luteum. This structure releases progesterone and estrogen, which keeps the uterine lining thick and ready for fertilized egg implantation → if conception occurs, human chorionic gonadotropin (hCG) will be produced to maintain the corpus luteum and thick uterine lining → if conception does not occur, the corpus luteum will shrink and be reabsorbed. This leads to decreased levels of estrogen and progesterone, which causes the onset of menstruation
- Menstruation
  - The thickened lining of the uterus is no longer needed to support a pregnancy, so it sheds through the vaginal canal → low hormone levels stimulate the hypothalamus, and the cycle starts again

Routine Health Maintenance and Laboratory Procedures

Mammogram

- The American Cancer Society screening recommendations for women at average breast cancer risk:
  - 40 to 44: option to begin annual mammography
  - 45 to 54: annual mammography
  - 55 and older: annual or biannual mammography
  - 75 and older: a woman and her provider should share in the decision regarding her screening based on her health history, individual concerns, and priorities

Cervical Cytology ("Pap Test")

- The U.S. Preventive Services Task Force (USPSTF) and the American College of Obstetricians and Gynecologists screening recommendations for women at average risk of cervical cancer:
  - < 20: do not screen (regardless of age of onset of sexual activity)
  - 21 to 29: screen with cytology alone every 3 years
  - 30 to 65: screen with cytology alone every 3 years OR co-testing with cytology and human papillomavirus (HPV) testing every 5 years
  - 65 and older: can stop screening unless at high risk for cervical cancer
  - Note: HIV-positive women and those with a history of cervical cancer or diethylstilbestrol exposure may require more frequent screening and should not follow the routine guidelines.

Human Papillomavirus DNA Test

- HPV types 16 and 18 cause nearly all cases of cervical cancer. Women are exposed to high-risk HPV through sexual intercourse.
- HPV vaccine: "Gardasil"
  - If given between the ages of 9 and 14, a two-dose series is required; the second dose is given 6 to 12 months after the initial dose.
  - If given between the ages of 15 to 26, vaccination is given in a three-dose series.
  - Vaccine doses do not have to be repeated if the vaccine schedule is interrupted.
  - Vaccination is not recommended for those older than 26 years, but some adults 27 years or older may benefit from HPV immunization (e.g., no history of sexual intercourse)

The Bethesda System

- Standardized system for reporting cervical cytology results
- Atypical Squamous Cells of Undetermined Significance (ASCUS)
  - Cells appear mildly abnormal, but the cause cannot be identified (e.g., infection, irritation, precancer)
  - Ages 21 to 24: repeat Pap test in 12 months
  - Ages 25 to 29: complete reflex HPV test
  - 30 and older: co-test for high-risk HPV; if HPV is positive, refer for colposcopy
- Atypical Squamous Cells and Cannot Exclude a High-Grade Squamous Intraepithelial Lesion (ASC-H)
  - Cells appear abnormal. A possible precancer is present and requires more testing and possible treatment.
  - Age 21 and older: refer for colposcopy
- Atypical Glandular Cells
  - More common in women 40 to 69 years old. Associated with premalignancy or malignancy in 30 percent of cases; risk of cancer increases with age.
  - Follow-up tests include colposcopy, endocervical sampling, and endometrial sampling.

- Low-Grade Squamous Intraepithelial Lesions (LSILs)
  - Presence of mildly abnormal cells, usually caused by HPV infection
  - Age 21 to 24: repeat Pap test in 12 months
  - Age 25 to 29: refer for colposcopy
  - 30 and older: repeat Pap in 12 months or refer for colposcopy
- High-Grade Squamous Intraepithelial Lesions (HSILs)
  - More serious changes in the cervix than LSILs. More likely to be associated with precancer or cancer
  - Age 21 to 24: refer for colposcopy
  - 25 and older: refer for immediate excisional treatment or colposcopy. It can be done by loop electrosurgical excision procedure (LEEP) with cervical conization or surgery of the cervix.

Clinical Pearls

- Applying a small amount of lubricant jelly to the tips of a speculum before performing a pelvic exam will not affect Pap test results. This will provide comfort to women with atrophic vaginitis (e.g., reduces pain and vaginal bleeding)
- Cervical ectropions may be present or larger in adolescents and adult women on birth control pills
- Cervical cancer 5-year survival rate: localized = 92 percent, regional spread = 56 percent, distant metastasis = 17 percent

Exam Success Tips

- If a reproductive-age female presents with acute abdominal or pelvic pain, always order a pregnancy test first.
- A palpable ovary in a menopausal female is never normal. Order an intravaginal ultrasound to rule out ovarian cancer.
- If a hard, irregular, immobile breast mass is palpated, order a mammogram and refer the patient to a breast specialist to evaluate for breast cancer.
- Annual mammograms begin at 45 years old, but evaluate risk in patients between 40 to 44 years.
- Pap and HPV testing are not recommended before the age of 21 years, even if the patient is sexually active, has an STI, or has multiple sex partners.
- A colposcopy is a test used to visualize the cervix and obtain cervical biopsy.

Colposcopy

- A colposcope is a specialized "microscope" used to visualize the cervix, obtain cervical biopsies, and gain access to the cervix during cryotherapy or laser ablative therapy.
- The diagnostic test for cervical cancer is a biopsy of the cervix, which is obtained during a colposcopy.

Contraception

Combined Hormonal Contraceptives

Overview

Combined hormonal contraception (estrogen and progesterone) works by stopping ovulation (inhibiting the LH surge) and thickening the cervical mucus plug.

Combined Oral Contraceptives (*typical use failure rate: 9 percent*)

- Dosed Monophasic Pills
  - Loestrin FE 1/20: 21 days of estrogen/progesterone and 7 days placebo pills (contain iron supplementation)
- Biphasic Pills
  - Ortho-Novum 10/11: contains two different progesterone doses; the dose increases halfway through the cycle
- Triphasic Pills
  - Ortho Tri-Cyclen: 21 days of active pills and 7 days of placebo pills; the dose of hormones varies weekly for 3 weeks
- Ethinyl Estradiol and Drospirenone
  - Yaz 28/Yasmin: 24 days of active pills and 4 days of placebo pills. Results in lighter menses and lower rates of unscheduled bleeding. Consider for women with acne, PCOS, hirsutism, or premenstrual dysphoric disorder. However, there is a higher risk of deep vein thrombosis (DVT) and hyperkalemia.
- Extended-Cycle Oral Contraceptive Pills
  - Seasonale: contains 84 consecutive days (3 months) of estrogen/progesterone with a 7-day pill-free interval. This method results in four periods per year, although breakthrough bleeding is not uncommon during the first few months.

Non-Oral Forms (*typical use failure rate: 7 percent*)

- Cervical Ring
  - Transparent, flexible ring of a polymer that is infused with etonogestrel. The ring is inserted vaginally for 21 days and removed for a

1-week ring-free period when the woman will have her menses.
- Ortho Evra Transdermal Contraceptive Patch
  - A thin, flexible patch that is effective for 7 days. The woman will use each patch for 7 days and replace it weekly for 3 weeks. In the 4th week of her cycle, she goes without a patch for 7 days, and her menses occurs.
  - The patch results in higher levels of estrogen exposure compared with oral contraceptives (e.g., higher risk of blood clots, DVT).

Contraindications to Combined Hormonal Contraceptive Use

- Any condition (past or present) that increases the risk of blood clotting:
  - History of thrombophlebitis or thromboembolic disorders
  - Genetic coagulation defects
  - Major surgery with prolonged immobilization
- Person who smokes and is older than the age of 35, greater than 15 cigarettes per day
  - Note: A person who smokes and is younger than the age of 35 is considered a relative risk.
- Any condition that increases the risk of strokes
  - Migraine with aura or focal neurological symptoms
  - History of cerebrovascular accidents (CVAs) or transient ischemic attacks (TIAs)
  - Hypertension (Systolic Blood Pressure [SBP] >160 mmHg or Diastolic BP [DBP] >100 mmHg)
- Inflammation and/or acute infections of the liver with elevated liver function tests (LFTs)
  - Hepatocellular adenomas or hepatomas
  - Cholestatic jaundice of pregnancy
  - When LFTs are back to normal, the patient can go back on birth control pills.
- Known or suspected cardiovascular disease
  - Moderately to severely impaired cardiac function
  - Complicated valvular heart disease
  - Coronary artery disease
  - Diabetes with a vascular component
  - Systemic lupus erythematosus
  - Hypertension if SBP ≥160 or DBP ≥ 100 mmHg
    - Note: Adequately controlled hypertension is considered a relative risk.
- Some reproductive system conditions or cancers
  - Known or suspected pregnancy
  - Undiagnosed genital bleeding or breast mass
  - Breast, endometrial, or ovarian cancer (or any estrogen-dependent cancer)
  - Less than 21 days postpartum

Advantages of Combined Hormonal Pill (After 5 or More Years of Use)

- Decreased risk of ovarian and endometrial cancer
- Decreased incidence of dysmenorrhea and cramps, pelvic pain for patients with endometriosis, heavy and/or irregular periods, acne, and hirsutism

Disadvantages of Combined Hormonal Contraceptives

- Unscheduled bleeding
  - Spotting may occur during the first few weeks after starting the contraceptive; for most, this will resolve spontaneously in 3 months.
  - If the patient has continued spotting, an option is to switch to an oral contraceptive with a higher dose of estrogen (e.g., from 10 mcg EE to 30 mcg EE)
- Nausea and breast tenderness
  - Occurs during the first few days; symptoms should resolve spontaneously in 1 month
- Potential to miss pills
  - Missed 1 day → take two pills now and continue with the same pill pack ("doubling up"); continue taking remaining pills at the usual time
  - Missed 2 consecutive days → take the most recent missed pill as soon as possible (even if it means taking two pills the same day); discard any leftover missed pills; continue taking remaining pills at the usual time; use backup contraception (condoms) or avoid sex until hormonal pills have been taken for 7 days
  - Pill missed on the last week of hormonal pills → omit hormone-free (or placebo) pills by finishing the hormonal pills in the current pack and starting a new pill pack the next day; use backup contraception until hormonal pills have been taken for 7 consecutive days
- Drug interactions with oral contraceptives
  - These drugs can decrease the efficacy of oral contraceptives. Advise patients to use an alternative form of birth control (condoms) when taking these drugs and for one pill cycle afterward:
    - Anticonvulsants: phenobarbital, phenytoin
    - Antifungals: griseofulvin (Fulvicin), ketoconazole (Nizoral)

- HIV/hepatitis C virus (HCV) protease inhibitors: indinavir, boceprevir
- Certain antibiotics: ampicillin, tetracyclines, rifampin, clarithromycin
- St. John's wort: may cause breakthrough bleeding

Prescribing a Contraceptive

- Rule out pregnancy.
- Perform a thorough health history to determine if the patient has any contraindications.
- Check blood pressure (BP) to rule out hypertension.
- A physical/pelvic examination, Pap test, STI testing, and laboratory blood testing are not required for initiating contraception in most healthy patients.
  - Exception is a pelvic exam before insertion of an IUD (to rule out an abnormal uterus or cervicitis) and when fitting a patient for a diaphragm
- Oral contraceptives can be started anytime in the menstrual cycle:
  - Quick start: start taking the pill on the day prescribed
  - Day 1 start: take the first pill during the first day of the menstrual period
  - Sunday start: take the first pill on the first Sunday after the menstrual period starts
- Instruct the patient to use backup methods during the first week of the first pill pack.
- A follow-up visit is needed within 2 to 3 months to check blood pressure, assess side effects, and answer patient questions.

> **Red Flag**
>
> **Pill Danger Signals**
> These signs indicate a possible thromboembolic event. Advise patient to report these or call 911 if symptoms "ACHES":
> - **A**bdominal pain → ischemic pain of the mesenteric artery caused by a blot clot
> - **C**hest pain → blood clot in a coronary artery
> - **H**eadaches → stroke, TIA
> - **E**ye problems or change in vision → blood clot in the retinal artery of affected eye
> - **S**evere leg pain → blood clot on a deep vein of the leg

Progesterone-Only Contraceptives

Depo-Provera *(typical use failure rate: 4 percent)*

- Injectable hormonal contraceptive that is given intramuscularly every 3 months
- Check for pregnancy before starting the dose
- May be given to breastfeeding patients if administered in the 6th postpartum week
- If on Depo-Provera for > 1 year, amenorrhea may occur due to severe uterine atrophy from lack of estrogen.
- If on Depo-Provera for > 2 to 5 years, the patient is at risk for osteopenia and osteoporosis.
  - Do not prescribe to women with a history of anorexia nervosa.
  - Recommend calcium with vitamin D and weight-bearing exercises.
- Avoid in women who want to become pregnant in 12 months (causes delayed return of fertility and may take up to 1 year to start ovulating).
- Other adverse effects: weight gain, acne, depression

Etonogestrel Contraceptive Implant *(typical use failure rate: 0.1 percent)*

- A thin, plastic rod inserted on the inner aspect of the upper arm subdermally (nondominant arm) contains a long-acting form of progestin (etonogestrel).
- Nexplanon (one rod) is effective for up to 3 years; Norplant II (two rods) is effective for up to 5 years.
- Initially, unscheduled bleeding is common, but when the endometrial lining atrophies, amenorrhea results.
- 1 out of 10 women stop using the implant due to unfavorable changes in menstrual bleeding.
- Ovulation may not occur for a few weeks to 12 months after removal.

Progestin-Only Pills *(typical failure rate: 7 percent)*

- Also known as the "mini-pill"; Micronor (norethindrone 0.35 mg), start pill on day 1 of menstrual cycle
- Safe for women who have higher body mass and are breastfeeding.
- It is important to take the pill at the same time each day; if the dose is late (> 3 hours) or a day is missed, the woman should use condoms or abstain from sexual intercourse for 2 days.
- If a patient vomits or has severe diarrhea within 3 hours of taking a dose, take another pill as soon

as possible; continue taking pills at the same time each day and use backup contraception.

Emergency Contraception ("Morning-After Pill") (*89 percent effective*)

- Most effective if taken within 72 hours after unprotected sexual intercourse or if 2 consecutive days of birth control pills are skipped
- Women and men of all ages can get emergency contraceptive pills (except ulipristal acetate) without a prescription in the United States.
- Levonorgestrel (Plan B)
  - Take the first dose as soon as possible (up to 72 hours after) and the second dose in 12 hours.
  - The medication may cause nausea (because of the estrogen); encourage over-the-counter antiemetics (antihistamine drug class); if the patient vomits a tablet within 1 hour of ingestion, she may need to repeat the dose.
- Advise patient that if she does not have a normal period in the next 3 weeks, she should return for follow-up to rule out pregnancy.

Advantages

- Preferred for those who cannot take combination options (e.g., breastfeeding mothers, age greater than 35, and a person who smokes or has migraines with aura, or diabetics with vascular disease)

Disadvantages

- There is a continuous need for compliance; must be taken at the same time every day (3-hour window)
- Still should not be used in those with active cancers or liver disease

Other Contraceptive Methods

Intrauterine Device

Levonorgestrel (LNG) 0.1% to 0.4%/Copper; typical use failure rate: 0.8 percent
- A small device is inserted into the uterus through the cervix by a trained healthcare provider. A baseline pelvic examination, Pap test, pregnancy test, and STI screening must be performed before insertion.
- Two types
  - Hormonal: Levonorgestrel intrauterine device (IUD, Mirena), effective up to 5 years, slightly more effective than copper-bearing IUD
  - Nonhormonal: Copper IUD (ParaGard), effective up to 10 years, can cause heavy menstrual bleeding and cramping the first few months of use
- Advantages
  - Long-term protection from pregnancy
  - Immediate return to fertility upon removal of the IUD
  - The patient may have lighter periods or amenorrhea within 1 year (Mirena IUD).
- Disadvantages
  - Needs to be inserted by a healthcare provider
  - Potential perforation of the uterus when inserted
  - Possible unintentional expulsion of IUD
  - Increased risk of STIs if the woman or her partner has multiple partners
  - Increased risk of endometrial or pelvic infections in the first few months after insertion
  - Heavy or prolonged periods (Cu-IUD)
- Contraindications
  - Active pelvic inflammatory disease (PID) or history of PID within the past year
  - Suspected or confirmed pregnancy or has an STI
  - Uterine or cervical abnormality
  - Undiagnosed vaginal bleeding or uterine/cervical cancer
  - History of ectopic pregnancy
- Patient Education
  - Patients should periodically check for missing or shortened string, especially after each menstrual period. Order a pelvic ultrasound if the patient or clinician does not feel the string.

Barrier Methods

Condoms

- Male Condoms (*typical use failure rate: 18 percent*)
  - More effective than female condoms
- Female Condoms (*typical use failure rate: 21 percent*)
  - Do not use with any oil- or silicone-based lubricants or creams
- Advantages
  - Convenient and relatively inexpensive
  - Able to purchase without a healthcare provider's prescription
  - Offers protection from STIs

- Disadvantages
  - May interrupt foreplay
  - Can cause irritation if the patient has a latex allergy
  - Must be applied and removed correctly to prevent spilling of semen into the vagina

Diaphragm with Contraceptive Gel and Cervical Cap (typical use failure rate: 17 percent)

- Overview
  - Both the diaphragm and cervical cap require a prescription and must be fitted.
  - The diaphragm must be used with spermicidal gel. After intercourse, leave the diaphragm inside the vagina for at least 6 to 8 hours (it can remain inside the vagina for up to 24 hours). The cervical cap can be left in the vagina for up to 2 days.
  - Need additional spermicide application before every act of intercourse. Apply the spermicidal foam/gel inside the vagina without removing the diaphragm.
- Disadvantages
  - Not as effective as hormonal forms of contraception. The cervical cap is less effective than a diaphragm. After vaginal birth, the failure rate of the cervical cap increases to 29 percent.
  - The cervical cap may cause abnormal cervical cellular change (abnormal Pap).
  - Vaginal and cervical irritation increases the risk of HIV infection, urinary tract infections, and toxic shock syndrome (rare).

Sponge (typical use failure rate: nulliparous 14 percent/ multiparous 27 percent)

- Overview
  - Purchased OTC. Made from a soft foam that contains spermicide. It is inserted inside the vagina so that it covers the cervix.
  - It can be inserted up to 24 hours before sex, and it should be left in place at least 6 hours after sexual intercourse. The sponge should not be worn for more than 30 total hours.

Clinical Pearls

- Yaz/Yasmin contains estrogen and drospirenone. It has a higher risk of blood clots, stroke, heart attacks, and hyperkalemia.
- Do not recommend Depo-Provera for women who want to become pregnant in 12 to 18 months because it may cause delayed return of fertility. It can take up to 1 year for some women to start ovulating.
- Cu-IUD has the broadest indication for use as a contraceptive for women with medical conditions (e.g., diabetics, person who smokes for more than 35 years, patients on anticonvulsant or antiretroviral therapy, and those with ovarian cancer, ischemic heart disease, or liver tumors).

Exam Success Tips

- Minors do not need parental consent for STD treatment, contraception, or pregnancy care.
- Rule out pregnancy prior to prescribing contraception.
- Desogen, Ortho-TriCyclen, and Yaz/Yasmin are all indicated for treatment of acne.
- If a patient misses 2 consecutive pills, take the most recent missed pill as soon as possible. Discard any leftover missed pills. Continue taking remaining pills at the usual time and use backup contraception for 7 consecutive days.
- Avoid using Depo-Provera in anorexic and/or bulimic patients (very high risk of osteoporosis).
- Women taking Seasonale (84 days hormones/7 days placebo pill) will have only four periods per year.
- Mefenamic acid (Ponstel) is an NSAID that is very effective for menstrual pain.
- Plan B is most effective if taken within 72 hours of unprotected sexual intercourse.
- Cu-IUD lasts 10 years. Mirena IUD lasts 5 years.
- Some questions will ask for the best birth control method for a case scenario. Remember the contraindications or adverse effects of each method (e.g., combined hormonal contraceptives or Depo-Provera).

Disease Review

Fibrocystic Changes of the Breast

Etiology

- Definition
  - Fibrocystic changes of the breast are a benign condition. There is a thickening of breast tissue and the development of fluid-filled cysts in one or both breasts.
- Incidence
  - Commonly occurs in reproductive-aged women between 25 to 50 years old

- Risk Factors
  - Related to the menstrual cycle (will enlarge right before menses and shrink after)
  - Increased stress, a diet high in saturated fat, and excessive caffeine intake may potentiate symptoms.

Clinical Presentation

- History of Present Illness
  - Premenstrual, cyclic breast pain and breast lumps with tenderness, swelling, and fullness to touch that has occurred for several years
  - Once menstruation starts, the tenderness lessens, and the size of the breast lumps decreases.
- Physical Assessment Findings
  - The breast tissue may feel dense, with thicker tissue areas having an irregular, nodular, or ridge-like surface.
  - If a mass is present, it is mobile with discrete edges, not attached to the skin, and feels rubbery to firm texture.
  - The nipple and/or breast may feel tender.

Clinical Management

- Laboratory and Diagnostic Studies
  - Diagnostic mammogram and breast ultrasound (to exclude breast cancer)
- Pharmacologic
  - First line
    - Analgesics and anti-inflammatory medication to reduce breast pain and swelling (e.g., oral and topical NSAIDs or acetaminophen)
  - Second line
    - Oral contraceptives with low estrogen content to modulate symptoms
- Nonpharmacologic
  - Cool compresses, avoiding trauma to breasts, wearing a well-fitting, supportive brassiere, reduction in caffeine, supplementation of vitamin E and primrose oil
- Indication for Referral
  - Refer to a breast surgeon for fine-needle aspiration/biopsy if indicated by mammogram/ultrasound.

Evaluation and Follow-Up

- Follow-up times are variable; depends on the clinical situation and pertinent family history

Breast Cancer

Etiology

- Definition
  - Malignant neoplasm of cells native to the breast: epithelial, glandular, or stroma
- Incidence
  - Incidence rates have increased by 1 percent between 2012 and 2021
  - It is the most diagnosed cancer in women and the second most common cause of cancer death for women in the United States.
- Risk Factors
  - Nonmodifiable risk factors: age > 50 years, genetic mutations (BRCA 1/2), early menarche (< 12 years), late menopause (> 55 years), dense breast tissue, personal or family history of breast cancer, radiation therapy to the chest/breast before age 30, mother took diethylstilbestrol (DES) between 1940–1971
  - Modifiable risk factors: not being physically active, overweight or higher weight after menopause, hormones taken during menopause for more than 5 years, pregnancy at age 30 years or older, not breastfeeding, nulliparity, moderate-to-high alcohol intake

Clinical Presentation

- History of Present Illness
  - Fixed, nonmoveable, painless lump in breast or axilla
  - Swelling, thickening, redness, or dimpling of the skin
  - Nipple discharge (bloody), erosion, or retraction
  - Symptoms of metastases include back or leg pain (bone), nausea, jaundice, anorexia (liver), shortness of breath, cough (lung), or headache (brain)
- Physical Assessment Findings
  - Visualize breasts and axillary region, looking for masses, skin dimpling, peau d'orange, and asymmetry.

Clinical Management

- Laboratory and Diagnostic Studies
  - Age > 30: order diagnostic mammogram and breast ultrasound (to determine if cystic or solid); if abnormal, refer to a breast specialist.
  - Age < 30: order breast ultrasound with/without diagnostic mammogram; if there is low clinical suspicion, may observe for one or two menstrual cycles.

- Present skin changes (peau d'orange, dimpling): order a diagnostic mammogram and refer the patient to a breast specialist for a biopsy.
- Treatment
  - Chemotherapy, radiation therapy, surgery (lumpectomy, mastectomy)
- Patient Education
  - Maintain a healthy weight, limit alcohol use, and consider vitamin D supplementation.

Evaluation and Follow-Up
- Follow-up every 4 to 6 months for 5 years and then annually

Galactorrhea
Etiology
- Definition
  - Milky nipple discharge that is not associated with gestation or present for longer than 1 year after weaning
  - Does not include serous, purulent, or bloody nipple discharge
- Incidence
  - Predominantly occurs in ages 20 to 35
- Risk Factors
  - Physiologic causes: pregnancy, nipple stimulation, piercing
  - Pathophysiologic causes: hyperprolactinemia, chest wall trauma, herpes zoster
  - Pharmacologic causes: opioids, psychiatric medications, oral contraceptives

Clinical Presentation
- History of Present Illness
  - Spontaneous or induced bilateral nipple discharge that may appear milky white or brown
- Physical Assessment Findings
  - Look for physical signs of associated conditions (e.g., acromegaly, adrenal insufficiency, chest wall conditions, hypogonadism, hypothyroidism, polycystic ovarian syndrome, pituitary macroadenoma, etc.)

Clinical Management
- Laboratory and Diagnostic Studies
  - Labs: pregnancy test, prolactin level, thyroid-stimulating hormone (TSH), liver and renal function; consider FSH and LH levels if amenorrheic; consider growth hormone levels if acromegaly suspected
- Treatment Goals
  - Identify and treat the underlying cause.
  - Discontinue causative agents, if possible.
- Pharmacologic
  - Dopamine agonists (e.g., cabergoline, bromocriptine) work to reduce prolactin levels and shrink tumor size.
  - Treatment is discontinued when tumor size has been reduced/regressed or after pregnancy has been achieved.
- Nonpharmacologic
  - Ingestion of peppermint, parsley, or sage
  - Topical application of cabbage leaves over breast tissue
- Patient Education
  - Avoid excess nipple stimulation
  - Warn about symptoms of mass enlargement in the pituitary gland (e.g., vision changes, headaches)
  - Offending medications should be discontinued long term
- Indication for Referral
  - Consider surgery or radiotherapy for patients not responding to medication

Evaluation and Follow-Up
- Check prolactin levels every 6 weeks until normalized and then every 6 to 12 months.
- Monitor visual fields and/or obtain annual MRI until stable for prolactinoma.

Atrophic Vaginitis
Etiology
- Definition
  - Inflammation, drying, and thinning of vaginal tissues caused by decreased estrogen levels
- Incidence
  - Predominantly occurs in postmenopausal women
- Risk Factors
  - Estrogen-deficient states (including lactation), smoking, alcohol use, sexual abstinence or decreased frequency of coital activity, lack of exercise, absence of vaginal childbirth, chemotherapy, radiation therapy

Clinical Presentation
- History of Present Illness
  - Vaginal burning and itching, dyspareunia, vulvar or vaginal bleeding after intercourse,

increased urinary frequency, urinary incontinence, recurrent UTIs
- Physical Assessment Findings
  - Loss of pubic hair; decreased vulvar and vaginal fullness; fusion of labia minora; vulvar erythema or ecchymosis; decreased vulvar subcuticular fat and moisture; pale-appearing, shiny, smooth vaginal and urethral epithelium; vaginal shortening (pain with speculum examination); loss of vaginal rugation; pelvic organ prolapse; urethral atrophy; Bartholin gland atrophy; cervical atrophy; and stenosis of os

Clinical Management

- Laboratory and Diagnostic Studies
  - Generally unnecessary to determine a diagnosis, but the following may be obtained: FSH and estrogen levels, evaluation for infections via wet preparation and vaginal pH, urinalysis if suspected urinary tract infection (UTI), and transvaginal ultrasound.
- Pharmacologic
  - Mild symptoms: nonhormonal, vaginal moisturizers and lubricants (e.g., "Replens"); use 2 to 3 days per week routinely
  - Moderate to severe symptoms: local endocrine therapy (vaginal estrogen) → comes in several forms (cream, tablet, capsule, or vaginal ring); progesterone supplementation is also needed if using long term to decrease the risk of endometrial hyperplasia.
  - Vasomotor symptoms in addition to atrophic vaginitis: systemic hormonal therapy (use in lowest possible dose for shortest duration of time)
  - Not responsive to therapy or contraindications to vaginal estrogen: nonestrogen therapy (e.g., ospemifene)
- Nonpharmacologic
  - Wear loose-fitting, undyed cotton underwear; avoid prolonged pad use, especially scented pads; avoid feminine deodorant sprays and douching; increase coital activity; smoking cessation
- Patient Education
  - Symptoms should improve within 30 to 60 days; if they do not, reevaluate and reexamine for other causes.
  - Lactating postpartum women are in a hypoestrogenic state; these women should be instructed to use lubrication for symptoms of dyspareunia.
- Indication for Referral
  - Refer to urogynecologist for evaluation if symptomatic due to pelvic organ prolapse and/or refractory stress and urge urinary incontinence.
  - Recurrent UTIs should be further evaluated and may require referral to urogynecology and/or urology.

Lichen Sclerosus

Etiology

- Definition
  - Benign, chronic, progressive, dermatologic condition characterized by marked inflammation, epithelial thinning, and distinctive dermal changes that may be accompanied by pruritus or pain
- Incidence
  - It can occur at any age but most commonly occurs during the prepubertal period and the perimenopause to postmenopausal period.
- Risk Factors
  - Family history, history of autoimmune conditions, hypoestrogenic states

Clinical Presentation

- History of Present Illness
  - Vulvar pruritus, anal discomfort, dyspareunia, dysuria
- Physical Assessment Findings
  - Classic lichen sclerosus presents as white, atrophic papules and macules that may coalesce into plaques; it can also be hemorrhagic, purpuric, hyperkeratotic, bullous, eroded, or ulcerated.
  - Scratching may result in excoriations and secondary, mild lichenification, which is often associated with edema of the labia minora and the prepuce.

Clinical Management

- Laboratory and Diagnostic Studies
  - Diagnosis can often be made upon recognizing clinical manifestations.
  - When necessary, a biopsy can be performed to confirm a diagnosis.
- Pharmacologic
  - Superpotent topical corticosteroid (e.g., clobetasol propionate)

- Nonpharmacologic
  - Avoid scratching, implement good vulvar hygiene practices, daily use of a fragrance-free emollient, use of a vaginal lubricant during intercourse
- Patient Education
  - Proper application technique for topical treatments
  - Risk for malignancy and need for reassessment if new, hyperkeratotic plaques, ulcers, or erosions present or failure to improve with treatment in 2 weeks
  - Resources for psychological support or sexual counseling
- Indication for Referral
  - Referral to a vulvar specialist is beneficial for patients with a disease that responds poorly to topical corticosteroids or patients with a history of vulvar intraepithelial neoplasia or vulvar squamous cell carcinoma.

Evaluation and Follow-Up

- Patients with well-controlled disease and a stable treatment plan should be examined at least once yearly.

Vulvovaginal Candidiasis

Etiology

- Definition
  - Overgrowth of *Candida albicans* yeast in the vulva/vagina
- Incidence
  - *Candida albicans* are normal oral and GI tract flora present in more than 70 percent of the U.S. population.
- Risk Factors
  - Immune suppression, corticosteroid use, smoking, alcoholism, broad-spectrum antibiotic therapy, birth control pills, intrauterine devices, uncircumcised men

Clinical Presentation

- History of Present Illness
  - White, "curd-like" vaginal discharge that is accompanied by severe vulvovaginal pruritus, swelling, and redness
- Physical Assessment Findings
  - Thick, whitish, cottage cheese-like discharge; vaginal or perineal erythema

Clinical Management

- Laboratory and Diagnostic Studies
  - 10 percent potassium hydroxide (KOH) slide preparation (a condition associated with normal vaginal pH [< 4.5])
  - Pseudohyphae and spores with a large number of white blood cells (WBCs) are present. See **Figure 17-1**.
- Pharmacologic
  - First line
    - Miconazole (Monistat) 2% cream or clotrimazole (Gyne-Lotrimin) intravaginal

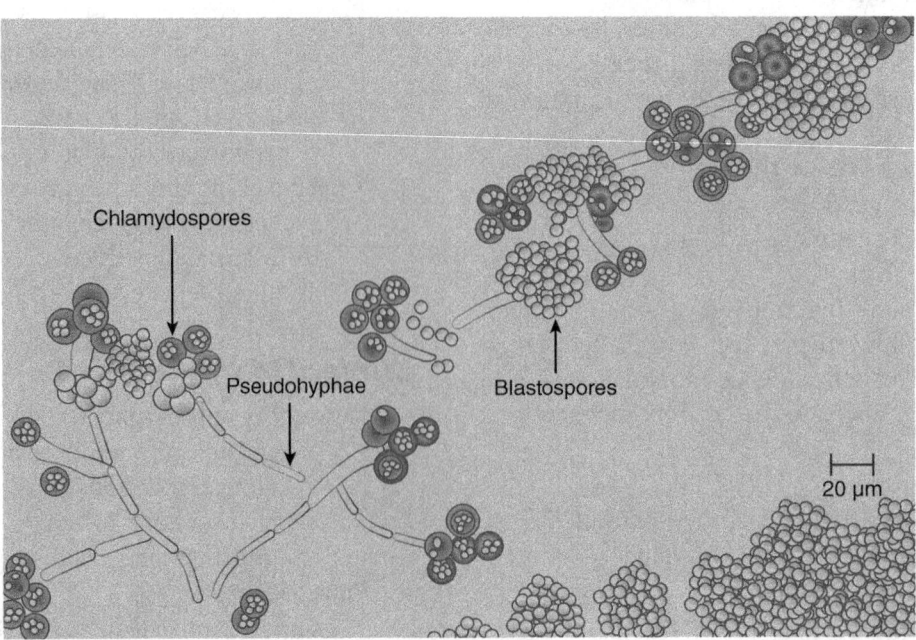

Figure 17-1 Pseudohyphae.

suppository or fluconazole (Diflucan) 150 mg PO single dose
- Severe symptoms or immunocompromised
    - Fluconazole (Diflucan) 150 mg PO in 2 doses given 3 days apart
- Asymptomatic women and sexual partners do not need treatment.
- Nonpharmacologic
  - Use antibiotics and steroids judiciously, avoid douching, minimize perineal moisture, and optimize glycemic control in people with diabetes; active culture yogurt or other live lactobacillus may decrease colonization.
- Patient Education
  - Vaginal antifungal creams and suppositories can weaken condoms and diaphragms.
  - Oral "azole" medications should be avoided in the first trimester because they are teratogenic.
- Indication for Referral
  - Evaluate patients with recurrent superficial candidal infections for immunodeficiency.

Evaluation and Follow-Up

- Immunocompromised patients may benefit from regular evaluation and screening.

Bacterial Vaginosis
Etiology
- Definition
  - The disease process of the vagina caused by an overgrowth of anaerobic bacteria
- Incidence
  - It is the most common cause of vaginal discharge in reproductive-aged women.
- Risk Factors
  - Smoking, receptive oral sex, women who have sex with women, vaginal douching, multiple sexual partners

Clinical Presentation
- History of Present Illness
  - Unpleasant, fish-like vaginal odor with thin, homogeneous vaginal discharge
  - Discharge may worsen after intercourse or menses.
  - Pain and pruritus are uncommon.
- Physical Assessment Findings
  - Thin, watery discharge that can range from clear to gray to tan colored

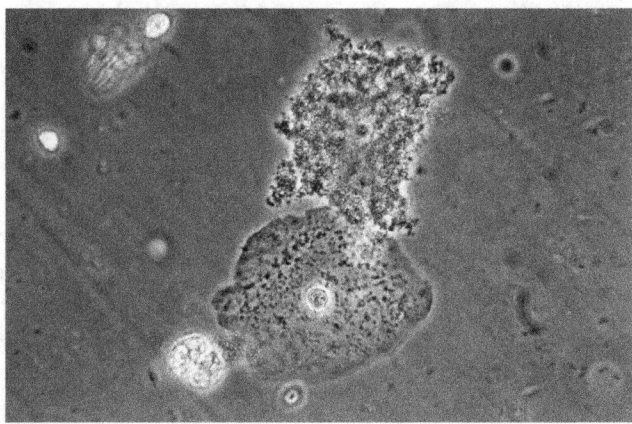

Figure 17-2 Clue Cells.
Courtesy of Center for Disease Control and Prevention.

  - An amine or "fishy" smell may be present.
  - The vaginal epithelium should appear normal and noninflamed.

Clinical Management
- Laboratory and Diagnostic Studies
  - At least three Amsel criteria are necessary:
    - Thin, gray, homogeneous discharge that smoothly coats the vaginal wall
    - Vaginal pH > 4.5
    - Positive amine or "whiff" test with the use of KOH solution added to discharge
    - > 20 percent clue cells on saline wet mount (these are vaginal epithelial cells with blurred margins). See **Figure 17-2**.
- Pharmacologic
  - Oral metronidazole (Flagyl) 500 mg PO BID x 7 days or metronidazole gel 0.75% 5 g intravaginally for 4 days or clindamycin cream 25% 5 g intravaginally nightly for 7 days
- Nonpharmacologic
  - Avoid douching and tight-fitting clothes
- Patient Education
  - Sexual partners do not need to be treated.
  - Abstain from sexual intercourse or use condoms until treatment is complete.
  - Advise patients to avoid alcohol during treatment with oral metronidazole and for 72 hours after treatment (risk for disulfiram-like reaction).
  - Asymptomatic pregnant women generally do not require treatment.

Evaluation and Follow-Up
- No specific follow-up is needed; if symptoms persist or recur within months, repeat pelvic exam and culture.

Dysmenorrhea

Etiology

- Definition
  - Pelvic pain occurring at or around the time of menses
  - Primary: pelvic pain without pathologic physical findings
  - Secondary: more severe pelvic pain; results from specific pelvic pathology (e.g., endometriosis) and is often resistant to typical treatments
- Incidence
  - Primary: predominant age is teens to early 20s
  - Secondary: predominant age is 20s to 30s
- Risk Factors
  - Primary: cigarette smoking, alcohol use, early menarche, age < 30 years, family history, irregular/heavy menstrual flow, nonuse of oral contraceptives, sexual abuse/history of sexual assault, nulliparity
  - Secondary: pelvic infection, use of IUD, structural pelvic malformation, family history of endometriosis

Clinical Presentation

- History of Present Illness
  - Primary: onset 6 to 12 months after menarche; may have associated nausea, vomiting, diarrhea, headache, fatigue, insomnia, and pain radiating into the lower back or inner thighs; usually responds well to NSAIDs
  - Secondary: chronic pelvic pain, midcycle pain, dyspareunia, abnormal uterine bleeding; lack of response to NSAIDs/hormonal treatment
- Physical Assessment Findings
  - Primary: physical exam is typically normal; pelvic exam recommended if the patient is sexually active to rule out infection.
  - Secondary: evaluate for cervical discharge, uterine enlargement, tenderness, irregularity, or fixation.

Clinical Management

- Laboratory and Diagnostic Studies
  - Pregnancy test, urine testing for infection, gonorrhea/chlamydia testing (especially in women < 25 years old)
  - Primary: consider pelvic ultrasound to rule out secondary abnormalities
  - Secondary: ultrasound and/or laparoscopy to define anatomy for severe/refractory cases
- Pharmacologic/Surgical
  - First line
    - NSAIDs (e.g., ibuprofen, naproxen sodium, celecoxib, mefenamic acid) or hormonal contraceptives
  - Second line
    - Acetaminophen or acetaminophen with caffeine
  - Surgery
    - Laparoscopic uterosacral nerve ablation and presacral neurectomy
- Nonpharmacologic
  - Acupuncture therapy, aromatherapy, regular exercise
- Patient Education
  - Reassure the patient that primary dysmenorrhea is treatable with the use of NSAIDs, oral contraceptives, exercise, or local heat and that it will usually ablate with age and parity.
  - Secondary is likely to require therapy based on the underlying cause.

Amenorrhea

Etiology

- Definition
  - Primary: no menses by age 13 with absence of secondary sexual characteristics or no menses by age 15 with normal secondary characteristics
  - Secondary: cessation of menses for 3 months if previously normal menstrual cycle or cessation of menses for 6 months if history of irregular cycles
  - Absence of menses can be temporary, intermittent, or permanent due to dysfunction of the hypothalamus, pituitary, uterus, ovaries, or vagina.
- Risk Factors
  - Obesity, excessive exercise ("female athlete triad"), eating disorders, malnutrition, stress, family history of amenorrhea or early menopause, treatment with antipsychotic medication

Clinical Management

- Laboratory and Diagnostic Studies
  - Labs: pregnancy test, prolactin, FSH, and TSH
- Treatment Goals
  - Identify and correct underlying pathology if possible

- Pharmacologic
  - Progesterone challenge and replacement with medroxyprogesterone (Provera): 10 mg/day for 10 days will result in withdrawal bleed within 7 days of the last dose if the hypothalamic-pituitary-gonadal axis is intact.
  - Estrogen replacement with oral contraceptives
- Nonpharmacologic
  - Maintenance of proper body mass index and healthy lifestyle
- Patient Education
  - Educate on the circumstances/complications of the condition and its underlying etiology.
  - Discuss the expected duration of amenorrhea, its effect on fertility, and the long-term sequelae of untreated amenorrhea.
- Indication for Referral
  - Many causes of amenorrhea require referral to specialists in OB-GYN, endocrine, surgery, and/or psychiatry.

Evaluation and Follow-Up

- Depends on the cause and treatment chosen
- If hormonal replacement is used, discontinue after 6 months to assess spontaneous resumption of menses.

Abnormal Uterine Bleeding

Etiology

- Definition
  - Irregular uterine bleeding (heavy, prolonged, or frequent)
  - May be acute or chronic (> 6 months)
- Incidence
  - Adolescent and perimenopausal women are most often affected.
- Risk Factors
  - Unopposed estrogen therapy, increasing age, obesity, PCOS, diabetes mellitus, nulliparity, early menarche or late menopause, chronic anovulation or infertility, history of breast cancer or endometrial hyperplasia, tamoxifen use, family history, thyroid disease

Clinical Presentation

- History of Present Illness
  - Obtain the patient's menstrual history over the last 6 months: onset, severity, timing
  - Assess association with other factors: coitus, contraception, weight loss/gain
  - Obtain GYN history
- Physical Assessment Findings
  - Evaluate physical and pelvic examination

Clinical Management

- Laboratory and Diagnostic Studies
  - Labs: pregnancy test, complete blood count (CBC)
  - Consider prothrombin time (PT), partial thromboplastin time (PTT), and activated partial thromboplastin time (aPTT); thyroid stimulating hormone (TSH), prolactin level, follicle stimulating hormone (FSH), sexually transmitted infection (STI) screening, potassium hydroxide (KOH) prep, vaginitis panel, transvaginal ultrasound, Papanicolaou test (Pap test)
- Pharmacologic
  - Acute, emergent, nonovulatory bleeding
    - Conjugated equine estrogen
  - Acute, nonemergent, nonovulatory bleeding
    - Monophasic combined oral contraceptive pills (OCPs) or medroxyprogesterone acetate
  - Nonacute, nonovulatory bleeding
    - Levonorgestrel IUD (Mirena)
- Nonpharmacologic
  - Antiemetics if prescribing a high-dose estrogen or progesterone
  - Iron supplementation if anemia is identified
- Patient Education
  - Pad counts and clot size can help determine and monitor the amount of bleeding.
  - Women treated with estrogen or OCPs should keep a menstrual diary to document bleeding patterns and their relation to therapy.
- Indication for Referral
  - If an obvious cause for vaginal bleeding is not found, refer to endocrinologist or gynecologist.

Evaluation and Follow-Up

- Once stable from acute management, follow up in 4 to 6 months.

Endometriosis

Etiology

- Definition
  - Common but potentially painful and debilitating estrogen-dependent condition
  - Tissue that normally grows within the uterus grows in different places: the uterine wall,

around the ovaries, fallopian tubes, and the intestines.
- Incidence
  - Found in 6 to 10 percent of fertile women and 20 to 50 percent of infertile women
  - Found in 71 to 87 percent of women with chronic pelvic pain
- Risk Factors
  - Family history, nulliparity, prolonged exposure to endogenous estrogen, late menopause, shorter menstrual cycles, heavy menstrual bleeding, obstruction of menstrual outflow, taller height, lower body mass index

Clinical Presentation
- History of Present Illness
  - Moderate-to-severe pelvic pain during menses, heavy cramping, dyspareunia, dyschezia, hematochezia, cycle nausea, abdominal distension
- Physical Assessment Findings
  - Focal pain/tenderness on pelvic exam, pelvic mass may be present, immobile pelvic organs, rectovaginal exam reveals uterosacral nodules or tenderness

Clinical Management
- Laboratory and Diagnostic Studies
  - Labs are only useful to rule out other diagnoses.
  - A definitive diagnosis is made with tissue biopsy.
- Pharmacologic
  - First line
    - NSAIDs
  - Second line
    - Low-dose OCPs or low-dose progestins or levonorgestrel IUD
- Nonpharmacologic
  - Increased exercise, increased intake of fruits and vegetables
- Patient Education
  - Excellent prognosis if diagnosis and treatment plans are initiated early in the disease
- Indication for Referral
  - Refer to specialist for definitive diagnosis; failure to respond to conservative or first-line therapy, chronic pelvic pain, delayed fertility

Evaluation and Follow-Up
- Routine gynecological follow-up
- Complications: chronic pelvic pain, reduced quality of life, repetitive surgical intervention, depression, medication side effects and costs, infertility

Uterine Fibroids
Etiology
- Definition
  - Well-circumscribed, benign tumors composed mainly of smooth muscle with varying amounts of fibrous connective tissue
- Incidence
  - Increases with each decade during reproductive years
- Risk Factors
  - African American heritage, early menarche, oral contraceptive use before 16 years old, nulliparity, hypertension, familial predisposition, obesity, alcohol use

Clinical Presentation
- History of Present Illness
  - Usually asymptomatic; 30 percent of patients present with abnormal symptoms: abnormal uterine bleeding, infrequent pain, suprapubic discomfort, urinary frequency, low back pain, constipation
- Physical Assessment Findings
  - Firm, smooth nodules/masses arising from the uterus; masses are mobile without tenderness.

Clinical Management
- Laboratory and Diagnostic Studies
  - Pregnancy test, hemoglobin level, pelvic ultrasound
- Treatment Goals
  - Treatment must be individualized and based on symptoms, fertility desires, and time until menopause.
- Nonpharmacologic
  - Use of progesterone-only contraceptives
  - Diet (fruits, veggies, low-fat dairy)
- Indication for Referral
  - Surgical options should be considered if symptomatic or worrisome fibroids are unresponsive to conservative/medical management.

Evaluation and Follow-Up
- Pelvic examination and ultrasound every 2 to 3 months for newly diagnosed symptomatic/excessively large fibroids
- Once uterine size and symptoms stabilize, monitor every 6 to 12 months.

Polycystic Ovarian Syndrome

Etiology

- Definition
  - Endocrine disorder that is characterized by hyperandrogenism, insulin resistance, and anovulation, typically presenting as amenorrhea or oligomenorrhea
- Incidence
  - Occurs in 6 to 10 percent of reproductive-aged females
- Risk Factors
  - Commonly associated conditions: infertility, obesity, obstructive sleep apnea, hypertension, diabetes mellitus, endometrial hyperplasia/carcinoma, fatty liver disease, mood disturbances and depression, hirsutism

Clinical Presentation

- History of Present Illness
  - Menstrual dysfunction, infertility, hirsutism, acne, obesity, and metabolic syndrome
- Physical Assessment Findings
  - Central obesity, hirsutism, acne, male hair patterns, balding, acne, seborrhea, acanthosis nigricans, ovarian enlargement, clitoromegaly

Clinical Management

- Laboratory and Diagnostic Studies
  - Rotterdam criteria (2 out of 3 need to be present for diagnosis):
    - Anovulation (oligo- or amenorrhea)
    - Increased androgen levels
    - Multiple cysts seen on the ovaries
  - Transvaginal ultrasound: enlarged ovaries seen with multiple small follicles ("ring of pearls" appearance)
  - Labs: TSH, fasting glucose, and lipid levels; serum testosterone, dehydroepiandrosterone (DHEA), and androstenedione are elevated; FSH levels are normal or low.
- Treatment Goals
  - Depends on the patient's symptoms and goals for fertility
- Pharmacologic
  - Can be divided into four main categories:
    - Restore menses → OCPs and progestins
    - Decrease insulin resistance → glucophage (Metformin)
    - Ameliorate androgen excess → spironolactone (Aldactone)
    - Assist in fertility
- Nonpharmacologic
  - Weight loss through diet and exercise
- Patient Education
  - Discuss the chronic nature of this condition and the risks/benefits and side effects of potential treatments
- Indication for Referral
  - Refer to a reproductive endocrinologist for all women who cannot achieve pregnancy with medication alone.

Evaluation and Follow-Up

- Six-month intervals to evaluate response to therapy and to monitor weight and medication side effects
- Complications: infertility, insulin resistance, diabetes mellitus, cardiovascular disease, increased anxiety, mood disorder, eating disorder, depression

Ovarian Cancer

Etiology

- Definition
  - Malignancy that arises from the epithelium, sex cord-stromal, or germ cells of the ovary, as well as tumors metastatic to the ovary
- Incidence
  - Leading cause of GYN cancer death in women
- Risk Factors
  - Older age, white race, infertility, nulligravida, early menarche or late menopause, endometriosis, postmenopausal estrogen replacement therapy, residence in an industrialized Western country

Clinical Presentation

- History of Present Illness
  - Acute presentation: shortness of breath (pleural effusion), nausea, vomiting, decreased oral intake (bowel obstruction), calf pain, shortness of breath (venous thromboembolism), severe abdominal or pelvic pain (ovarian torsion or rupture)
  - Subacute presentation: abdominal or pelvic pain/cramping, bloating, sense of abdominal fullness, ascites, early satiety, anorexia, dyspepsia, dyspareunia, urinary frequency/urgency, fatigue, weight loss, precocious puberty
- Physical Assessment Findings
  - General appearance: cachexia, hirsutism
  - Lymphatics: lymphadenopathy; firm, immobile, enlarged lymph nodes

- Pulmonary: decreased breath sounds
- Abdominal: fluid wave, mass, omental caking
- Pelvic: solid, irregular, fixed mass

Clinical Management
- Laboratory and Diagnostic Studies
  - CBC, LFT, urinalysis, serum albumin, tumor markers, transvaginal ultrasound, abdominal CT, and pelvis with contrast, chest x-ray or chest CT
- Treatment Goals
  - Surgical exploration with staging and debulking is critical.
- Patient Education
  - Patients should be educated on signs and symptoms of recurrence, including pelvic or abdominal pain/discomfort, bloating, and early satiety
- Indication for Referral
  - Although the USPSTF does not recommend routine screening for ovarian cancer in the general population (Grade D), high-risk women with suspected BRCA 1/2 mutations should be referred for genetic counseling and testing.

Evaluation and Follow-Up
- Surgical patients should follow up within 4 weeks for postoperative assessment for further treatment planning.
- Patients undergoing chemotherapy should have regular visits to assess toxicity and disease progression.

Menopause
Etiology
- Definition
  - Natural menopause: 12 consecutive months of amenorrhea in a nonpregnant woman > 40 years of age, resulting from loss of ovarian activity
  - Perimenopause/menopausal transition: the period from the onset of irregular menses to the final menstrual cycle
  - Primary ovarian insufficiency: irregularity of cessation of ovulatory cycles before age 40 years
- Incidence
  - The median age of menopause is 51 years old.
- Risk Factors
  - Aging, oophorectomy/hysterectomy, sex chromosome abnormalities, family history of early menopause, smoking, chemotherapy and/or pelvic radiation, low body mass index

Clinical Presentation
- History of Present Illness
  - Cessation of menses (generally preceded by a period of irregular cycles with heavy vaginal bleeding followed by diminished vaginal bleeding), vasomotor symptoms, vulvovaginal atrophy, anxiety/depression, sleep disturbance, change in intensity and severity of migraines, skin thinning, mild hirsutism, brittle nails
- Physical Assessment Findings
  - Decrease in breast size and change in breast texture, atrophic vulva, and vaginal mucosa; increased risk for uterine prolapse

Clinical Management
- Laboratory and Diagnostic Studies
  - Lab testing for menopause is not required; the patient's age and symptoms establish the diagnosis.
  - Lab tests are appropriate in patients younger than 45 if premature/early menopause is suspected or to rule out other causes of oligomenorrhea.
- Pharmacologic
  - First line
    - Hormone therapy
      - Broad term to describe any hormone supplementation; typically combination estrogen-progesterone
      - Most effective for vasomotor symptoms (e.g., hot flashes, night sweats), GU syndrome of menopause (e.g., loss of vaginal elasticity), and prevention of fracture and bone loss
      - If the patient does not have a uterus (e.g., hysterectomy), estrogen therapy alone is appropriate.
      - If the patient still has a uterus, progesterone is required to prevent cancer.
      - Low-dose, topical estrogen therapy may be indicated for patients with vaginal dryness, recurrent UTIs, or dyspareunia.
      - Risks involved: heart disease, blood clots, breast cancer

- Contraindications: history or first-degree family member history of breast or endometrial cancer, heart disease, venous thromboembolic event (VTE), cerebrovascular accident (CVA), transient ischemic attack (TIA), liver disease, unexplained vaginal bleeding; not recommended if patient is older than 60 years due to risk of CV/vascular event
        - Patients should be on hormone therapy for the least amount of time possible (ideally less than 3 to 5 years).
    - Second line
        - Nonhormonal treatment
            - Paroxetine is approved for the treatment of vasomotor symptoms.
            - Gabapentin is shown to lower hot flashes compared to placebo.
- Nonpharmacologic
    - Hypnotherapy and mindfulness meditation, acupuncture, yoga
- Patient Education
    - Smoking cessation; reduce alcohol intake; exercise > 30 minutes, 3 times weekly; healthy diet to maintain appropriate weight; address cardiovascular risk factor modification
- Indication for Referral
    - May refer to urogynecology for pelvic floor physical therapy

Evaluation and Follow-Up

- If hormone replacement therapy is initiated, consider decreasing or discontinuing after 3 to 5 years to minimize risks.
- Complications: osteoporosis, increased risk of CVD following menopause

Osteoporosis

Etiology

- Definition
    - A skeletal disease characterized by low bone mass, with disruption of bone architecture leading to compromised bone strength and risk of fracture
- Incidence
    - Predominantly occurs in older females > 60 years of age
- Risk Factors
    - Modifiable: low body weight, calcium/vitamin D deficiency, inadequate physical activity, cigarette smoking, excessive alcohol intake, various medications (e.g., chronic steroids)
    - Nonmodifiable: age > 65 years, female and menopause, White or Asian, family history of osteoporosis, history of fragility fracture

Clinical Presentation

- Physical Assessment Findings
    - Thoracic kyphosis, poor balance, deconditioning
    - Historical height loss > 4 cm

Clinical Management

- Laboratory and Diagnostic Studies
    - Dual-energy x-ray absorptiometry (DEXA) of the lumbar spine/hip is considered the gold standard for measuring bone mineral density and diagnosing osteoporosis
        - Osteoporosis: T-score of −2.5 or lower standard deviation (SD) at the lumbar spine, femoral neck, or total hip region
        - Osteopenia: T-scores between −1.5 and −2.4 SD
- Treatment Goals
    - Treat postmenopausal women who have osteoporosis (T-score of −2.5 or less) or a history of hip/vertebral fracture
- Pharmacologic
    - First line
        - Bisphosphonates (e.g., alendronate, risedronate, zoledronic acid)
            - Side effects: inflammation of the esophagus and stomach
            - Educate the patient to take them immediately upon awakening in the morning with a full glass of plain water; take tablets sitting or standing and wait at least 30 minutes before lying down; swallow tablets whole; do not take these medications with other medications, juice, coffee, antacids, or vitamins
    - Second line
        - Monoclonal antibody therapy (e.g., denosumab, romosozumab)
        - Side effects: dermatologic reactions, musculoskeletal pain, hypocalcemia, atypical femur fracture
    - All patients
        - Vitamin D 2,000 to 4,000 IU/day

- Nonpharmacologic
  - Weight-bearing exercises 30 minutes, 3 times per week
    - Weight-bearing exercises are walking, jogging, aerobic dance classes, most sports, yoga, and tai chi; swimming and biking are not considered a weight-bearing exercise (but are good for severe arthritis)
  - Smoking cessation (smoking cigarettes accelerates bone loss)
- Indication for Referral
  - Endocrinology for recurrent bone loss/fracture or atypical cases of osteoporosis
  - Dental professional for oral examinations

Evaluation and Follow-Up

- Yearly height measurement assesses treatment efficacy
- Repeat DEXA 2 years after starting bisphosphonate therapy.

Exam Success Tips

- Mefenamic acid (Ponstel) is an NSAID that is very effective for menstrual pain.
- There will be questions on all the types of vaginitis (bacterial vaginosis, trichomoniasis, candidal, atrophic vaginitis); the questions range from diagnosis and lab workup to treatment plans.
- Women who have persistent vaginal infections and UTIs, despite hygiene measures, adequate hydration, and in the absence of sexual exposures from partner(s), should be screened for underlying glucose metabolism disorders and diabetes.
- Become familiar with bacterial vaginosis: "clue cells" are squamous epithelial cells that have blurred edges due to the large number of bacteria on the cell's surface.
- The "female athlete triad" is menstrual disturbance, restricted/disordered eating, and low bone mineral density.
- The bone density score for osteoporosis is T-score of > −2.5, and for osteopenia, it is T-score of −1.0 to −2.5.
- Contraindications to bisphosphonate therapy include delayed esophageal emptying, inability to stand/sit upright for 30 to 60 minutes after taking the bisphosphonate, hypocalcemia, and severe renal impairment.
- Take bisphosphonates with a full glass of water in the morning on an empty stomach and sit upright for at least 30 minutes.

Pregnancy and Prenatal Care

Obstetric History

GTPAL

- Gravida (G): number of pregnancies (twins or multiples counts as one)
- Term (T): number of deliveries after 37 weeks
- Preterm (P): number of deliveries after 20 weeks (up to 38 weeks)
- Abortion (A): number of deliveries before 20 weeks (induced or spontaneous)
- Living (L): number of living children

Signs of Pregnancy

Presumptive

- Subjective symptoms reported by the woman:
  - Amenorrhea, nausea, vomiting, breast changes (swollen, tender), fatigue, urinary frequency, "quickening" (mother feels the baby's movements for the first time)

Probable

- Physiologic and anatomic changes noted by the provider:
  - Positive pregnancy test
  - Abdominal/uterine enlargement
  - Ballottement (a technique for confirmation of pregnancy by feeling the rebound of the fetus following a quick digital tap on the wall of the uterus)
  - Braxton-Hicks contractions
  - Goodell's sign (4 weeks): cervical softening
  - Chadwick's sign (6 to 8 weeks): blue coloration of the cervix and vagina
  - Hegar's sign (6 to 8 weeks): softening uterine isthmus
  - Skin hyperpigmentation (chloasma, linea nigra)

Positive

- Objective signs attributed to the presence of the fetus
  - Fetal outline and/or movement by practitioner
  - Fetal heart rate heard at 10 to 12 weeks with a Doppler; at 20 weeks with a fetoscope
  - Embryo/fetus seen on ultrasound

Exam Success Tips

- Memorize the three signs of pregnancy; by process of elimination, you can rule out (or in) the correct answer choice.
- The signs with surnames (Goodell, Chadwick, Hegar) are all probable signs.
- Palpation of fetal movements by the mother is not considered a positive sign of pregnancy ("quickening"); it is classified as a presumptive sign.
- Urine/serum pregnancy tests are considered probable signs (do not confuse them as positive signs); beta HCG also presents in molar pregnancy and ovarian cancer.

Prenatal Care

Goals of Prenatal Care

- Ensure the well-being of the mother and baby using the best available evidence and a patient-centered approach.
- General concepts include estimating the gestational age accurately, identifying risk for complications, encouraging and empowering the patient for motherhood, newborn care, breastfeeding, and intervening when fetal complications are present to prevent morbidity and mortality.

Prenatal Care Visit Schedule

- First Prenatal Visit
  - Should be completed as soon as possible after the woman suspects she may be pregnant
  - Education topics include anticipatory teaching of what to expect with pregnancy, visit schedule, nutritional guidance, sexuality, contraceptive methods, choice of newborn nutrition
  - Ensure the patient is taking one prenatal vitamin daily with the addition of folic acid 400 to 800 mcg by mouth daily to reduce neural tube abnormalities of the fetus.
  - Appropriate follow-up and referrals should be made.
- Return Prenatal Visits
  - Every 4 weeks until 28 to 30 weeks gestation
  - Every 2 weeks until 36 weeks gestation
  - Every week until delivery
  - At each return visit, evaluate vital signs; urine for protein, ketones, and glucose; weight; fetal heart rate; fetal presentation and activity; and fundal height measurement.
  - Depending on the practice, a cervical exam may be indicated at 36, 38, and 40 weeks.

Laboratory Testing/Expected Changes During Pregnancy

First Prenatal Visit

- Lab tests
  - Hemoglobin and hematocrit
  - Blood type
  - Rhesus type
  - Antibody screen
  - Hemoglobin electrophoresis
  - Urine culture
  - Ab titers for Rubella and Varicella
  - STI screen: Rapid Plasma Reagin/Venereal Disease Research Laboratory (RPR/VDRL), Gonorrhea-Chlamydia (GC/C), Hepatitis B (Hep B), Human Immunodeficiency Virus (HIV)
- Carrier screening
  - Cystic fibrosis
  - Spinal muscular atrophy
  - Hemoglobinopathies
- Screening for fetal aneuploidy
  - All women should be offered screening or diagnostic testing, regardless of maternal age.
  - Triple marker screening combines the alpha-fetoprotein (AFP), beta HCG, and estriol serum levels.
    - AFP Overview
      - Glycoprotein is synthesized by the fetus beginning in early gestation; production occurs initially in the yolk sac, then the GI tract, and then the fetal liver (majority located here).
    - Low AFP
      - Down syndrome
    - High AFP
      - Multiple gestation, neural tube defects (e.g., spina bifida)
  - Quadruple marker screening combines the triple screening hormones plus inhibin-A (a hormone released by the placenta).
- Cervical cancer screening

Subsequent Prenatal Visits

- Urinalysis to check protein, leukocytes, nitrites, blood, and glucose
- If 20 weeks gestation or more, rule out preeclampsia if protein is 1+ or higher

24 to 28 Weeks Prenatal Visits

- Gestational diabetes screen
- Repeat hemoglobin and hematocrit

35 to 37 Weeks Prenatal Visits

- Group B streptococcus culture; if positive, administer intrapartum antibiotic prophylaxis with penicillin G IV, followed by IV every 4 hours until delivery; use clindamycin if allergic

Clinical Method for Dating Pregnancy

Naegele's Rule

- Determines the woman's estimated date of delivery (EDD); last menstrual period (LMP) is determined by the first day of the last normal menses
- Method 1: LMP + 9 months + 7 days
- Method 2: LMP – 3 months + 7 days

Uterine Sizing

- For fundal heights, see **Figure 17-3**.
  - 12 weeks (3rd month)
    - Uterine fundus first rises above the symphysis pubis
  - Fetal heart tones (FHTs) are heard by Doppler by 10 to 12 weeks
- 16 Weeks (4th month)
  - Uterine fundus between the symphysis pubis and the umbilicus
- 20 Week (5th month)
  - Uterine fundus at the level of the umbilicus
  - FHTs heard with a fetoscope or stethoscope
- 20 to 25 Weeks
  - Measure the distance between the upper edge of the pubic symphysis and the top of the uterine fundus using a paper tape measure. Fundal height in centimeters equals the number of weeks of gestation, ±2 cm. For example, a 32-week-gestation fetus should have a fundal height between 30 and 34 cm.
  - If the uterine fundus is ≤ 2 cm (fetus smaller than expected), it can be caused by dating errors, intrauterine growth restriction (IUGR), or other problems. If the fundus size is ≥ 2 cm (fetus larger than expected), it can be due to dating errors, macrosomia, or other problems. Order an ultrasound.

Physiologic Changes During Pregnancy

Weight Gain and BMI

- Healthy weight (BMI 18.5 to 24.9): gain a total of 25 to 35 lb or 11.34 to 15.88 kg
- Underweight (BMI <18.5): gain a total of 28 to 40 lb or 12.7 to 18.14 kg
- Obese (BMI >30): gain a total of up to 11 to 20 lb or 4.9 to 9.07 kg
- After delivery: loss of up to 15 to 20 lb or 6.8 to 9.07 kg in the first few weeks is appropriate.
- Twins: increased weight gain (37 to 54 lb) or 16.78 to 24.49 kg is appropriate, but weight gain should not be double that for a single fetus.

Vital Signs

- Temperature may be a high normal of 99.2°F to 99.6°F.
- Pulse may be elevated by 10 to 15 beats per minute.
- Respiratory rate (RR) increases up to 15 percent later in pregnancy due to pressure of the uterus on the diaphragm.

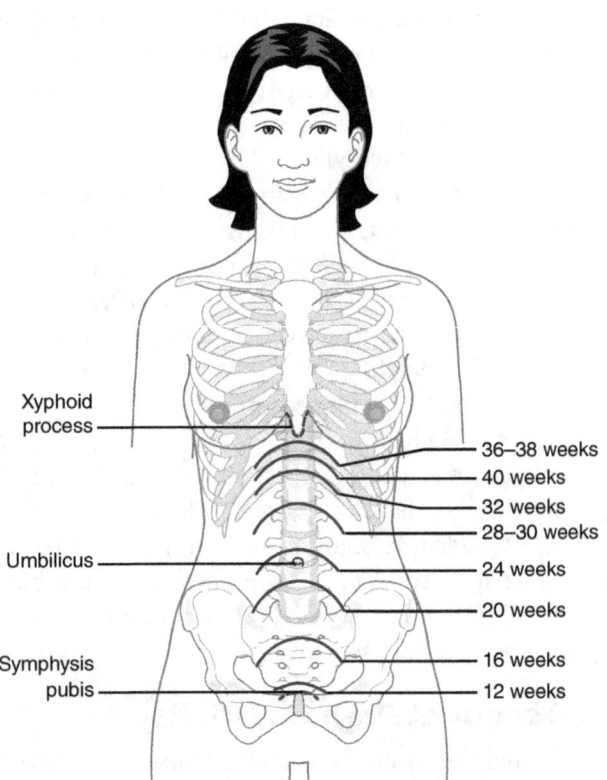

Figure 17-3 Fundal Heights.

- BP decreases in the second trimester and returns to prepregnancy levels by the third trimester.

Cardiovascular

- Heart position: the heart is shifted anteriorly toward the left; it rotates toward a transverse position as the uterus enlarges.
- Heart sounds: louder in pregnancy; S3 heart sound also known as a ventricular gallop is common.
- Murmurs: a systolic ejection murmur (grade II/IV) over the pulmonary and tricuspid areas is common.
- Cardiac output increases by 30 to 50 percent and peaks at about 28 to 34 weeks gestation.
- Preload increases because of higher blood volume.
- Afterload decreases because of the decrease in peripheral vascular resistance during pregnancy.
- Plasma volume increases by almost 50 percent by the end of the second trimester; hemodilution results in physiologic anemia during pregnancy (most obvious from 6 to 9 months).
- The inferior vena cava compresses due to an enlarged uterus, decreasing the blood return to the brain and resulting in orthostatic hypotension (postural hypotensive syndrome). Advise women to lie on the left side and change positions slowly.
- Coagulation factors: pregnancy is a hypercoagulable state (clotting factors go up), especially after labor.
- Varicose veins become more severe during pregnancy.
- Peripheral edema is considered normal in pregnancy; mild edema of the lower extremities and the feet is most noticeable in the third trimester.

Respiratory

- Presence of basal rales that disappear with coughing or deep breathing
- Feeling of breathlessness ("innocent hyperpnea") and decreased exercise tolerance
- Physiologic dyspnea in pregnancy has a slow onset; sudden-onset dyspnea is abnormal; rule out pulmonary emboli (e.g., pleuritic chest pain, tachypnea, hemoptysis).
- The gravid uterus pushes up the diaphragm as it gets larger; the diameter of the thorax is increased.
- There is no change in forced expiratory volume (FEV1) in one second, but total lung capacity drops slightly.

Integumentary

- Pigmentary changes: an increase in melanocyte-stimulating hormone from higher levels of estrogen causes the linea nigra (dark pigmented "line" that extends from the mons pubis to the umbilicus located midline) and the nipples/areola to darken.
- Chloasma ("melasma"): blotchy hyperpigmentation on the forehead, cheeks, nose, and upper lip seen in pregnant women and some birth control pill users; usually gets lighter and regresses within 1 year; however, in some women, hyperpigmentation may be permanent.
- Striae gravidarum ("stretch marks"): most common locations are the abdomen, breasts, and thighs; other less common areas are the upper arms, lower back, and buttocks.
- Telogen effluvium (hair loss): during the postpartum period, hair loss may accelerate, but it is temporary.

Endocrine

- Diffusely enlarged, with higher metabolic activity

Gastrointestinal

- Decreased peristalsis from progesterone effects (e.g., constipation, heartburn)

Renal

- Kidney size increases during pregnancy; the ureters and renal pelvis dilate (physiologic hydronephrosis).
- Glomerular filtration rate is much higher in pregnancy because of higher cardiac output and renal blood flow.

Ears, Nose, Throat

- Some women develop nasal congestion and/or epistaxis due to increased blood flow to the nasopharynx during pregnancy.
- Rule out acute sinusitis if purulent mucus is seen in the posterior pharynx.

Musculoskeletal

- Weight gain, enlarged uterus, and hormonal changes contribute to joint ligamentous laxity and exaggerated lordosis of the lumbar spine.

- Up to 60 percent of pregnant women experience back pain (not related to labor).
- Gait changes to a wider stance.

Drugs and Vaccines During Pregnancy

FDA Classification System of Medication Use During Pregnancy

- A → multiple studies showed no risk to the fetus in the first trimester
    - Prenatal vitamins, insulin, thyroid hormone, folic acid, pyridoxine
- B → caution is advised because no adequate studies have been done on pregnant women; animal studies show no risk
    - Antacids, docusate sodium, acetaminophen, antibiotics (e.g., penicillin, cephalosporins, macrolides, nitrofurantoin), antihypertensives (e.g., methyldopa, calcium channel blockers, labetalol)
- C → animal studies show adverse fetal effects, but no controlled human studies or no controlled human or animal studies; to be used only if benefits outweigh the risks
    - Sulfa drugs, trimethoprim–sulfamethoxazole, pseudoephedrine
- D → positive evidence that human fetal risk/maternal benefit may outweigh fetal risk in serious or life-threatening situations; some significant risks associated
    - Angiotensin enzyme inhibitors (ACEIs), angiotensin receptor blockers (ARBs), fluoroquinolones, tetracyclines, NSAIDs
- X → always contraindicated unless using the medication outweighs the risks because animal or human studies have found evidence of human fetal risk
    - Accutane, methotrexate, anticancer drugs, Proscar, misoprostol, tamoxifen

Vaccines

- The inactivated influenza injection can be given during any trimester.
- Tdap during each pregnancy should be given between 27 and 36 weeks.
- Mumps, measles, and rubella (MMR), oral polio, varicella, and FluMist are contraindicated in pregnancy.
- After a live virus vaccine, advise reproductive-aged women not to get pregnant (and use reliable birth control) in the next 4 weeks (e.g., MMR) or 3 months (e.g., varicella and shingles vaccine).
- A mother who has a negative rubella titer can be immunized even if breastfeeding.

Teratogens

- Agents that can cause structural abnormalities during pregnancy
    - Paroxetine (Paxil): taking the drug during the first trimester increases the risk of congenital disabilities (particularly heart defects)
    - Fluoxetine (Prozac): causes heart wall defects and craniosynostosis
    - Other SSRIs (citalopram, escitalopram, sertraline): first-trimester exposure may be associated with a low risk of teratogenicity
    - Alcohol: fetal alcohol syndrome
    - Aminoglycosides: deafness
    - Cigarettes: intrauterine growth retardation, prematurity
    - Cocaine: cerebrovascular accidents, cognitive deficits, abruptio placentae
    - Isotretinoin (Accutane): central nervous system (CNS)/craniofacial/ear/cardiovascular defects
    - Lithium: cardiac defects

Patient Education

- Dietary supplements
    - 400 to 800 mcg/day of folic acid beginning at least 1 month before attempting conception and continuing throughout pregnancy
    - 1,000 to 1,3000 mg/day of calcium may be beneficial for women with a high risk for gestational hypertension or communities with low dietary calcium intake
    - Caffeine should be limited to < 200 mg/day
    - Screen for anemia and order extra iron supplementation
- Airline travel is generally safe until week 35; longer than 2 hours without ambulation increases the risk of thrombosis.
- Healthy women with uncomplicated pregnancies should continue to exercise.
- Wear lap and shoulder seat belts.
- Intercourse while pregnant is not associated with adverse outcomes; avoiding sex may be necessary in cases of low-lying placenta, placenta previa, or vasa previa.
- Alcohol, cigarettes, and illicit drugs are injurious to fetal and maternal health.

- Avoid large fish such as shark, tuna, swordfish, and mackerel (high levels of mercury).
- Avoid soft cheeses (blue cheese, brie), raw milk, uncooked hot dogs, and "deli" meat (Listeria bacteria).
- Do not use hot tubs or saunas or expose oneself to excessive heat.
- Be aware of the Zika virus (spread by mosquitoes), which can cause severe congenital disabilities and neurodevelopmental abnormalities; avoid travel to areas with Zika outbreaks; use condoms or avoid sex with someone who has recently traveled to a risk area; if travel is necessary, consult guidelines by Centers for Disease Control and Prevention.

Exam Success Tips

- Understand how to utilize Nagele's rule by method 1: LMP + 9 months + 7 days or method 2: LMP − 3 months + 7 days.
- S3 heart murmur is a normal finding in pregnancy; S4 is not.
- Chloasma/melasma is due to high estrogen levels.
- Fundus at 12 weeks is above symphysis pubis.
- Fundus at 16 weeks is between the symphysis pubis and the umbilicus.
- Fundus at 20 weeks is at the umbilicus.
- Sexually active females with hypertension who do not use birth control who get pregnant should avoid ACEIs and ARBs to treat hypertension.
- Preferred medications for hypertension in pregnancy are methyldopa (Aldomet), labetalol (beta blocker), hydralazine, and long-acting nifedipine.
- For methyldopa, check LFTs at baseline and periodically (contraindicated if active hepatic disease); discontinue if jaundice, abnormal LFTs, or unexplained fever occur.

Disease Review During Pregnancy

Oligohydramnios vs. Polyhydramnios

- Oligohydramnios
  - Amniotic fluid volume that is less than the minimum expected for gestational age. It is diagnosed by ultrasound and measured as the amniotic fluid index (AFI < 5 cm) or the deepest vertical pocket (DVP).
  - Fetal malformation, pulmonary hypoplasia, umbilical cord compression, and fetal or neonatal death are at a higher risk.
  - It may occur in the first, second, or third trimester. It can be idiopathic or have maternal, fetal, or placental causes.
- Polyhydramnios
  - Amniotic fluid volume is more than expected for gestational age.
  - It is mostly caused by fetal anomalies (usually associated with genetic abnormality or syndrome).
  - Occurs in approximately 1 percent of pregnancies.
- Refer to an obstetrician for management in both cases.

RH-Incompatibility

Etiology

- Definition
  - Antibody-mediated destruction of red blood cells that bear Rh surface antigens in individuals who lack the antigens and have become sensitized to them
- Incidence
  - Predominantly affects fetuses/neonates of sensitized, childbearing females
- Risk Factors
  - Any Rh-positive fetus in an Rh-negative pregnant person can result in sensitization.
- General Prevention
  - Blood typing (ABO and Rh) on all pregnant women and before blood transfusions
  - Antibody screening early in pregnancy

Clinical Presentation

- Physical Assessment Findings
  - Jaundice of the newborn
  - Kernicterus signs and symptoms

Clinical Management

- Laboratory and Diagnostic Studies
  - Positive indirect Coombs' test (antibody screen) during pregnancy
    - Coombs' test detects the presence of Rh antibodies in the mother (indirect Coombs' test) and the infant (direct Coombs' test).

- Treatment Goals
  - Depending on the severity of involvement, treatment of the fetus may include intrauterine transfusion and early delivery (no later than 37 to 38 weeks).
  - Treatment of newborns may include exchange transfusion, transfusion after delivery, and phototherapy.
  - Give anti-D immune globulin (RhoGAM) for all pregnancies of Rh-negative mothers, even if they terminate in miscarriages, abortions, or tubal or ectopic pregnancies.
    - RhoGAM is made from pooled IgG antibodies against the Rh factor. It is an immunoglobulin that helps prevent maternal isoimmunization (self-immunization) or alloimmunization (immunity against another individual of the same species). If RhoGAM is not given to Rh-negative pregnant women, this will result in fetal hemolysis and fetal anemia in future pregnancies.
    - Give RhoGAM 300 mcg IM first dose at 28 weeks; give the second dose within 72 hours (or sooner) after delivery.
- Indication for Referral
  - Pregnancies in Rh-sensitized women are usually managed at tertiary care facilities with maternal-fetal medicine specialists.

Evaluation and Follow-Up

- Complications: pregnancy loss from umbilical blood sampling, pregnancy loss from intrauterine transfusion, fetal distress requiring emergency delivery

Gestational Diabetes

Etiology

- Definition
  - Gestational diabetes mellitus (GDM) is diabetes diagnosed in the second or third trimester that was not overt diabetes before conception.
  - Among the main consequences of GDM are increased risks of preeclampsia, large-for-gestational-age newborns, cesarean birth, and their associated morbidities.
- Incidence
  - Prevalence has been increasing over time, likely due to an increase in mean maternal age and BMI.
- Risk Factors
  - GDM in a previous pregnancy, obesity, ethnicity (Asian, American Indian, Pacific Islander, African American, Hispanic), macrosomic infant (> 9 lbs), age (older than 35 years)

Clinical Presentation

- History of Present Illness
  - Commonly asymptomatic

Clinical Management

- Laboratory and Diagnostic Studies
  - Screen at the first visit if there is a history of GDM and/or the presence of risk factors.
  - If not at high risk for GDM, screen at 24 to 28 weeks gestation.
  - There are two methods of testing for GDM:
    - One-Step Method (Preferred)
      - Administer 75-g oral glucose tolerance test (check fasting, 1 hour, and 2 hours)
      - Diagnostic criteria:
        - Fasting: ≥ 92 mg/dL
        - 1 hour: ≥ 180 mg/dL
        - 2 hours: ≥ 153 mg/dL
      - If one value is elevated in this test, it is diagnostic of GDM.
    - Two-Step Method
      - Screening: 50-g glucose load (nonfasting), check plasma glucose at 1 hour
      - If ≥ 140 mg/dL: rule out GDM. Order 100-g oral glucose tolerance test (OGTT) (fasting, 1 hour, 2 hours, and 3 hours)
      - Diagnostic criteria:
        - Fasting: ≥ 95 mg/dL
        - 1 hour: ≥ 180 mg/dL
        - 2 hours: ≥ 155 mg/dL
        - 3 hours: ≥ 140 mg/dL
- Nonpharmacologic
  - The first-line treatment is lifestyle. Eat three meals per day plus two or three snacks; limit carbohydrates; exercise 30 minutes per day at least 5 days a week.
- Pharmacologic
  - If medication is needed, human insulin is the preferred agent; however, oral antihyperglycemic drugs, such as glyburide and metformin, can also be used.

- Patient Education
  - Glucose monitoring: check blood glucose at least four times per day (fasting, 1 or 2 hours after the first bite of each meal)
  - Glycemic targets in pregnancy are:
    - Preprandial: ≤ 95 mg/dL
    - 1 hour postmeal: ≤ 140 mg/dL
    - 2 hour postmeal: ≤ 120 mg/dL
    - A1C goal: < 6%
- Indication for Referral
  - Consult with an obstetrician if the estimated fetal weight is ≥ 4,500 g or if the nonstress test or amniotic fluid index is abnormal.
  - Obstetricians should consult with maternal–fetal medicine if early induction of labor is being considered (at 38 weeks gestation or earlier).

Evaluation and Follow-Up

- Check for prediabetes or diabetes at 4 to 12 weeks postpartum and advise lifelong screening at least every 3 years; patients with GDM are at high risk of developing type 2 diabetes later in life.

Preeclampsia (Pregnancy-Induced Hypertension)

Etiology

- Definition
  - A disorder of pregnancy occurring after 20 weeks gestation characterized by new onset hypertension, new onset proteinuria, and/or impaired organ function.
  - It may progress from mild to life-threatening in hours to days; it is reversible by delivery.
  - Most postpartum cases of preeclampsia occur within 48 hours of delivery but can occur up to 4 weeks postpartum.
- Incidence
  - Occurs in 5 to 8 percent of all pregnancies.
- Risk Factors
  - Nulliparity, age > 40 years, family history of preeclampsia, high BMI, diabetes, chronic hypertension, chronic renal disease, multifetal pregnancy, previous pregnancy with preeclampsia, systemic lupus erythematosus, in vitro fertilization

Clinical Presentation

- History of Present Illness
  - May be asymptomatic; in some cases, rapid excessive weight gain (> 5 lb per week)
  - Headache, visual disturbance, and epigastric or right upper quadrant (RUQ) pain may be present in more severe cases and often precede seizure.
- Physical Assessment Findings
  - BP criteria:
    - Preeclampsia without severe features: > 140/90 mmHg
    - Preeclampsia with severe features: > 160 systolic mmHg or > 110 mmHg diastolic
    - Eclampsia: tonic-clonic seizure activity
    - Normal BP (even in response to treatment) does not rule out the potential for seizures.

Clinical Management

- Laboratory and Diagnostic Studies
  - Blood pressure
    - New-onset elevated BP: SBP > 140 mmHg or DBP > 90 mmHg (on two occasions at least 4 hours apart) or > 160/110 mmHg after 20 weeks gestation (within a shorter interval)
  - Proteinuria
    - Proteinuria > 300 mg/24 hr
- Or without proteinuria and new onset of any of these features:
  - Platelets > 100,000/uL
  - Liver transaminase levels > 2 times normal
  - Creatinine > 1.1 mg/dL or doubling of serum creatinine
  - Pulmonary edema
  - Cerebral or visual symptoms
- Eclampsia diagnosis:
  - New-onset tonic-clonic, focal, or multifocal seizures
  - No history of neurologic diseases
- Treatment Goals
  - Preeclampsia without severe features:
    - Outpatient care
    - Maternal: daily home BP monitoring, daily weights, weekly labs (CBC, creatinine, LFTs)
    - Fetal: patient-measured daily "kick counts," Nonstress test/biophysical profile/ultrasound (NST/BPP/US), delivery at 37 weeks, steroids for gestation < 37 weeks
  - Preeclampsia with severe features:
    - Inpatient care

- Maternal: daily labs, IV magnesium sulfate for seizure prophylaxis, antihypertensive therapy (labetalol or hydralazine) titrated to keep SBP < 160 mmHg and DBP < 100 mmHg
- Fetal: continuous heart monitoring, daily ultrasound (US) with biophysical profile (BPP), check amniotic levels and fetal growth
- Patient Education
  - Without severe features: restricted activity and close monitoring
  - With severe features: restricted activities in hospital

Urinary Tract Infection

Etiology
- Definition
  - UTIs are common in pregnancy.
  - Acute cystitis can occur alone or may be complicated by acute pyelonephritis.
- Incidence
  - The incidence of bacteriuria in pregnant women is approximately the same as in nonpregnant women; however, recurrent bacteriuria is more common during pregnancy.
- Risk Factors
  - The most common organism is *Escherichia coli* (75 to 95 percent).

Clinical Presentation
- History of Present Illness
  - Asymptomatic bacteriuria: asymptomatic
  - Acute cystitis: sudden onset of dysuria and urinary urgency and frequency
  - Acute pyelonephritis: fever, flank pain, nausea, vomiting, and/or costovertebral angle tenderness
- Physical Assessment Finding
  - Urine dipstick:
    - WBCs (leukocyte esterase): positive
    - Nitrites: may be positive or negative

Clinical Management
- Laboratory and Diagnostic Studies
  - Send midstream urine for urinalysis and urine culture and sensitivity (C&S)
- Pharmacologic
  - Pregnant women with asymptomatic bacteriuria are always treated because they are at high risk for acute pyelonephritis.
  - Nitrofurantoin (Macrobid) BID × 5 to 7 days
    - Do not use nitrofurantoin or sulfa drugs (e.g., Bactrim) near term because of the risk of hyperbilirubinemia; it causes hemolysis if the mother (or both mother and baby) has G6PD anemia.
  - Or amoxicillin–clavulanate (Augmentin) BID x 3 to 7 days or amoxicillin BID x 3 to 7 days or cephalexin BID x 3 to 7 days
- Patient Education
  - Take antibiotics as directed; drink plenty of fluids.
- Indication for Referral
  - If pyelonephritis is suspected, refer to ED or a physician.

Evaluation and Follow-Up
- Document resolution of infection by ordering posttreatment urine C&S 1 week after completing antibiotic therapy
- UTIs increase the risk of preterm birth, low birth weight, and perinatal mortality.

Uncomplicated Chlamydia Infection (Cervicitis, Urethritis)

Etiology
- Definition
  - Treating *Chlamydia trachomatis* infection in the mother will help to prevent the transmission of the infection to the newborn through the birth canal.
- Risk Factors
  - New or multiple sex partners, a sex partner with concurrent partners, a sex partner who has a UTI

Clinical Management
- Laboratory and Diagnostic Studies
  - Obtain nucleic acid amplification test (NAAT)
- Pharmacologic
  - First line
    - Azithromycin 1 g orally (single dose)
  - Alternative
    - Amoxicillin 500 mg PO TID × 7 days (lower cure rate than azithromycin)
- Sexual Partners
  - Azithromycin 1 g orally (single dose) or doxycycline 100 mg PO BID × 7 days (do not use if breastfeeding → stains tooth enamel, category D)

- Patient Education
  - Avoid sexual activity for 7 days, avoid unprotected intercourse until both partners are treated, and test for other STDs (gonorrhea, syphilis, HIV)

Evaluation and Follow-Up
- Test of cure needed in 3 weeks after completing antibiotic treatment.

Abortion
Overview
- Spontaneous: "miscarriage"; spontaneous loss of the fetus before it is viable (< 20 weeks)
- Threatened: vaginal bleeding occurs, but cervical os remains closed; most of these cases will result in an ongoing pregnancy.
- Inevitable: cervix is dilated and unable to stop the process; the fetus will be aborted.
- Complete: vaginal bleeding with cramping occurs; placenta and fetus are expelled completely; cervical os will close and bleeding stops.
- Incomplete: vaginal bleeding with cramping occurs; placental products remain in the uterus; cervical os remains dilated, and bleeding persists; pieces of tissue may be seen at the cervical os; vaginal discharge

Exam Success Tips

- There are two methods of screening for GDM: one-step method uses the 75-g OGTT (both for screening and diagnosis) and the two-step method uses 50-g OGTT test (nonfasting) as the screening test.
- First-line treatment for GDM is lifestyle change (diet and exercise).
- Risk factors for GDM include a history of GDM in a previous pregnancy, obesity, ethnicity (Asian, American Indian, Pacific Islander, African American, Hispanic), macrosomic infant (> 9 1bs), and age (older than 35 years).
- Action of RhoGAM: Rh antibodies hemolyze Rh-positive fetal RBCs.
- Always treat asymptomatic bacteriuria and UTIs in pregnant women.
- UTIs in pregnant women are classified as "complicated UTIs."
- A count of 10^3 cfu/mL or higher in a symptomatic pregnant person is considered a UTI; in a nonpregnant healthy adult, a UTI is defined as 100,000 CFU, or 10^5 CFU, of one organism.
- Signs and symptoms of UTI in pregnant women are the same as in those in a nonpregnant state.
- Amoxicillin is not the first-line drug for empiric UTI treatment (high resistance rates).

Red Flag

Ectopic Pregnancy
- Definition: implantation of the egg outside of the uterine cavity
- Risk factors: history of pelvic inflammatory disease, previous ectopic pregnancy, use of an IUD, tobacco use, age > 35
- History of present illness: reproductive-age, sexually active female with sudden onset of abdominal pain coupled with cessation of/or irregular menses and acute vaginal bleeding
- Physical assessment: abdominal tenderness with/without rebound tenderness associated with vaginal bleeding, palpable mass on pelvic exam, cervical motion tenderness
- Diagnostic studies: definite diagnosis is by serum quantitative chorionic gonadotropin level and transvaginal ultrasonography.
- Treatment: refer to the emergency department; patient needs methotrexate or a surgical procedure; these are nonviable pregnancies.

Placenta Abruption (Abruptio Placentae)
- Definition: premature partial to complete separation of a normally implanted placenta from the uterine bed; mostly occurs after 20 weeks (between 27 to 40)
- Risk factors: females with history of placenta abruption, hypertension (HTN), preeclampsia/eclampsia, smoking, trauma, cocaine use
- History of present illness: pregnant woman who is in the last few weeks of pregnancy with sudden onset of vaginal bleeding (mild to hemorrhage) with abdominal and/or back pain; painful uterine contractions; uterus is rigid (hypertonic) and very tender
- Treatment: refer to the emergency department; requires emergency treatment and cesarean section.

(continues)

Placenta Previa
- Definition: the placenta implants too low either on top of the cervix or on the cervical isthmus/neck
- Risk factors: previous history of placenta previa or C-section, multipara, older age, smoking, fibroids, or cocaine use
- History of present illness: a multipara woman who is in the late second to third trimester complains of new onset of painless vaginal bleeding that is worsened by intercourse; blood is bright red in color; uterus is soft and nontender
- Treatment: refer to the emergency department.
  - If cervix is not dilated:
    - Treatment is strict bed rest.
    - Administer IV magnesium sulfate if there is uterine cramping.
    - Uterus will usually reimplant itself if mild.
    - Vaginal or rectal insertion/stimulation is an absolute contraindication.
  - If cervix is dilated or hemorrhaging:
    - Fetus is delivered by C-section.

HELLP (Hemolysis, Elevated Liver Enzymes, and Low Platelets) Syndrome
- Definition: serious but rare complication of preeclampsia/eclampsia
- History of present illness: multipara woman older than 25 years of age who is in the third trimester of pregnancy; presents with the signs and symptoms of preeclampsia accompanied by RUQ (or midepigastric) abdominal pain with nausea/vomiting and malaise; symptoms can present suddenly
- Physical assessment findings: elevated AST, ALT, bilirubin, and lactate dehydrogenase (LDH) with decreased number of platelets and disseminated intravascular coagulation (DIC), peripheral smear with schistocytes and burr cells, and hemoglobin and hematocrit; if severe, RUQ/epigastric pain may have hepatic bleed or swelling, which may be signs of impending hepatic rupture.

Preterm Labor
- Definition: labor prior to 37 weeks
- Risk factors: multiple gestation pregnancy, smoking, infections, UTIs
- Treatment:
  - Betamethasone: used in preterm labor to reduce neonatal morbidity/mortality associated with respiratory distress syndrome (improves lung function and gas exchange in fetal lungs)
  - Surfactant: administered to newborn infants with respiratory distress syndrome to help gas exchange in the alveoli of the lungs

---

- is foul smelling (bacterial vaginosis); treatment is dilation and curettage (D&C) and antibiotic.
- Stillbirth or fetal death: pregnancy loss that occurs at 20 weeks gestation or later, or weight of 350 grams or greater

Postpartum

Occurs immediately after delivery and generally lasts about 6 weeks.

Uterine Involution

- It is normal for postpartum women to have uterine contractions (spontaneous or with breastfeeding) during the first 2 to 3 days after giving birth.
- After delivery, the uterus is the size of a 20-week pregnancy (fundi at the umbilicus).
- A soft boggy uterus accompanied by heavy vaginal bleeding is a sign of atony (inadequate contraction).
- Uterine involution takes about 6 weeks.

Breastfeeding

- Colostrum and breast milk
  - During the first 1 to 2 days of breastfeeding, colostrum is produced (thick yellow color), which contains maternal antibodies (passive immunity).
  - By days 3 to 4, mature breast milk is produced; the full-term healthy infant can be exclusively breastfed for the first 6 months, with no supplemental fluids unless ill or dehydrated.

- Vitamin D
  - All breastfed infants need vitamin D supplementation started within the first few days.
  - Formula-fed infants should only be given iron-fortified formula (has vitamin D).
- Iron
  - All exclusively breastfed infants require iron (ferrous sulfate) supplementation starting at 4 months at 1 mg/kg of body weight; breast milk contains very little iron.
  - At about 6 months, infants' iron needs can be met through introducing iron-rich foods, iron-fortified cereals, or iron supplement drops.
  - Infants on iron-fortified formula do not need additional iron supplementation.
- Breastfeeding Technique
  - Breastfeeding within the first hour of birth gives the baby colostrum and helps the uterus contract.
  - A new mother should be taught proper breastfeeding techniques. Refer to a lactation specialist if having problems; follow up at home.
  - If noisy, assess for improper latch-on (check positioning, sucking, clicking noises); swallowing noises are normal, but not clicking noises.
  - For clicking, advise the mother to use her index finger to pull down the baby's chin so that the baby's lower lip will be outside; the baby should have the entire nipple and most of the areola inside their mouth.

Lactational Mastitis
Etiology
- Definition
  - Painful, localized inflammation of the breast, generally caused by a clogged duct or a bacterial infection such as *Staphylococcus aureus*.
- Risk Factors
  - Breastfeeding, milk stasis, nipple trauma, maternal diabetes, maternal HIV, smoking
- General Prevention
  - Regular emptying of both breasts and nipple care to prevent fissures when breastfeeding.
  - Good hygiene includes hand washing and washing breast pumps after each use.

Clinical Presentation
- History of Present Illness
  - Fever, malaise, myalgia, nausea and/or vomiting, localized breast tenderness, firmness, heat, swelling, redness, possible breast mass
- Physical Assessment Findings
  - Breast tenderness, localized breast induration, redness, and warmth, peau d'orange appearance to overlying skin

Clinical Management
- Laboratory and Diagnostic Studies
  - Usually not needed; this is a clinical diagnosis.
- Pharmacologic
  - Low risk of MRSA
    - Dicloxacillin 500 mg PO QID *or* cephalexin (Keflex) 500 mg PO QID for 10 to 14 days
    - Do not use sulfas during the newborn period due to the increased risk of kernicterus.
  - High risk of MRSA
    - Trimethoprim–sulfamethoxazole (Bactrim) 1 to 2 tablets PO BID (can be used if a healthy infant is 1 month or older, no jaundice) *or* clindamycin 300 mg PO QID for 10 to 14 days
    - Continue to breastfeed on the affected breast during antibiotic treatment. If unable to breastfeed, pump milk from the infected breast (and discard) to prevent engorgement. Complete emptying of the breast is important during the infection.
    - If a breast abscess is suspected, order an ultrasound and refer for incision and drainage.
    - NSAIDs for pain and fever as needed. Apply cold compresses on the indurated breast area.
    - Refer to a lactation consultant if poor breastfeeding technique is suspected.
- Nonpharmacologic
  - Supportive care includes analgesia, warm compress, and effective, frequent milk removal from the affected breast via breastfeeding, pumping, or hand expression.
  - Smoking cessation is necessary for patients with periductal mastitis.
- Patient Education
  - To prevent fissures, encourage oral fluids and nipple care (simply with breast milk or with hypoallergenic nipple balm).

Postpartum Contraception
- Women who exclusively breastfeed (at least every 4 hours daily) with amenorrhea and who are less than 6 months postpartum are much less likely to ovulate than a woman who does not breastfeed exclusively.

- In women who do not breastfeed, ovulation resumes around 39 days postpartum.
- During the postpartum period and with breastfeeding, birth control pills or any contraceptive method containing estrogen (pregnancy category X) is contraindicated.
- Postpartum women or women who cannot take estrogens can use methods such as IUDs (copper or levonorgestrel) or progesterone-only contraception, such as etonogestrel (Nexplanon); depot medroxyprogesterone (Depo Provera); progestin-only pills; or barrier methods (condoms, diaphragm, cervical cap).

Postpartum Depression
- Can occur up to 1 year postpartum.
- Screening: Edinburgh postnatal depression scale; screen before patient leaves the hospital at every follow-up appointment.
- Management: Cognitive behavioral therapy (CBT), antidepressants

Exam Success Tips
- Swallowing noises may be heard in breastfeeding, especially in younger babies.
- If clicking noises are heard during breastfeeding, it is abnormal; advise the mother to use her index finger to pull down the baby's chin so that the baby's lower lip will latch better onto the areola.
- If a question describes a mother who complains of sore nipples, do not advise her to stop breastfeeding, to supplement with formula, or to use formula at nighttime feedings; the best answer is to advise the mother that it is a common problem during the first 2 weeks and will resolve and to continue breastfeeding.

CASE STUDY
Read the case study and consider the following questions:
- A 32-year-old female (G3P1) presents to the family nurse practitioner (FNP) at 25-weeks gestation. She complains of bright red vaginal bleeding that occurs after intercourse. She thought she noticed spotting earlier in the week, but over the last 2 days, she has had bleeding that lasts for several hours and soaks through one peripad. She denies abdominal pain, cramping, nausea, vomiting, or trauma. She is scared that something has happened to her baby.
  - How should the FNP first respond to this clinical situation?
  - What diagnosis does the FNP suspect is causing the vaginal bleeding?
  - What testing is indicated to evaluate or confirm the diagnosis?
  - What steps should the FNP take to manage this condition?

Rationale:
- The FNP should tell the patient that experiencing painless vaginal bleeding can be a troublesome sign. She should not be told that this is a normal finding, as vaginal bleeding after intercourse is never normal. If the patient were bleeding due to labor, there would usually be other signs, such as low back pain, cramping, or dark red bleeding.
- The FNP suspects that this patient has a placenta previa. Placenta previa presents with the classic signs of painless, bright red vaginal bleeding, especially in the second trimester. A placental abruption presents with abdominal pain and dark red bleeding and is generally unrelated to intercourse. A friable cervix would generally not present with bleeding that lasts several hours and has soaked through a peripad. An STI could potentially cause cervical friability but would not cause this level of vaginal bleeding.
- The first course of action is to order a transvaginal ultrasound to ascertain if placenta previa is the diagnosis. If there is no partial or complete placenta previa, the FNP will rule out other potential causes, such as a friable cervix.
- Management for placenta previa includes assessing fetal well-being by auscultating fetal heart rate for at least 1 minute and conducting an ultrasound to assess fetal well-being and placental location, putting the woman on bedrest as appropriate, educating to refrain from intercourse or putting anything inside the vaginal canal and to record accurate documentation of these findings and steps, and referral to an OB-GYN.

Review Questions

1. A woman at 38 weeks gestation has been setting up her baby's nursery over the weekend. This was done with a lot of bending and lifting. Today, Tuesday, she calls the family nurse practitioner's (FNP) office to get clearance to use ibuprofen for body aches. She denies fever or chills but complains of "sore muscles." The FNP advises her against using this medication because ibuprofen is what?
   A. Pregnancy category A drug
   B. Pregnancy category B drug
   C. Pregnancy category C drug
   D. Pregnancy category X drug

2. A 15-year-old adolescent who is 12 weeks pregnant with her first child comes for a prenatal visit. The FNP notes that the adolescent had been taking Ortho Tri-Cyclen 28 for acne. Upon questioning, the adolescent reports, "I only took the medication when my acne was really bad. I want to continue it because my skin has had a bad breakout for the past month." The FNP's best response is:
   A. "Feel free to continue the Ortho Tri-Cyclen 28 as it will help your acne."
   B. "Do not continue the Ortho Tri-Cyclen 28 because it won't help reduce your acne during pregnancy."
   C. "Ortho Tri-Cyclen 28 should not be taken during pregnancy because it can affect the baby's development."
   D. "Ortho Tri-Cyclen 28 should not be taken during pregnancy because it can increase your incidence of morning sickness."

3. A woman reports having her last menstrual period (LMP) on August 13. The FNP knows that using Naegele's rule will give this woman an estimated due date (EDD) of which of the following?
   A. May 20
   B. May 6
   C. November 20
   D. November 6

4. A woman comes to the FNP for her fifth prenatal visit and is 34 weeks by date and size. She shares with the FNP that she fears being alone at home with her partner. The best response from the FNP would be which of the following?
   A. "He doesn't hit you, does he?"
   B. "Many women feel that way at this point in their pregnancies."
   C. "Would you like to tell me more about this?"
   D. "That is silly since he is the father of your baby."

5. A woman comes for her first prenatal visit and reports she has a 3-year-old with spina bifida. The FNP knows that this is a neural tube problem and decides to put the woman on folic acid daily. This is done to:
   A. reduce the chances of a neural tube defect in this pregnancy.
   B. increase the risk of neural tube defects.
   C. increase the woman's hematocrit.
   D. decrease the woman's hematocrit.

6. A woman comes to her prenatal visit at 38 weeks gestation and reports regular fetal movement until this morning. She reports that she has not felt the baby move since last night. She reports having a full breakfast today as well. The FNP's priority action is to do which of the following?
   A. Calm the woman with soothing words
   B. Take the woman's vital signs
   C. Listen to the fetal heart rate with a Doppler
   D. Measure the woman's fundal height

7. An adolescent girl comes to the FNP with vesicular lesions around her vaginal introitus that burn and hurt. She reports having intercourse with her romantic partner 2 weeks before. The FNP knows this is a primary case of which of the following?
   A. Genital chlamydia
   B. Genital herpes
   C. Vulvovaginitis
   D. Monilial vaginitis

8. A 57-year-old woman who went through menopause 6 years ago comes to see the FNP today. She tells the FNP that she has been having vaginal bleeding for the last 5 days. She denies intercourse in the past few weeks. The FNP decides to investigate this further by ordering which of the following tests?
   A. Uterine ultrasound
   B. Complete blood count to rule out anemia
   C. An endometrial biopsy
   D. A mammogram

9. A woman comes to the FNP for her first prenatal appointment. Based on her dates and LMP, the FNP believes she is at 12 weeks gestation. The FNP assesses the uterine size and finds it consistent with the woman's dates at what size/location?
   A. Uterine size of a lemon
   B. Uterine size of a baseball
   C. Uterine fundus at the umbilicus
   D. Uterine fundus at symphysis pubis

10. The best time for the genetic assessment of an alpha-fetoprotein (AFP) screening test is which of the following?
    A. 12 to 14 weeks gestation
    B. 16 to 18 weeks gestation
    C. 22 to 24 weeks gestation
    D. 28 to 30 weeks gestation

11. The FNP is caring for a pregnant person who reports her obstetric history as having three children, all of whom are living. One was born at 39 weeks gestation, another at 34 weeks gestation, and another at 35 weeks gestation. How will the FNP document the patient's gravity and parity using the GTPAL system?
    A. G3 T1 P2 A0 L3
    B. G3 T0 P3 A0 L3
    C. G4 T1P 1A 1 L3
    D. G4 T 1P 2 A0 L3

12. The FNP is caring for a woman in the prenatal clinic in her 6th week of pregnancy. The patient reports urinary frequency and asks if this will continue throughout the pregnancy. Which response by the FNP is MOST accurate?
    A. "If you decrease your fluid intake, the problem will be less bothersome."
    B. "Urinary frequency persists until the 12th week but may continue if you have poor bladder tone."
    C. "It is difficult to predict how long this will last for individuals."
    D. "This may last until the 12th week of your pregnancy as the baby sits high in your uterus but will return as your due date approaches."

13. A 28-year-old woman who is 8 weeks pregnant comes to see the FNP with complaints of nausea, vomiting, and frequent urination. Based on this information, the FNP knows these are most indicative of which signs of pregnancy?
    A. Presumptive signs of pregnancy
    B. Positive signs of pregnancy
    C. Probable signs of pregnancy
    D. Signs of a urinary tract infection

14. A woman returns for her second prenatal visit at 14 weeks gestation. The FNP measures her fundal height at the woman's umbilicus. The FNP will order which diagnostic test to assess the situation?
    A. Amniocentesis to assess for fetal genetic abnormality
    B. Glucose challenge test (GCT) to assess for gestational diabetes
    C. Maternal serum AFP to assess for Down syndrome
    D. Ultrasound to assess for number of fetuses

15. The nurse practitioner (NP) works in an outpatient obstetric office and assesses four primigravida clients. Which of the following client findings would the nurse prioritize for a potential referral?
    A. 17 weeks gestation; denies feeling fetal movement
    B. 24 weeks gestation; fundal height at umbilicus
    C. 27 weeks gestation; complaints of excessive salivation
    D. 34 weeks gestation; complaints of hemorrhoid pain

16. Ashley comes to the FNP for her first prenatal appointment with this pregnancy. Using Naegele's rule and the woman's LMP date, the FNP determines she is at 12 weeks gestation. Ashley reports previous pregnancies; the FNP documents them as G3 T1, P1, A0, and L1. She reports having a fetal demise at 34 weeks gestation during her second pregnancy and states the autopsy revealed a male infant weighing 4300 grams with no evident cause of death. Upon questioning, the woman reports, "I think they told me my sugar testing was high, but they never did anything about it." What does the FNP know that could have contributed to Ashley's fetal demise?
    A. A second pregnancy
    B. A small-for-gestational-age fetus
    C. A normal-sized fetus
    D. An elevated blood sugar level

17. With Ashley's case in the earlier question, what will the FNP do to rule out a potential for gestational diabetes mellitus? (Select all that apply.)
    A. Order an ultrasound for gestational dating.
    B. Have the patient do fetal movement counts every day.
    C. Have the patient go for a glucose challenge test.
    D. Check her urine for ketones and glucos.

18. The FNP is caring for a patient at 24 weeks gestation, complaining of low back pain and increased watery vaginal secretions. She denies flu-like symptoms or other problems. What is the most likely diagnosis for this patient?
    A. Vaginal infection
    B. Premature rupture of membranes
    C. Preterm labor
    D. Back strain due to heavy lifting

19. A 22-year-old woman comes to the FNP to discuss her menstrual cycle. She reports irregular menses with light vaginal bleeding every 30 to 40 days. She also reports facial hair and an

increase in her weight. Based on this information, the FNP suspects what diagnosis for this patient?
A. Premenstrual syndrome (PMS)
B. Polycystic ovarian syndrome (PCOS)
C. Pregnancy
D. Perimenopause at an early age

20. The FNP knows there are several risk factors for breast cancer. Of the following conditions, which of these puts the woman at higher risk for breast cancer? (Select all that apply.)
A. History of late menarche
B. Pregnancy
C. Family history of breast cancer
D. Positive genetic workup for breast cancer

21. A 13-year-old girl is brought to the FNP for a discussion about preventing cancer. What things might the FNP suggest to protect the girl from various cancers? (Select all that apply.)
A. Do monthly breast self-exams (BSE).
B. Get the series of injections to reduce the chances of getting herpes.
C. Get the series of injections to reduce the incidence of human papillomavirus (HPV).
D. Avoid getting sunburned while on the beach.

22. The FNP knows that giving a teenager the three-injection vaccine series of Gardasil will reduce the teen's chances of contracting what?
A. Breast cancer
B. Rubella
C. HPV
D. Syphilis

23. The menopausal woman has many hormonal changes that may cause her to have dyspareunia. The FNP knows that to reduce dyspareunia, the woman could be put on hormone replacement therapy (HRT). What is an absolute contraindication to doing this?
A. History of hirsutism
B. History of fibrocystic disease
C. History of a mastectomy
D. History of mood changes

24. A patient who is 27 weeks gestation comes for her fourth prenatal appointment with the FNP. She reports no issues but asks, "Is it okay for me to use peripads to keep my panties dry? I have had wet panties since last week." What is the best response from the FNP?
A. "Peripads are fine to use. Just don't use tampons."
B. "Tell me more about this wetness that you are describing."
C. "Any wetness in your panties during pregnancy is due to what we call leukorrhea. It is normal in pregnancy."
D. "Don't worry about anything. I will make sure everything is okay with your pregnancy."

25. A woman who is at 32 weeks gestation comes to the FNP's office reporting leaking clear, odorless fluid since 2 days ago. The woman denies fever, chills, or reduced fetal movement. What test will give the FNP the best information to address this issue and form a diagnosis?
A. The first sonogram
B. Ferning test
C. Leopold's maneuver
D. HbA1C

Answers and Rationales

1. Answer D is correct. Ibuprofen is considered a pregnancy category X drug and should not be given in the third trimester. Category X drugs are contraindicated during pregnancy because studies in animals or humans have demonstrated fetal abnormalities, or there is strong evidence of fetal risk.

   Answer A is incorrect. Pregnancy Category A drugs have been shown to have no evidence of risk to the fetus when used during pregnancy. Examples of Category A drugs include Folic acid, Levothyroxine, Thiamine, and Senna.

   Answer B is incorrect. Category B drugs in pregnancy are those for which animal studies have not shown a fetal risk, but there are no adequate human studies in pregnant women. These medications are generally considered safe for use in pregnancy, especially if there is a clinical need for them. Examples of Category B drugs are Acetaminophen, Amoxicillin loratadine, and ondansetron.

   Answer C is incorrect. In Category C drugs there are no satisfactory studies in humans, but animal studies demonstrated a risk to the fetus; potential benefits of the drug may outweigh the risks. Examples of Category C drugs are amlodipine, trazadone and gabapentin.

2. Answer C is correct. Ortho Tri-Cyclen 28 should not be taken during pregnancy because it can affect the baby's development and is a pregnancy category X medication.

Answer A is incorrect. It is unsafe to use Ortho Tri-Cyclen during pregnancy because it is Category X and may be harmful to the fetus. The nurse practitioner should use a stepwise approach of using topical agents and oral antibiotics that are in Category B to treat acne during pregnancy.

Answer B is incorrect. While Ortho Tri-Cyclen may reduce acne it is contraindicated in pregnancy.

Answer D is incorrect. Ortho Tri-Cyclen is FDA-approved specifically for acne treatment in females who also need birth control and are not pregnant. It has not been proven to increase morning sickness.

3. Answer A is correct. Naegele's rule is used to determine an EDD based on the woman's reported LMP. To calculate the EDD, take the first day of the LMP + 7 days − 3 months + one year.

Answer B is incorrect. The clinician calculated the LMP − 7 days − 3 months & 1 year to get May 6.

Answer C is incorrect. The clinician calculated the LMP + 7 days + 3 months and − one year to get November 20.

Answer D is incorrect. The clinician calculated the LMP − 7 days + 3 months and − one year to get November 6.

4. Answer C is correct. In a pattern of intimate partner violence, the woman needs to understand she can tell someone whom she trusts about her violent situation. The best way for the FNP to react is to open the door for the woman to discuss it more.

Answer A is incorrect. The statement "He doesn't hit you, does he?" completely is a closed ended statement that shuts down any opportunity for the patient to freely express herself.

Answer B is incorrect. The statement "Many women feel that way at this point in their pregnancies." disregards the patient's feelings and condones the partner's behaviors.

Answer D is incorrect. The statement "That is silly since he is the father of your baby." makes the patient feel stupid and unheard.

5. Answer A is correct. Giving the woman oral folic acid has been shown to reduce the risk of neural tube defects, especially with those women who have had an infant with such a defect in the past.

Answer B is incorrect. Folic acid supplementation before and during early pregnancy can prevent about 70% of neural tube defects (NTDs).

Answers C and D are incorrect. Folic acid neither increases or decreases the hematocrit in pregnancy but it does play a role in cell growth and the production of red blood cells, which are important for both the mother and the developing fetus.

6. Answer C is correct. The priority action is assessing the fetal heart rate and well-being. Once a fetal heart rate has been auscultated, other things can be done.

Answer A is incorrect. Acknowledging the patient's anxiety and providing reassurance is important but the first priority is to measure fetal heart rate.

Answer B is incorrect. Assessing the fetal heart rate is the priority given the patient's reported history; checking the patient's vital signs would be an additional assessment to follow.

Answer D is incorrect. Assessing the fetal heart rate is the priority here; while measuring the patient's fundal height may be important it is not the first step.

7. Answer B is correct. The most likely diagnosis is genital herpes, which occurs 2 to 7 days after exposure and presents with painful, burning vesicles.

Answer A is incorrect. Genital chlamydia typically presents with dysuria, vaginal discharge, or pain in the lower abdomen. Chlamydia may also be asymptomatic.

Answer C is incorrect. Vulvovaginitis is characterized by inflammation of the vulva and vagina, often accompanied by symptoms like itching, burning, and abnormal vaginal discharge. Bacterial vaginosis, a shift in the vaginal flora, is often considered the most prevalent cause.

Answer D is incorrect. Monilial vaginitis is a common fungal infection caused by the overgrowth of Candida yeast. It's characterized by symptoms like itching, burning, and a white, curdy vaginal discharge.

8. Answer C is correct. A woman who has been postmenopausal and presents with vaginal bleeding needs to have an endometrial biopsy to rule out endometrial cancer.

Answer A is incorrect. A uterine ultrasound will be beneficial to help detect and diagnose conditions like uterine fibroids, ovarian cysts, polyps, and endometrial hyperplasia but an endometrial biopsy is the gold standard to evaluate for endometrial cancer cells.

Answer B is incorrect. If a patient had profuse prolonged vaginal bleeding a complete blood count would be useful to evaluate for microcytic anemia.

Answer D is incorrect. A mammogram is used to screen for breast cancer.

9. Answer D is correct. The normal uterine size and location for 12 weeks gestation is just above the symphysis pubis.

Answer A is incorrect. Eight-week gestation is the uterine size of a lemon.

Answer B is incorrect. Ten-week gestation is the uterine size of a baseball.

Answer C is incorrect. The uterine fundus at the umbilicus is 20–22 weeks gestation.

10. Answer B is correct. The best time to get the most accurate reading of an AFP test is at 16 to 18 weeks gestation. The fetal liver produces alpha-fetoprotein and can be tested for it via maternal blood. It is a screening test to assess the risk for neural tube defects in each pregnancy. This test is best performed between 16 and 18 weeks gestation for increased reliability. If the test is abnormal, follow-up procedures to rule out neural tube defects include genetic counseling for families with a history of neural tube defects, repeated AFP, high-resolution ultrasound, and potentially an amniocentesis.

Answer A is incorrect. At 12 to 14 weeks gestation the nurse practitioner may order a nuchal translucency scan, assess fetal growth, confirm due date, and check for structural abnormalities. The scan can assess the placenta and amniotic fluid.

Answer C is incorrect. At 22 to 24 weeks gestation the nurse practitioner may order a 2nd-trimester growth scan or fetal well-being ultrasound, which is a routine part of prenatal care.

Answer D is incorrect. At 28 to 30 weeks gestation the nurse practitioner may order an early 3rd-trimester growth scan or late pregnancy ultrasound. It is used to assess fetal growth, well-being, and position, and to check for any potential complications or abnormalities. It can estimate fetal weight and monitor amniotic fluid levels.

11. Answer D is correct. The pregnant person is now experiencing her fourth pregnancy, which is documented as G4. One child was full term, and two children were born prematurely at less than 38 weeks. All three children are living. She is a G4, P = 1 full-term, 2 premature, 0 abortions, and 3 living.

Answer A is incorrect. G3 T1 P2 A0 L3 (patient is in her G 4th pregnancy; the others are correct)

Answer B is incorrect. G3 T0 P3 A0 L3 (patient is in her G 4th pregnancy, she had 1 Term birth, 2 premature and 3 living)

Answer C is incorrect. G4 T1P 1A 1 L3 (patient is in her G 4th pregnancy, she had 1 Term birth, 2 premature and 3 living. She had no abortions or miscarriages)

12. Answer D is correct. Urinary frequency usually disappears around week 12 of gestation (the fetus takes up more space higher in the uterus with less pressure on the bladder), but as the enlarging uterus puts pressure on the bladder, the problem returns near the due date.

Answer A is incorrect. The patient should be instructed to maintain adequate hydration throughout pregnancy without excessive fluid intake before bed. Also limiting or avoiding caffeine, which can be a diuretic and exacerbate frequent urination, should be advised.

Answer B is incorrect. Urinary frequency is a normal part of pregnancy due to hormonal changes and increased blood volume. Kegel exercises should be taught to strengthen the pelvic floor muscles and improve bladder control.

Answer C is incorrect. Urinary frequency during pregnancy follows a predictable pattern beginning in the first trimester and continuing through the third trimester. It's primarily caused by hormonal changes, a growing uterus pressing on the bladder, and increased blood volume, which leads to increased kidney filtration.

13. Answer A is correct. Presumptive signs of pregnancy are breast changes, amenorrhea, nausea, vomiting, urinary frequency, and quickening.

Answer B is incorrect. Positive signs of pregnancy are visualization of the fetus via ultrasound and the auscultation of fetal heart tones.

Answer C is incorrect. Probable signs of pregnancy include a positive pregnancy test, Goodell's, Hegar's, and Chadwick's signs, and ballottement.

Answer D is incorrect. Signs of a urinary tract infection are burning, pain in urination, and strong, malodorous urine.

14. Answer D is correct. At approximately 16 weeks gestation, the maternal uterine size will be greater than dates if there is more than one fetus. An ultrasound will assist in the determination of the number of fetuses in the woman's uterus.

Answer A is incorrect. Amniocentesis is an invasive procedure used at 15-20 weeks in women who are at greater risk for fetal genetic abnormality. This test does not assess for larger-than-normal uterus size.

Answer B is incorrect. The Glucose challenge test (GCT) is typically done between 24 and 28 weeks of pregnancy to assess gestational diabetes and will not assess the larger-than-normal uterus size.

Answer C is incorrect. Maternal serum AFP is typically done between 15 and 20 weeks gestation to assess Down syndrome and does not address the larger-than-normal uterus size.

15. Answer B is correct. A normal fundal height for 24 weeks gestation is 1 to 2 fingerbreadths above the umbilicus/24 cm from the symphysis pubis to the uterine fundus. Since this is smaller than expected, the FNP will consider a referral to an OB-GYN.

Answer A is incorrect. During the first pregnancy patients typically begin feeling fetal movement between 18 and 20 weeks and sometimes later so not feeling fetal movement at 17 weeks gestation is normal.

Answer C is incorrect. Complaints of excessive salivation is a normal finding during pregnancy.

Answer D is incorrect. Complaints of hemorrhoid pain is a common normal change that can occur during pregnancy.

16. Answer D is correct. A woman who has "high sugar" levels is possibly a person with gestational diabetes (GDM). With these pregnancies, the woman will have a large-for-gestational-age infant, with the potential for fetal demise due to uncontrolled maternal blood sugar levels. Other risk factors for fetal demise include high blood pressure, tobacco use, obesity, advanced maternal age, and post term pregnancy.

Answer A is incorrect. A second pregnancy has nothing to do with the fetal demise.

Answer B is incorrect. While a small-for-gestational-age fetus has an increased risk of fetal demise the patient's fetus was a large-for-gestational-age fetus, being over 4,000 g.

Answer C is incorrect. A normal-sized fetus has nothing to do with fetal demise.

17. Answers A, C, and D are correct. The FNP is considering that Ashley has GDM. The initial screenings must be done ASAP to rule this out and ascertain the correct gestational age. Checking her urine for ketones and glucose assists the FNP to further evaluate for GDM.

Answer B is incorrect. Daily fetal movement counts cannot be done until the fetus can be felt moving around 16 to 18 weeks gestation for a multigravida.

18. Answer C is correct. A 24-week gestation pregnancy with these symptoms should alert the FNP to potential signs of preterm labor. The FNP will need to do a thorough history and vaginal exam to rule all of this out or to confirm the diagnosis.

Answer A is incorrect. A vaginal infection during pregnancy would present with abnormal vaginal discharge findings suggestive of bacterial vaginosis, vaginal trichomoniasis, chlamydia, gonorrhea or vaginal candidiasis, e.g., dark yellow, brown, green, grey, white curd-like discharge and/or malodorous discharge. There may be abdominal pain, fever, and chills. This patient's vaginal secretions are watery.

Answer B is incorrect. Premature rupture of membranes (PROM) is a sudden gush or continuous leakage of clear amniotic fluid. It can occur at or after 37 weeks of gestation (term PROM) or before 37 weeks (preterm PROM).

Answer D is incorrect. The patient's history does not indicate any trauma or heavy lifting that would contribute to back strain.

19. Answer B is correct. These symptoms reported by this woman are consistent with PCOS. The symptoms that support this diagnosis are light, irregular periods, weight gain, and androgenic changes.

Answer A is incorrect. The symptoms of Premenstrual syndrome (PMS) may include breast tenderness, fatigue, and mood swings due to hormonal fluctuations. This is not consistent with this patient's presenting complaints.

Answer C is incorrect. Presenting symptoms of pregnancy are often associated with nausea and vomiting (morning sickness), a missed period, and frequent urination.

Answer D is incorrect. Early perimenopause generally starts in the late 30s or early 40s, but some women experience it as early as their mid-30s; this patient is only 22 years of age and getting her periods on a 30-40 day cycle.

20. Answers A, C, and D are correct. A family history of breast cancer, a positive genetic workup for breast cancer, and a history of late menarche have been correlated to an increased risk of breast cancer in women.

Answer B is incorrect. Pregnancy, particularly early pregnancies, is associated with a lower lifetime risk of breast cancer. This is thought to be due to the fact that pregnancy interrupts exposure to estrogen and reduces the total number of menstrual cycles a woman experiences.

21. Answers A, C, and D are correct. Doing monthly BSE empowers the teen to be aware of the potential breast changes that can occur as her body matures. Gardasil is a recombinant HPV vaccine used to prevent certain strains of HPV, specifically HPV types 6, 11, 16, and 18. It also reduces the potential for getting cervical cancer by reducing HPV, which is correlated to cervical cancer. Avoiding the sun and/or using sunscreen will reduce the potential for skin cancers in the future.

    Answer B is incorrect. There is no Herpes vaccine.

22. Answer C is correct. Gardasil is a recombinant HPV vaccine used to prevent certain strains of HPV, specifically HPV types 6, 11, 16, and 18. It also reduces the potential for getting cervical cancer by reducing HPV, which is correlated to cervical cancer.

    Answer A is incorrect. There is no vaccine for the prevention of breast cancer.

    Answer B is incorrect. Rubella occurrences are reduced by giving a single-dose vaccine against that virus.

    Answer D is incorrect. There is no vaccine for the prevention of breast cancer or syphilis.

23. Answer C is correct. A history of breast cancers for which a mastectomy was done is an absolute contraindication to HRT. Other absolute contraindications include the risk of developing estrogen-sensitive cancers and a history of thromboembolic events.

    Answer A is incorrect. History of hirsutism is not an absolute contraindication to HRT.

    Answer B is incorrect. History of fibrocystic disease is not an absolute contraindication to HRT.

    Answer D is incorrect. Mood changes may be a side-effect of HRT but is not an absolute contraindication.

24. Answer B is correct. The best response is this therapeutic one.

    Answer A is incorrect. "Peripads are fine to use. Just don't use tampons." This statement is judgmental.

    Answer C is incorrect. It is clear that the discharge the patient describes is a normal physiologic change of pregnancy and no further explanation is needed.

    Answer D is incorrect. The statement "Don't worry about anything. I will make sure everything is okay with your pregnancy." dismisses the patient's question and is paternalistic.

25. Answer B is correct. The ferning test will evaluate whether the woman has a spontaneous rupture of membranes (SROM). Amniotic fluid will have a characteristic fern-like pattern under a microscope when a vaginal fluid sample is air-dried.

    Answer A is incorrect. The first sonogram cannot be compared to anything to assess if amniotic fluid volume is reduced.

    Answer C is incorrect. The Leopold's maneuver does not evaluate for spontaneous rupture of membranes (SROM). It is a series of four systematic abdominal palpations used during pregnancy to determine the fetal position, presentation, and engagement.

    Answer D is incorrect. Glycated Hemoglobin A1c (HbA1C) measures the average level of blood sugar (glucose) over the previous 2–3 months and does not evaluate for spontaneous rupture of membranes (SROM).

Resources

American Cancer Society. (2023). *American cancer society recommendations for the early detection of breast cancer.* https://www.cancer.org/cancer/types/breast-cancer/screening-tests-and-early-detection/american-cancer-society-recommendations-for-the-early-detection-of-breast-cancer.html

Arnold, S. J., & Kreuser-Genis, I. M. (2023). *Vulva lichen sclerosus: Clinical manifestations and diagnosis.* UpToDate. https://www.uptodate.com/contents/vulvar-lichen-sclerosus-clinical-manifestations-and-diagnosis

Cash, J. C. (2023). *Family practice guidelines* (6th ed.). Springer Publishing.

Domino, F. J. (2023). *The 5-minute clinical consult* (31st ed.). Wolters Kluwer.

Joe, B. N. (2023). *Clinical features, diagnosis, and staging of newly diagnosed breast cancer.* UpToDate. https://www.uptodate.com/contents/clinical-features-diagnosis-and-staging-of-newly-diagnosed-breast-cancer

Lawrence, L. R. (2022). *Breastfeeding: A guide for medical professionals* (9th ed.). Elsevier.

Leik, M. T. (2020). *Family nurse practitioner certification intensive review* (4th ed.). Springer Publishing.

Sabel, M. S. (2023). *Overview of benign breast diseases.* UpToDate. https://www.uptodate.com/contents/overview-of-benign-breast-diseases

Secor, M. R., & Holland, A. C. (2023). *Advanced health assessment of women: Clinical skills and procedures* (5th ed.). Springer Publishing.

Watson, S. (2023). *Stages of the menstrual cycle.* Healthline. https://www.healthline.com/health/womens-health/stages-of-menstrual-cycle

CHAPTER 18

Men's Health

Nancy L. Dennert, MS, MSN, FNP-BC, CDCES, BC-ADM

Anatomy of the Male Reproductive System

- **Male penis:**
  - Two parallel cylinders of erectile tissue
  - Corpora cavernosa
  - Corpus spongiosum, which is a single ventrally placed cylinder that surrounds the urethra and distally forms the glans penis
- **Testes**: makes and stores sperm and produces testosterone
- **Scrotum**: functions to protect the two testes and keeps the temperature below body temperature
- **Vas Deferans**: connects the epididymis and the urethra, stores sperm, and moves it from the scrotum to the urethra
- **Epididymis:** moves the sperm out of the testicles
- **Seminal vesicles**: produces seminal fluid
- **Prostate**: walnut sized; surrounds the neck of the bladder and urethra
- Eighty percent smooth muscle tissue; 20 percent glandular
- Secretes alkaline fluid to form part of the seminal fluid

Urethritis

- Urethritis is more commonly seen in young, sexually active men.
- Urinary tract infections occur in older men with prostatic hypertrophy or a history of prior catheterization.
- Dysuria is also reported in most men with symptomatic gonorrhea and over half of patients with nongonococcal urethritis (NGU).
- NGU: Inflammation of the urethra not caused by gonorrhea but characterized by a mucopurulent discharge
- Twenty-five to 55 percent of cases are caused by chlamydia.
- Other causes include trichomonas, herpes simplex virus (HSV), ureaplasma, and mycoplasma.
- Symptomatic males: urethral discharge (yellow, white, or cloudy), dysuria, and itch
- White blood cells (WBCs) found in urine.

Dysuria

- The incubation period for gonorrhea is shorter (less than 2 weeks).
- The incubation period for chlamydia has a variable onset of 2 to 35 days.
- Urethral discharge that is described as acute and frankly purulent is suggestive of gonorrhea.
- Patients with dysuria alone are more likely to have chlamydial infection.
- Dysuria that is accompanied by painful genital ulcers is probably due to genital HSV.

Prostate Disorders

- Acute bacterial prostatitis, chronic bacterial prostatitis
- Inflammation or infectious process of the prostate gland
- Occurs in 50 percent of men in their lifetime

Prostatitis

- Both acute and chronic prostatitis can occur in young and middle-aged men.
- Chronic prostatitis can occur as a complication of acute prostatitis or without any recognized initial infection.
- Urethral instrumentation, prostatic surgery, pelvic trauma, **men who have sex with men** (MSM), and human immunodeficiency virus (HIV) are risk factors for prostatitis.
- Gonorrhea and chlamydia
- E-coli (the primary organism implicated in prostatitis)
- Members of the *Enterobacteriaceae* family

Common Symptoms of Prostatitis

- Both obstructive and irritative symptoms
- Difficulty initiating urination
- Decreased force of stream and urinary flow
- Frequency, dysuria, and nocturia
- Arthralgias, myalgias
- Pain in perineal and rectal areas that extend to the tip of the penis

Acute Bacterial Prostatitis

- Acute bacterial prostatitis is an acute infection of the prostate.
- Etiology
  - E. coli: 80 percent
  - Pseudomonas, Serratia, Klebsiella, Proteus: 10 to 15 percent;
  - Enterococci: 5 to 10 percent

Clinical features
- Men of all ages
- Acute onset of fever, malaise, arthralgia, myalgia
- Pelvic area pain
- Dysuria, frequency, urgency
- Digital rectal exam (DRE): tender, warm prostate
- Complete blood count (CBC): Elevated WBC
- Urinalysis (U/A) Pyuria
- May have elevated PSA

Possible Complications
- Prostatic abscess, acute urinary retention, septicemia
- Rarely: vertebral osteomyelitis, chronic prostatitis

Treatment
- Toxic patients: in-hospital IV therapy
- Nontoxic patients: oral therapy (fluoroquinolones or trimethoprim-sulfamethoxazole or tetracycline derivatives), treatment for 2 to 4 weeks
- Other therapy: antipyretics, analgesics, stool softeners, bed rest, increased fluid intake

> **Clinical Pearls**
>
> Avoid prostate massage if acute prostatitis is expected to minimize inducing bacteremia. **Prostate massage can disseminate infected fluid and cause sepsis**.

Pharmaceutical Treatment
- Fluoroquinolones (Cipro 500 mg PO q 12 hrs or Levaquin 500 mg QD PO x 4 weeks or trimethoprim-sulfamethoxazole
  - Treatment for 4 weeks is recommended but may require a longer duration.
  - It is very important to choose antibiotics that can penetrate the prostate.
  - The cure rate at 1 year is ~60 percent when treated with fluoroquinolones and ~ 40 percent when treated with trimethoprim-sulfamethoxazole.
    - Possible complications include repeated urinary tract infections and a possible decrease in fertility.

Chronic Bacterial Prostatitis

- Recurrent infection of the prostate
- Etiology
  - Same organisms as acute bacterial prostatitis (E coli: 80 percent)

Clinical features
- Older men
- Recurrent urinary tract infection or asymptomatic bacteriuria
- Urinary symptoms and pelvic area pain
- DRE: variable prostate exam; enlarged, tender, boggy, or firm
- Abdominal exam: distended bladder
- Treat empirically

Benign Prostatic Hypertrophy

- Benign prostatic hypertrophy (BPH) is the noncancerous enlargement of the prostate gland.
- The most common prostate problem for men over the age of 50.

- Incidence: 90 percent of men have some degree of hyperplasia by 8th decade.
- Risk factors:
  - First-degree relatives
  - BPH is more prevalent in African Americans than Caucasians.
  - Obesity, Type 2 diabetes mellitus (DM), cardiovascular (CV) disease
- There is no straightforward relationship between signs and symptoms of obstruction and prostate size.
  - The majority of men with prostate enlargement never develop significant obstruction.
  - Slow, gradual progression
  - Slightly increased chance of prostate cancer if prostate-specific antigen (PSA) velocity increases more than 0.75 ng/ml per year.
- Symptoms of obstructive BPH:
  - decreased force of stream
  - incomplete emptying with a weak or interrupted stream
  - difficulty starting a stream
  - hesitancy
  - dribbling

History and Physical Examination (PE)

- DRE reveals enlargement of the prostate without nodules; boggy, spongy feeling
- Increased postvoid residual greater than 100 ml

Complications

- Most men do not develop these more severe complications.
  - Acute urinary retention
  - Hematuria
  - UTIs
  - Bladder stones
  - Kidney damage

Diagnostic Tests

- Serum creatinine and Blood Urea Nitrogen (BUN) may be elevated if obstruction affects renal function.
- Urodynamic testing
- Cystoscopy
- Transrectal ultrasound
- Biopsy of the prostate if a strong suspicion of prostate cancer

Clinical Pearls

PSA levels are not diagnostic in themselves because levels may become elevated with aging, prostate infections, and inflammation. However, PSA may be useful in diagnosing and monitoring cancer progression.

Age-Specific Prostate Specific Antigen Levels

Normal PSA levels

40–49	< 2.5 ng/mL
50–59	< 3.5 ng/mL
60–69	< 4.5 ng/mL
70–79	< 6.5 ng/mL

As a patient ages, the prostrate hypertrophies, and more PSA is produced, which increases levels.

Treatment

- Small frequent amounts of water and decreased fluid intake after evening meal
- Void frequently throughout the day
- Avoid over-the-counter (OTC) cold preparations because of the anticholinergic effects
- Frequent intercourse to decrease obstruction

Pharmaceutical Treatment

- Alpha-adrenergic blockers (Terazosin = Hytrin; Cardura = Doxazosin) relax smooth muscle.
- Tamsulosin= Flomax
  - Side effects: palpitation, tachycardia, hypotension, headache (h/a)
- 5-alpha-reductase inhibitors (Finasteride = Proscar; Dutasteride = Avodart) are antiandrogens that deprive the prostate of growth-enhancing factors
- Saw Palmetto herbal remedy for symptom relief
- Urologist for persistent worsening symptoms
- Surgery

Prostate Cancer

- Risk factors
  - Increasing age (80 percent of men who are diagnosed are older than 65)

- Race (African American males have a higher incidence of prostate cancer vs. all Black people)
- Occupational exposure to carcinogens
- Vasectomy as a risk factor is controversial.
- Unpredictable course
- Prostate Cancer Screening
  - The American Cancer Society (ACS) recommends that men who are at an average risk for prostate cancer should start a discussion with their provider at age 50 whether to have screening performed (age 45 if high risk such as African American males or those with a family history of prostate cancer). Screening is typically done with a PSA blood test along with a digital rectal exam (DRE).
  - The United States Preventative Services Task Force (USPSTF), in contrast to the American Cancer Society (ACS), explicitly recommends against PSA-based screening for prostate cancer.

Evaluation of Patient

- Obtain a thorough urological history
- Assess for unexplained weight loss
- Urinary obstruction, UTI
- Pelvic heaviness/fullness
- Low back pain (may be symptomatic of metastasis to the spine)
- Anemia, bone pain
- DRE at age 40 to assess for asymmetric, nodular, localized painful prostate (DRE does not decrease morbidity or mortality)
- PSA levels are not specific for cancer but may help guide treatment and diagnosis
- Biopsy may be recommended for symptomatic patients with PSAs greater than 4 to 10.
- Check for elevated Alk Phos levels for metastases.

Management

- Refer to a urologist for management and treatment.
- Younger patients will receive more aggressive treatment.
- Patients and providers may select watchful waiting for older patients.
- Surgery: radical prostatectomy
- Radiation: External beam and seeds
- Hormonal (metastatic): Flutamide and Lupron; androgen deprivation therapy (ADT) lowers androgen levels

Disorders of the Scrotum/Testes

Epididymitis

- Secondary to bacterial infection (i.e., gonorrhea (GC), chlamydia); most common cause in men under 35.

Symptoms

- Scrotal pain, swelling, and induration
- Urinary frequency, hematuria, and cloudy urine
- Fever, chills
- Positive Prehn's sign (lifting the testicle relieves pain)
- Pyuria, increased WBC in urine

Treatment for Epididymitis

- Ice packs and elevation of the scrotum
- Bed rest for 1 to 2 days
- Increase fluid
- Antibiotic treatment for underlying cause
- Pain management with NSAIDs
- Follow up (F/U) in 48 hrs
- Possible urology referral

Antibiotic Treatment Regimens for Epididymitis

- Single Dose Ceftriaxone 250 mg to 500 mg IM x 1 plus Doxycycline 100 mg BID for 10 days
- Levofloxacin 500 mg PO daily for 10 days
- Ciprofloxacin 300 mg BID for 10 days
- Trimethorprim-Sulfamoxazole 160 mg PO BID x 14 days
- Treat sexual partners

Testicular Cancer

- Accounts for 1 percent of all cancers in men in the United States.
- Men age 15 to 34 years old.
- Risk is 5 times higher in White men compared to African Americans and double that of Asian men.

Risk Factors for Testicular Cancer

- Scrotal trauma
- Atrophy
- Exogenous estrogen hormone exposure
- Cryptorchidism
- Family history
- > 50 years old with a history of lymphoma

Symptoms
- Nodular swelling, heavy sensation, dull ache, painless mass
- Metastatic: back pain, dyspnea, gynecomastia

Diagnostics
- Ultrasound
- CT Abdomen and Pelvis
- MRI

Treatment
- Surgery, radiation, and may need chemotherapy if advanced
- F/U appts include PE and labs to check tumor markers
- Teach monthly testicular self exam (TSE)

Testicular Torsion
- Twisting of the spermatic cord that results in compromised testicular blood flow
- May occur spontaneously after activity or trauma
- Commonly occurs during puberty
- Congenital "Bell Clapper" deformity puts the patient at higher risk for developing testicular torsion.

History and Diagnostics
- Sudden onset of testicular pain that radiates to the groin
- Nausea and vomiting in 50 percent of patients
- May have lower abdominal pain

Clinical Pearls
Absence of cremasteric reflex, negative Prehn's sign, no urethral discharge, or dysuria but may have increased frequency of urination.
Ultrasound may be used to confirm diagnosis and check blood flow.

Treatment
- **Urologic emergency**: Surgery within 4 to 8 hours is preferred to save the testicle. The spermatic cord needs to be untwisted to restore the blood supply.
- Ischemic injury and necrosis if no surgery
- Salvage rate < 75 percent if surgery not done within 12 hours

Cryptorchidism
- Failure of the testes to descend into the scrotum
- Testes normally descend in utero at around 36 weeks.
- If testes are undescended by 6 months old, they are unlikely to descend spontaneously.
- Mechanical failure (i.e., hernia sac, shortened spermatic artery)
- Lack of androgenic hormones during fetal development
- Deterioration of the testicle begins around 1 year old
- Correlates with poor semen quality and infertility.
- Increased risk for malignancy, testicular torsion, emotional stress, trauma, and hernia
- Refer all children to a pediatric urologist for surgical repair.

Varicocele
- It affects 15 to 20 percent of men and is more likely to occur on the left side (97 percent).
- Varicose veins secondary to incompetent venous valves may cause testicular atrophy.
- It is the most common cause of identifiable infertility in men.
- Palpation may feel like "a sack of worms."
- Unilateral right-sided varicocele may be associated with malignancy affecting the retroperitoneum (obstructing venous flow) and warrants further imaging and referral to a urologist.
- No treatment for small veins
- Surgery for large veins

Hydrocele
- Symptoms
  - Painless swelling in the scrotum occurs when fluid collects in the tunica vaginalis (thin sheath) surrounding a testicle.
  - It is common in newborns and usually disappears without treatment by age 1.
  - Older boys and adult men can develop a hydrocele due to inflammation or injury within the scrotum.
- Diagnostics
  - Ultrasound
  - CBC
  - GC/Chlamydia
  - HIV
  - Erythrocyte sedimentation rate (ESR)
  - C-reactive protein (CRP)

Treatment:

- Watchful waiting, NSAIDs, scrotal support
- Surgical aspiration, sclerotherapy, or resection

Spermatocele

- It is a common occurrence that affects nearly 1 in 3 men, occurring most commonly in midlife in the 40 to 50 age range.
- A benign, painless cystic accumulation of milky fluid that may contain sperm.
- It is not a sexually transmitted infection.
- It may be discovered incidentally while performing a TSE.
- Usually, it does not go away on its own without treatment.
- It presents as a painless cystic mass.
- Moveable, firm, and painless
- Distinct borders
- Transilluminates easily
- Check ultrasound, urinalysis (U/A)
- Symptomatic treatment, scrotal support
- Surgery for excision if large

CASE STUDY 1

A 25-year-old male presents to the clinic complaining of groin pain and heavy sensation in his scrotum. History reveals unprotected intercourse within the past few weeks. On exam, his scrotum is swollen (twice the normal size). The right testicle is firm, hard, and very tender. His inguinal area was not tender, and no bulge was found. He denies any nausea or vomiting. The pain had come on gradually over the past 2 days. He could still go to work, but his major complaint is "tenderness." He has a positive Prehn's sign, and an ultrasound revealed increased intratesticular blood flow.

a. Epididymitis
b. Testicular cancer
c. Orchitis
d. Testicular torsion

Answer: Epididymitis

CASE STUDY 2

A 24-year-old sexually active male is seen in the college health clinic with complaints of heaviness in the scrotum. He denies any pain or trauma. He does state that he had an undescended testicle until he was 8 months old. The nurse practitioner (NP) should have a high index of suspicion for:

a. Epididymitis
b. Testicular cancer
c. Orchitis
d. Testicular torsion

Answer: Testicular Cancer

CASE STUDY 3

A 25-year-old male soccer player presents to your clinic for an urgent visit. Last evening, he experienced a slight groin discomfort after soccer practice. Later that night, he was awakened by intense unilateral (left side) abdominal and groin pain. His parents brought him into the clinic first thing in the morning. He denies sexual activity or recent sports injury/trauma. This morning, he was nauseated and vomited once. On exam, his scrotum is edematous; he has an absent cremasteric reflex, negative Prehn's sign, and the left testicle is high and extremely tender. The nurse practitioner should have a high index of suspicion for:

a. Epididymitis
b. Testicular cancer
c. Orchitis
d. Testicular torsion

Answer: Testicular Torsion

Erectile Dysfunction

- Erectile Dysfunction (ED) is defined as the consistent inability to achieve and/or maintain an erection sufficient for satisfactory sexual activity.
- Most common vascular disease that decreases blood flow to the penis.
- ED Statistics:
- Erectile dysfunction is very common and affects between 30 and 50 million men in the United States. It is more common as people get older.
  - Age 40–40 % of males are affected
  - Age 70–70% of males are affected
  - Most men have occasional episodes of erectile failure
  - Caused by stress, fatigue, distraction
  - Current evidence suggests that up to 80 percent have an organic origin
  - Hispanic men were nearly twice as likely to have ED and develop the condition at younger ages.
  - 1 percent of men younger than 35 are affected.

Physiology of Erections

- Erection is a hemodynamic process mediated by neurogenic, endothelial, endocrinologic, and cortical/psychogenic influences.
- Flow varies according to the contractile state of the smooth muscle lining.
- Impaired venous outflow
- Autonomic and parasympathetic nerve innervation
- Corpus cavernosal smooth muscle tissue relaxation and penile erection

Types of Erectile Dysfunction

The **first** thing to do is figure out the etiology of the problem.

- Psychogenic
- Rapid onset
- Associated with morning erections
- Associated with REM sleep
- Physiologic (Organic)
- Impaired erections at all times
- Vascular, neurogenic, hormonal
- Men with diabetes are 2 to 3 times more likely to develop ED.

Medications for ED

- PDE5 inhibitors
  - It enhances the production of nitric oxide in the body, causing vasodilation, which increases blood flow to the penis.

> **Clinical Pearls**
>
> 1. PDE5 inhibitors cannot be taken if the patient is taking nitrates due to the risk of severe hypotension.
> 2. PDE5 inhibitors may cause a priapism. The patient should be instructed to call a healthcare provider or EMS if an erection lasts longer than 4 hours (develops a priapism), which may cause damage to the penis.

Examples of PDE5 Inhibitors

- Avanafil (Stendra)
- Sildenafil (Viagra)
- Tadalafil (Cialis)
- Vardenafil

Inguinal Hernias

- Protrusion of intra-abdominal contents through a defect in the abdominal wall or scrotal tissue
- Risk factors to football players, weightlifters, men who have obesity, family history of hernia
- Painful groin bulge that comes and goes
- It appears after exercise, coughing, or lifting a heavy object.
- Surgical repair of the abdominal wall
- Incarcerated hernias (which cannot be reduced by pushing the hernia back in) can lead to severe pain, nausea, vomiting, and an inability to have a bowel movement due to bowel obstruction.
- Incarcerated hernias can become strangulated, which is a surgical emergency due to cutting off the blood supply to the intestine and is considered life threatening.

Diagnosis

- Most hernias can be easily diagnosed with a physical exam. Standing and coughing will make an inguinal hernia more prominent.
- Less often, the patient may need an abdominal ultrasound, CT scan, or MRI if the diagnosis isn't readily apparent.

Chapter 18 Men's Health

Review Questions

1. A nurse practitioner (NP) suspects the patient may have testicular torsion. As part of the assessment, the patient is asked to lie supine, and the NP strokes the medial part of the thigh in a downward direction. This technique is done to assess for:
   A. a positive Prehn's sign.
   B. the cremasteric reflex.
   C. cryptorchidism.
   D. bell clapper deformity.

2. A 45-year-old male patient is experiencing erectile dysfunction (ED). He states it is occurring about 50 percent of the time. He is asking for a prescription for Sildenafil or Tadalafil. The NP reviews his current medications. Which of the following medications would prevent the NP from ordering Sildenafil or Tadalafil?
   A. Metoprolol
   B. Isosorbide
   C. Finasteride
   D. Semaglutide

3. A 20-year-old male patient has been experiencing dysuria for the past 3 days, which has progressed in intensity. He reports that he had unprotected sex with a woman approximately 3 to 4 weeks ago. The urine has no odor but a slight milky penile discharge. No visible lesions or open areas. With this information, the NP suspects:
   A. gonorrhea.
   B. HSV-2.
   C. syphilis.
   D. chlamydia.

4. A 22-year-old sexually active male arrives at the clinic with complaints of scrotal pain, swelling, fever, and chills. He does not use condoms. He has a positive Prehn's sign. The clinician suspects the patient has:
   A. acute bacterial prostatitis.
   B. epididymitis.
   C. testicular torsion.
   D. chronic bacterial prostatitis.

5. A 50-year-old male patient is experiencing erectile dysfunction, and the NP reviews his medications while taking his history. She observes that the patient is on the following medications: Allopurinol 150 mg daily, Semaglutide 0.5 mg weekly, Finasteride 5 mg daily, and metformin 500 mg BID. Which of those medications may be contributing to his ED?
   A. Allopurinol
   B. Semaglutide
   C. Finasteride
   D. Metformin

6. A 71-year-old male patient has a history of benign prostatic hypertrophy (BPH). He does not experience any urinary obstructive symptoms. During his annual physical exam, he asks the NP to order a prostate-specific antigen (PSA) test. He states that his last PCP ordered it for him 5 years ago, which was 3.0. There is no personal or family history of prostate cancer. What is the most appropriate response by the NP?
   A. "It would not be appropriate because the PSA test is no longer recommended as a screening test for prostate cancer."
   B. "I can order it for you, but if it is elevated, you will need to see a urologist."
   C. "The PSA test result always gets higher as you get older."
   D. "The PSA test is no longer considered to be a valid test. You will need a prostate biopsy."

7. A 25-year-old male patient presents to the clinic with a complaint of heaviness in the scrotum. He states that during a testicular self exam (TSE), he felt a painless lump on his testes. The NP reviews his medical history. Which of the following conditions may alert the NP to the possibility of testicular cancer?
   A. Parotitis (mumps) as a child
   B. Cryptorchidism
   C. Urethritis
   D. Varicocele

8. The clinician is assessing for Prehn's sign when determining a patient's etiology of testicular pain. What maneuver does the clinician do to determine the Prehn's sign?
   A. Stroke the inside of the medial thigh in a downward motion.
   B. Lift the scrotum and determine if the pain worsens or improves.
   C. Have the patient stand and place one hand in the patient's groin area. Ask the patient to cough.
   D. The examiner places the index finger in the patient's rectum and palpates the prostate gland.

9. The clinician notes a negative Prehn's sign elicited from a patient complaining of testicular pain. The clinician now has a higher index of suspicion for:
   A. epididymitis.
   B. testicular cancer.
   C. urethritis.
   D. testicular torsion.

10. While performing a physical exam on a 25-year-old male patient, the clinician notes that the patient has a bell clapper deformity. This is observed by the fact that:
    A. the testicles hang in the scrotum and swing freely.
    B. the left testicle hangs lower in the scrotum than the right testicle.
    C. only one testicle can be palpated in the scrotum.
    D. there is a distinct feeling of a "sack of worms" noted in one of the testes when palpated.

11. A male patient has an identified bell clapper deformity. This puts the patient at a higher risk for:
    A. orchitis.
    B. testicular cancer.
    C. epididymitis.
    D. testicular torsion.

12. A 60-year-old male patient states that he feels his enlarged prostate is getting worse. He has to get up at least three times a night lately, and in the past, he only needed to get up once at night. The patient does not want surgery and states he already takes too many medications. With this information, what is the best intervention for the NP to recommend to address his problem?
    A. Discuss with the patient that he needs to be evaluated by a urologist.
    B. Discuss with the patient that he can try strategies such as limiting fluids 2 hours before bedtime and decreasing or eliminating alcohol, caffeine, red meat, and salt.
    C. Obtain a PSA test to determine if the patient has prostate cancer.
    D. Advise the patient that he likely has acute bacterial prostatitis and should be placed on a 10-day course of antibiotics.

13. A patient comes to the clinic and complains of worsening ED. The NP obtains a complete history. While assessing the patient's medications, she notes that the patient's ED may be worsened by the fact that he is taking:
    A. lisinopril.
    B. saw palmetto.
    C. rosuvastatin.
    D. paroxetine (Paxil).

14. The NP is assessing a patient's medications. The patient states he feels well overall but has noticed that he is experiencing ED more than 50 percent of the time. The NP is aware that the following classifications of which medications may worsen ED:
    A. Antidepressants, diuretics, tranquilizers, and anti-ulcer medications
    B. Herbal supplements, multivitamins, over-the-counter (OTC) cold remedies
    C. GLP-1 RAs and SGLT-2s (Sodium-glucose cotransporter-2)
    D. Anti-obesity drugs, statins, and anti-anginal medications

15. A 30-year-old male patient presents to the clinic with complaints of pelvic area pain, dysuria, fever, and body aches. The NP notes that his U/A is positive for pyuria. The NP then gently performs a digital rectal exam (DRE) and palpates a warm prostate that is very tender. The NP suspects that the patient has:
    A. urethritis.
    B. orchitis.
    C. acute bacterial prostatitis.
    D. epididymitis.

16. A 40-year-old male patient verbalizes that he and his spouse have been trying to get pregnant for a year without success. After taking a thorough history, the NP performs a physical exam. The NP notes that the left testicle feels like it has a "sack of worms." The NP suspects the patient may have:
    A. cryptorchidism.
    B. a varicocele.
    C. a hydrocele.
    D. testicular torsion.

17. A 40-year-old male is having a scrotal ultrasound performed. The examiner notes that the mass transilluminates easily. The patient had palpated a movable, firm, and painless mass while doing a TSE. The NP suspects that the patient likely has:
    A. a varicocele.
    B. a hydrocele.
    C. a spermatocele.
    D. testicular cancer.

18. A patient is complaining that the symptoms of his BPH have worsened recently, and he has been having some difficulty urinating. He explains that he does not have any other systemic symptoms. His history indicates that he only takes medications for his seasonal allergies. Which of the following medications or treatments is the patient taking that is likely causing his worsening symptoms?
    A. Fluticasone (Flonase)
    B. Nasal saline rinse with a netty pot
    C. Diphenhydramine (Benadryl)
    D. Loratidine (Claritin)

19. A 30-year-old male patient presents to the walk-in clinic with complaints of continuous pain in his left groin area. This morning, he developed nausea and vomiting, and he has not had a bowel movement (BM) for 3 days. He states that he normally has a BM daily in the morning. He states that he has a history of a left inguinal hernia but that it usually "comes and goes." During the exam, the NP notes that the skin area surrounding the hernia appears dusky. What is the next best course of action?
    A. Advise the patient not to lift anything heavy for the next four weeks. He may return home and remain in bed for the rest of the day, and he should apply ice to reduce swelling.
    B. Advise the patient that there is a concern for strangulation of the hernia and activate EMS.
    C. Administer ondansetron (Zofran) in the office and advise watchful waiting over the next week.
    D. Provide the patient with prescriptions for oxycodone to control the pain and ondansetron to alleviate the nausea and vomiting.

20. A 65-year-old male patient with a history of BPH since age 55 presents to his PCP's office with complaints of worsening ED. Which of the following medications that the patient takes for his BPH is likely causing worsening symptoms of his ED?
    A. PDE5 inhibitors such as sildenafil or tadalafil
    B. Alpha blockers such as alfuzosin
    C. 5a-reductase inhibitors such as finasteride
    D. Herbal remedies such as saw palmetto

21. A 24-year-old male patient presents to the clinic with complaints of a sudden onset of testicular pain. He has not been sexually active for the past 6 months. While performing a physical exam on the patient's genitals, the NP notes that the Prehn's sign is negative. This is one indicator that the patient may have:
    A. epididymitis.
    B. testicular cancer.
    C. testicular torsion.
    D. a bell clapper deformity.

22. A 40-year-old male patient presents to the clinic with concerns that he has been experiencing ED with a female partner that he has recently been dating. Information elicited during the history includes information that the patient does not take any medications and awakens most mornings with a firm erection. The clinician suspects that:
    A. the patient may have diabetes since males with diabetes are two to three times more likely to develop ED.
    B. there may be a psychogenic etiology.
    C. the patient is likely using alcohol or illicit drugs that are causing the ED.
    D. the patient has a low testosterone level.

23. A male patient is taking a PDE5 inhibitor several times a week before sexual intercourse. While reviewing the patient's medication list, the NP observes that the patient has been prescribed NTG S.L. prn for angina. The patient reports having the medication on hand but does not need to use it. The NP is aware that:
    A. the combination of nitrates with PDE5 inhibitors can predispose the patient to severe hypertension and lead to a major cardiovascular event.
    B. the combination of PDE5 inhibitors with nitrates may cause a priapism to develop.
    C. the combination of PDE5 inhibitors with nitrates may cause severe hypotension, which could lead to an myocardial infarction (MI) or stroke.
    D. the combination of PDE5 inhibitors with nitrates will cause increased penile flaccidity.

24. A 45-year-old male has been diagnosed with a spermatocele. He states that he is in a monogamous relationship with his wife. He verbalizes a concern that his spouse has not been monogamous and that an STI has caused him to develop this condition. What is the most appropriate response by the NP to address his concern?
    A. "A spermatocele is not a sexually transmitted infection."
    B. "You should consider using condoms whenever you are having sexual intercourse with your spouse."
    C. "You should verbalize your concerns to your wife and seek counseling if necessary."
    D. "Most men experience a spermatocele at some point in their life."

25. The NP performs a digital rectal exam (DRE) on a patient with suspected BPH. The NP has a higher index of suspicion that the patient does have BPH if the prostate feels:
    A. enlarged with several firm nodules.
    B. enlarged with a boggy, spongy feeling.
    C. round and firm like the tip of a nose.
    D. enlarged, warm, and tender during the DRE exam.

Answers With Enhanced Rationales

1. Answer B is correct. The cremasteric reflex is elicited by stroking the inner medial thigh, which causes contractions of the cremaster muscle that then elevates the testes.

    Answer A is incorrect. A positive Prehn's sign is elicited by lifting the scrotum to evaluate the effect on testicular pain.

    Answer C is incorrect. Cryptorchidism is when one or both testes are undescended into the scrotum.

    Answer D is incorrect. The bell clapper deformity is a condition where the testes hang freely in the scrotum and can swing freely, much like the clapper inside a bell. This increases the risk of testicular torsion.

2. Answer B is correct. Isosorbide is a medication in the nitrate class and is contraindicated for use with PDE5 inhibitors, such as sildenafil or tadalafil, due to a potential for extreme hypotension.

    Answer A is incorrect. Metoprolol is a beta blocker and may contribute to ED. However, it is not contraindicated with the PDE5 inhibitors.

    Answer C is incorrect. Finasteride is a medication used to treat BPH. It is a 5-alpha reductase inhibitor and can cause ED. It is safe to use with the PDE5 inhibitors.

    Answer D is incorrect. Semaglutide is a medication prescribed for diabetes in the GLP1-RA class. It is safe to use with sildenafil or tadalafil.

3. Answer D is correct. Patients with chlamydia commonly present with dysuria and may have a slightly milky penile discharge. Generally, symptoms of chlamydia take longer to develop than gonorrhea, with a variable incubation period of up to 35 days.

    Answer A is incorrect. Gonorrhea symptoms in a male usually appear within a week of infection, and the discharge is mucopurulent in appearance.

    Answer B is incorrect. It is unlikely that the dysuria is due to HSV-2 since there are no visible lesions.

    Answer C is incorrect. Symptoms of early syphilis are usually a chancre, which is one or more painless open ulcers on the genital area.

4. Answer B is correct. Scrotal pain, swelling, fever, chills, and a positive Prehn's sign are all consistent with epididymitis.

    Answer A is incorrect. Acute bacterial prostatitis presents with urinary symptoms and pain in the perineal or rectal area that may extend to the tip of the penis.

    Answer C is incorrect. With testicular torsion, the patient has a negative Prehn's sign. This means that lifting the scrotum provides no pain relief. Testicular torsion is a surgical emergency.

    Answer D is incorrect. Prostatitis symptoms are primarily urinary, such as urgency, frequency, and dysuria. Pain is more common in the groin and lower abdominal area.

5. Answer C is correct. Finasteride is an effective treatment for BPH; however, it may contribute to ED. Finasteride is a 5 alpha-reductase inhibitor and may decrease androgens by decreasing the conversion of testosterone to dihydrotestosterone (DHT).

    Answer A is incorrect. Allopurinol is a treatment for gout prevention. It is not known to contribute to ED.

    Answer B is incorrect. Semaglutide, A GLP-1 RA, is not known to contribute to ED. It is possible that the patient has type 2 DM and, therefore, would be at an increased risk because of the impact that diabetes has on the vasculature.

    Answer D is incorrect. Metformin is not known to contribute to ED. However, if the patient has type 2 DM, this may be responsible for the patient's ED.

6. Answer A is correct. Per the USPSTF, men aged 70 and older should not undergo PSA screening tests. There is a lack of evidence that the benefits of PSA testing would be beneficial and may cause harm through further testing, such as biopsy. It is a Grade D recommendation per the USPSTF.

    Answer B is incorrect. It is inappropriate to order the test and not "own" the results but pass the patient off to a urologist.

    Answer C is incorrect. While it is true that the PSA test will likely get higher as the patient ages, this answer does not explain to the patient why the NP should not order the test.

    Answer D is incorrect. The PSA test may be used to guide treatment for those with known prostate cancer. The patient does not need a prostate biopsy.

7. Answer B is correct. A male with a history of cryptorchidism is at greater risk for developing

testicular cancer. Testicular cancer is the most common cancer in males aged 15 to 34.

Answer A is incorrect. A history of mumps may cause orchitis in males when they are infected. It should not have any effect on the male later in life. In extreme cases, it may cause a decrease in fertility, but this is not common.

Answer C is incorrect. Urethritis is an inflammation of the urethra that is mostly associated with an STI, such as chlamydia or gonorrhea. It is not related to scrotal heaviness.

Answer D is incorrect. A varicocele (varicosity of the veins surrounding the testes) may cause mild symptoms such as swelling or aching pain in the testicle. Palpation of the testicles feels like "a sack of worms" and is most commonly on the left side.

8. Answer B is correct. Lifting the scrotal sack to determine if pain improves or worsens can assist in diagnosing some disorders. This is known as the Prehn's sign.

Answer A is incorrect. This maneuver is known as the cremasteric reflex test. The cremasteric reflex test assists the clinician in diagnosing reasons for testicular pain, such as testicular torsion.

Answer C is incorrect. Having the patient stand and cough while the examiner palpates the groin area is a test to identify the presence of an inguinal hernia.

Answer D is incorrect. This is a DRE that assesses the condition of the prostate gland.

9. Answer D is correct. A negative Prehn's sign means that lifting the scrotal sac does not affect the patient's testicular pain. This is one indication of testicular torsion.

Answer A is incorrect. A patient with epididymitis will likely have a positive Prehn's sign, which indicates some relief of pain when the scrotal sac is lifted.

Answer B is incorrect. Testicular cancer is often found during a TSE since it is usually a painless lump palpated on the testicle.

Answer C is incorrect. Urethritis does not cause testicular pain and would not warrant the clinician performing the test for Prehn's sign.

10. Answer A is correct. When the testicles hang in the scrotum and can swing freely, the bell clapper deformity puts the patient at higher risk for testicular torsion.

Answer B is incorrect. The left testicle often hangs lower than the right testicle. This is a normal finding.

Answer C is incorrect. If only one testicle can be palpated in the scrotum, the patient may have cryptorchidism and need a referral to a urologist.

Answer D is incorrect. The "sack of worms" is associated with a varicocele, and 97 percent occur on the left testicle.

11. Answer D is correct. A bell clapper deformity, where the testes hang freely in the scrotal sac, can predispose a patient to testicular torsion, where the spermatic cord twists and cuts the blood supply to the testicle.

Answer A is incorrect. Orchitis is an inflammation of the testicles. It can be caused by parotitis (mumps) or a bacterial infection, such as an STI.

Answer B is incorrect. Testicular cancer is the most common cancer in young males; however, it is not associated with the bell clapper deformity.

Answer C is incorrect. Epididymitis is an inflammation of the epididymis and is usually related to a bacterial infection. It is not associated with a bell clapper deformity.

12. Answer B is correct. The patient is looking for interventions other than surgery or medication. Therefore, recommendations that involve strategies the patient can implement on his own would be preferred to address the problem.

Answer A is incorrect. The patient does not want surgery or medications. A referral to a urologist would likely lead to one of these recommended interventions.

Answer C is incorrect. A PSA is one test that may assist in the diagnosis of prostate cancer; however, this does not answer the question about interventions that the patient can try to help alleviate some of the symptoms he is experiencing.

Answer D is incorrect. Treating the patient with antibiotics is not an appropriate intervention since there is no indication that the patient has acute bacterial prostatitis.

13. Answer D is correct. Any of the medications in the SSRI class of antidepressants may cause ED. Paroxetine is one of the SSRIs that frequently causes ED.

Answer A is incorrect. Lisinopril is not associated with causing ED. Any BP medication may cause ED; however, it is more commonly associated with thiazide diuretics and beta blockers, which may decrease blood flow to the penis.

Answer B is incorrect. Saw palmetto is an herbal medication taken by some men to reduce the symptoms of BPH. It is not associated with ED.

Answer C is incorrect. Rosuvastatin is used to reduce cholesterol and is not associated with causing ED. Statins may possibly improve erectile function since LDL-C is associated with improved endothelial function.

14. Answer A is correct. Medications such as SSRIs, benzodiazepines, diuretics, beta blockers, PPIs, and H2 blockers have been implicated in causing ED symptoms to worsen.

    Answer B is incorrect. Herbal supplements and multivitamins are not implicated in ED. Cold remedies with antihistamine properties, especially first-generation antihistamines such as diphenhydramine, may cause ED.

    Answer C is incorrect. GLP-1RAs and SGLT-2 class of medications do not cause ED. The patient on these medications has type 2 DM, which is known to contribute to ED.

    Answer D is incorrect. Anti-obesity drugs (such as GLP-1 RAs) are not implicated in ED. Statins are not implicated in ED. Anti-anginal medications, such as nitrates, do not cause ED, but they cannot be taken with tPDE5 inhibitors due to the risk of severe hypotension.

15. Answer C is correct. The patient is having symptoms that are consistent with acute bacterial prostatitis.

    Answer A is incorrect. The patient who is complaining of urethritis will complain of pain with urination and possibly a urethral discharge.

    Answer B is incorrect. Orchitis presents as testicular pain and swelling. An STI likely causes it but may have a viral origin, such as parotitis (mumps)

    Answer D is incorrect. The patient does have symptoms that are associated with epididymitis, such as pelvic pain, fever, and pyuria. However, the warm, tender prostate is more indicative of acute bacterial prostatitis.

16. Answer B is correct. A varicocele, when palpated, feels like a "sack of worms." A varicocele can cause reduced sperm quality, production, and motility. Theoretically, it is likely due to the varicocele causing increased temperature around the testes and possibly a reduced blood supply.

    Answer A is incorrect. Cryptorchidism can cause male infertility, but the examiner would not palpate a "sack of worms," which is consistent with a varicocele.

    Answer C is incorrect. A hydrocele is a painless swelling of fluid that surrounds the testicle within the tunica vaginalis. The testes would feel smooth; pain generally only exists if considerable swelling occurs.

    Answer D is incorrect. Testicular torsion is a surgical emergency. The patient would be complaining of severe testicular pain, often radiating to the groin and/or lower abdominal area.

17. Answer C is correct. A spermatocele transilluminates easily. It is a fluid-filled cyst consisting of sperm and is visualized when a light is shown directly at the scrotum in a darkened room. Spermatoceles develop above or behind the testicles.

    Answer A is incorrect. A varicocele does not transilluminate and feels like a "sack of worms" when palpated.

    Answer B is incorrect. A hydrocele is a collection of fluid that surrounds the testes. It does not transilluminate. It is most common in newborns and rarely occurs in older males unless there is trauma or injury.

    Answer D is incorrect. The palpable mass transilluminating is significant in this question because testicular cancer may present as a painless but solid mass, so the light will not shine through.

18. Answer C is correct. First-generation antihistamines are implicated in causing worsening symptoms of BPH.

    Answer A is incorrect. Fluticasone is a nasal spray containing a corticosteroid. It is used intranasally to relieve allergy symptoms. It does not harm the prostate gland.

    Answer B is incorrect. Using nasal saline rinse or a Neti Pot would not negatively affect the patient's BPH.

    Answer D is incorrect. Loratidine is a second-generation antihistamine. It may negatively affect the patient's ability to urinate due to weakened bladder contractions; however, the effects are not as severe as with first-generation antihistamines, such as diphenhydramine. However, it is notable that *any* antihistamine may negatively affect BPH.

19. Answer B is correct. The patient is demonstrating symptoms of an incarcerated hernia with strangulation, and this is a surgical emergency.

    Answer A is incorrect. Advising a patient not to lift anything heavy or to rest may be appropriate with a minor and reducible inguinal hernia.

    Answer C is incorrect. Administering an anti-emetic, such as ondansetron (Zofran), is inappropriate as it does not recognize that the patient is experiencing a surgical emergency and the N/V is likely related to bowel obstruction and lack of blood supply to the bowel.

Answer D is incorrect. Providing the patient with narcotic pain relievers and an anti-emetic will mask the patient's symptoms and worsen the patient's prognosis for recovery. The patient has symptoms of a strangulated bowel.

20. Answer C is correct. 5A-reductase inhibitors, such as finasteride, may cause a decrease in androgen production.

    Answer A is incorrect. PDE5 inhibitors, such as sildenafil or tadalafil, are used for ED and are not prescribed as medications to treat BPH.

    Answer B is incorrect. Alpha blockers may be used for BPH and hypertension. They generally do not cause the side effect of ED. Caution should be taken if alpha blockers are used with PDE-5 inhibitors due to an enhanced hypotension effect.

    Answer D is incorrect. Herbal remedies, such as saw palmetto, are often used by patients who prefer "natural" treatments to reduce prostate enlargement. Some small studies have shown that there may be some ED associated with the use of saw palmetto, but the most likely medication that is implicated in this question is the 5A-reductase inhibitor.

21. Answer C is correct. With testicular torsion, the Prehn's sign will be negative. Lifting the scrotum will not provide any relief.

    Answer A is incorrect. With epididymitis, the patient will have a positive Prehn's sign, and the inflammation of the epididymis is often associated with an STI. (Patient reports that he has not been sexually active for 6 months.)

    Answer B is incorrect. Testicular cancer does not present with a sudden onset of testicular pain but rather a gradual development of a "heaviness" or dull ache in the scrotal area.

    Answer D is incorrect. A bell clapper deformity does not in and of itself cause pain; however, it is important that the NP is aware the bell clapper deformity does put the patient at risk for testicular torsion, which is a surgical emergency.

22. Answer B is correct. Often, ED has a psychogenic origin. This is particularly true if the patient is awakening most mornings with a spontaneous erection.

Answer A is incorrect. There is no evidence that this patient has diabetes, which would have been elicited in the history, and he takes no medications.

Answer C is incorrect. There is no evidence in the question that indicates the patient is using alcohol or illicit drugs.

Answer D is incorrect. The question does not contain information that would lead the clinician to believe the patient has a low testosterone level. The fact that he gets morning erections likely indicates he has adequate testosterone levels.

23. Answer C is correct. The use of nitrates with PDE5 inhibitors is contraindicated. The patient would need to be educated regarding this dangerous combination of medications.

    Answer A is incorrect. The combination of PDE5 inhibitors with nitrates may cause severe hypotension as they both cause vasodilation. The combination of these two medications does not cause hypertension.

    Answer B is incorrect. A priapism may develop at any time when using PDE5 inhibitors. The patient needs to be informed regarding contacting a medical professional if an erection lasts longer than 4 hours. The combination of the two medications does not increase the risk of priapism.

    Answer D is incorrect. Both PDE5 inhibitors and nitrates cause vasodilation. An erect penis is the result of blood filling the chambers of the penis. Vasodilation allows for increased blood flow to these chambers.

24. Answer A is correct. The NP should explain to the patient that a spermatocele is not a sexually transmitted infection. This addresses the concern of the patient.

    Answer B is incorrect. A spermatocele is not a sexually transmitted infection. Telling the patient that he should use condoms when having intercourse with his spouse will reinforce his concerns that his spouse is not monogamous.

    Answer C is incorrect. The patient needs to understand that a spermatocele is not an STI and that it is a very common occurrence in men aged 40 to 50. Telling the patient to seek counseling is inappropriate for this condition.

    Answer D is incorrect. While it is true that a large percentage of men will develop a spermatocele at some point during their lifetime (roughly 33 percent), this does not address the patient's concern that his wife has not been monogamous.

25. Answer B is correct. An enlarged, boggy, spongy-feeling prostate is consistent with BPH.

    Answer A is incorrect. A prostate that feels enlarged with one or more firm nodules present needs further evaluation by a urologist who will likely perform a prostate biopsy to assess if prostate cancer is present.

    Answer C is incorrect. A round, firm prostate that feels like the tip of a nose is a normal prostate.

    Answer D is incorrect. During DRE, the prostate of a patient with acute bacterial prostatitis will feel enlarged, warm, and tender.

Resources

Benner, J. S., & Ojo, A. (2020). *Causes of scrotal pain in children and adolescents*. UptoDate. https://www.uptodate.com/contents/causes-of-scrotal-pain-in-children-and-adolescents#:~:text=The%20most%20common%20causes%20of,and%20epididymitis%20(table%201)

Bourke, M. M., & Silverberg, J. Z. (2019). Acute scrotal emergencies. *Emergency Medicine Clinics of North America Volume, 37*(4). https://doi.org/10.1016/j.emc.2019.07.002

Devlin, C. M., Simms, M. S., & Maitland, S. J. (2020). Benign prostatic hyperplasia—what do we know? *BJU International, 127*(4). https://doi.org/10.1111/bju.15229

Gurung P., Yetiskul, E., & Jialal, I. (2023). *Physiology, male reproductive system*. In: StatPearls (Internet). StatPearls Publishing. https://www.ncbi.nlm.nih.gov/books/NBK538429/

Khera, M., & Cunningham, G. R. (2019). *Treatment of male sexual dysfunction*. UpToDate. https://www.uptodate.com/contents/treatment-of-male-sexual-dysfunction

Leslie, S. W., & Sooriyamoorthy, T. (2024, January 9). *Erectile dysfunction*. In: StatPearls (Internet). StatPearls Publishing. PMID 32965924

Morrison, Z., Kashyap, S., & Nirujogi, V. L. (2023). *Adult inguinal hernia*. In: StatPearls (Internet). StatPearls Publishing. https://www.ncbi.nlm.nih.gov/books/NBK537241/#:~:text=An%20inguinal%20hernia%20is%20one,year%20in%20the%20United%20States.

Ringdahl, E., & Teague, L. (2006). Testicular torsion. *American Family Physician, 74*(10).

CHAPTER 19

Pediatrics

Christopher Kennedy, DNP, FNP-BC, PMHNP-BC, CNE, APRN

This chapter is not intended to be a comprehensive review of pediatrics, but it does review some of the more commonly tested items.

Growth and Development

Growth and development in children encompasses the physical, learning, language, and behavioral development of a child monitored at every well-child visit. One in six children, or about 17 percent, between the ages of 3 and 17, live with at least one developmental delay (CDC, 2022a). Nurse practitioners (NPs) must focus efforts on identifying children at risk, implementing early interventions, and providing up-to-date and comprehensive care for those children with disabilities and their families.

The American Academy of Pediatrics (AAP) provides many screening tools and resources identifying core components of pediatric screening goals and measures. Bright Futures is an online tool that is useful to identify key areas of wellness assessment for children from birth through 21 years of age (AAP, 2022).

Bright Futures/American Academy of Pediatrics Periodicity Schedule

Bright Futures (n.d.) provides guidelines for clinicians, including all key assessment areas for children.

Physical Growth and Development

Newborn and Infant Through 3 Months of Age

- Initial loss of 5 to 10 percent of birth weight is within normal limits, with expected regain within 10 to 14 days
- Average expected weight gain = 0.5 to 1 ounce per day or about 2 pounds (1 kg) per month
- Average expected gain in length = 1.4 inches (3.5 cm) per month
- Average increase in head circumference = 0.8 inches (2 cm) per month

Infant 4 to 5 Months

- Birth weight should be doubled, and weight gain slows to approximately 5 ounces per week.
- Average expected gain in length = 0.8 inches (2 cm) per month
- Average increase in head circumference = 0.4 inches (1 cm) per month

Infant 6 to 8 Months

- Average expected weight gain = 3 to 4 ounces per week or 1 pound per month
- Average expected gain in length = 0.5 to 0.6 inches (1.2 to 1.5 cm) per month
- Average increase in head circumference = 0.2 inches (0.5 cm) per month
- Birth weight doubles by six months.

Infant 9 to 12 Months

- Average expected weight gain = 1 pound (0.5 kg) per month
- Average expected gain in length = 0.5 to 0.6 inches (1.2 to 1.5 cm) per month
- Average increase in head circumference = 0.2 inches (0.5 cm) per month
- Birth weight triples by the end of the first year.

Toddler to Preschool

- Birth weight quadruples by the end of the second year.
- Average height increases by 5 inches in the second year.
- Average height increases by 3 to 4 inches in the third year.
- Average height increases by 2 to 3 inches yearly from year 4 until puberty.

School-Age

- The average weight gain is 5 pounds per year.

Adolescent

- During adolescence, for males and females, weight doubles, and height increases by 15 to 20 percent.
- Pubertal growth spurt begins, on average, 2 years earlier for females and lasts approximately 2 years for females and longer for males.
- Sexual Maturity Rating (SMR), also known as Tanner stages, assesses pubertal growth and maturation by identifying the presence or absence of secondary sexual characteristics. Scales range from I–V and measure breast development in females, testes and scrotum development in males, and pubic hair development in females and males. In females, Tanner staging may be used to estimate the time of menarche. In the United States, the average age of menarche is between 12 and 13 years.

Gross Motor Development

- 1 month—Turns head when prone
- 4 months—Sits with support; able to roll over
- 6 to 7 months—Sits independently; may rock on hands and knees
- 7 to 8 months—Supports weight standing
- 7 to 9 months—May begin to crawl
- 9 to 10 months—Cruising
- 12 months—Walks holding hand, stands alone
- 18 months—Able to throw at a target, walks well independently
- 24 months—Runs well, kicks a ball, walks up and down stairs
- 30 months—Jumps with both feet off the ground
- 36 months—May pedal a tricycle, hop on one foot, balance on one foot for a few seconds
- 60 months—Skips, stands on one foot for 7 to 8 seconds, catches bounced ball
- School-age—Balance and coordination improve; skills continue to develop with practice

Fine Motor Development

- 4 months—Reaching, ulnar/palmer grasp
- 7 to 8 months—Digital grasp
- 12 months—Pincer grasp
- 18 months—Drinks well from a cup, scribbles, makes a tower of four cubes
- 24 months—Makes a tower of seven cubes, unbuttons or unzips clothing
- 30 months—Makes a tower of nine cubes, imitates a circle, may hold a fork
- 36 months—Able to use scissors, starts to hold and use a toothbrush, puts on shoes
- 48 months—Dresses self, can string small beads
- 60 months—May be able to print names, cut out shapes, and pour from a small pitcher
- School-age—Continued improvement in self-care skills, better control with handheld instruments, improvement in eye-hand coordination

Language Development

- 0 to 3 months—Startles to sound, attends to voice
- 3 to 6 months—Turns to sound, babbles, laughs
- 6 to 9 months—Imitates sounds, may begin nonspecific "mama" and "dada"
- 9 to 12 months—May have one or two words with meaning, imitates sounds
- 12 to 18 months—Approximately 10 words, names, identifies pictures and body parts
- 18 to 24 months—Names self, begins to combine words
- 24 to 30 months—Two- to three-word sentences
- 36 to 42 months—Three- to four-word sentences
- 48 to 60 months—Uses past and future tenses, asks "how" questions

Social and Emotional Development

- 0 to 3 months—Turns to voice, smiles briefly, ability to quiet
- 3 to 6 months—Smiles when hears parental voice

- 6 to 9 months—Enjoys social play; stranger anxiety may emerge
- 9 to 12 months—Stranger anxiety, fears of new experiences, interactive social games
- Toddler and Preschooler—Development of a strong sense of autonomy and independence
- School-Age—Development of social and emotional maturity. Peer group mastery
- Adolescence—Abstract thinking, judgment, self-discipline, ethical behavior, control of emotions

Social and Developmental Theorists

- Freud
- Kohlberg
- Piaget
- Maslow
- Erikson

Erikson's Stages of Development for Children

- 0 to 12 months: Trust vs. mistrust
- 12 to 36 months: Autonomy vs. shame and doubt
- 3 to 6 years: Initiative vs. guilt
- 6 to 11 years: Industry vs. inferiority
- 12 to 17 years: Identity vs. role confusion

Body Mass Index

Body mass index (BMI) measures a person's weight in kilograms divided by the square of height in meters. It is recommended that this measure be calculated at each well-child visit. The BMI for children and teens is both age and gender specific and indicates body fat. The BMI allows for categorizing weight that may indicate potential health problems. BMI calculators and information may be accessed on the CDC (2024c) website.

Immunizations

Many factors influence the ability of the primary care provider to administer vaccines, such as shortages of vaccines, parent refusal, changing recommendations, complicated catch-up schedules, and so on. The Center for Disease Control has child and adolescent immunization guidelines easy-to-read schedules and is a resource to answer common questions (CDC, 2024a).

Vital Signs

Tables 19-1, 19-2, and 19-3 illustrate normal heart rates (HR), respiratory rates, and blood pressures, respectively.

(Reference: Pediatric Advanced Life Support Guidelines)

Heart Rate

Table 19-1 Normal Heart Rates by Age (beats/minute)

Age	Awake Rate	Sleeping Rate
Newborn to 3 months	85–205	80–160
3 months to 2 years	100–190	75–160
2 to 10 years	60–140	60–90
>10 years	60–100	50–90

Respiratory Rate

Table 19-2 Normal Respiratory Rate by Age (breaths/minute)

Age	Normal Respiratory Rate
Infants (<12 months)	30–60
Toddler (1–3 years)	24–40
Preschool (4–5 years)	22–34
School age (6–12 years)	18–30
Adolescence (13–18 years)	12–16

Blood Pressure

Table 19-3 Hypotension Reference Ranges

Age	Systolic BP in mmHg
Term Neonates (0–28 days)	< 60
Infants (1–12 months)	< 70
Children 1–10 years	< 70 + (age in years × 2)
Children >10 years	< 90

Clinical Pearls

Routine blood pressure screening in otherwise healthy children should begin at the 3-year well-child visit.

Table 19-4 Assessment of the Newborn

APGAR Score: Done at 1 and 5 Minutes After Birth. Each Area Scores 0, 1, or 2 Points			
	0	1	2
A – Appearance (Color)	blue/pale	acrocyanosis	pink
P – Pulse (Heart Rate)	absent	< 100	> 100
G – Grimace (Reflex/Irritability)	no response	grimaces	cries on stimulation
A – Activity (Tone)	none	some flexion	flexed arms and legs
R – Respirations	absent	weak, gasping	strong cry

History

- Maternal history—Age, preexisting illness, medications, infertility, tobacco/drug/alcohol use, previous pregnancy outcome(s)
- Family History
- Obstetrical history—Screening tests, ultrasounds, genetic testing, multiple gestation
- Labor and delivery—Abnormality of the fetal heart rate/rhythm, premature labor, maternal fever, meconium-stained fluid, obstetrical anesthesia/analgesia, and placental abnormalities (blood vessels, size). See **Table 19-4** for the assessment of a newborn at the time of delivery.

Physical Exam

This should be done within the first 24 hours of birth. Maintain the infant's body warmth. Use a systematic head-to-toe approach. See normal vital signs shown earlier.

- Measurements: weight, length, head circumference, abdominal circumference
- Observe the infant's overall appearance, posture, and movements. It should be pink, with no rashes, symmetrical, and extremities flexed.
- If quiet, assess the heart and lungs.

Heart

S1, louder at apex, S2 louder near base

- S3 may be heard near the apex—considered normal
- S4 NEVER normal. Rapid HR, difficult to distinguish gallop sound

Lungs

Signs of distress—Flaring, grunting, retractions. Assess chest wall symmetry.

Skin

May find milia, congenital dermal melanocytosis (also known as slate gray nevi), jaundice, erythema toxicum, café au lait spots

Head

- Two fontanelles: anterior and posterior
- There are two frontal bones, two parietal bones, and one occipital bone.
- Sutures allow the bones to move during the birth process and the head to grow as the brain expands, and these include the metopic, coronal, sagittal, and lambdoid.
- The posterior closes the first few months to 1 year; the anterior by 18 months.

Cephalohematoma

Cephalohematoma occurs in 1.5 to 2.5 percent of deliveries, causing an injury to blood vessels in the subperiosteal area. It may take several days or weeks to resolve.

Clinical Pearls

Cephalohematoma does not cross suture lines.

Caput Succedaneum
- Edema due to pressure, typically from vacuum-extraction
- Boggy, ill-defined
- Resolves within 48 hours

> **Clinical Pearls**
>
> Caput succedaneum crosses suture lines.

Primitive/Primary Reflexes

These reflexes are present at birth due to an immature nervous system and gradually disappear over the first year of life:

- Palmer grasp—disappears by 4 months
- Stepping reflex—disappears by 4 months
- Tonic neck—disappears by 4 months
- Sucking reflex—disappears by 4 months
- Rooting reflex—disappears by 4 months
- Moro startle reflex—disappears by 6 months
- Plantar grasp reflex—disappears by 12 months
- Babinski reflex—disappears by 10 months

> **Clinical Pearls**
>
> Persistence of primitive reflexes beyond their expected duration needs further neurological evaluation.

Important Terms

- *Epstein pearls*—whitish-yellow cysts in the roof of the mouth and gums
- *Retinoblastoma*—most common (1/17,000) malignant intraocular tumor in childhood (30 percent bilateral) (*presents with leukocoria)
- *Nystagmus*—transient rapid, involuntary oscillating of eyes; normal finding in newborns resolving by 6 months
- *Hypospadias*—urethral opening on the underside of the penis
- *Hydrocele*—fluid-filled sac around the testes; common; usually resolves within the first year without any intervention
- *Varicocele*—edema of the veins in the testes appearing as a "bag of worms"; similar to varicose vein
- *Barlow maneuver* (posterior displacement)—the examiner gently moves hips into mild adduction, then applies slight forward pressure to assess for hip dysplasia
- *Ortolani's test* (anterior displacement)—the examiner puts hands on knees and places thumb on the middle of the thigh. Apply gentle upward stress with fingers on the hip and then slow abduction. A positive test will result in a "clunking" sound.
- *Wilm's tumor*—most common kidney cancer in children; typically affects 3 to 4 years old; generally, prognosis is good.
- *Talipes equinovarus*—clubfoot; adduction, supination, and varus of the foot
- *Genu varum*—Bowed legs; should resolve by age 3 or 4 years

Breastfeeding

The gold standard (Baby Friendly Hospital Initiative) recommends frequent sessions (8 to 12 times per day for 15 to 20 minutes on each breast). Contraindications include galactosemia, human immunodeficiency virus (HIV), cytotoxic drugs, and radioactive compounds. Encourage exclusive breastfeeding for 4 to 6 months.

Anticipatory Guidance Topics

- Car Seat
- Sudden Infant Death Syndrome (SIDS) prevention
  - Crib safety
- Place infant on back to sleep
- Immunizations
- "Babywearing"—decreases fussiness and increases learning
- Water safety
- Sunscreen (beginning at 6 months) and insect repellant (beginning at 2 months, depending on ingredients)

Congenital Heart Defects

A congenital heart defect is a cardiac lesion present in neonates.

Acyanotic Defects—Left to Right Shunts

Results in increased pulmonary blood flow

- **Atrial-septal defect** (ASD): 50 percent more common in females, accounting for 7 to 10 percent of congenital heart defects (CHD). The child may be asymptomatic or may fatigue easily. May get frequent upper respiratory tract infections (URTIs) and lower respiratory tract infections (LRTIs). The small defects may close on their own. Large defects require intervention. Murmur grade I–III/VI is auscultated best in the pulmonic area. S2 is split widely and is fixed in relation to respirations.

- **Ventricular-septal defect** (VSD): The most common congenital heart defect, accounting for 25 percent of all CHD. Associated with Down syndrome. Up to 50 percent are very small and may close on their own by the time the child is 4 years old. Murmur: Holosystolic murmur at lower left sternal border (LLSB). The murmur may be louder when the VSD is smaller since there will be more turbulent blood flow across the defect.
- **Atrioventricular septal defect** (AVSD): Accounts for only 2 percent of congenital heart defects; however, up to 40 percent of patients with AVSD have Down syndrome. Children with complete canal defects may exhibit signs and symptoms of congestive heart failure (CHF)—difficulty feeding, pale skin, poor weight gain, and increased respiratory rate and effort. Murmur grade II–V/VI low-pitched, holosystolic at LLSB. The murmur may not be present until 2 to 8 weeks when pulmonary vascular resistance falls and blood is shunted across the ASD and VSD.
- **Patent ductus arteriosis** (PDA): Normally, functional closure of the ductus arteriosis occurs 12 to 72 hours after birth. PDA accounts for 9 to 12 percent of all CHD. The ratio of females to males is 2:1. Infants and children may be asymptomatic if the PDA is small. For large PDAs, children may manifest symptoms of CHF. A murmur is typically a grade II–V/VI harsh, rumbling, continuous murmur heard in the pulmonic area. Most infants with a small PDA are followed for 2 years to determine if there is a spontaneous closure. Patients with larger PDAs may have their ductus ligated. Interventional radiologists may close a PDA by placing coils into the ductus in the cardiac catheterization lab.

Cyanotic Defects—Right to Left Shunts

- **Transposition of the great arteries** (TGA): Accounts for 5 to 8 percent of CHD. It is more common in males by 60 to 70 percent. With TGA, the aorta arises from the right ventricle, receives deoxygenated blood, and returns it to systemic circulation. The pulmonary artery arises from the left ventricle and sends oxygenated blood back through the pulmonic circulation. For the neonate or infant to survive, there must be another heart defect (either an ASD, VSD, or PDA) present to allow for the mixing of the oxygenated and deoxygenated blood. Without treatment, there is a 90 percent mortality rate within the first year of life. Cyanosis is usually evident shortly after birth, and CHF symptoms develop rapidly.
- **Tetralogy of Fallot** (TOF): Accounts for 10 percent of all CHD. Also referred to as TET, tetralogy of Fallot consists of four defects: pulmonic valve stenosis, right ventricular hypertrophy, VSD, and overriding aorta that crosses the ventricular septum. TOF is the most common of the cyanotic defects, accounting for up to 9 percent of the cases of CHD. The severity of the cyanosis usually depends on the degree of right ventricular obstruction due to pulmonic stenosis. The child may present with dyspnea and cyanotic mucous membranes. Murmur: grade III–V/VI harsh systolic ejection murmur is heard at the left second intercostal space. VSD murmur will be a holosystolic murmur at the LLSB.
- **Tricuspid atresia:** Accounts for less than 3 percent of all CHD and results in no communication between the right atrium and the right ventricle. TGA also occurs in approximately 50 percent of these patients. The infant with tricuspid atresia presents with cyanosis, dyspnea, easy fatigue, and poor growth. The right ventricle is usually hypoplastic (small).

Obstructive Lesions

- Aortic stenosis (AS): AS accounts for 5 percent of all cases of CHD and is more common in males. Depending on the severity of the defect, growth may be normal, or there may be activity intolerance, fatigue, chest pain, CHF, and syncope that may increase in severity as the child ages. The apical impulse may be pronounced. A grade II–IV/VI loud, harsh systolic ejection murmur in the heart at the upper right sternal border with radiation to the neck, LLSB, and apex. Treatment depends on the severity of the stenosis and may be unnecessary or require valve replacement surgery.
- **Pulmonic stenosis**: Accounts for 6 to 8 percent of CHD. Due to the stenosis of the pulmonic valve, right ventricular pressure increases, and RVH occurs. Murmur: A grade II–IV harsh mid-late systolic ejection murmur is heard over the upper-left sternal border in the pulmonic region and may radiate to the neck and back regions. Cyanosis and

symptoms of right-sided CHF may occur with severe pulmonic stenosis.
- **Coarctation of the aorta**: Accounts for 5 percent of CHD. A narrowing of the portion of the aorta. The severity of the coarctation, location, and degree of obstruction determine the symptoms' manifestation. Both systolic and diastolic pressures are high in the vessels above the narrowed area, and hypotension exists in the vessels below the area of narrowing. Physical exam often reveals hypertension in the upper extremities and hypotension in the lower extremities (LEs). In severe cases, poor perfusion to the LEs may present with mottling or pallor. Bounding brachial, radial, and carotid pulses may be evident. Surgical resection of the constricted area and anastomosis of the upper and lower segments yield an excellent prognosis.
- **Innocent murmurs**: Innocent heart murmurs, also known as functional or physiologic murmurs, are harmless and can be common during infancy and childhood and often disappear by adulthood. They usually are grade I–II/VI, and the murmur may change with position changes. The Valsalva maneuver may cause the innocent murmur to disappear. Typically, vital signs are normal, and the echocardiogram (ECG) is normal. The ECG reveals no pathology.
- **Hypertrophic obstructive cardiomyopathy (HOCM)**: Symptoms of hypertrophic cardiomyopathy may be any or all of the following: dyspnea, syncope, angina, palpitations, orthopnea, paroxysmal nocturnal dyspnea, CHF, dizziness, and sudden cardiac death. Sudden cardiac death has the highest incidence in preadolescent and adolescent children and is particularly related to extreme exertion. The risk of sudden death in children is as high as 6 percent per year. In more than 80 percent of cases, the arrhythmia that causes sudden death is ventricular fibrillation. The murmur is a systolic crescendo-decrescendo murmur that is best heard between the apex and left sternal border and radiates to the suprasternal notch. The murmur increases markedly with the Valsalva maneuver and any increase in preload, such as squatting.

Clinical Pearls

HOCM is often genetic. Ask about any history of unexplained accidents or drownings in the family, which may have resulted from undiagnosed HOCM.

Primary Care for Congenital Heart Defects

- Adequate nutrition
- Optimal psychosocial development
- Optimal preventive and primary care
- Prevention of complications (ensure good cardiology follow-up)
- Optimal fitness
- Optimal neurodevelopment

Chest Pain in Children

Two types of chest pain:

- Acute onset, severe chest pain
  - Most likely seen in pediatric emergency department (ED)
  - Only 4 percent due to cardiac causes
  - One-third idiopathic
- Chronic and recurrent episodes of less severe chest pain
  - Most likely seen in the office.
  - The patient is unlikely to have pain at the time of the visit.
  - The exam is likely to be normal.
  - Most "chest pain" complaints are not caused by cardiac disease.
  - The most common cause of chest pain is costochondritis (20 to 75 percent).
  - The most common arrhythmia associated with chest pain is supraventricular tachycardia (SVT).
  - Twenty-one to 39 percent of children and adolescents with chest pain are thought to be idiopathic.
  - Thirty percent are a result of musculoskeletal causes.
  - Anxiety and emotional causes account for 9 to 20 percent of chest pain in adolescents.
- Assess for associated symptoms
  - Fever
  - Coughing
  - Vomiting
  - Lightheadedness
  - Syncope
  - Palpitations
  - Shortness of breath
  - Diaphoresis
- Common Causes of Chest Pain in Children (Cardiac and Noncardiac)
  - Cardiac: Predisposing medical conditions: Marfan syndrome, CHD, Kawasaki disease, mitral valve prolapse, pericarditis, endocarditis,

juvenile rheumatoid arthritis, dysrhythmias (usually SVT)
- Noncardiac: Spontaneous pneumothorax (absent or decreased breath sounds, chest pain, and splinting), pleural irritation, bacterial pneumonia/empyema, sickle cell crisis, pulmonary embolism, exercise-induced asthma/chronic asthma, hyperventilation syndrome, a "stitch," musculoskeletal inflammation, GERD, esophageal spasm, foreign body, achalasia, splenic or pancreatic pain, trauma, stress, depression

> **Clinical Pearls**
>
> All cardiac causes of chest pain need a referral to a pediatric cardiologist and/or emergency department.

Pediatric Hypertension

Hypertension in the pediatric population can be primary idiopathic or secondary (with the most common cause being renal disease). Nearly 5 percent of all children have hypertension, with a higher incidence in Black or African American children. Risk factors for primary idiopathic hypertension are similar to those for adult hypertension.

Treatment and Referral

- History and physical exam; diagnostic testing
- Diet
- Exercise
- Antihypertensive medications
- Diuretics
- ACE inhibitors
- Beta blockers
- Calcium channel blockers

Respiratory Conditions in the Pediatric Population

Asthma

The respiratory chapter of this review book provides a comprehensive review of the pathophysiology and treatment of asthma.

The Global Initiative for Asthma (GINA) has separate guidelines for managing asthma in children under 5 years of age. Diagnosing asthma in this age group is difficult because wheezing can occur from other causes. Diagnosis is based on symptom patterns, frequency, history, and physical examination findings. Full information on diagnosis and management of asthma in all age groups can be found at www.ginasthma.org.

- Close to 4.7 million American children (under 18 years old) have asthma, according to the CDC (2023).
- Asthma is the most common cause of missed school days and emergency department visits and is the leading chronic disease of children.
- Asthma is more common in boys than girls.
- Factors that may aggravate asthma, causing increased or returning symptoms, include exercise, stress, smoke, viral respiratory infections, and allergens, such as dust mites, cockroaches, and pollens.
- History: The patient (or parent) gives a history, including symptoms such as wheezing, chest tightness, cough, and/or shortness of breath.
- Physical examination: May be normal; may hear wheezing.
- Diagnostic testing: Forced expiratory volume in one second/forced vital capacity (FEV_1/FVC) less than 0.90 in children, and after bronchodilator treatment, the child's FEV_1 increased by more than 12 percent of the predicted value.

Description of Asthma Levels

- **Intermittent**: Symptoms of wheezing and coughing occur no more than twice/week. Nighttime flares no more than twice a month.
- **Mild Persistent**: Symptoms occur more than twice/week but not once/day; symptoms may affect activity level; nighttime flares more than twice/month but not weekly; lung function is approximately 80 percent normal if not treated.
- **Moderate Persistent**: Symptoms occur daily, and flare-ups may last days. Coughing and wheezing affect activity. Nighttime symptoms interrupt sleep. Lung function is between 60 and 80 percent less than normal without treatment.
- **Severe Persistent**: Wheezing and coughing occur daily and often disrupt activities and sleep. Lung function is less than 60 percent without treatment.

According to the guidelines from the National Asthma Education and Prevention Program, these steps should be followed:

- **Initial Visit**: This includes diagnosing asthma, assessing its severity, prescribing and educating about medication and use, developing an action

plan in writing with the patient and parent/guardian, and scheduling a follow-up.
- **Follow-Up Visits**: Assess asthma control, review how to use prescribed medications, and assess adherence, as well as how well environmental factors are being controlled; any changes in medication dosage (increased or decreased) should be reviewed; review the asthma action plan and schedule a follow-up appointment.

> **Clinical Pearls**
>
> Asthma management aims to maintain treatment at the lowest effective dose. The clinician should consider stepping down treatment if asthma is well-controlled for at least 3 months.

Croup

Croup (also known as laryngotracheobronchitis) is a syndrome of acute edema and obstruction of the subglottal area.

- **Etiology**: Most often caused by viruses such as parainfluenza, influenza A&B, respiratory syncytial virus (RSV), and COVID-19, but it can also be caused by allergies or acid reflux.
- **Occurrence**: Late fall to early spring
- **Manifestations**: Upper respiratory infection (URI) for 3 to 5 days, "seal's bark" sounding cough more apparent with recumbency at night; inspiratory stridor; Steeple sign (or wineglass) on X-ray—tapering of the upper trachea on a frontal chest X-ray, which appears like that of a church steeple.
- **Treatment/Education**:
  - Cool fluids/air
  - Upright positioning
  - Needs to run its course over several days
  - Keep children calm
  - Albuterol/Xopenex
  - Systemic corticosteroids
  - Hospitalization may be necessary
  - Danger signs: drooling, circumoral cyanosis, stridor, dyspnea
  - Children with moderate to severe croup with labored breathing requiring hospitalization may need oxygen and racemic epinephrine.

Bronchiolitis

Acute inflammation of the bronchioles causing increased mucus secretion, bronchial constriction/obstruction, necrosis of the respiratory epithelium, air trapping, atelectasis

- **Etiology**: Viral, usually RSV or parainfluenza
- **Occurrence**: Late winter/early spring; usually less than 2 years old but can range from 3 months to 3 years
- **Risk Factors**
  - Premature or low birth weight
  - Crowded living conditions and/or daycare
  - Parental smoking
  - CHD, respiratory, neurologic, or immune disease
- **Manifestations**
  - Abrupt onset of fine wheezing and dyspnea
  - Tachycardia, tachypnea
  - Low-grade fever
  - Apnea
  - Poor feeding
  - Hypoxia
  - Retractions
- **Treatment**
  - Primarily supportive therapy
  - Oxygen
  - Chest PT/cool mist therapy
  - Antivirals (when indicated)
  - Nutrition/rest/electrolyte replacement
  - May require hospitalization with more serious signs and symptoms

> **Clinical Pearls**
>
> The American Academy of Pediatrics recommends against using cough suppressants/decongestants in children under 4 years old with extreme caution advised until after age 6.

Respiratory Syncytial Virus

Respiratory syncytial virus (RSV) affects people of all ages. Nearly 40 percent of cases of RSV lead to infections of the lower respiratory tract, leading to more than 120,000 hospitalizations each year.

- **Etiology**: Viral
- **Occurrence**: It occurs usually from November to April. By age 2, 80 to 90 percent of all children have had this highly contagious illness, with the median age being 3.3 months.
- **Risk Factors**
  - Premature or low birth weight
  - Daycare

- **Manifestations**
  - Nasal congestion
  - Fever
  - Cough
  - Sore throat
  - Fatigue
  - Irritability
  - Feeding problems
- **Complications**
  - Long-term pulmonary sequelae/wheeze/asthma
  - Respiratory failure, apnea, secondary bacterial infections
- **Treatment**
  - Primarily supportive therapy
  - Oxygen
  - Nutrition/rest/electrolyte replacement
  - May require hospitalization with more serious signs and symptoms
- **Prevention**: The American Academy of Pediatrics recommends nirsevimab (a monoclonal antibody) vaccination in neonates and infants born during or entering their first RSV season. If the mother received the vaccine more than 14 days before birth, most infants will not need the vaccine after birth. The CDC (2024d) provides more details.

Acute Bronchitis

Acute bronchitis is a temporary inflammatory condition that affects the distal trachea and the major bronchi.

- **Etiology**: It usually occurs as a secondary infection while the airways are vulnerable, causing thickened bronchial walls and mucous gland hypertrophy. Ninety percent of cases are viral.
- **Occurrence**: Winter to early spring
- **Manifestations**
  - Cough
  - Rhinitis
  - Wheezing
  - Low-grade fever
- **Treatment/Follow-Up for Otherwise Healthy Children**
  - Primarily supportive therapy
  - Bronchodilators for wheezing; oral corticosteroids may be needed if there is no improvement.
  - Antibiotics for bacterial infection (bacterial infections uncommon)

> **Clinical Pearls**
>
> What appears to be chronic bronchitis in children is often actually asthma.

Pneumonia

Pneumonia is the leading infectious disease cause of death in children worldwide (WHO, 2022). Prevention by vaccines is available in developed countries, but vaccines and antibiotics are not available in many developing countries. Pneumonia is spread by respiratory droplets from person to person and through contact via fomites.

- **Etiology**: Pneumonia is caused by viruses, bacteria (chlamydia, mycoplasma, strep), fungi, chemical exposure, and aspiration.
- **Occurrence**: Neonates are more likely to have bacterial pneumonia; otherwise, most are viral. Children over 5 years are less likely to have mycoplasma pneumonia.
- **Risk Factors**
  - Living in a home with smokers
  - Wood-burning stoves
  - Boys are more commonly affected than girls.
- **Clinical Manifestations**
  - Sputum-producing cough
  - Tachypnea
  - Crackles
  - Pulse oximetry < 90 percent
  - Viral generally has a gradual onset, lower-grade fever, and less acute symptoms, frequently preceded by upper respiratory infection.
  - Bacterial has a more acute onset, lethargy, green- or blood-tinged sputum, and higher fever.
- **Diagnostics**
  - Clinical presentation
  - X-ray
  - Sputum culture
- **Treatment**
  - Inpatient care is required if pulse oximetry is less than 92 percent and if the patient is younger than 3 to 6 months, if there is a concern for compliance and/or appropriate assessment of signs/symptoms, or if other complicating factors exist.
  - Antibiotics for outpatients: Amoxicillin, Augmentin, azithromycin, or alternatives for atypical infections per guidelines.

- Antibiotics for inpatients: IV penicillin G, ampicillin, IV azithromycin, or alternatives for atypical infections per guidelines.
- Supportive care, fluids, rest, oxygen
- **Complications**: pneumothorax, pleural effusion, abscess, acute respiratory failure, carditis, meningitis, sepsis

*See Head, Eyes, Ears, Nose, and Throat (HEENT) chapter for upper respiratory infections, including pharyngitis.

Sports Physical/Preparticipation Physical Evaluation

The sports physical aims to assess general health and detect potential life-threatening disorders. In addition, the screening aims to detect any medical and/or musculoskeletal issues that could cause injury. Each state determines what type of provider may perform this physical examination. Be sure to check this to be assured of practicing within the legal scope of practice.

Sudden Death

Sudden death affects males more than females 3:1. Approximately 75 percent of cases of sudden death occur during mild physical activity, with 10 to 15 percent occurring during competitive athletics. The most common symptoms before death are syncope and chest pain.

Causes

Myocarditis (20 to 40 percent), hypertrophic cardiomyopathy (25 percent and higher in Black people or African American people), congenital coronary artery anomalies (18 percent), coronary artery disease (14 percent), conduction system abnormalities, mitral valve prolapse, aortic dissection, and Marfan syndrome.

History

A comprehensive personal and family history must be taken. Specific questions related to syncope, family history of cardiovascular problems, seizures, palpitations, and shortness of breath should be included.

Physical

A comprehensive full physical exam is essential. General appearance notes should include any indication of Marfan syndrome, and the cardiac exam must include listening for murmurs while the patient is standing, sitting, and during the Valsalva maneuver. A robust musculoskeletal exam may indicate issues needing further evaluation.

The American Academy of Pediatrics (2021) provided the PPE 5 guidelines with monographs and forms for history and physical.

> **Clinical Pearls**
>
> States have varying requirements for the sports physical. Familiarize yourself with the requirements of the state in which you practice.

Pediatric Infectious Diseases Not Covered Elsewhere in Review Book

Parvovirus B19 (Erythema Infectiosum, Fifth Disease)

Symptoms are usually mild and include fever, coryza, and headache. After a few days, the child may get the hallmark "slapped cheek" appearance. This can spread to the back, chest, and rest of the body, lasting 7 to 10 days.

- **Incubation**: 4 to 14 days, but can be as long as 21 days
- **Transmission**:
  - Contact with respiratory secretions
  - Percutaneous exposure to blood or blood products
  - Vertical transmission from mother to fetus
- **Viral shedding**: No longer contagious once the rash appears
- **Complications**: Aplastic crisis may occur after 7 days (at-risk children, e.g., sickle cell)

> **Clinical Pearls**
>
> People who are pregnant should avoid contact with Fifth disease, although approximately 50 percent are immune. If the disease develops, there is a risk of miscarriage.

Measles (Rubeola)

Measles is one of the most contagious infectious diseases. Approximately 7 to 10 days after infection, the patient will develop coryza, conjunctivitis, cough, and a high fever. Two to 3 days after symptoms begin, the patient may develop Koplik's spots in the mouth. Three to 5 days after symptoms start, the patient will develop a rash with flat red spots near the hairline, which spreads down the body. The flat spots may develop raised red bumps. The rash and symptoms will disappear a few days later. Suspect measles in patients with a fever and rash and those with international travel or contact with international visitors in the preceding 3 weeks.

- **Incubation**: 7 to 21 days
- **Transmission**
  - Contact with respiratory secretions
  - Contact with contaminated surfaces via fomites
  - Airborne (sharing the same air as infected persons)
- **Viral shedding**: Four days before rash onset through 4 days after
- **Complications**
  - Otitis media with potential hearing loss
  - Pneumonia
  - Encephalitis
  - Premature delivery
  - Low birth weight
  - Death

> **Clinical Pearls**
>
> Vaccine status should be evaluated for all children presenting with symptoms of measles. Although as many as 3 percent of vaccinated individuals can still get measles if exposed, the two-vaccine series is highly protective.

Impetigo

Caused by bacterial infections (usually strep or staph) via cuts and scrapes or other forms of skin breakdown. This infection occurs most often in the 2- to 5-year-old age group and is highly infectious. There are two forms: bullous and nonbullous. Typically, a honey-colored crust forms. The entire process usually lasts about 7 days.

- A staph infection causes bullous impetigo. A toxin causes cell adhesion, which separates the epidermis and dermis layers. A clear, yellow-colored liquid fills the blisters, which break easily.
- Either strep or staph can cause nonbullous impetigo. Small red papules turn into blisters, which then become pustules.

Gentle cleansing and application of Bactroban (mupirocin) typically help resolve the infection and prevent secondary infections. Oral antibiotics, such as amoxicillin or Augmentin, may be indicated in case of a severe infection.

> **Clinical Pearls**
>
> Impetigo remains contagious until 24 to 48 hours after treatment has begun, and direct physical contact should be avoided until after this time.

Coxsackievirus (Hand, Foot, and Mouth Disease)

Hand, foot, and mouth disease is one of the enteroviruses that commonly affects young children. This is a respiratory virus with dermatological manifestations. Complications, while rare, can be severe.

- **Incubation**: 2 to 6 days
- **Transmission**
  - Contact with respiratory secretions
  - Fecal-oral
- **Viral shedding**: The virus sheds for 1 week via the respiratory tract but several weeks in feces.
- **Manifestations**
  - Fever
  - Malaise
  - Rash
  - Painful blisters (commonly in the mouth, palmar surface of hands, and plantar surface of feet)
- **Treatment**
  - Supportive care
  - Analgesics
  - Diphenhydramine
- **Complications**
  - Encephalitis
  - Endocarditis

Child Maltreatment and Abuse

Child abuse is defined as a nonaccidental injury to a child, which, regardless of motive, is inflicted or

Child Maltreatment and Abuse

allowed to be inflicted by the person responsible for the child's care. This includes:

- any injury that is at variance with the history given.
- maltreatment, such as, but not limited to, malnutrition, sexual molestation, deprivation of necessities, emotional abuse, or cruel punishment.

Child Abuse in the United States (U.S. Department of Health & Human Services, 2022)

- 1,990 children died from abuse and neglect in 2022.
- Children under the age of 1 year have the highest rate of child maltreatment.
- Boys have a higher fatality rate from child abuse.
- Black or African American children who are abused have 3.3 times higher rates of fatality than White or Hispanic children who are abused.
- Females represent more than 50 percent of abuse perpetrators.
- Seventy-six percent of perpetrators were a parent to the child abuse survivors.

Physical Abuse

Physical abuse refers to any injury inflicted other than by accidental means, any injury at variance with the history given of them, or a child's condition that is the result of maltreatment, such as malnutrition, deprivation of necessities, or cruel punishment.

- **Examples of injuries that may result from physical abuse**
  - Head injuries
  - Bruises, cuts, or lacerations
  - Internal injuries
  - Burns, scalds
  - Reddening or blistering of the tissue through the application of heat by fire, chemical substances, cigarettes, matches, electricity, scalding water, friction, and so on.
  - Injuries to bone, muscle, cartilage, ligaments, fractures, dislocations, sprains, strains, displacements, hematomas, and so on.
  - Death

Emotional Abuse

Emotional abuse is the result of cruel or unconscionable acts and/or statements made, threatened to be made, or allowed to be made by the person responsible for the child's care who has a direct effect on the child. The observable and substantial impairment of the child's psychological, cognitive, emotional, and/or social well-being and functioning must be related to the behavior of the person responsible for the child's care.

Sexual Abuse

Sexual abuse is any incident of sexual contact involving a child that is inflicted or allowed to be inflicted by the person responsible for the child's care.

- **Normal or Nonspecific Findings**
  - Hymenal tags, bumps, or mounds
  - Labial adhesions
  - Clefts or notches in the anterior half (between the 9- and 3-o'clock position) of the hymen
  - Vaginal discharge
  - Erythema of the genitalia or anus
  - Perianal skin tags
  - Anal fissures
  - Anal dilatation with stool in the ampulla
- **Concerning But Not Diagnostic Findings**
  - Notches or clefts in the posterior half of the hymen
  - Condylomata acuminata in a child older than 2 years who gives no history of sexual contact
  - Immediate, marked anal dilatation
  - Anal scarring
- **Diagnostic Positive Physical Findings**
  - Acute laceration or ecchymosis of the hymen
  - Absence of hymenal tissue in the posterior half
  - Healed hymenal transection or a complete cleft
  - Deep anal laceration
  - Pregnancy without a history of consensual intercourse

Most exams are "normal," with no signs of abuse due to a variety of reasons:

- The nature of the abuse was not damaging.
- Abuse may have occurred days or weeks before.
- Complete healing may have occurred.
- Children who have not been abused may have findings that seem "not normal" but are variations of normal.

Contact the specialty team for evaluation, interview, and examination.

The Role of the Family Nurse Practitioner

- Recognize signs and symptoms of abuse.
- Perform a thorough history and physical exam and **document** accurately (separate interviews for child and caregiver).

- Try not to be judgmental.
- Ensure the child's safety is the priority.
- Collect evidence.
- REPORT suspicions in good faith.
- Remember that minor injuries are common and often witnessed by others.
- A child or adolescent needs an exam if there is/are:
  - any suspicion of abuse.
  - suspicion of sexual abuse, even if it is sexual play.
  - physical signs and symptoms of genitourinary problems.
  - a history of pain, injury, or possible trauma.
  - a need for child/adolescent and family reassurance.
- Key Steps
  - Gather and document pertinent information.
  - Determine the safety and welfare of the child/adolescent.
  - Determine who should examine the child/adolescent and when.
  - Determine if you are mandated to report this situation.
- TIPS
  - Suspect injuries that do not "fit" with the explanation.
  - Suspect unexplained injuries, especially to protected body parts (buttocks, thighs, torso, frenulum, ears, neck, retina).
  - Consider the child's behavior and developmental ability:
    - Bruises are rare in infants who do not cruise.
    - Analyze the shape/pattern of injury (handprint, belt buckle, cord loops, glove or sock, etc.).
    - Transverse long-bone fracture in a 3-month-old is highly suspicious for abuse yet may be unremarkable in an 8-year-old child.
    - A complete skeletal survey is needed in any child under 2 years of age when physical abuse is suspected.

Differential Diagnoses

- **Hematologic**: Hemophilia, idiopathic thrombocytopenic purpura (ITP), Von Willebrand's
- **Dermatologic**: Phytophotodermatitis, slate gray nevi, vascular malformations, subcutaneous fat necrosis
- **Infectious**: Bullous impetigo, staph-scalded skin syndrome, petechiae/purpura from systemic infections
- **Metabolic**: Osteogenesis imperfecta, rickets

Additional Clinical Resources

In addition to Bright Futures, several additional clinical screening resources are available to help practitioners assess, diagnose, and treat pediatric patients. A partial list of the most common is available below:

- Ages & Stages Questionnaires, Third Edition (ASQ-3)
- Modified Checklist for Autism in Toddlers, Revised with Follow-Up (M-CHAT-R/F)
- HEADSSS Assessment: Risk and Protective Factors
- Personal Health Questionnaire—Modified for Adolescents (PHQ-A)
- Screen for Child Anxiety Related Disorders (SCARED)
- Vanderbilt ADHD Diagnostic Rating Scale

Review Questions

1. A 7-year-old male child is brought to the clinic by his parents for evaluation. The child has no significant past medical history (PMH). Approximately 5 days ago, he developed a cold and has developed a persistent cough and fever since then. His older sister was also ill with cold symptoms at the same time. The nurse practitioner (NP) performs a physical exam and notes that the child has mild tachypnea, crackles in both bases and an oxygen saturation of 96 percent. His temperature is 100.8°F. There is no wheezing auscultated. What is the best course of action for the NP?
   A. This is likely bacterial pneumonia. The NP should prescribe amoxicillin and order a chest x-ray (CXR) with a follow-up in 24 hours.
   B. This is likely viral pneumonia. The NP should educate on supportive care and recommend the patient return to the office in 1 week and call if symptoms worsen.

C. This is bronchiolitis. The NP should prescribe a bronchodilator and corticosteroids.
D. This is bronchitis. The NP should refer the child to the emergency department for further evaluation.

2. A 6-month-old male is being seen with his caretaker for a cough that sounds like a "seal's bark," which is making the caretaker anxious. The baby seems to have mild respiratory distress, and the pulse oximeter reads 94 percent. The FNP sends the baby for a CXR. What findings are likely to be reported?
   A. Ground glass appearance over affected lung field(s)
   B. Pneumothorax of an upper lung field
   C. Steeple-shaped appearance with narrowing in the upper airway
   D. CXR will be unremarkable

3. When not contraindicated, amoxicillin is the first-line treatment for acute bacterial otitis media because of susceptibility of which most common causative organism?
   A. *Haemophilus influenzae*
   B. Adenovirus
   C. *Streptococcus pneumoniae*
   D. *Staphylococcus aureus*

4. A 19-year-old mother brings her 2½-month-old boy to the clinic with a concern that the baby has become less interested in his feedings over the past 2 or 3 days, taking in only about half the normal amount of formula before becoming tired and falling asleep. His birth history is normal, and he has normal development and weight gain. His temperature is 100.4°F (axillary) now. He has no respiratory symptoms, and his physical examination reveals no identifiable source of fever. Which of the following questions/observations would be **most** helpful in establishing a diagnosis?
   A. "Does he have any known ill contacts?"
   B. "How sick do you think he is?"
   C. "Has he ever had a temperature before?"
   D. "Did you have any infection or rash when you were pregnant?"

5. Which of the following recommendations should the NP give regarding the respiratory syncytial virus (RSV) vaccine?
   A. "All adults who will care closely for the infant should be vaccinated."
   B. "Pregnant people should be vaccinated from 32 weeks through 36 weeks gestation."
   C. "Infants should be vaccinated for RSV at the first sign of infection."
   D. "Only premature infants qualify for the RSV vaccine."

6. Which of the following represent(s) language developmental red flags that warrant further evaluation? Select all that apply.
   A. No single words by 16 months
   B. A 2-year-old who only uses 2-word combinations that are intelligible to 50 percent of strangers
   C. A 2-year-old with a vocabulary of approximately 30 words
   D. A 4-year-old who is unintelligible to approximately 25 percent of strangers

7. A 9-year-old child experiences wheezing four times a week during the day and three times during the night, with an FEV1 of 80 percent. What would be the classification of his asthma severity?
   A. Severe persistent
   B. Moderate persistent
   C. Mild persistent
   D. Mild intermittent

8. An 8-year-old male has mild persistent asthma. Appropriate daily preventive medication should include which of the following?
   A. An inhaled low-dose corticosteroid
   B. Short-acting beta-2 agonists
   C. An oral systemic corticosteroid
   D. A cough suppressant

9. A 4-month-old female is brought to the office for a routine examination, and numerous bruises in varying stages are noted on the infant's arms and legs. The mother explained that she got the bruises from crawling around and bumping into things. A necessary next step for this scenario is which of the following?
   A. Explain to the mother that she has to leave the baby with the office staff for the Department of Children and Families to come and get her.
   B. Discuss with the mother that sometimes congenital bleeding issues can cause these types of bruises and make an appointment for her to return with the baby in 2 days for bloodwork.
   C. Explain to the mother that bruises such as these are uncommon in a 4-month-old, and further assessment, including a skeletal body scan, is required.
   D. Ask the mother to call the baby's father to come to the office so that the family can be interviewed regarding child abuse.

10. According to Erikson's developmental theory, if the infant's needs are not met consistently, the infant will develop which of the following?
    A. Trust
    B. Guilt
    C. Mistrust
    D. Love

11. An infant's birth weight is 7 pounds, 5 ounces. What would the NP expect the infant to weigh at 6 months?
    A. 12 pounds
    B. 15 pounds
    C. 18 pounds
    D. 22 pounds

12. A father brings his 2-year-old to the clinic. He verbalizes frustration with the child's willfulness and states that he wants to know the best form of discipline for his child. The nurse practitioner responds that based on evidence:
    A. a gentle spanking works best because it is the most effective.
    B. a 5-minute time-out is most effective.
    C. a 2-minute time-out is most effective.
    D. discipline should be individualized to the child and family based on social and cultural preferences.

13. The nurse practitioner provides anticipatory guidance to parents/guardians at every well-child visit to help prevent which leading cause of death in infants and children?
    A. Accidents
    B. Suicide
    C. Malignant neoplasms
    D. Vaccine-preventable illnesses

14. A parent is frustrated with her 2-year-old's inability to share her toys with siblings or playmates. The NP explains to the parent that a toddler has difficulty seeing anyone else's point of view, that this is a normal part of development, and that it is referred to as _____.
    A. industry.
    B. identity
    C. egocentric thinking.
    D. autonomy.

15. The NP observes that a 3-year-old has amblyopia. The NP recommends the following:
    A. Patch the weaker eye for 2 to 6 hours every day
    B. Patch the stronger eye for 2 to 6 hours every day
    C. Patch the weaker eye overnight
    D. Patch the stronger eye overnight

16. The NP is evaluating a 3-month-old infant at the well-baby clinic. The NP discovers positive Barlow and Ortolani tests. The NP should prepare the parent for which of the following interventions?
    A. Surgery
    B. Amputation
    C. Bracing/harnessing
    D. Injections

17. A 16-year-old engages in risky behavior, such as driving while drunk. The parent asks the adolescent, "Why would you do something you know is so stupid?" The 16-year-old replies, "I don't know." One possible explanation for this answer is that most adolescents:
    A. do not think of the repercussions of getting caught.
    B. believe that bad things only happen to other people.
    C. have not formed the physiological connections within the brain that connect the prefrontal cortex with the limbic system.
    D. have not developed the ability to perform concrete operational thinking.

18. The mother of a 14-year-old female child verbalizes concern that her daughter is losing weight and exercising for several hours a day. The NP performs a complete history and physical exam on the 14-year-old adolescent. Which of the following is *not* a characteristic associated with anorexia nervosa?
    A. Amenorrhea that may last 3 months or longer
    B. Low self-esteem
    C. Improvement in body image as weight loss occurs
    D. Feelings of helplessness

19. The NP is performing a physical assessment on a 3-year-old child and notes that pulses in the upper extremities are stronger than those in the lower extremities. The next best course of action would be to:
    A. check for anemia.
    B. check pulse oximetry.
    C. compare the blood pressure in the upper extremities with that of the lower extremities.
    D. refer the child to the emergency department.

20. An NP is performing a sports physical on a 15-year-old male entering high school who wants clearance to play on the high school football JV

team. The NP auscultates a systolic murmur between the apex and the LLSB when he performs the Valsalva maneuver. The NP asks the patient to squat and then stand. When standing after squatting, the murmur becomes markedly louder. The NP suspects which of the following?
   A. An innocent murmur
   B. Hypertrophic obstructive cardiomyopathy
   C. Pulmonic stenosis
   D. Coarctation of the aorta

21. Which of the following screening tools, if used at the 18- and 24-month visits, can lead to early identification and intervention of autism spectrum disorder?
    A. PHQ-A
    B. M-CHAT-R/F
    C. SCARED
    D. Vanderbilt rating scale

22. The NP is evaluating a 5-year-old female child who has been brought into the clinic by her mother for a sick visit. The mother states that the child has had a "cold" for approximately one week. The NP observes coryza and conjunctivitis; the child's temperature is 103°F. The NP performs an oral exam and observes Koplik's spots in the child's mouth. Which of the following questions will be most helpful to assist the NP in formulating a diagnosis?
    A. "What medications have you tried up to this point to treat the child?"
    B. "Can you supply me with your child's immunization records?"
    C. "Is there anyone else sick at home?"
    D. "Does the coughing awaken your child during the night?"

23. An acyanotic heart condition can be characterized as a condition where:
    A. there is a shunting of blood from the left side of the heart to the right side of the heart.
    B. spontaneous closure of the congenital heart malformation will commonly occur.
    C. there is a shunting of blood from the right side of the heart to the left side of the heart.
    D. open heart surgery is commonly performed after the child reaches the age of 1 year.

24. A 7-year-old child is brought into the office for a sick visit evaluation by her parents. The child's parents state that the child has had a cold for 4 days that has been associated with fever and a headache. The NP observes that the child's cheeks are reddened and appear as if the child was recently slapped on both sides of the face. With this information, the NP:
    A. suspects child abuse and files a report in good faith with the Department of Family and Children's Services.
    B. suspects meningitis and refers the child to neurology for further workup.
    C. prescribes liquid amoxicillin 80 mg/kg/day divided into Q12 hour doses for 7 days.
    D. explains to the parents that only supportive therapy is necessary to treat her symptoms and that the condition will resolve on its own.

25. Which of the following represent motor developmental red flags that warrant further evaluation? Select all that apply.
    A. Not walking independently at 18 months
    B. Unable to sit unsupported at 9 months
    C. The persistence of primitive reflexes at 3 months
    D. Unable to skip at 36 months

Answers and Rationales

1. Answer B is correct. Viral pneumonia often develops after a viral illness. If the patient is stable, supportive care and watchful waiting are indicated.

   Answer A is incorrect. This clinical presentation is more consistent with viral pneumonia. Antibiotics are not indicated.

   Answer C is incorrect. The diagnostic criteria and age of the patient suggest pneumonia rather than bronchiolitis. Bronchodilators and steroids are not indicated in the treatment of bronchiolitis.

   Answer D is incorrect. The diagnostic criteria suggest pneumonia. Oxygen saturation levels are normal, and the fever is not excessive. Referral to the emergency department is not warranted.

2. Answer C is correct. The baby has laryngotracheobronchitis (croup), which is associated with a "steeple sign" on the X-ray. This is caused by glottic and subglottic narrowing.

   Answer A is incorrect. A ground-glass appearance of the lungs suggests several other etiologies, but not croup, which affects the trachea.

   Answer B is incorrect. Pneumothorax is a condition of the lung that results in a linear shadow without lung markings.

Answer D is incorrect. If croup is severe enough to affect oxygen saturation levels, a "steeple sign" would be expected.

3. Answer C is correct. *Streptococcus pneumoniae* is the most common causative organism responsible for bacterial otitis media and usually responds to amoxicillin.

   Answer A is incorrect. *Haemophilus influenzae* is vaccine-preventable and not a common cause of bacterial ear infections. Fewer than 100 children in the United States get *Haemophilus influenzae* annually.

   Answer B is incorrect. Otitis media, which is associated with adenovirus, is most likely viral and will not respond to antibiotics.

   Answer D is incorrect. *Staphylococcus aureus* is the most common cause of skin infections, not ear infections.

4. Answer A is correct. The child's symptoms are consistent with the prodromal phase of a viral or bacterial infection. Asking if there are sick contacts would provide the most valuable information.

   Answer B is incorrect. Asking how sick the mother thinks the child is will not add beneficial information to the NP's assessment.

   Answer C is incorrect. Whether the child has had a temperature before is irrelevant to the current illness.

   Answer D is incorrect. This question is only relevant for a fever that appears within the first 30 days after birth.

5. Answer B is correct. All pregnant people should receive the RSV vaccine between 32 and 36 weeks gestation.

   Answer A is incorrect. This recommendation is for the Tdap vaccine, not the RSV vaccine.

   Answer C is incorrect. Infants should be vaccinated at birth if their mother was not vaccinated between 32 and 36 weeks gestation.

   Answer D is incorrect. All infants are now eligible for the RSV vaccine.

6. Answer A is correct. A 16-month-old should have a vocabulary of 10 to 15 words.

   Answer C is correct. A 2-year-old should have a vocabulary of at least 50 words.

   Answer D is correct. A 4-year-old should no longer be unintelligible to strangers.

   Answer B is incorrect. This 2-year-old has reached expected language developmental milestones.

7. Answer B is correct. The child's symptoms are consistent with the diagnosis of moderate persistent asthma.

   Answer A is incorrect. Severe persistent asthma would have symptoms throughout the day rather than once per day, and nighttime awakenings would occur almost every night.

   Answer C is incorrect. Mild persistent asthma would not have daily symptoms.

   Answer D is incorrect. Mild intermittent asthma has symptoms 2 or fewer days per month with two or fewer nighttime awakenings per month.

8. Answer A is correct. A child with mild persistent asthma should use the stepwise approach to management. Per GINA guidelines, the child should be using an inhaled low-dose corticosteroid to control symptoms.

   Answer B is incorrect. A short-acting beta-2 agonist is a rescue medication rather than a preventive one. Ideally, it should not be needed daily.

   Answer C is incorrect. Oral systemic corticosteroids have many side effects and should not be used long-term or as a preventive measure.

   Answer D is incorrect. A cough suppressant will not treat asthma symptoms and can be detrimental.

9. Answer C is correct. Any child under the age of 2 with unexplained bruises is required to have a full skeletal body scan. Since this child is not yet mobile, the mother's story is inconsistent.

   Answer A is incorrect. While a call to the proper authorities is mandated in this case, it is not the office's responsibility to detain the child.

   Answer B is incorrect. Congenital bleeding issues would be more systemic and would likely involve joint pain, swelling, nosebleeds, petechiae, and so on.

   Answer D is incorrect. It is not the responsibility of the office to conduct interviews where child abuse is suspected. Proper authorities should be notified.

10. Answer C is correct. According to the developmental theorist Erikson, if an infant's needs are not met, they develop a mistrust of the world around them (Trust vs. Mistrust stage).

    Answer A is incorrect. According to the developmental theorist Erikson, infants develop trust in the world around them when their needs are met (Trust vs. Mistrust stage).

    Answer B is incorrect. Guilt develops if a preschooler does not successfully navigate Erikson's third stage of psychosocial development.

Answer D is incorrect. Love is not one of Erikson's stages of psychosocial development.

11. Answer B is correct. At 6 months of age, an infant is expected to double their body weight.

    Answer A is incorrect. This infant would be underweight.

    Answer C is incorrect. This infant would exceed weight gain expectations.

    Answer D is incorrect. This infant would exceed weight gain expectations.

12. Answer C is correct. The recommended form of discipline for a child is to use the "timeout" strategy. Most young children can sit in "timeout" for the same number of minutes that is equal to what their age is in years.

    Answer A is incorrect. Spanking is not an effective form of punishment, and the American Academy of Pediatrics recommends against it.

    Answer B is incorrect. While timeout is the most effective form of punishment, 5 minutes exceeds the recommended time for a child of this age.

    Answer D is incorrect. Timeouts are the recommended discipline for toddlers, independent of social and cultural preferences.

13. Answer A is correct. Per U.S. national statistics, accidents remain the number one cause of death in children.

    Answer B is incorrect. Suicide is a leading cause of death but is surpassed by accidents as leading causes.

    Answer C is incorrect. While cancer is one of the leading causes of death in children, it is surpassed by accidents as the leading cause.

    Answer D is incorrect. Vaccine-preventable illnesses are not a leading cause of death in children.

14. Answer C is correct. Egocentricity is commonly seen in toddlers, who develop a sense of self that is separate from their primary caregivers and see themselves as the center of their universe.

    Answer A is incorrect. Industry develops when a preschooler successfully navigates Erikson's third stage of psychosocial development.

    Answer B is incorrect. Identity develops during the teen years.

    Answer D is incorrect. Autonomy develops when a toddler successfully navigates Erikson's second stage of psychosocial development as they head into the preschool years.

15. Answer A is correct. Patching the stronger eye reinforces connections between the brain and the weaker eye. Occlusion therapy has been the mainstay of treatment for amblyopia. The endpoint goal of occlusive therapy is equal visual acuity in both eyes. Once visual acuity has stabilized, patching may be decreased slowly, and the child should be monitored for reoccurrence.

    Answer B is incorrect. Patching the weaker eye would be of no benefit as the other eye is already stronger.

    Answer C is incorrect. The weaker eye should never be patched.

    Answer D is incorrect. Patching overnight offers no benefit as neither eye is used for strengthening.

16. Answer C is correct. The infant demonstrates a positive Ortolani test and needs further evaluation for hip dysplasia. First-line treatment in a child under 6 months usually involves bracing/harnessing first.

    Answer A is incorrect. Surgery is reserved for the most severe cases and those not caught before 6 months.

    Answer B is incorrect. Amputation is not a treatment for developmental dysplasia of the hip.

    Answer D is incorrect. Injections are not useful in treating developmental dysplasia of the hip.

17. Answer C is correct. Behavioral neuroscientists have speculated that the "pruning" of neurons in the prefrontal cortex occurs gradually over the period between childhood and adulthood. This "pruning" allows for greater behavior control, less impulsivity, and poor decision-making.

    Answer A is incorrect. Most adolescents fear getting caught more than other repercussions for negative actions.

    Answer B is incorrect. Most schools still teach the dangers of alcohol intoxication before adolescents are old enough to drive.

    Answer D is incorrect. Piaget's concrete operational stage of cognitive development is usually reached by 11 years of age.

18. Answer C is correct. Anorexia nervosa is an eating disorder with a high mortality rate. The patient demonstrates an intense fear of weight gain, obsession with weight, and persistent behavior to prevent weight gain. Most patients are unable to recognize or appreciate the severity of the situation, even in the presence of severe starvation and

impending death. Body image does not improve no matter how much weight is lost.

Answer A is incorrect. Amenorrhea can last indefinitely with anorexia nervosa.

Answer B is incorrect. Low self-esteem is a common trait among those who experience anorexia nervosa.

Answer D is incorrect. Most individuals with anorexia nervosa experience feelings of helplessness at some point during their illness.

19. Answer C is correct. A child with coarctation of the aorta will exhibit a higher blood pressure above the area of coarctation and a lower pressure below the area of coarctation. Occasionally, the arterial flow to the lower extremities can be severe enough to cause mottling.

Answer A is incorrect. Checking for anemia is not a priority step in evaluating for coarctation of the aorta.

Answer B is incorrect. While low blood oxygen levels can be associated with coarctation of the aorta, the next best course of action after discovering weaker pulses in the lower extremities is to check blood pressure.

Answer D is incorrect. Coarctation of the aorta that is discovered incidentally during a physical assessment at age 3 should be referred for urgent evaluation by a pediatric cardiologist. Still, it would not warrant a referral to the emergency department in the absence of other life-threatening symptoms.

20. Answer B is correct. It is essential that the NP can distinguish an innocent or functional murmur from the murmur of HOCM. While many of the characteristics are similar, a person with HOCM will have an increase in the intensity of the murmur during both the Valsalva maneuver and when standing after squatting.

Answer A is incorrect. An innocent murmur becomes softer when standing.

Answer C is incorrect. Pulmonic stenosis would be best auscultated over the pulmonic area at the left side of the sternum, the second intercostal space.

Answer D is incorrect. The murmur most associated with coarctation of the aorta is auscultated on the back below the left shoulder blade, although a murmur is not always heard with this condition.

21. Answer B is correct. The Modified Checklist for Autism Spectrum Disorder in Toddlers, Revised with Follow-up (M-CHAT-R/F) is an evidence-based screening tool for autism spectrum disorder administered at the 18- and 24-month well-child visits.

Answer A is incorrect. The Patient Health Questionnaire for Adolescents (PHQ-A) is a screening tool for depression.

Answer C is incorrect. The Screen for Child Anxiety-Related Disorders is a screening tool for anxiety disorder symptoms.

Answer D is incorrect. The Vanderbilt scale measures the core symptoms of attention-deficit hyperactivity disorder (ADHD).

22. Answer B is correct. The child presents with symptoms of the measles. It would be essential for the NP to ascertain if the child has received the MMR vaccine and missed any doses of the recommended vaccination schedule.

Answer A is incorrect. While asking which medications have been tried is always appropriate, the answer to this question will not help rule out the primary differential of measles.

Answer C is incorrect. While an important question, whether anyone else is sick at home will not provide the information needed to diagnose this illness.

Answer D is incorrect. In the presence of Koplik's spots, the severity of nighttime cough is not information that will impact the diagnosis.

23. Answer A is correct. The shunting of blood from an area of high pressure (left side of the heart) to an area of lower pressure (right side of the heart) occurs when an opening between the two sides allows for a mixing of deoxygenated and oxygenated blood.

Answer B is incorrect. While some mild congenital heart malformations may spontaneously resolve, this is not the usual.

Answer C is incorrect. Right-to-left shunting represents a cyanotic heart defect.

Answer D is incorrect. Surgery is most often completed before 1 year of age.

24. Answer D is correct. The child has a classic presentation of parvovirus B19 (Fifth disease). The parents should be educated that it is a viral disease that requires only supportive therapy while allowing the virus to run its course. The parents should also be told that the child may develop a rash on the trunk or back within a few days. Most adults are immune to the disease. However, pregnant people should be cautioned to avoid

exposure to a child with known parvovirus as it has been associated with spontaneous abortion in pregnant people who do not have immunity.

Answer A is incorrect. A good history and physical quickly rule out child abuse as a cause for the reddened cheeks.

Answer B is incorrect. At this point, additional symptoms suggesting meningitis, such as stiff neck, light sensitivity, and nausea/vomiting, are lacking.

Answer C is incorrect. The presenting symptoms are consistent with viral illness; therefore, the prescription of antibiotics is not indicated.

25. Answer A is correct. A child who is not walking independently by 18 months exhibits a developmental delay.

    Answer B is correct. A child unable to sit unsupported at 9 months represents a developmental delay.

    Answer C is incorrect. Many primitive reflexes are still present at 3 months of age.

    Answer D is incorrect. Many children are unable to skip until 4 to 6 years of age.

Resources

American Academy of Pediatrics (AAP). (2022). *Bright futures*. https://brightfutures.aap.org/materials-and-tools/tool-and-resource-kit/Pages/default.aspx

American Academy of Pediatrics (AAP). (2021). *Preparticipation physical evaluation*. Retrieved from https://www.aap.org/en/patient-care/preparticipation-physical-evaluation/

Botash, A. (2015). *Child abuse evaluation and treatment for medical providers*. http://www.childabusemd.com

Bright Futures. (n.d.). *Practice management*. American Academy of Pediatrics (AAP). https://www.aap.org/en/practice-management/bright-futures

Carolan, P. (2023). *Pediatric bronchitis*. Medscape. http://emedicine.medscape.com/article/1001332-medication#showall

CDC. (2022a). *CDC's work on developmental disabilities*. https://www.cdc.gov/child-development/data-research/?CDC_AAref_Val=https://www.cdc.gov/ncbddd/developmentaldisabilities/about.html

CDC. (2022b). *About child and teen BMI*. https://www.cdc.gov/bmi/faq/?CDC_AAref_Val=https://www.cdc.gov/healthyweight/assessing/bmi/childrens_bmi/about_childrens_bmi.html

CDC. (2024). *Parvovirus B19 and Fifth disease*. https://www.cdc.gov/parvovirus-b19/about/index.html

CDC. (2024a). *Child and adolescent immunization schedule by age*. Retrieved from https://www.cdc.gov/vaccines/hcp/imz-schedules/child-adolescent-age.html

CDC. (2024b). *Respiratory syncytial virus: For health professionals*. Retrieved from https://www.cdc.gov/rsv/hcp/clinical-overview/?CDC_AAref_Val=https://www.cdc.gov/rsv/clinical/

CDC. (2024c). *Child and Teen BMI calculator widget*. https://www.cdc.gov/bmi/child-teen-calculator/widget.html?CDC_AAref_Val=https://www.cdc.gov/healthyweight/bmi/calculator.html

CDC. (2024d). *RSV in infants and young children*. https://www.cdc.gov/vaccines/vpd/rsv/public/child.html

Chumlea, W. C., Schubert, C. M., Roche A. F., Kulin, H. E., Lee, P. A., Himes, J. H., & Sun, S. S. (2003). Age at menarche and racial comparisons in U.S. girls. *Pediatrics, 111*(1), 110–113.

Garzon, D. L., Starr, N. B., Brady, M. A., Gaylord, N. M., Driessnack, M., & Duderstadt, K. G. (2019). *Pediatric primary care* (7th ed.). Elsevier.

Global Initiative for Asthma. (2023). *Global strategy for asthma management and prevention*. https://ginasthma.org/wp-content/uploads/2023/07/GINA-2023-Full-report-23_07_06-WMS.pdf

Haines, C., Soon, A., & Mercurio, D. (2013). Community acquired pneumonia in pediatric populations. *Emergency Medicine Reports, 34*(17), 197–207.

U.S. Department of Health and Human Services; Administration for Children and Families; Administration on Children, Youth and Families; Children's Bureau. (2022). *Child maltreatment 2022*. Retrieved from https://acf.gov/cb/report/child-maltreatment-2022

World Health Organization (WHO). (2022). *Pneumonia in children*. Retrieved from http://www.who.int/mediacentre/factsheets/fs331/en/

CHAPTER 20

Geriatrics

Nancy L. Dennert, MS, MSN, FNP-BC, CDCES, BC-ADM

Considerations for the Older Patient

Advances in medicine and technology have enabled older adults to live longer and healthier lives. Since the start of the 20th century, the average life expectancy in the United States has increased considerably.

Family nurse practitioners (FNPs) must be prepared to provide comprehensive care to older adults across the continuum of healthcare delivery services (e.g., primary care, subacute rehabilitation care, long-term care, assisted living facilities), including the management of geriatric syndromes and health maintenance, as well as have a solid foundation and understanding of the physiology of aging based on scientific underpinnings. **Table 20-1** describes the physiologic changes and their clinical implications in older adults. FNPs must also be well-informed about reimbursement and regulatory issues that guide advanced practice nursing.

Geriatric Fast Facts: A Profile of Older Adults

Older adults are often divided into groups:

- Young-old, 65 to 75 years
- Middle-old, 75 to 84 years
- Old-old, 85 plus
- Centenarians, 100+

Oldest Old Is the Fastest Growing Segment of Older Adults

The 85+ population is projected to more than double from 6.5 million in 2022 to 13.7 million in 2040 (a 111% increase).

Multiple Chronic Care Needs

Older adults—4 out of 5—live with one or more chronic conditions (e.g., diabetes, hypertension, chronic obstructive pulmonary disease [COPD], congestive heart failure [CHF]).

Marital Status

- Men are more likely to be married than women.
- Forty percent of older women are widows.

Leading Causes of Death

- Heart disease
- Cancer
- Chronic lower respiratory disease

Income

- Income—Almost 15.9 percent of older adults were below the poverty level due to out-of-pocket medical expenses in 2011.

Table 20-1 Age-Related Changes

Organ/System	Physiologic Change	Clinical Implications
Body	Decrease in lean body mass Decrease in skeletal mass Decrease in total body H_2O Increase in adipose tissue until age 60, then decreases	Increased risk of dehydration Decreased strength Alteration in drug levels
Ears	Hearing loss (high frequency) Sensorineural/conductive	Presbycusis Inability to understand speech and tone
Eyes	Increase in cataracts Pupil reflex—increased time Decrease in lens flexibility Decrease in tear production Increase in intraocular pressure Cell breakdown in macula of the retina—loss of central vision	Changes in visual acuity Difficulty adjusting to light Increased glare Presbyopia Dry eyes Glaucoma Macular degeneration
Olfactory	Alterations in smell	Decrease in appetite Varied taste sensation
Oropharyngeal	Decrease in salivation Decrease in muscle strength for mastication	Dry mouth (xerostomia) Dysphagia
Cardiac	Change in intrinsic heart rate Diminished baroreflex in response to change in blood pressure	Increase in syncopal events Increase in atrial fibrillation Decrease in ejection fraction Rise in diastolic heart failure and dysfunction
Pulmonary	Increase in residual volume Decrease in vital capacity Decrease in FEV1	Increased incidence of pneumonia Complications related to chronic lung disease Increased shortness of breath
Gastrointestinal	Changes in motility Alteration in splanchnic blood flow	Constipation or diarrhea
Musculoskeletal	Decrease in bone density Demineralization Fibrosis Cartilage degeneration Compression of spine	Increased risk of fractures Progression to osteoarthritis Joint tightening Loss of height
Renal	Decrease in glomerular filtration Decrease in renal mass Renal blood flow decrease Decrease in reabsorption and secretion of renal tubular	Increased risk of dehydration Alterations in drug levels Risk of adverse effects
Hepatic	Activity decrease of P-450 system Decrease in hepatic mass	Alterations in drug levels
Integumentary	Decrease in elasticity Decrease in collagen and subcutaneous fat tissue	Shearing and skin tears Prolonged wound healing
Immune System	Decrease in T-cells Atrophy of thymus	Risk of developing infections
Central Nervous System	Slowdown in cognitive processing Decrease in dopamine receptors	Parkinson's disease

Major Source of Income Is Derived from

- Social Security
- Private pensions
- Assets
- Earnings
- Government-related pensions

Prescription, Over-the-Counter, and Alternative Therapy Use

- Many take multiple medicines at the same time. A recent survey of 17,000 Medicare beneficiaries found that 2 out of 5 patients reported taking five or more prescription medicines.
- Account for 30 percent of total over-the-counter (OTC) usage and 34 percent of prescription drug consumption.
- Older adults are at increased risk of serious adverse drug events, including falls, depression, confusion, hallucinations, and malnutrition, which are an important cause of illness, hospitalization, and death among these patients.
- Drug-related complications have been attributed to the use of multiple medicines and associated drug interactions, age-related changes, human error, and poor medical management (e.g., incorrect medicines prescribed, inappropriate doses, lack of communication and monitoring).
- Almost 40 percent of older people cannot read prescription labels, and 67 percent cannot understand the information given to them.

Goals of Geriatric Care

Geriatric care aims to provide safe, comprehensive, and cost-effective quality health care based on evidence-based practice (EBP) to maintain and/or optimize function and improve the quality of life. To achieve this aim, the FNP must create an environment that provides a private and quiet face-to-face encounter away from noise and other distractions in a well-lit, ventilated area. The face-to-face interaction (interview) between the FNP and patient is key to obtaining a thorough and comprehensive health history that will guide the care plan and formulate a differential diagnosis.

Key elements essential to the health history include all the components in the adult health history, with an additional focus on the following:

- **Family history**—Review of parent and sibling health history, including the cause of death if appropriate
- **Work history**—To include previous exposures to occupational or environmental toxins
- **Medication use**—OTC, prescription, herbals, alternative modalities, as well as medications prescribed for family or friends
- **Allergies or sensitivities**—Foods, medication, latex
- **Smoking status**—Including present and past smoking history
- **Substance use**—Alcohol use and history of illicit drug use
- **Nutritional assessment**—Includes the ability to shop for and prepare food, change in appetite, alteration in taste, and attitude toward eating. A sudden weight loss of 5 percent total body weight is a red flag and warrants further assessment and evaluation.
Note: The Mini-Nutritional Assessment Short Form is a six-question screening tool used to identify older adults (65+) who are at risk of malnutrition or who are malnourished. The test takes about 5 minutes to complete and can be integrated into the comprehensive geriatric assessment.
- **Sleep hygiene**—Hours of sleep? Need for nonpharmacological or pharmacological sleep aids. Sleep patterns. Naps? The location where sleep takes place.
Note: **The Epworth Physical Activity**—Including exercise (e.g., walking, swimming, dancing).
- **Health maintenance**—Screenings (e.g., mammograms, prostate-specific antigen, colonoscopy, ophthalmology exams), dental exams, and immunizations
- **Past medical history**—A compilation of information relevant to the patient's past health and illness. The information obtained will provide the FNP with vital clues related to contributing factors or underlying etiology pertinent to the patient's current health status, including the following:
  - **Childhood and adult illnesses**—Document the date of diagnosis and treatment, and whether they are ongoing or resolved.
  - **Immunizations**—Document dates of last immunizations (e.g., influenza, pneumovax, varicella, Prevnar 13, tetanus, diphtheria, pertussis). Documentation of Mantoux tuberculin skin test or Bacilli Calmette-Guerin (BCG).
  - **Hospitalizations** (medical, surgical, and mental health)—Record basis for admission, course of treatment, and resulting complications.
  - **Accidents, injuries, or falls**
  - **Religious beliefs and health practices**

Health Maintenance

The U.S. Preventive Services Task Force (USPSTF) recommends clinical services for adults 65 and over. The evidence-based practice guidelines target preventive health services pertinent to older adults. (See health promotion chapter for details.) They include:

- Abdominal aortic aneurysm,
- Breast cancer screening,
- Carotid artery stenosis screening,
- Cervical cancer screening,
- Colorectal cancer screening,
- Coronary heart disease screening,
- Dementia screening,
- Fall prevention in older adults,
- Hearing loss in older adults,
- Hormone replacement in older adults,
- Immunizations (Adult),
- Osteoporosis screening,
- Ovarian cancer screening,
- Peripheral artery disease screening,
- Prostate cancer screening,
- Thyroid disease screening, and
- Vision screening in older adults

The decision to screen for any or all recommended preventive services should be individualized to the patient and circumstances. The USPSTF has assigned a letter grade to each recommendation that reflects the certainty and strength of the evidence supporting the provision of a specific preventive service and guides the healthcare provider and patient in clinical decision-making. Only services with a letter grade of "A" or "B" should be discussed with appropriate patients.

Communication Techniques

- Sit face to face, maintain eye contact. Do not stand over the patient.
- Be an attentive listener.
- Show genuine concern for the patient.
- Do not shout. Speak slowly.
- Know your personal biases.
- Be cognizant of ethnic and cultural differences.
- Observe for signs of distress (e.g., exhaustion, anxiety, confusion).
- Ask specific, open-ended questions to elicit important healthcare information.
- Address one issue at a time.

Creating the Relationship

- Recognize communication barriers and make appropriate changes.
- Be cognizant of cultural and ethnic diversities.

Eliciting the Health History

The primary objective—If the patient is unable to provide history, it may be necessary to gather history from another responsible individual (e.g., family member, friend, conservator, or power of attorney for the person). Key elements essential to the health history include, but are not limited to, the following:

- Biographical data
  - Similar to other populations. Be sure to include emergency contact information.
- Family history
  - Provide family history for parents and siblings. If applicable and available, include the cause of death.
  - List history of any major medical problems (e.g., mental health issues, cancer, diabetes, substance use, cardiac disease, neurocognitive disorders).

Geriatric Health Maintenance

Health maintenance initiatives, including preventive measures, are key to promoting optimal health and well-being for older adults. As with other populations (e.g., pediatrics, adolescents, adults), optimizing the management of acute and chronic morbidities in older adults will improve quality of life and physical function. In addition to scheduled follow-up or interval visits, which are determined by the FNP and are multifactorially dependent on presenting symptomatology and management of the underlying disease, the Centers for Medicare and Medicaid (CMS), as a result of the Affordable Care Act signed into law in 2010, has implemented preventive visits.

Welcome to Medicare Preventive Visit

- Goals of initial preventive physical examination (IPPE)—Health promotion, disease prevention, and detection
- Medicare allows for one IPPE during the beneficiary's lifetime.
- Provided within the first 12 months of enrollment of the beneficiary in Medicare Part B.

The Seven Components

- **Review of medical and social history** (e.g., past medical and surgical history, medication and supplement use, family history, use of alcohol or other substance use, tobacco use, diet, and physical activity)

- **Review potential risk factors for depression and other mood disorders**
- **Review safety and functional ability** (e.g., fall risk, activities of daily living, hearing acuity, home safety) utilizing standardized questionnaires or screening tools
- **Exam** includes height, weight, body mass index (BMI), blood pressure, visual acuity screening, additional elements pertinent to the beneficiary's medical and social history, congruent with current standards of practice
- **End-of-life planning**—To include written or verbal information relevant to the beneficiary's ability to prepare an advance directive in the event of an injury or illness that impacts the beneficiary's capacity to make healthcare decisions, as well as whether the healthcare provider is willing to follow the wishes of the beneficiary as stated in the advance directive
- **Educate, counsel, and refer**—Based on the previous five components
- **Educate, counsel, and refer for other preventive services**—To include written plan of care (e.g., appropriate **screenings** and Medicare-covered preventive services), as well as once-in-a-lifetime screening and electrocardiogram, as appropriate

Medicare Annual Wellness Visit

- Review of medical and family history
- Recent medical events (i.e., siblings, children)
- Personal medical and surgical history
- Illness and hospital stays
- Medication use, including nonprescription medications (i.e., OTC or herbals)

Role of FNP

- Routine body measurements and assessments
- Height, weight, BMI (**Note:** Significant weight loss [5 percent] or significant weight gain in the past year may indicate underlying comorbidities.)
- Vital signs including blood pressure, pulse, and temperature
- Detection of cognitive impairment (**Note:** CMS does not specify a tool or test to be used. Examples include the Mini-Mental Status Exam [MMSE], the Saint Louis University Mental Status Exam [SLUMS], and Mini-Cog.)
- Depression screening (only during the initial annual wellness visit). **Note:** There is no specified tool or instrument. (Examples of tools include Geriatric Depression Scale [GDS], Patient Health Questionnaire 9 [PHQ-9], Patient Health Questionnaire 2 [PHQ-2].) Document alterations in sleep or appetite, expressed feelings of social isolation, anhedonia (loss of ability to experience pleasure), suicidal thoughts, and so on.
- Functional capacity and level of safety at home (Timed Get Up and Go test), risk of falls
- Assess hearing and vision
- Assess the ability to perform activities of daily living (ADLs). Examples of instruments are the Katz Index of Independence in Activities of Daily Living. The Katz ADL index assesses the six functions of bathing, dressing, toileting, transferring, continence, and feeding. Each item gets a score of 1 (yes) or 2 (no). A score of 6 is a fully functional person independent in performing ADL's and Instrumental Activities of Daily Living which was developed by Lawton and Brody in 1969 and assesses a person's ability to perform everyday tasks such as shopping, housekeeping, medication, and finances. It is a self-reported questionnaire which takes about 15 minutes. Its limitation is that there may be an over or under estimation of their own ability to perform these tasks.
- Assess identified risk factors and maladies.
- Establish individual screenings and preventive services (every 5 to 10 years, as appropriate).
- Develop personalized health advice and referrals as indicated.

Medicare Basics

Medicare was signed into law by President Lyndon B. Johnson on July 30, 1965. The initial intent of this program was to provide basic health coverage for those who did not have health insurance. Medicare continues to provide coverage to older adults and individuals with disabilities. Enrollment and eligibility requirements for Medicare services are not based on income level. Medicare has evolved from the cost and charge reimbursement fee for service toward value-based payment. At this time, Medicare has four distinct entities that cover different services. They include:

Medicare Part A—Referred to as hospital insurance

- Covers *most* medically necessary hospital, skilled nursing, home health care, or hospice services.
- Individuals who are 65 and older who are eligible for Social Security are automatically enrolled, whether retired or not.
- Criteria—Must have worked and paid Social Security taxes for at least 40 calendar quarters (10 years), or if worked less, will be required to pay a monthly fee.

- Individuals who are younger than 65 and are permanently and totally impaired may enroll in Medicare Part A upon receiving disability benefits from Social Security for 2 years.
- **Note:** Advanced practice nurses in the hospital will not be paid directly for their services.

Medicare Part B—Referred to as medical insurance (supplemental)

- Requires a monthly premium payment by the beneficiary
- Medicaid may cover it for low-income individuals who meet the eligibility criteria.
- Covers **most** medical services to 80 percent of approved services when the annual deductible is met, including preventive (e.g., mammograms, influenza, pneumococcal, hepatitis), physician services, X-rays, laboratory services, durable medical equipment, physical therapy, speech therapy, occupational therapy

Medicare Part C—Referred to as Medicare Advantage Plans

- Not a separate benefit
- Allows private insurance companies to provide Medicare benefits
- Provided through health maintenance organizations (HMOs) and preferred provider organizations (PPOs)
- Additional services and screenings may be provided.
- The beneficiary pays a monthly premium.

Medicare Part D—Outpatient prescription drug coverage

- Provided by private insurance companies that have contracts with the government
- Not included in "original" Medicare
- Allows older adults to receive prescriptions at lower out-of-pocket expenditures
- Each plan has its own formulary of covered drugs.
- Formulary changes may occur; the beneficiary must receive written notice at least 60 days prior.
- Deductibles vary by drug plan. No Medicare drug plan can have a deductible of more than $545 (a $40 increase from 2023), and some Medicare Part D plans have no deductible.
- The ACA gradually closed the "donut hole." Beginning in January of 2025, Part D coverage will have three phases: the deductible phase, the initial coverage phase, and the catastrophic phase. All Medicare Part D plans will also have a $2,000 out-of-pocket cap.

Prescribing Practices in Older Adults

Polypharmacy is a common problem among older adults regardless of where they reside. The use of multiple medications is common due to multiple co-morbidities. Age-related physiological changes place older adults at increased risk for adverse events and poor outcomes. Polypharmacy becomes problematic when multiple providers are prescribing medications without the knowledge of other healthcare providers. FNPs must thoroughly understand pharmacodynamics (what the drug does to the body), pharmacokinetics (what the body does to the drug), drug interactions, adverse effects, and so on, to ensure safe and effective practice when prescribing for older adults.

Pharmacokinetics

Every drug has a specific pharmacokinetic profile based on given parameters (e.g., sex, age, BMI, renal and hepatic function). Based on the pharmacokinetic profile, proper dosing can be established for each individual.

Pharmacodynamics

Absorption

Gastrointestinal changes can occur in aging and impact drug absorption.

- Aging can decrease gastric motility.
- Gastric acid secretion is reduced, causing an increase in gastric pH.
- Decreased gastric blood flow and increased pH can reduce drug absorption, whereas decreased gastric motility may increase drug absorption.
- Absorptive changes may be influenced by concurrent use of medications and fluctuating pH.
- Using proton pump inhibitors (PPIs) and antacids can alter gastric pH.
- Drugs that utilize first-pass metabolism may be affected (e.g., lipophilic beta blockers, propranolol, and nitrates).
- **Note:** Absorption of drugs can be influenced by other factors (e.g., use of feeding tubes, dysphagia, and nutritional status).

Distribution

Begins after the drug enters the bloodstream (e.g., into the brain after crossing the blood–brain barrier, body fluids, or tissues).

Factors influencing distribution include:

- Molecular size
- pH
- Protein binding of the drug (only the unbound drug is distributed)
- Solubility of the drug (hydrophilic or lipophilic)
  - Example—Dilantin (phenytoin); highly protein bound; can lead to adverse effects in older adults with reduced albumin levels (check free Dilantin and pre-albumin levels to monitor for toxicity)
- Decrease in muscle mass, along with increased proportion of body fat, resulting in greater volume of distribution in older adults
- For drugs distributed in muscle tissue, the volume of distribution may be decreased.
  - Example—Valium (diazepam) dosing changes may be required until the desired outcome is achieved. Not frequently used in older adults.
- Other factors to consider—Reduction in total body water

Metabolism

The primary organ responsible for metabolism is the liver.

- Alterations in the normal metabolic process can significantly impact the pharmacokinetics of the drug.
- Significant adverse events are increased if the metabolic process is slowed, thereby prolonging the drug's half-life.
- In contrast, if the process is sped up, the drug's half-life is reduced, and the drug's efficacy is changed.
- Other factors impacting drug metabolism include genetics, nutritional status, diet, sex, and alcohol consumption.

Excretion

Drugs are primarily eliminated in the renal system. Renal function decreases with age, which may increase a drug's half-life.

- Physiological changes (e.g., decrease in kidney mass, reduced blood flow to the kidneys, reduction in number and size of nephrons)
- Renal changes can be predictive to some degree.
- Several tools available to calculate (e.g., Cockcroft–Gault)

Adverse Drug Events in the Older Patient

Adverse drug events (ADEs) occur in 15 percent or more of older adults seen in primary care, extended care facilities, and hospital settings. They are the result of inappropriate prescribing practices, medication errors, drug-to-drug interactions, drug-to-disease interactions, and poor compliance. Physiological changes of aging in older adults increase the probability of an ADE. The annual cost associated with ADEs is reported to be $70 to 80 billion annually. An estimated 35 percent of ambulatory older adults experience an ADE; 29 percent of these reactions require intervention from a healthcare provider or hospital admission. Many of them can be prevented.

Serious ADEs include:

- Delirium
- Falls
- Orthostatic hypotension
- Heart failure
- Gastrointestinal hemorrhage
- Intracranial bleed
- Renal failure
- Death

Common adverse drug reactions attributed to older adults include:

- Anorexia
- Dizziness
- Gastrointestinal complaints (e.g., nausea, vomiting, constipation, diarrhea)
- Edema
- Urinary incontinence

Commonly Prescribed Drug Categories for Older Adults Resulting in Potential Side Effects

- Cardiovascular agents
- Antibiotics
- Diuretics
- Anticoagulants
- Hypoglycemics
- Steroids
- Opioids
- Anticholinergics
- Nonsteroidals
- Benzodiazepines

Associated Problems With Medication Use

- Visual impairment—Difficulty reading labels and instructions may result in improper medication use.
- Manual dexterity—Physical changes (e.g., osteoarthritis, gout, hemiplegia), unable to open bottles, difficulty handling small pills, administer injectables, or use an inhaler
- Insufficient knowledge—Inadequate health information provided by a healthcare provider, language barrier, illiteracy, hearing deficit
- Costs—Prescription not filled due to costs and limited financial resources
- Cognitive deficit—May forget to take med or take more than the actual dose; may not understand the rationale for taking
- Multiple healthcare providers—Prescribing additional meds or duplication of current meds (generic/brand names), using both local and mail-order pharmacies

Assessment Tools to Reduce Medication Risks in Older Adults

- The Beers Criteria for potentially inappropriate medication use in older adults
  - Indexes medications that cause side effects in older adults due to physiologic changes of aging
  - Used by healthcare providers for older adults residing in the community, hospitalized older adults, and those residing in long-term care such as skilled nursing facilities and post-acute care settings.
- Medications to be used cautiously in older adults include:
  - Tertiary tricyclic antidepressants
  - First-generation antihistamines
  - Muscle relaxants
  - Benzodiazepines
  - Digoxin >0.125 mg, and so on

STOPP/START Tool

Screening Tool of Older Persons' Potentially Inappropriate Prescriptions (STOPP)

- Medication review to identify risks versus benefits of prescription drugs
- Criteria are organized by system
- Emphasis on drug–drug interaction and duplicate drug class prescriptions

Screening Tool to Alert Doctors to the Right Treatment (START)

- Focus on prescribing omissions and identifying undertreatment in older adults

Psychiatric

Delirium

- Incidence in older people: 14 to 56 percent of hospitalized older adults
- Present in 10 to 22 percent of older adults at the time of hospital admission
- 10 to 30 percent develop after admission to the hospital for other causes
- Postoperative delirium accounts for 5 to 10 percent following general surgery. Orthopedic surgery has the highest risk: up to 42 percent.

There is no specific laboratory test to diagnose delirium. The diagnosis is based on clinical assessment. According to *The Diagnostic and Statistical Manual of Mental Disorders*, 5th edition (DSM-5), diagnostic criteria for delirium include:

- A disturbance in attention (i.e., reduced ability to focus, direct, sustain, or shift attention) and awareness (a reduced orientation to the environment)
- Alteration in cognition (e.g., disorientation, memory deficit, language, and/or perceptual disturbance not founded upon preexisting, established, or evolving dementia)
- Acute in onset. Develops over a short interval of time (hours to days). It changes from the patient's baseline behavior and varies in severity during the day.
- Supporting evidence from patient history, physical examination, or laboratory findings that the disturbance is triggered by a direct physiological consequence of an underlying medical condition, medication use (e.g., initiation of drug therapy or withdrawal; see Beers Criteria for inappropriate drug use in older adults), exposure to a toxin, as well as multiple etiologies.
- The goal of treatment is to determine the underlying cause and reverse or stop symptoms. Avoid physical restraints. Maintain a stable, quiet, and well-lit environment.
- Correct sensory deficits with the use of hearing aids and eyeglasses.

Neurocognitive Disorders

FNPs play a critical role in the treatment, management, and care of patients diagnosed with Alzheimer's disease and other related dementias. No treatment intervention (e.g., pharmacological or nonpharmacological) is available to reverse the process. The goal is to preserve functional and cognitive ability, minimize associated behavioral issues, and impede disease progression. Failure to diagnose and inadequate treatment lead to rapid deterioration for the patient and severely impact the lives of the patient and family.

Replaces dementia in DSM-5. Diagnostic criteria are as follows:

- **Mild**—Cognitive impairment in one or more cognitive domains (moderate decline; e.g., language, judgment, abstract thinking, and executive functioning). Deficits do not impair the ability to live independently.
- **Major**—Presents significant cognitive decline in one or more cognitive domains. Impairs the ability to live independently. Documented by standard neuropsychological testing.

Neurocognitive Disorders include:

- Alzheimer's disease
- Frontotemporal lobar degeneration
- Lewy Body dementia
- Parkinson's disease
- Vascular dementia
- Other neurocognitive disorders (e.g., Huntington's disease, traumatic brain injury, human immunodeficiency virus [HIV])

Classify: Mild, Moderate, or Severe

Document with or without behavioral disturbance.

Neurocognitive Domains

- **Language**—Naming, word finding, expressive language
- **Social cognition**—Recognition of emotions, inappropriate social behavior
- **Perception**—Visual-motor, praxis
- **Learning and memory**—Long-term memory, short-term memory, and recent memory
- **Executive functioning**—Planning and decision-making
- **Complex attention**—Sustained attention, divided attention, selective attention

Treatment Interventions

- Nonpharmacologic: complementary therapies, aromatherapy, creative arts expression (e.g., art therapy, music therapy), behavioral therapy, reality orientation, reminiscence, pet therapy
- Goal of therapy: Patient-centered focus to improve the patient's quality of life
- Pharmacologic: Cholinesterase inhibitors are utilized as first-line therapy in patients diagnosed with mild to moderate dementia.
- In patients diagnosed with moderate to severe dementia, a glutamate antagonist is used.
- Other treatment modalities are in development at this time.

Treatment Options

Cholinesterase Inhibitors

- **Aricept (Donepezil)**—Approved for mild to moderate dementia
  - Side effects—Nausea, vomiting, diarrhea, increase in agitation; resolves after several weeks
  - Note: Gastrointestinal reported complaints may be reduced if taken with food.
- **Razadyne (Galantamine)**—Approved for mild to moderate dementia
  - Side effects—Gastrointestinal complaints (e.g., nausea, vomiting, or diarrhea)
  - Note: Gastrointestinal effects can be reduced by taking with meals and gradual dose titration.
- **Exelon (Rivastigmine)**—Approved for mild to moderate dementia
  - Available in capsule and patch form
  - Side effects—Abdominal pain, weight loss, headaches, nausea, vomiting, diarrhea
  - Note: Gastrointestinal effects are less likely to occur with the use of the patch.

N-methyl-D-aspartate (NMDA) Antagonist

- **Namenda (memantine)**—Approved for moderate to severe dementia
  - Available in short-acting oral tablets, extended-release tablets, and oral suspension
  - Side effects—Dizziness, fatigue, somnolence, back pain, headache, constipation, hypertension

Combination Pill

- **Namzaric (donepezil/memantine)**
  - Available in tablet

- Side effects—Similar to the profile for donepezil and memantine
- Not indicated for first-line therapy
- Goal of therapy: To preserve cognitive and functional ability, maintain patient's and caregiver's quality of life, slow disease progression, and decrease behavioral disturbances.
- Additional pharmacological modalities may be necessary to target specific behaviors and symptoms.

Depression

Depression is a medical condition that impacts the lives of many older adults and can be treated successfully. It is estimated that up to 5 percent of community-dwelling older adults meet the diagnostic criteria for major depression. In comparison, the prevalence of a major depressive episode for older adults residing in long-term care is approximately 12.4 percent. An additional 30 percent of older adults residing in long-term care present with significant depressive symptoms. This is in contrast to a reported 15 percent of community dwellers with symptomatology indicative of significant depression. It is important to note that depression is not a normal process of aging.

Symptoms of Depression

- Depressed mood or change in affect
- Feelings of worthlessness
- Difficulty concentrating or making decisions
- Changes in sleep patterns
- Weight gain or loss
- Talk of hurting oneself
- Lack of energy
- Loss of interest in activities once enjoyed

Risk Factors for Depression

- Unresolved grief
- Loss of independence
- Chronic pain
- Chronic medical issues
- Past episodes of depression
- Cognitive changes
- Medications
- Financial and social stressors
- Progressive sensory losses

Criteria for Diagnosis of Depression in Long-Term Care

- **Major depressive disorder**—The individual must present with at least five out of nine depressive symptoms for at least 2 weeks, along with impaired social function.
  - **Psychotic depression**—A subtype of major depression more commonly found in older adults residing in long-term care
  - Characterized by major depressive symptoms, along with delusions and/or hallucinations
  - Delusions are persecutory and somatic.
- **Minor depression**—Not meeting the preceding criteria for presence of subthreshold symptoms (e.g., poor self-reported health, impaired physical functioning, marital status)
- **Dysthymia**—Low-grade depression symptoms that are chronic >2 years
- **Depression in Alzheimer's disease**—Must present with three symptoms specific to the criteria
  - Irritability is a qualifying symptom.
  - Additional symptomatology includes:
    - Anhedonia (inability to experience pleasure)
    - Poor sleep
    - Poor appetite
    - Social isolation (not a symptom of major depressive disorder)
    - Fatigue
    - Feelings of worthlessness

Workup for Depression in Long-Term Care

- Screening for depression with the Geriatric Depression Scale
- Past medical history, including past trials of antidepressant medications
- Present illness history, including medications and report of suicidal ideation
- Cognitive evaluation—Mini Mental Status Exam or other tools
- Laboratory tests (e.g., basic metabolic profile, thyroid profile, complete blood count, serum B12, and albumin if poor nutritional status is suspected)
- Additional workup may include an electrocardiogram, sleep studies, or an MRI of the brain.
- Treatment modalities include:
  - **Nonpharmacological treatment** (e.g., cognitive behavioral therapy, light therapy)

- Electroconvulsive therapy (ECT) is used only in severe cases when medication therapies have failed or rapid deterioration of the patient is evident.

Pharmacological Treatment

- Selective Serotonin Reuptake Inhibitors [SSRI]
  - Lexapro (escitalopram)
  - Celexa (citalopram)
- Serotonin norepinephrine reuptake inhibitors [SNRI]:
  - Effexor (venlafaxine)
  - Cymbalta (duloxetine)
  - Tricyclic antidepressants
  - Dopamine norepinephrine reuptake inhibitor (buproprion)
  - Serotonin modulator (trazadone)
  - Norepinephrine serotonin modulator (mirtazapine)
  - Psychostimulants
- Treatment strategies and pharmacological treatment choices based on provider selection and targeting symptoms
- Start low, go slow

Adverse Effects Associated with Pharmacological Treatment—*Class-Dependent*

- SSRIs
  - Decreased appetite
  - May cause hyponatremia in older adults
  - Agitation
  - Insomnia
  - Initial weight loss
  - Somnolence
- Tricyclic antidepressants
  - Constipation
  - Urinary retention
  - Dry mouth
  - Orthostatic hypotension
  - Delirium
  - Change in cognition
  - Blurred vision
  - Dry mouth
  - Arrhythmia
- Buproprion
  - Hypertension
  - Dry mouth
  - Seizures (do not stop abruptly)
- SNRIs
  - Dry mouth
  - Increased risk of hypertension at higher doses (> 150 mg to 225mg/day), including adverse events similar to SSRIs
- Serotonin modulator (trazodone)
  - Priapism (rare but reported)
  - Sedation
  - Postural hypotension at increased doses
- Psychostimulants
  - Anorexia
  - Insomnia
  - Elevated blood pressure
  - Arrhythmias
  - Anxiety
  - Weight loss

Clinical Pearls

It may be necessary for the healthcare provider to adjust doses of other medications due to the potential for interactions and possible adverse effects of antidepressant medications to achieve therapeutic success.

Chronic Disease and Older Adults

Older adults account for the fastest-growing population in this country. These numbers will continue to rise over the next several decades. Older adults are more vulnerable to chronic disease than other populations.

The consequences of living with and/or caring for an older adult with a chronic illness impacts not only health care services and expenditures, it places undue burdens on the patient and their family support system, which manifests in myriad somatic, physical, and psychological complaints, in addition to an enhanced likelihood of social isolation as a result.

Stats at a Glance

- More than 50 percent of older adults live with one chronic condition.
- It is estimated that 11 million older adults live with five or more chronic conditions.
- Older adults with a diagnosis of hypertension are projected to be at greater than 40 percent.
- Dyslipidemia accounts for 1 out of 4 older adults.

- Mental illness of varying degrees impacts almost 20 percent of older adults.
- Diabetes is a growing concern in older adults, with approximately 29.2 percent of people over 65 living with diabetes (approximately 1 of 3 adults 65 and older).
- Other chronic illnesses include osteoarthritis, osteoporosis, hypothyroidism, and so on.

Hypertension

- Current American College of Cardiology (ACC) and American Heart Association (AHA) guidelines recommend treating older adults with blood pressure (BP) readings of 130/80 or higher with medications.
- Pharmacological treatment should be initiated if the BP goal has not been achieved using nonpharmacological interventions (e.g., diet, exercise, meditation).
- First-line treatment modalities for older adults include:
  - Thiazide diuretics
  - Calcium channel blockers
  - ACE or ARBs
- Caution when initiating therapy due to the increased risk of orthostatic BP.
- Close follow-up until the target BP is achieved.
- Renal artery stenosis should be considered if a new onset of diastolic hypertension occurs in a previously well-controlled patient, despite pharmacological treatment with three or more antihypertensive agents at maximum doses.
- Treatment goals should be individualized for each patient and the family nurse. The practitioner should consider underlying comorbidities.

Diabetes

The criteria for diagnosis are discussed in Chapter 12, The Endocrine System.

Goals of treatment developed by the American Diabetes Association and American Geriatrics Society:

- **Healthy** older adults should have an HgbA1c goal of 7.0 to 7.5.
  - Consider the BP target of <130/80 and statin therapy.
- **Complex** older adults should achieve an $HgbA_{1c}$ goal of 7.5 to 8.0.
  - Fasting or postprandial goals: 90–150
  - Bedtime goal of 90–150
  - Use of statins and target BP goal as discussed.
  - Complex patients may have multiple comorbidities, a diagnosis of mild-to-moderate cognitive impairment or a deficit in 2+ Instrumental activities of daily living.
- Older adults who are very complex or in poor health should achieve an $HgbA_{1c}$ of 8.5 to 9.0.
- Careful consideration must be given when choosing treatment. Sulfonylureas, although inexpensive, can increase mortality, putting the patient at high risk for severe hypoglycemia.

Osteoarthritis

Osteoarthritis (OA) can include:

- Inflammatory—Morning stiffness of more than 30 minutes and complaints of night pain
- Findings from diagnostic X-rays may reveal a joint effusion.
- Noninflammatory—General findings include crepitus, joint tenderness, and bony prominence. Complaints of pain and disability.

Physical examination includes:

- Gait—Difficulties in maintaining balance or other gait abnormalities should be further evaluated.
- Range of motion—Should be performed effortlessly
- Evaluation of joint pain
- Osteoarthritis of the knee may present with crepitus, knee locking, and unsteadiness of gait.
- Patients with suspected OA of the hip may present with a limp to avoid pain on the affected side. This is known as an antalgic gait.
- Diagnosis can be made with or without X-rays. Findings include subchondral cyst formation, osteophytosis, and joint space narrowing.

Treatment Modalities Include Pharmacologic and Nonpharmacologic Therapies

- Nonpharmacologic therapies—Aqua therapy and walking
- Pharmacology treatment modalities—Acetaminophen is the drug of choice. Risk of toxicity.
- Limit acetaminophen to <3,000 mg/day. Educate patients about the risks of toxicity and that acetaminophen is found in many OTC products.
- Use COX 2 inhibitors (e.g., Celebrex [celecoxib]). Contraindicated for some.
- Lidocaine patches
- Capsaicin cream
- Diclofenac (e.g., gel, patch, or tablet)
- Corticosteroid injections

Osteoporosis

- A progressive, chronic disease characterized by bone fragility and a microarchitecture (National Osteoporosis Foundation, 2014).
- Black adults have a lower risk of developing the ailment. Those diagnosed have a similar risk of fractures compared to other groups.
- The risk of developing osteoporosis in White women over a lifetime is 1 in 3; in White men, it is 1 in 5.
- USPSTF recommends screening for all women >65+
- USPSTF reports insufficient evidence to screen all men >70
- Workups for newly diagnosed older adults with osteoporosis should include:
  - Thyroid-stimulating hormone
  - Vitamin D 25-hydroxyl
  - Creatinine
  - Evaluation for secondary osteoporosis (e.g., epilepsy, Parkinson's disease, COPD, celiac)

FRAX WHO Fracture Risk Assessment Tool

Treatment interventions should include:

- Smoking cessation
- Fall risk assessment
- Exercise
- Moderation of alcohol intake
- Consideration of OTC pharmacological interventions
- Initiation of bisphosphonate therapy (Careful consideration should be given to previous jaw osteonecrosis or atypical hip fracture.)
- Other treatment modalities—Hormone replacement therapy; use of denosumab or teriparatide
- The continuation of bisphosphonate therapy after 5 years should be weighed considering benefits versus risks.

Falls

It is estimated that one-third of community-dwelling older adults and nearly 60 percent of nursing home residents fall each year. Falls account for multiple emergency room visits and hospitalizations, annually resulting in expenditures of nearly $30 billion and possibly resulting in brain injuries, hip fractures, physical decline, social isolation, and death. Falls are not a normal expectation of aging.

Risk Factors

- History of previous falls
- Parkinson's disease
- Gait deficit
- Vertigo
- Balance deficit
- Depression
- Medication use (e.g., benzodiazepines, antipsychotics, antiarrhythmics, antihypertensives, diuretics, muscular skeletal relaxants, SSRIs, monoamine oxidase inhibitors [MAOIs], tricyclic antidepressants [TCAs])
- Cognitive impairment
- Pain
- Visual or sensory deficits, and so on.

USPSTF recommends assessing the risk of falling annually and at episodic visits. Three factors should be considered:

- Poor performance on the timed "Get Up and Go" test (How long it takes to stand up from a chair, walk 10 feet, turn around, walk back, and sit down. Healthy older adults should be able to complete this test in 10 seconds or less.
- History of mobility issues
- Prior history of falls

A multidisciplinary approach should be utilized. Home safety should be evaluated.

Atypical Presentation of Disease in Older Adults

Atypical presentation of acute illness in older adults is complicated by underlying comorbidities, along with the physical changes of aging. The FNP must recognize the more common atypical presentations seen in this population. Subtle changes from an individual's baseline (physical or cognitive) may be the first sign of illness. These may include increased confusion, decreased appetite, weakness, and so on. Older adults greater than 85+ and on multiple medications and with multiple comorbidities are at increased risk, as well as other older adults who have underlying physical and cognitive impairments.

The FNP must incorporate strategies to assess for atypical presentation of illness in older adults. The ability to differentiate between true pathology and age-related changes is key.

Urinary Tract Infections

- Use of McGeer criteria for infection surveillance
- Worsening or new onset of incontinence

- Increased urgency or frequency
- Falls
- Increased confusion

Acute Abdomen
- Vague respiratory symptoms
- Mild discomfort
- Complaint of diarrhea or constipation

Pneumonia
- No fever
- General malaise or weakness
- Nausea or vomiting
- Minimal cough
- Symptom of a new cardiac arrhythmia
- No leukocytosis on CBC

Other Atypical Presentations
- Myocardial infarction
- Malignancy
- Diabetes
- Hypothyroidism

End-of-Life Care/Advance Care Planning

FNPs have long established the capacity to provide patients with quality, safe, and cost-effective health care in multiple healthcare environments. Advance care planning is essential to primary, acute, and long-term care institutions. Advance care planning encourages patients, families, and loved ones to reflect on their values and beliefs when considering end-of-life care. It is a process that requires the FNP to have an open and honest discussion with the patient and family regarding end-of-life preferences should the time come when the patient cannot speak for themselves or can no longer make medical decisions. It is not simply about completing an advance directive; it is a very sensitive matter that has the potential to impact the patient and family on multiple levels. Advance care planning needs to begin in the primary care setting and, at minimum, be discussed annually or any time there is a change in the patient's condition.

Review Questions

1. An 89-year-old man has recently relocated from the West Coast to be closer to his daughter. He wants to establish a new primary care physician (PCP). His daughter, who was not present for the exam, calls at the end of the day to discuss his visit. She is concerned that her father did not provide her with all the details. What should be the next step?
   A. Provide her with a summary of the visit.
   B. Ask her to come into your office to discuss it.
   C. Tell her that the information can only be discussed with the patient.
   D. Request a copy of his advanced directives.

2. All the following are covered under Medicare Part A EXCEPT:
   A. inpatient hospital care.
   B. hospice services.
   C. durable medical equipment.
   D. short-term rehab.

3. Delirium in older people is associated with functional decline, increased use of chemical and physical restraints, prolonged delirium posthospitalization, and increased mortality. Predisposing risk factors for delirium include older age, multiple comorbidities, a recent severe illness, past ETOH abuse, hearing or vision impairments, and a history of delirium. Which of the following is the best tool to assess a patient for delirium?
   A. Geriatric Depression Scale
   B. MMSE (Mini-Mental State Exam)
   C. CAGE Test
   D. CAM (Confusion Assessment Method)

4. An 85-year-old female patient lives independently in her own house. Her spouse died about 3 years ago. Her two daughters live approximately 30 minutes from her. Although she talks to them daily, she has not seen them in over 2 weeks. On her most recent visit to the office, she reports that she continues to experience considerable pain from her left hip and has been more disabled by this for the past 6 months. She states that she is on a waiting list for a hip replacement. She states, "I feel miserable and no longer enjoy reading or

gardening. I have no energy and everything is an effort." What is the most appropriate response or intervention for this patient?
A. Tell her that the symptoms she is experiencing are likely due to old age.
B. Check a urinalysis (UA) and if positive, C (culture) and S (sensitivity).
C. Perform a Geriatric Depression Scale.
D. Recommend that she move to an assisted living facility because there will be staff who can assist her as needed and other persons her age to increase her socialization.

5. A 76-year-old male had a total knee replacement with a planned discharge for the following morning. Before his discharge, the nurse reports increased confusion overnight. He has been trying to climb out of bed, is agitated and calling out for his family. He is not responding to attempts at re-orientation. His labs are within normal limits (WNL), and his vital signs are stable. The most likely cause is:
A. he is agitated that he can't go home as promised.
B. he likely developed an infection postsurgery.
C. he has developed depression, which he should be screened for.
D. he has developed hospital-acquired delirium.

6. Which of the following statements is the most accurate description of Alzheimer's disease (AD)?
A. The disease is reversible with pharmacological treatment modalities, including Aricept (donepezil) and Namenda.
B. The disease is progressive.
C. The disease is characterized by remissions and exacerbations.
D. Over 50 percent of older adults will develop AD at some time.

7. The *only* acetyl cholinesterase inhibitor (ACHI) approved to treat moderate to severe dementia is:
A. Exelon (rivastigmine).
B. Aricept (donepezil).
C. Namenda (memantine).
D. Razadyne (galantamine).

8. The FNP is preparing to do a round on hospital patients in the morning before going to the office. Which of these hospitalized patients should be checked first?
A. A 67-year-old male who had a right below the knee amputation (BKA) yesterday, following a motor vehicle accident who is complaining of phantom pain
B. A 76-year-old female, who is less than 24 hours post surgery, complaining of back pain with a new onset of urinary incontinence
C. An 80-year-old male who received two units of packed red blood cells (PRBCs) the previous day for a suspected upper gastrointestinal (GI) bleed
D. A 90-year-old nursing home patient who is scheduled for an endoscopy later in the day, who demands that she have her breakfast

9. The FNP has just seen an older patient in the practice with suspected osteoarthritis (OA) of the hip. What is the most distinguishing characteristic of the physical examination?
A. Gait abnormality
B. Pain with external or internal rotation
C. Joint instability
D. Crepitus

10. Recommended immunizations for adults 65+ include:
A. an annual influenza vaccine, TDAP vaccine every 5 years, shingles vaccination, pneumococcal vaccines 13 and 23.
B. TDAP vaccine every 10 years, annual influenza vaccine, shingles vaccine after age 60, pneumococcal vaccines 13 and 23.
C. an annual influenza vaccine, annual pneumococcal vaccines, TDAP every 10 years, and the shingles vaccine after age 60.
D. the shingles vaccine—2 doses given 6 months apart, TDAP every 10 years, annual influenza vaccine, and pneumococcal vaccines 13 and 23.

11. A patient with several comorbidities who is taking multiple prescription medications to manage his chronic diseases presents to the office. He is concerned about the rising cost of his medications and will soon enroll in Medicare. Which Medicare Plan would help cover his prescription drugs?
A. Medicare A
B. Medicare B
C. Medicare C
D. Medicare D

12. Therapeutic communication with older adults includes:
A. talking to family members who are present to elicit a comprehensive health history.
B. speaking slowly in a deep tone and addressing your questions to the patient.
C. standing close to ensure they will hear you.
D. addressing the patient by their first name to create a "friendly atmosphere."

13. When prescribing for an older adult, all should be considered EXCEPT:
    A. Beers criteria.
    B. pharmacodynamics.
    C. McGeer criteria.
    D. pharmacokinetics.

14. According to the American Geriatrics Society, the hemoglobin A_{1C} ($HgbA_{1C}$) goal for an older adult with three multiple comorbidities or mild to moderate cognitive impairment should be:
    A. individualized for each patient.
    B. HgbA1C < 6.0.
    C. HgbA1C between 6.5 and 7.0.
    D. HgbA1C between 7.5 and 8.0.

15. Which class of drug should be used cautiously in older adults with diabetes, due to the increased risk of hypoglycemia?
    A. Biguanides
    B. Sulfonylureas
    C. Dipeptidyl peptidase inhibitor (DPP-IV inhibitor)
    D. Sodium glucose cotransporter 2 inhibitor (SGLT-2 inhibitor)

16. The United States Preventive Services Task Force (USPSTF) recommends primary, secondary, and tertiary preventive services. Which of the following is not considered a primary preventive service?
    A. Smoking cessation
    B. Mammogram
    C. Immunizations
    D. Physical activity

17. Which of the following is the most common form of anemia diagnosed in older adults?
    A. Iron (Fe) deficiency anemia
    B. Cooley's anemia
    C. Anemia of chronic kidney disease
    D. Vitamin B12 deficiency

18. Which of the following statements is true regarding suicide rates?
    A. Nonmarried women are more at risk.
    B. White men 85 and older are more at risk.
    C. Hispanic men of any age are more at risk.
    D. Black widowers are more at risk.

19. The FNP is seeing a 65-year-old male for the "Welcome to Medicare" exam. As Medicare guidelines require, the FNP begins the discussion regarding end-of-life planning. The patient states, "I plan on being around for a while. Look at me. I am as fit as a teenager." Which of the following responses is best?
    A. "End-of-life care planning is mandatory in all 50 states once you go on Medicare."
    B. "You are right, you are a healthy man. We can discuss this at a later time."
    C. "We need to do this today and put it in writing."
    D. "End-of-life care planning ensures that your preferences for end-of-life care are specified if you cannot make medical decisions or speak for yourself."

20. The FNP is seeing an older female patient accompanied by her son. Over the past 2 weeks, the patient had two visits to the ER after falling and using her Life Alert to call for help. The FNP reviews her ER discharge summary, including consults, labs, and other diagnostics. What should the FNP do next?
    A. Instruct the patient to keep a "fall diary."
    B. Order durable medical equipment (e.g., bedside commode, walker).
    C. Perform the "Get Up and Go" test.
    D. Refer her to Social Services to assess if she can care for herself.

21. The underlying characteristics of Alzheimer's disease include:
    A. atrophy of the brain.
    B. atherosclerotic changes in the cerebral and carotid arteries.
    C. amyloid plaques and neurofibrillary tangles.
    D. multi-microvascular infarcts of the cerebellum.

22. Contributing factors associated with an increased risk of falls in older adults include all of the following EXCEPT:
    A. osteoporosis.
    B. auditory changes.
    C. urinary incontinence.
    D. cardiovascular disease.

23. Osteoporosis is a disease in which decreased bone mass increases the risk of bone fracture and bone frailty. What is the most common fracture associated with osteoporosis?
    A. Hip fracture
    B. Vertebral fracture
    C. Distal radial fracture (Colles fracture)
    D. All of the above have the same incidence of occurrence.

24. Hearing loss impacts an estimated one-third of older adults between the ages of 61 and 74 and continues to rise as one ages. Which of the following is presbycusis most associated with?
    A. Cholesteatoma
    B. Ototoxic drugs
    C. Cerumen impaction
    D. Loss of high-frequency sounds

25. Physiological and anatomical changes related to normal aging can present atypically with symptomatology not observed in other populations. Older adults with a UTI may exhibit:
    A. urinary incontinence and dehydration.
    B. a change in mental status, falls, and dehydration.
    C. complaints of pain, urinary incontinence, and a change in appetite.
    D. dementia, weight gain, and a change in appetite.

Answers With Enhanced Rationales

1. Answer C is correct. The Health Insurance Portability and Accountability Act (HIPAA) protects healthcare consumers concerning their private health information. A patient with the mental capacity to make their medical decisions is not required to agree to sharing personal/medical information with family members.

   Answer A is incorrect. The patient's daughter is not allowed access to her father's medical record without written permission allowing her access.

   Answer B is incorrect. It is illegal to discuss another patient's private medical information without specific written permission from the patient.

   Answer D is incorrect. An advanced directive allows another person or persons to have control over healthcare decisions if the individual cannot communicate their decisions.

2. Answer C is correct. Durable medical equipment is covered under Medicare Part B.

   Answers A, B, and D are incorrect. Inpatient hospital care, hospice services, and short-term rehabilitation are all covered under Medicare Part A.

3. Answer D is correct. The best way to assess for delirium is the CAM.

   Answer A is incorrect. The Geriatric Depression Scale is a screening tool that helps assess depression in older people.

   Answer B is incorrect. The MMSE is used to assess cognition in older adults.

   Answer C is incorrect. The CAGE questionnaire is used to assess ETOH abuse.

4. Answer C is correct. The Geriatric Depression Scale is a valid and reliable assessment tool to screen for depression in the clinical setting. It is available in short and long forms. It does not assess for suicide risk.

   Answer A is incorrect. A patient who states they feel miserable and no longer enjoy activities that they had previously enjoyed is demonstrating symptoms of depression. This is not a normal part of the aging process.

   Answer B is incorrect. UTIs manifest differently in older patients. However, this patient is not experiencing any symptoms consistent with UTIs in older people, such as confusion, falls, incontinence, or decreased appetite.

   Answer D is incorrect. The patient is currently living alone and does not need assistance with ADLs, nor is she expressing feelings of loneliness.

5. Answer D is correct. Hospital-acquired delirium is the most likely cause. Older patients who are hospitalized are at increased risk of delirium. Precipitating factors include medications, psychological stressors, sensory overload, nutritional deficiencies, and so on.

   Answer A is incorrect. The patient's symptoms are more serious than simple frustration of not being discharged home.

   Answer B is incorrect. There is no evidence that the patient has developed an infection. His labs are WNL, and his vital signs are stable.

   Answer C is incorrect. Depression in older people does not manifest as agitation or inability to be reoriented.

6. Answer B is correct. AD is progressive. There is no cure available. It is a severe and progressive cognitive impairment, and decline is eventually fatal.

Answer A is incorrect. AD is not reversible, and pharmacological interventions may only slow the disease's progress.

Answer C is incorrect. Alzheimer's disease is progressive. It does not have remissions or exacerbations.

Answer D is incorrect. The risk of developing AD is 1 in 13 for people aged 65 to 84 and 1 in 3 for people aged 85 and older.

7. Answer B is correct. The only acetyl cholinesterase inhibitor approved to treat moderate to severe dementia is Aricept (donepezil).

    Answer A is incorrect. Rivastigmine (Exelon) is a medication that treats mild to moderate dementia caused by AD.

    Answer C is incorrect. Memantine (Namenda) is used to treat moderate to severe dementia related to AD. However, it belongs to a class of drugs called NMDA receptor antagonists.

    Answer D is incorrect. Galantamine is used to treat mild to moderate dementia.

8. Answer B is correct. The patient that should be evaluated first is the 76-year-old female who is less than 24 hours post op, complaining of back pain with a new onset of urinary incontinence. This is a red flag and should be further evaluated.

    Answer A is incorrect. It is common for a patient to experience phantom pain after an amputation of a limb.

    Answer C is incorrect. The patient received two units of PRBCs the day before. A transfusion reaction will occur immediately during the transfusion.

    Answer D is incorrect. The 90-year-old patient who is NPO and demanding breakfast does not have an urgent need for a visit and only requires further education regarding the reason for the NPO status.

9. Answer A is correct. The most distinguishing characteristic of the physical examination for suspected hip OA is gait abnormality. Patients with hip OA routinely present with an antalgic gait to avoid pain in the affected hip.

    Answer B is incorrect. The patient may exhibit pain with internal or external manipulation, but the most telling characteristic is the gait abnormality.

    Answer C is incorrect. Joint instability occurs when the tissues, such as muscles, ligaments, and tendons, weaken. They can no longer hold the joint in the correct position, potentially leading to dislocation.

    Answer D is incorrect. Crepitus is the crackling sound made when two fragments of bones rub together when moving a joint. It may be a symptom of joint damage, injury, inflammation, or infection. Since crepitus has many causes (including OA), it is not a distinguishing characteristic.

10. Answer D is correct. Recommended immunizations for adults 65+ include TDAP every 10 years, an annual influenza vaccine, the Shingrix vaccine (two doses given 4 to 6 months apart) after age 50, and pneumococcal vaccines 13 and 23.

    Answer A is incorrect. The TDAP vaccine is recommended every 10 years unless the patient has not had the TDAP for more than 5 years and has recently been exposed to a puncture wound.

    Answer B is incorrect. The CDC recommends the Shingrix vaccine (two doses given 4 to 6 months apart) for those aged 50 and older, even if the patient already had shingles.

    Answer C is incorrect. Annual pneumococcal vaccines are not appropriate. Shingles vaccines are recommended for any adult over the age of 50.

11. Answer D is correct. Medicare Part D is the Medicare prescription drug benefit and helps offset the costs associated with outpatient drug coverage.

    Answer A is incorrect. Medicare Part A covers hospitalization, skilled nursing services, and hospice care. Enrolling is free if the beneficiary has worked and paid Social Security taxes for a minimum of 40 calendar quarters. If the beneficiary has not contributed, a monthly premium may be required.

    Answer B is incorrect. Medicare Part B covers outpatient services (e.g., diagnostics, visits to healthcare providers) and durable medical equipment.

    Answer C is incorrect. Medicare Part C allows private insurance companies to provide health benefits (e.g., Medicare Advantage plans).

12. Answer B is correct. The most appropriate response is to speak slowly in a deep tone and address your questions to the patient.

    Answer A is incorrect. Addressing questions to family members about the patient is inappropriate, and it sends a message to the patient that the clinician does not think the patient is competent to answer.

Answer C is incorrect. When interviewing the patient, the FNP should be seated face to face with the patient.

Answer D is incorrect. The clinician should not assume that the patient wants to be called by their first name. It is important to ask how the patient wishes to be addressed.

13. Answer C is correct. McGeer criteria is not a consideration for prescribing. The FNP utilizes McGeer criteria to provide guiding principles that define infections (e.g., UTIs) using specific benchmarks in the long-term care setting.

    Answers A, B, and D are incorrect. Each criteria (Beers, pharmacodynamics, and pharmacokinetics) should be considered when prescribing for the older adult.

14. Answer D is correct. The American Geriatric Society supports the HgbA$_{1c}$ recommendation of the American Diabetes Association for older adults with three or more comorbidities or mild to moderate cognitive impairment.

    Answer A is incorrect. While each patient's decision should involve patient and provider goals, the AGS has recommendations concerning HgbA1c in an older patient with multiple comorbid conditions.

    Answer B is incorrect. An Hgb A1c of < 6.0% is inappropriate for this older patient and would likely lead to severe and dangerous hypoglycemia.

    Answer C is incorrect. A HgbA1c of 6.5 to 7.0% is a goal for a healthy, young adult with no cognitive impairment and little risk for severe hypoglycemia.

15. Answer B is correct. Sulfonylureas should not be used as a first choice for treating diabetes. First-generation sulfonylureas have been shown to increase the risk of hypoglycemia in older adults. Many other treatment options are available that do not increase the risk of severe hypoglycemia and should be selected first.

    Answer A is incorrect. Biguanides (metformin) do not typically cause hypoglycemia. However, they must be used cautiously in older people due to the accumulating effects if there is any renal impairment (risk of lactic acidosis)

    Answer C is incorrect. DPP-IV inhibitors such as sitagliptin (Januvia) or saxagliptin (Onglyza) do not cause hypoglycemia. They must be used cautiously and be dose adjusted for patients with renal impairment.

    Answer D is incorrect. SGLT-2 inhibitors, such as empagliflozin (Jardiance), canagliflozin (Invokana), and dapagliflozin (Farxiga), cause the kidneys to remove glucose from the bloodstream and excrete it in the urine. They do not cause hypoglycemia unless they are used in conjunction with a medication that can cause hypoglycemia, such as a sulfonylurea or insulin.

16. Answer B is correct. A mammogram is a secondary form of prevention. Primary prevention intends to implement measures to avert the onset of disease or illness. Secondary preventive practices include activities aimed at early detection to prevent or slow down the disease process and disability.

    Answer A is incorrect. Smoking cessation classes or treatments are a form of primary prevention.

    Answer C is incorrect. Immunizations are a form of primary prevention.

    Answer D is incorrect. Increasing physical activity is a form of primary prevention that aims to prevent the onset of disease or illness associated with a sedentary lifestyle.

17. Answer C is correct. Anemia of chronic kidney disease is the most common anemia in older adults.

    Answer A is incorrect. Iron deficiency anemia can occur in older adults. It is a microcytic anemia that can result from acute blood loss due to malignancy, gastrointestinal pathology, or malnutrition.

    Answer B is incorrect. Cooley's anemia is the most severe type of beta thalassemia, often requiring blood transfusions.

    Answer D is incorrect. Vitamin B12 deficiency is a macrocytic anemia. It is treatable and usually presents with another underlying medical illness.

18. Answer B is correct. The greatest suicide rate occurs in White males 85+.

    Answers A, C, and D are incorrect. Single women, Hispanic males, or Black widowers are not the highest groups at risk for suicide.

19. Answer D is correct. Advance care planning is an ongoing process that should begin in the primary care setting and be addressed periodically, whether the patient is young and healthy, is managing a chronic disease, or is living with a terminal illness. Advance care planning, or end-of-life care planning, ensures that the patient's preferences for end-of-life care treatment are specified and followed if they can no longer make healthcare

decisions or speak for themselves. Although the signing of an advance directive is encouraged, the role of the FNP should include providing education to ensure a clearer understanding of the process.

Answer A is incorrect. End-of-life care planning is highly recommended, as well as having a written advanced directive. Medicare does not mandate an advance directive.

Answer B is incorrect. End-of-life care planning should be done when the patient can make an educated decision about their treatment preference if they can no longer speak for themselves.

Answer C is incorrect. The patient should be given time to decide and discuss the decision with any significant persons in their life.

20. Answer C is correct. The best response is to perform the "Get Up and Go" test. The purpose of the test is to check mobility. A patient who scores 3 or more is at increased risk for falls.

Answer A is incorrect. Instructing a patient to keep a "fall diary" is inappropriate and would not be a recommended intervention.

Answer B is incorrect. Before ordering durable medical equipment for this patient, a full assessment must be performed to determine if the patient requires ambulatory aids, and so on. A "Get Up and Go" test is part of this assessment.

Answer D is incorrect. At this point in time, it is not appropriate to make a social service referral to determine her level of functioning. This referral may be needed later or if the patient or her son requests it.

21. Answer C is correct. Amyloid plaques and neurofibrillary tangles are the hallmark characteristics of AD.

Answer A is incorrect. The underlying characteristic of AD is not brain atrophy. Cerebral atrophy is a loss of connections between neurons. There are many reasons for brain atrophy, including cerebral palsy, infectious diseases, dementia, and aging.

Answer B is incorrect. Intracranial atherosclerosis is associated with cognitive decline due to impaired blood flow to the brain, but it is not a cause of AD.

Answer D is incorrect. Multi-microvascular infarcts to the cerebellum lead to impaired oxygenation and motor and balance control deficits. It is not a cause of AD.

22. Answer B is correct. Auditory changes do not increase the risk of falls.

Answers A, C, and D are incorrect. The risk for falls increases in older adults due to underlying comorbidities such as osteoporosis and cardiovascular conditions, which may cause syncope. Also, many medications can increase the risk of falls, such as diuretics, antihypertensives, hypnotics, and benzodiazepines, to name just a few classes of medications that contribute to the risk of falls.

23. Answer B is correct. The most common fracture associated with osteoporosis is a vertebral fracture. More than 1.5 million people in the United States are estimated to develop a new vertebral fracture annually. Mild vertebral fractures are associated with loss of height, while more severe vertebral fractures may cause significant pain and loss of mobility.

Answer A is incorrect. Hip fractures are considered fragility fractures, which are associated with osteoporosis. They occur as a result of low-level trauma, such as falling from a standing height. They are about half as common as vertebral fractures, which are known as compression fractures.

Answer C is incorrect. The Colles fracture occurs in people of all ages due to a fall landing on the hand while the wrist is in dorsiflexion. It may commonly occur in older women with osteoporosis. They are about half as common as vertebral fractures.

Answer D is incorrect. As previously identified, vertebral fractures are the most common cause of fractures associated with osteoporosis.

24. Answer D is correct. Presbycusis is a hearing loss in older adults. It is associated with a failure to hear high-frequency sounds.

Answer A is incorrect. Cholesteatoma is an abnormal noncancerous skin growth behind the tympanic membrane. It may cause hearing loss, but it is generally confined to one ear and is not common.

Answer B is incorrect. Ototoxic drugs may cause hearing loss and tinnitus. The most common ototoxic drugs are aminoglycoside antibiotics, macrolide antibiotics, salicylates, chemotherapeutic agents, and loop diuretics. Presbycusis is hearing loss associated with aging.

Answer C is incorrect. Cerumen impaction may occur when cerumen accumulates and causes hearing loss, itching, pain, or tinnitus. Cerumen impaction is not the most common cause of presbycusis.

25. Answer B is correct. Atypical presentations of acute illness in older adults are common, given the physiological changes of aging complicated by underlying comorbidities. Changes in cognition and/or physical function provide the FNP with "clues" of an acute illness. Atypical symptoms associated with a UTI in an older adult can include increased confusion, falls, lethargy, cough, weakness, abdominal pain, anorexia, and dehydration.

Answer A is incorrect. Urinary incontinence and dehydration may occur with a UTI in an older adult. Still, more commonly, the older adult with a UTI exhibits a change in mental status, delirium, dizziness, falls, and weakness.

Answer C is incorrect. The classic symptoms of a UTI, such as burning pain and frequency, may not manifest in the older adult. Instead, the older adult more commonly manifests UTI symptoms with behavioral changes such as confusion.

Answer D is incorrect. Older adults with a UTI may exhibit a change in mental status along with lethargy and a decrease in appetite. They do not experience weight gain, and the confusion is related to the UTI, not dementia. The mental status changes resolve when the UTI resolves.

Resources

Administration on Aging. (2024). *2023 Profile of Older Americans.* U.S. Department of Health and Human Services, Administration for Community Living. Retrieved from https://acl.gov/sites/default/files/profileofoa/acl-profileolderamericans2023/508.pdf

Alagiakrishnan, K., & Ahmed, I. (2014). *Delirium.* https://emedicine.medscape.com/article/288890-overview

American Geriatrics Society Core Writing Group of the Task Force on the Future of Geriatric Medicine. (2005). *Caring for older Americans: The future of geriatric medicine.* https://www.caretransitions.org/documents/Caring%20for%20older%20Americans%20-%20JAGS.pdf

American Geriatric Society. (2014). *Geriatrics at Your Fingertips.* American Geriatric Society.

American Geriatric Society. (2012). *Identifying medications that older adults should avoid or use with caution: The 2012 American geriatrics updated Beers criteria.* https://www.americangeriatrics.org/files/documents/beers/BeersCriteriaPublicTranslation.pdf

Berkow, R., & Beers, M. H. (2000). *Merck manual of geriatrics* (3rd ed.). Merck Research Laboratories.

Boult, C., Counsell, S., Leipzig, R., & Berenson, R. (2010). The urgency of preparing primary care physicians to care for older people with chronic illnesses. *Health Affairs, 29*(5), 811–815. https://pubmed.ncbi.nlm.nih.gov/20439866/

Centers for Disease Control and Prevention. 2025. *Older Adult Falls Data.* CDC. Accessed May 4, 2025. https://www.cdc.gov/falls/data-research/index.html

Centers for Disease Control and Prevention. (2013). *The state of aging and health in America.* Atlanta, GA: Centers for Disease Control and Prevention, U.S. Dept. of Health and Human Services.

Center for Mental Health Services. (2011). *Treatment of depression in older adults evidence-based practices (EBP) KIT.* HHS Publication No. SMA-11-4631. Rockville, MD: Substance Abuse and Mental Health Services Administration. http://store.samhsa.gov/product/Treatment-of-Depression-in-Older-Adults-EvidenceBased-Practices.

Cheslock, M., & DeJesus, O. (2023) Presbycusis. In: *StatPearls* (Internet). StatPearls Publishing. https://www.ncbi.nlm.nih.gov/books/NBK559220/

Donnally III, C. J., DiPompeo, C. M., & Varacallo, M. A. (2023, August 4). Vertebral compression fractures. In: *StatPearls* [Internet]. StatPearls Publishing. PMID: 28846351.

ElSayed, N. A., Aleppo, G., Aroda, V. R., Bannuru, R. R., Brown, F. M., Bruemmer, D., Collins, B. S., Cusi, K., Das, S. R., Gibbons, C. H., Giurini, J. M., Hilliard, M. E., Isaacs, D., Johnson, E. L., Kahan, S., Khunti, K., Kosiborod, M., Leon, J., Lyons, S. K., Murdock, L., ... on behalf of the American Diabetes Association (2023). Introduction and Methodology: Standards of Care in Diabetes-2023. *Diabetes Care, 46*(Suppl 1), S1–S4. https://doi.org/10.2337/dc23-Sint

Gill, J., & Moore, M. J. (2013). *The state of aging & health in America 2013.* https://stacks.cdc.gov/view/cdc/19146

Golan, D. E., Tashjiaaaaan, A. H., Armstrong, E. J. & Armstrong, A. (2012). *Principles of pharmacology: The pathophysiologic basis of drug therapy* (3rd ed.). Wolters Kluwer/Lippincott Williams & Wilkins.

Halloran, L. (2013). Prescribing for the elderly. *Medscape Medical Students.* https://www.medscape.com/viewarticle/779494

James, P., Oparil, S., Carter, B., Cushman, W., Dennison-Himmelfarb, C., Handler, J., ... & Ortiz, E. (2014). 2014 evidence-based guideline for the management of high blood pressure in adults: Report from the panel members appointed to the eighth joint national committee (JNC 8). *JAMA, 311*(5), 507–520. https://jama.jamanetwork.com/article.aspx?articleid=1791497

Jeremiah, M., Unwin, B., Greenawald, M., & Casiano, V. (2015). Diagnosis and management of osteoporosis. *American Family Physician,92*(4), 261–268.

Katz, S., Downs, T. D., Cash, H. R., & Grotz R. C. (1970) Progress in development of the index of ADL. *The Gerontologist, 10*(1), 20–30. https//doi.org/10.1093/geront/10.1 part 1.20

Kennedy–Malone, L., Fletcher, K., & Plank, L. (2014). *Advanced practice nursing care in the older adults.* F. A. Davis Company.

Koton, S., Shneider, A., Windham, G., Mosley, T., Gottesman, R., & Coresh, J. (2020). *Microvascular brain disease progression and risk of stroke.* https://doi.org/10.1161/StrokeAHA.120.030063

Lawton, M. P., & Brody, E. M. (1969, Autumn). Assessment of older people: self-maintaining and instrumental activities of daily living. *Gerontologist, 9*(3), 179–86. PMID: 5349366

Na, C. R., Wang, S., Kirsner, R. S., & Federman, D. G. (2012). Elderly adults and skin disorders: Common problems for non-dermatologists. *Southern Medical Journal, 105*(11), 600–606. https://www.medscape.com/viewarticle/774527_2

Namzaric. (2015). *Drug monograph.* https://www.empr.com/search/NAMZARIC/

National Center for Health Statistics. (2020, December 14). *Healthy People 2020*. Centers for Disease Control and Prevention. https://www.cdc.gov/nchs/healthy_people/hp20

National Council on Aging. (2015). *Falls prevention*. https://www.ncoa.org/resources/falls-prevention-fact-sheet/

National Institute on Aging. (2012, August 16). *Federal report details health, economic status of older Americans*. National Institutes of Health. https://www.nih.gov/news-events/news-releases/federal-report-details-health-economic-status-older-americans-0

National Osteoporosis Foundation. (2014). *Clinician's guide to prevention and treatment of osteoporosis*. National Osteoporosis Foundation.

Nelson, J., & Good, E. (2015). Urinary tract infections and asymptomatic bacteriuria in older adults. *The Nurse Practitioner, 40*(8), 43–50.

Nestle's Nutrition Institute. (n.d.). *MNA-Mini Nutritional Assessment*. https://www.mna-elderly.com/

Rhoads, J., & Petersen, S. W. (2014). *Advanced health assessment and diagnostic reasoning* (2nd ed.). Jones and Bartlett.

Rounds, L., Rappaport, B. A., & Mallary. L. L. (2013). Polypharmacy in senior adults. *Journal for Nurse Practitioners, 17*, 7–14.

Sadowsky, C., & Galvin, J. (2012). Guidelines for the management of cognitive and behavioral problems in dementia. *Journal of the American Board of Family Medicine, 25*(3), 350–366.

Taylor, W. (2014, September 25). Depression in the elderly. *New England Journal of Medicine, 371*, 1228–1236. https://www.nejm.org/doi/full/10.1056/NEJMcp1402180

USAging. 2025. "Home and Community-Based Services." *USAging*. Accessed May 4, 2025. https://usaging.org/hcbs.

U.S. Census Bureau. (2023, June 22). *America is getting older*. [Press release]. https://www.census.gov/newsroom/press-releases/2023/population-estimates-characteristics.html

U.S. Preventive Services Task Force. (2024). *Interventions to prevent falls in community-dwelling older adults: Recommendation statement*. JAMA. https://doi.org/10.1001/jama.2024.8481

Wolff, K., Johnson, R. A., & Saavedra, A. (2013). *Fitzpatrick's color atlas and synopsis of clinical dermatology* (7th ed.). McGraw-Hill.

Ward, K. T., & Ruben, D. B. (2013). *Comprehensive geriatric assessment*. UpToDate. https://www.uptodate.com/contents/comprehensive-geriatric-assessment

Zagaria, M. A. E. (2012). Potentially inappropriate medications for seniors: Focus on the 2012 Beers criteria. *American Journal for Nurse Practitioners, 16*, 26–28.

Zibel, S. (2011). *Advance care planning in primary care: An interventional approach to enhance patient understanding of treatment preferences at the end-of-life*. (Unpublished doctoral capstone). Chatham University.

CHAPTER 21

Mental Health in Primary Care

Melissa Scollan-Koliopoulos, EdD, DNP, FNP, PMHNP, CDCES

Primary care providers have an important role in identifying and managing mental health disorders, including:

- screening for and eliciting mental health and substance use concerns,
- facilitating referral to psychiatric care,
- initiating treatment pending transition to psychiatric care, and
- managing patients who are stable on medication with a confirmed diagnosis.

Mood Disorders

Etiology

Mood disorders are a group of diagnoses characterized by either prolonged periods of sadness, periods of excessive energy, or both. Some are chronic and lifelong disorders, such as bipolar disorder, while others, like major depressive disorder, may be a single episode, recurrent, or chronic. The mood disorders include unipolar major depressive disorder and bipolar disorder. Postpartum depression (PPD) and premenstrual dysphoria have a hormonal basis for their emergence. Premenstrual dysphoria is considered an excessive mood variation included under mood disorders and is a manifestation of premenstrual syndrome that occurs during two consecutive menstrual cycles (APA, 2013). Seasonal affective disorder is also a potential diagnosis, and if superimposed with preexisting depression, may be referred to as "double depression."

Major Depressive Disorder and Persistent Depressive Disorder Facts

- Death due to suicide occurs at a rate of approximately 14.5 per 100,000 population.
- The prevalence of adults with major depressive disorder is highest for 18 to 25-year-olds (NIMH, n.d.a).
- Around 60 percent of adults experiencing depression will not seek treatment.
- Symptoms of depression often present as unexplained physical problems such as fatigue, pain, or vague symptoms that result in frequent medical visits.
- Racial disparities in diagnosed depression: African Americans, Hispanics, and Asian Americans were less likely to receive depression diagnosis than non-Hispanic Whites.

Diagnosis of Depression

- Single episode is the first and only episode.
- Recurrent means at least two episodes.
- Bipolar disorder means depressive episodes alternating with manic symptoms.

Clinical Presentation/ Assessment Findings

- Poor concentration
- Feelings of excessive guilt or low self-worth

- Hopeless about the future
- Thoughts about dying or suicide
- Disrupted sleep
- Changes in appetite or weight
- Feeling very tired or low in energy

History of Present Illness

- For major depressive disorder, *symptoms must be present nearly every day* for at least 2 weeks.
- For persistent depressive disorder, symptoms are continuous for at least 2 years.
- Clinical judgment is needed to distinguish depression from a normal response to loss.
- Patients will likely report diminished interest or pleasure in activities they previously enjoyed, insomnia, changes in appetite or weight, fatigue and/or loss of energy, agitation, feelings of guilt and worthlessness, decreased ability to think or concentrate, and possibly thoughts of death or suicide.
- Patients may report socially withdrawing and may describe feeling indifferent to the world.
- In certain populations, depressive symptoms may vary.
  - In children and teenagers, depression may manifest as increased clinginess, increased physical complaints, poor attendance or school refusal, and avoidance of social interactions or loss of friendships.
  - In older adults, depression may manifest as problems with memory, personality changes, or social isolation.
  - The experience of depression across different cultures and ethnicities may lead to differing presentations as well, commonly presenting as increased physical health complaints.

Physical Assessment Findings

- A physical examination should include inspection of the patient's general appearance. Is the patient disheveled or tired looking? Is their affect flat?
- Assessments should include palpation of the thyroid gland, vital signs and auscultation of heart sounds. Additionally, the practitioner should observe for signs of self-harm such as scars, cut marks, or burns, and of hygiene deficits, such as body odor or soiled clothes.
- The mental status examination may depict the following: flat affect, impaired concentration, slow or monotone speech, a paucity of speech delayed reaction time, psychomotor retardation, minimal eye contact, downcast gaze.
- The patient may appear tearful or visibly despondent. They may fidget and/or show signs of restlessness or agitation.
- Emotional range may be blunted, constricted, or guarded.
- Thought process may include negative views, perseverations, thought blocking, or dearth of thought.
- If psychosis is present, the patient may have delusions, hallucinations, and other perceptual disturbances, such as incongruent mood and thoughts.
- Cognitive impairments, including impaired memory, learning, executive function, concentration, processing speed, or forgetfulness, may also be present.

Screening Recommendations

Several screening tools are available to help identify and manage depression. One of the most used in the primary care setting is the Patient Health Questionnaire 9 (PHQ-9).

- Screening with the PHQ-2 version can occur every 2 weeks.
- Routine screening is most beneficial in systems with resources to manage the condition once identified (O'Connor et al., 2023).

Differential Diagnosis

- Major depressive disorder
- Dysthymia
- Somatization or somatoform disorder
- Premenstrual dysphoria
- Attention-deficit/hyperactivity disorder
- Anxiety
- Hypothyroidism
- Anemia
- Chronic fatigue syndrome
- Fibromyalgia
- Diabetes
- Hypoglycemia

Clinical Management Laboratory and Diagnostic Studies

Labs would be used to differentiate other causes of symptoms:

- Rapid plasma reagin (RPR)
- Thyroid stimulating hormone (TSH)
- Triiodothyronine (T3)

- Adrenocorticotropic hormone (ACTH) and cortisol
- Complete blood count with differential (CBC-dif)
- Vitamin D 25-hydroxy
- Vitamin B-12
- Ferritin
- HIV test
- Calcium, phosphate, and magnesium levels
- BUN and Creatinine
- AST/ALT
- Blood and urine toxicology screens

Pharmacologic

- Serotonin reuptake inhibitors (SSRIs), such as citalopram, escitalopram, fluoxetine, and sertraline
- Selective norepinephrine reuptake inhibitors (SNRIs), such as venlafaxine and duloxetine.
- Norepinephrine dopamine reuptake inhibitor, such as bupropion.
- Atypical antidepressants, such as mirtazapine, nefazadone, and trazodone.
- Common side effects include headache, agitation, insomnia, and sexual side effects (bupropion excluded, which may even be used as an augmenting agent that can reduce sexual side effects).
- Antidepressants are selected with consideration for efficacy, tolerability, and target symptoms of the depressive episode's presentation.
- Antidepressants are usually selected based on the need to be "activating" or "calming." Other heuristics may include whether a family member tolerated one well because pharmacokinetics is inherited.
- Some providers may use pharmacogenetic testing before choosing, although this is not evidence based or economical.
- Screening tools are useful for determining dosage effectiveness. A common screening tool is the PHQ-9 or PHQ-2, which takes very little time and is easily administered during routine office visits (**Figure 21-1**).
- Tricyclic antidepressants, including nortriptyline and amitriptyline, should be monitored closely in patients with heart problems, risk of drug–drug interactions, or high risk of suicide.
- Monoamine oxidase inhibitors (MAOIs), such as imipramine, phenelzine, and selegiline, are typically restricted to patients who do not respond to other options. This is because of the MAOIs' many side effects and the risk of dangerously elevated blood pressure in patients when taken with certain foods or medications. Consider prescribing these medications in consultation with a psychiatric provider.
- Patients taking MAOIs should avoid foods containing tyramine, including:
  - aged cheese,
  - wine,
  - beer with yeast,
  - pickled and fermented products,
  - soy,
  - avocado,
  - dried fruits, and
  - organ meats.

Nonpharmacologic

- Treatment plans made in coordination with the patient must consider:
  - symptom severity,
  - level of functioning,
  - psychosocial stressors,
  - degree of support,
  - patient motivation, and
  - patient preferences.
- Psychotherapy, such as cognitive behavioral therapy (CBT), interpersonal therapy (IPT), and problem-solving treatment (PST), is the treatment of choice for mild to moderate depressive symptoms. In contrast, pharmacologic intervention and psychotherapy combined are first-line treatments for severe symptoms.
- Other strategies include mindfulness, behavioral activation, healthy sleep habits, stress management, and increased physical activity.

Patient Education

- Psychoeducation should include the benefits of psychotherapy, physical activity, and psychopharmacology.
- During prognosis, explain that depression can go into remission, which is the goal of treatment.
- Address concerns regarding stigma, medication action, side effects, and risks to monitor for.
- Advise not using St. John's wort or other homeopathic treatment that may potentiate serotonin syndrome when using SSRIs, SNRIs, or antipsychotics.
- There is a duty to warn and not maintain confidentiality if a patient is at risk for suicide or harming others.
- Teach families how to observe for signs of suicidality and how to remove the means to carry out a suicide plan effectively.

PATIENT HEALTH QUESTIONNAIRE (PHQ-9)

NAME: _____   DATE: _____

Over the last *2 weeks*, how often have you been bothered by any of the following problems?
(use "✓" to indicate your answer)

	Not at all	Several days	More than half the days	Nearly every day
1. Little interest or pleasure in doing things	0	1	2	3
2. Feeling down, depressed, or hopeless	0	1	2	3
3. Trouble falling or staying asleep, or sleeping too much	0	1	2	3
4. Feeling tired or having little energy	0	1	2	3
5. Poor appetite or overeating	0	1	2	3
6. Feeling bad about yourself—or that you are a failure or have let yourself or your family down	0	1	2	3
7. Trouble concentrating on things, such as reading the newspaper or watching television	0	1	2	3
8. Moving or speaking so slowly that other people could have noticed. Or the opposite—being so figety or restless that you have been moving around a lot more than usual	0	1	2	3
9. Thoughts that you would be better off dead, or of hurting yourself	0	1	2	3

add columns _____ + _____ + _____

(Healthcare professional: For interpretation of TOTAL, please refer to accompanying scoring card).   TOTAL: _____

10. If you checked off *any problems*, how *difficult* have these problems made it for you to do your work, take care of things at home, or get along with other people?	Not difficult at all _____ Somewhat difficult _____ Very difficult _____ Extremely difficult _____

Figure 21-1 Patient Health Questionnaire.

Copyright © 1999 Pfizer Inc. All rights reserved. Reproduced with permission. PRIME-MD© is a trademark of Pfizer Inc. A2663B 10-04-2005. Reproduced from SAMSHA. (2005). Suicide Prevention. Retrieved from http://www.samhsa.gov/suicide-prevention

PATIENT DEPRESSION QUESTIONNAIRE (PHQ-9)

For initial diagnosis:

1. Patient completes PHQ-9 Quick Depression Assessment.
2. If there are at least 4✓s in the shaded section (including Questions #1 and #2), consider a depressive disorder. Add score to determine severity.

Consider Major Depressive Disorder

- if there are at least 5✓s in the shaded section (one of which corresponds to Question #1 or #2)

Consider Other Depressive Disorder

- if there are 2–4✓s in the shaded section (one of which corresponds to Question #1 or #2)

Note: Since the questionnaire relies on patient self-report, all responses should be verified by the clinician, and a definitive diagnosis is made on clinical grounds taking into account how well the patient understood the questionnaire, as well as other relevant information from the patient. Diagnoses of Major Depressive Disorder or Other Depressive Disorder also require impairment of social, occupational, or other important areas of functioning (Question #10) and ruling out normal bereavement, a history of a Manic Episode (Bipolar Disorder), and a physical disorder, medication, or other drug as the biological cause of the depressive symptoms.

To monitor severity over time for newly diagnosed patients or patients in current treatment for depression:

1. Patients may complete questionnaires at baseline and at regular intervals (eg, every 2 weeks) at home and bring them in at their next appointment for scoring or they may complete the questionnaire during each scheduled appointment.
2. Add up✓s by column. For every ✓: Several days = 1 More than half the days = 2 Nearly every day = 3
3. Add together column scores to get a TOTAL score.
4. Refer to the accompanying **PHQ-9 Scoring Box** to interpret the TOTAL score.
5. Results may be included in patient files to assist you in setting up a treatment goal, determining degree of response, as well as guiding treatment intervention.

Scoring: add up all checked boxes on PHQ-9

For every ✓ Not at all = 0; Several days = 1; More than half the days = 2; Nearly every day = 3

Interpretation of Total Score

Total Score	Depression Severity
1–4	Minimal depression
5–9	Mild depression
10–14	Moderate depression
15–19	Moderately severe depression
20–27	Severe depression

Figure 21-1 (continued)

Indication for Referral
- Psychotherapy provider (psychiatric mental health nurse practitioner [PMHNP], licensed clinical social worker [LCSW], licensed mental health counselor [LMHC], doctoral degree [PhD])
- Psychiatric specialist (psychiatric mental health nurse practitioner/medical doctor/doctor of osteopathic medicine [PMHNP/MD/DO]) for psychosis, suicidal ideation, severe illness, or medications
- Emergency room or crisis activation if a suicide plan or attempt or homicidal ideation exists

Evaluation and Follow-Up
- Depends on severity, may be weekly or every 2 weeks until improvements are noted, then monthly
- Re-administer objective measures such as the PHQ-9

Clinical Pearls
Diagnostic Hint:
The mnemonic SIGECAPS (Carlat, 1998) may assist in remembering the symptoms of major depression and persistent depressive disorder:

Sleep disorder (increased or decreased)
Interest deficit (anhedonia)
Guilt (worthlessness, hopelessness, regret)
Energy deficit
Concentration deficit
Appetite disorder (increased or decreased)
Psychomotor retardation or agitation
Suicidality

Prescribing SSRIs, SNRIs, and Norepinephrine-Dopamine Reuptake Inhibitors (NDRIs)
- Adjustments usually occur after the initial 2 weeks if tolerated, allowing initial side effects to subside.
- Continue for 6 to 12 months after symptom remission.
- For older people, the rule is to go slow and stay low.
- For patients who do not respond to the maximum dosage or have intolerable side effects, consider switching agents.
- Consider maintenance therapy if a patient has experienced multiple episodes of depression, rapid recurrences, severe episodes, residual symptoms, or has a significant family history.

Serotonin Syndrome

Serotonin syndrome is a rare, potentially life-threatening condition associated with an increase in serotonin in the central nervous system. The risk is highest with MAOIs or when using multiple medications or adjusting medications, or with concurrent use of homeopathic medicines, such as St. John's wort or ginseng. This is a medical emergency and requires prompt treatment.

It may include:
- Confusion
- Agitation
- Dilated pupils
- Nausea/vomiting/diarrhea
- Shivering
- Fever
- Seizures
- Irregular or rapid heart rate

Postpartum Depression

PPD is thought to be due to changes in hormone levels. Women with a history of depression or premenstrual dysphoric syndrome are most at risk.

According to the Centers for Disease Control and Prevention, PPD affects 1 in 8 women (n.d.a). The recommended screening tool for PPD is the Edinburgh Postnatal Depression Scale (EPDS), administered 4 to 6 weeks after delivery. (The practitioner should always rule out underlying medical conditions before making the diagnosis of depression, including an evaluation for anemia and hypothyroidism.) The onset is 2 to 3 days after childbirth and can occur up to 1 year after giving birth.

Pediatric providers treating infants during routine well-child visits are in an optimal position to screen women for PPD, given the frequency of visits during the infant's first year of life.

Clinical Presentation and Assessment Findings
History of Present Illness
- The chief complaint may include anxiety and fear.
- The patient may cry for no reason.
- The HPI will closely resemble that of major depressive disorder.

Physical Assessment Findings
- Findings are the same as for major depressive disorder for both physical and mental status exams.

- Observe mother–infant interactions, including eye contact and affection, and her interaction with other children to determine if they are receiving adequate care.
- Observe for responsiveness to infant cries.

Differential Diagnosis
- Major depressive disorder
- Dysthymia
- Somatization or somatoform disorder
- Premenstrual dysphoria
- Attention-deficit/hyperactivity disorder
- Anxiety
- Hypothyroidism
- Anemia
- Chronic fatigue syndrome
- Fibromyalgia
- Diabetes
- Hypoglycemia

Clinical Management
- Laboratory and diagnostic studies
- Labs would be used to differentiate other causes of symptoms: RPR; TSH; T3; ACTH and cortisol; CBC-dif; Vitamin D 25 hydroxy; Vitamin B-12; ferritin; HIV test; calcium, phosphate, magnesium levels; BUN and creatinine; AST/ALT; and blood and urine toxicology screens.

Nonpharmacologic
For mild to moderate PPD, psychotherapy is considered first-line treatment.

Patient Education
- Provide education in adapting to parental role, attending to mother's own needs, sensitive responsiveness, crying patterns, and feeding and sleeping arrangements (Missler et al., 2020).
- Educate on the side effects of medications and the safety of lactation.
- Educate in adherence with the goal of remission.

Pharmacologic
- For moderate to severe PPD, pharmacotherapy should be considered using the adult depression heuristics, unless breastfeeding.
- A 14-day treatment of Zuranolone is the only FDA-approved treatment for PPD, but it has not yet been determined to be safe during breastfeeding.
- For women who are breastfeeding, antidepressants in general, such as sertraline, are considered relatively safe treatment, considering low transmission in breast milk and minimal adverse effects in neonates.
- Infants should be monitored for adverse effects or changes in behavior.
- Medication, when effective, should be used for no fewer than 12 weeks and maintained for 24 months and likely longer in women who have a history of depression.

Indication for Referral
- Refer to child protective services if signs of neglect or abuse exist.
- Refer to a psychiatrist, psychiatric nurse practitioner (NP), or emergency department if psychosis, suicidal or homicidal ideation, or self-harm behaviors occur.

Evaluation and Follow-Up
- Women with postpartum depression need to be evaluated closely and assessed for their ability to care for their newborn.
- A three-item version of the EPDS is predictive of PPD and should be relied on as PPD is difficult to ascertain by clinical interview alone (Kabir & Sheeder, 2008). Ask the patient if they:
  - "blamed themselves unnecessarily when things went wrong."
  - "have been anxious or worried for no good reason."
  - "have felt scared or panicky for no very good reason."

Bipolar Disorder

Bipolar disorder, also referred to as manic-depressive episodes, affects 2.8 percent of the American population aged 18 years and older (NIMH, n.d.b). With a median age of onset of 25, it can affect people as young as early adolescence and as old as their late 60s (NIMH, n.d.). It is characterized by intense mood, energy, and activity shifts that impact day-to-day functioning.

While routine screening for bipolar disorder is not generally recommended, many tools may help identify symptoms and encourage further evaluation. One of these tools is the Mood Disorder Questionnaire (MDQ). It is a brief self-report tool that takes approximately 5 minutes to complete. Two similar conditions that share the same diagnostic work-up and treatments include cyclothymic disorder and disruptive mood dysregulation disorder.

Cyclothymic Disorder

Cyclothymic disorder is a rare mood disorder in which a person experiences ups and downs in mood that are impairing but not as extreme as bipolar I or II disorder. Symptoms must occur persistently for 2 or more years with no more than two symptom-free months. Treatment management is consistent with that used for bipolar I and II disorder.

Disruptive Mood Dysregulation Disorder

While some children meet the full criteria for bipolar disorder, many children with chronic irritability may experience significant impairment but do not meet full criteria for bipolar disorder. This subset of children may be more likely to go on to develop major depressive disorder or generalized anxiety disorder in adulthood. *The Diagnostic and Statistical Manual of Mental Disorders*, Fifth Edition (DSM-5), defines disruptive mood dysregulation disorder as severe and recurrent temper outbursts over what is considered developmentally appropriate and out of proportion to the situation at hand. These tantrums must occur at least *three times a week for a minimum of 1 year.*

Clinical Presentation/ Assessment Findings

History of Present Illness

Bipolar disorder is typified by periods of mania or hypomania, or elevated, expansive, or irritable mood. Mania and hypomania are differentiated by degree of impairment, with mania being severely impairing and hypomania being mildly to moderately impairing. Bipolar disorder includes a history of mania, whereas bipolar II disorder includes a history of hypomania only. While many people also experience episodes of depression with bipolar disorder, it is mania that is diagnostic.

Patients typically have a chief complaint that they feel they do not need any sleep. They may appear very talkative, easily distracted, and usually feel on top of the world with high self-esteem. They will report high-risk behaviors, including sexual promiscuity, hypersexuality, gambling, and excessive spending.

Psychosis may or may not be present during episodes of severe mania. As many patients in the acute phase of mania or hypomania have poor insight into their symptoms, involving family members in their care may provide helpful collaborative information.

Physical Assessment Findings
Differential Diagnosis

- Schizophrenia
- Obsessive-compulsive disorder
- Major depressive disorder with psychotic features
- Hyperthyroidism
- Cushing's disease
- Addison's disease
- Vitamin B deficiency
- Personality disorders (histrionic or borderline)
- Brain tumors
- Dementia
- Cerebrovascular accident
- Encephalitis
- Lupus

Clinical Management
Laboratory and Diagnostic Studies

- There are no tests specific to the disorder, but rather to rule out other conditions. Labs would be used to differentiate other causes of symptoms: RPR; TSH; T3; ACTH and cortisol; CBC-dif; Vitamin D 25 hydroxy; Vitamin B-12; ferritin; HIV test; calcium, phosphate, magnesium levels; BUN and creatinine; AST/ALT; and blood and urine toxicology screens.

Nonpharmacologic

- Although medication is the mainstay of treatment, psychotherapy treats the core deficits of psychosocial impairment, low rates of medication adherence, interpersonal dysfunction, and cognitive impairment (Swartz & Swanson, 2014).

Patient Education

- Patients should be educated on medication adherence and the prediction of side effects.
- Sleep hygiene and the importance of sleep in preventing manic episodes should be reviewed.
- Educate patients to be aware of and to seek treatment early when they need less sleep and become very social or productive.
- Educate family on symptoms of mania, psychosis, and risks of suicide.

Pharmacologic

- Pharmacologic management is indicated for bipolar disorder and bipolar II disorder as a first-line treatment.
- Reoccurrence rates are high despite the use of prophylactic mood stabilizers, including lithium salts, mood-stabilizing anticonvulsants (carbamazepine, lamotrigine, and valproate), and second-generation antipsychotics (aripiprazole, asenapine, cariprazine, lurasidone, olanzapine, paliperidone, quetiapine, risperidone, ziprasidone, and so on.
- The most recent review by Oya et al. of RCTs on lithium and lamotrigine found both agents to be significantly superior to placebo in preventing new BD episodes of any mood polarity (Nestsiarovich et al., 2022).
- Antidepressant monotherapy for bipolar disorder is controversial, as antidepressants may exacerbate manic symptoms and/or lead to recurrence of symptoms in stable patients referred to as "manic switching" (Nestsiarovich et al., 2022). There are several classes of medication used to treat bipolar disorder, including lithium, anticonvulsants, and atypical antipsychotics. Often, multiple medications must be used to target the symptoms of depression and mania equally, as well as other presenting problems such as poor sleep.

Lithium

- Only medication that has a known protective mechanism against suicide
- Effects should occur in 1 to 3 weeks
- Requires frequent tests to monitor trough lithium plasma levels (should be between 0.5 and 1.2 mEq/L) to detect toxicity due to its narrow range between therapeutic dose and toxicity
- Caution with states of dehydration when using drugs that have renal clearance
- Potential side effects: ataxia, tremor, polyuria and polydipsia (nephrogenic diabetes), sedation, weight gain, diarrhea, nausea, goiter
- Drug monitoring: kidney function tests (creatinine and urine specific gravity), thyroid stimulating hormone (TSH), and electrocardiogram (EKG) for patients over age 50 on initiation; repeat 1 to 2 times a year
- Can cause severe acne.

Anticonvulsants

- Drug monitoring: CBC, LFTs, kidney function tests (creatinine and urine specific gravity), and TSH
- Potential side effects: sedation, weight gain, dizziness, headache, nausea, vomiting, diarrhea, blurred vision
- Effects should occur within a few weeks but may take several weeks to months to stabilize.

Carbamazepine (Tegretol)

- Rare aplastic anemia or agranulocytosis may occur (unusual bleeding or bruising, mouth sores, infections, fever, sore throat).
- Rare syndrome of inappropriate antidiuretic hormone secretion with hyponatremia may occur.
- Risk Category D pregnancy; Category D means that studies have shown that pregnant women who take this medication can develop birth defects in the developing fetus.

Valproate (Depakote)

- Rarely causes alopecia
- Requires frequent tests to monitor trough plasma levels (50 to 125 µg/ml)
- Risk Category D pregnancy—may cause neural tube defects, particularly when used in the first trimester

Lamotrigine (Lamictal)

- Generally tolerated well
- No monitoring of plasma levels
- Titration often takes 6 or more weeks due to the risk of Stevens-Johnson syndrome (SJS)
- Those at risk for SJS can be identified with genomic testing for the HLA-B*1502
- Gene carried most commonly by those of Asian descent

Atypical Antipsychotics

Refer to the section on psychotic disorders.

Indication for Referral

- A presentation of mania, particularly when accompanied by psychosis, is a medical emergency and often necessitates hospitalization.

Evaluation and Follow-Up

Due to high rates of medication nonadherence, patients should be monitored at least monthly.

Suicide Risk

The risk of suicide is 10 to 30 times higher in those with bipolar disorder than in the general population.

> **Clinical Pearls**
>
> A mnemonic that facilitates recalling the symptoms of hypomania/mania is DIG FAST:
>
> **D**istractibility
> **I**ndiscretion
> **G**randiosity
> **F**light of ideas
> **A**ctivity increase
> **S**leep deficit
> **T**alkativeness

Medication Nonadherence (*Experiencing Heightened Emotional States*)

- Because mood stabilizers are "dulling" and people generally feel "great" when they are experiencing heightened emotional states, some have the difficult feeling that they have lost their personality. Patients will say they do not like their personality change to less social, fun, or creative, and they feel less productive on mood stabilizers.

There is little diagnosis-specific clinical evidence regarding the most effective treatment. Treatment may include a combination of psychotherapy, such as parent therapy, cognitive behavioral therapy, and dialectical behavior therapy, and pharmacologic management with agents such as stimulant medication, antidepressants, atypical antipsychotics, and/or mood stabilizers (NIMH, n.d.b). Retrieved from NIMH website (National Institute of Mental Health [NIMH]—Transforming the understanding and treatment of mental illnesses).

Attention-Deficit/ Hyperactivity Disorder

Etiology

Attention-Deficit/Hyperactivity Disorder (ADHD) is a developmental disorder that first appears in childhood. It is characterized by functionally impairing symptoms of impulsivity, hyperactivity, and inattention across settings such as home, school, and work. The disorder is described as one of the following: ADHD predominantly inattentive presentation, ADHD predominantly hyperactive and impulsive presentation, or ADHD combined presentation.

ADHD Facts

- Affects about 9.8 percent of school-age children (CDC, n.d.b).
- For adults, the prevalence decreases to 4.4 percent (American Psychiatric Association, 2013).
- More severe cases are detected as early as age 4, with mild cases detected by age 7 (NIMH, n.d.e).
- Assessment of ADHD for children requires a report from a parent and a teacher. Routine collaboration in the form of standardized assessment tools, such as the Vanderbilt (Wolraich et al., 1998) or Conners Rating Scale (Conners, 2001), is critical for treatment management.

Diagnosis of ADHD

The following symptoms of each subcategory *must have been observed* before age 12 and present for at least 6 months.

Clinical Presentation/ Assessment Findings

- Inattention
- Easily distracted
- Difficulty with follow-through on work or activities
- Difficulty with organizational skills
- Avoidance of activities that require sustained attention
- Often forgetful
- Difficulty listening when spoken to
- Trouble sustaining attention
- Hyperactivity and impulsivity
- Fidgets with hands and feet
- Difficulty remaining seated
- Excessive running, climbing
- Difficulty enjoying or participating in quiet activities
- Excessive talking
- Behavior appears that person is "driven by a motor"
- Interrupts, intrudes on others
- Has difficulty waiting for a turn
- Blurts out answers before questions are finished

Screening Recommendations for ADHD

Routine screening for ADHD is not recommended. Screening tools are used in combination with a clinical interview.

Differential Diagnosis

- Hyperthyroidism
- Bipolar disorder
- Anxiety
- Autism spectrum
- Lead poisoning
- Depression
- Posttraumatic stress disorder
- Sleep–wake disorders
- Hearing loss

Clinical Management

Nonpharmacologic

- Recommended as first-line therapy for children under 6 years of age
- Includes parent training and recommendations for the classroom
- Used adjunctively with medications when appropriate and especially if a comorbid psychiatric disorder is present

Pharmacologic

Recommended for children ages 6 to 11 years

Stimulant Medications

- Methylphenidate (Ritalin, Concerta, Daytrana, Metadate CD, Methylin)
- Dexmethylphenidate (Focalin)
- Dextroamphetamine (Dexedrine)
- Mixed Amphetamine Salts (Adderall, Adderall XR)
- Lisdexamphetamine—Vyvanse
  - Controlled substances (C-II) with high abuse potential.
  - Monitor growth, including weight and height
  - Avoid if there is a family history of cardiac disease.
  - Side effects include insomnia, loss of appetite (weight loss), tics, hypertension, and tachycardia.
  - Controversial whether screening ECG for long QT syndrome should be a prerequisite to prescribing.

Nonstimulant Medications

- Atomoxetine (Strattera)—SNRI, once daily dosing
- Monitor for mood changes, gastrointestinal (GI) complaints, including decreased appetite.
- All antidepressants carry a black box warning for increased suicidal ideation.

Alpha-2 Agonists —Clonidine (Catapres) and Guanfacine (Tenex, Intuniv)

- Helpful with impulsive and hyperactive behaviors.
- Especially helpful if patients present with co-morbid Tourette's syndrome, anxiety, or other tic disorders
- Helpful at night for sleep disorders
- Monitor blood pressure, pulse, and potential sedation

Tricyclics—Desipramine (Norpramin) and Imipramine (Tofranil)

- For use when alternative therapies are ineffective or intolerable
- Recommended ECG at baseline and with increased dosage
- Blood levels help determine optimal dosing
- Monitor for anticholinergic effects, suicidal ideation (FDA Black Box Warning)

NDRI—Bupropion (Wellbutrin)

- Monitor for decreased appetite, sleeping difficulties
- Potential for lowered seizure threshold; contraindicated in those with bulimia

Evaluation and Follow-Up

- If the patient is using controlled and dangerous substances categorized as stimulants, a monthly visit is indicated with an exam on file, as medications are not refillable.
- Monthly psychoeducation for stimulant use should include executive function skills, accommodations, and ways to prevent developing a dependence and risk of addiction.
- Examination should include blood pressure, resting pulse, and heart rate variability.
- ECG before initial prescription of stimulants is controversial and within the provider's discretion to rule out long QT syndrome.
- Ongoing assessment on stimulants should include ruling out risks for seizure, eating disorders, electrolyte imbalances, and risks of psychosis, such as in patients with a comorbidity of bipolar disorder.

Psychotic Disorders

Etiology

Psychosis includes a range of abnormalities in thought from many possible causes. Psychosis is a potential result of illicit drugs, a psychiatric disorder such as schizophrenia, or an adverse effect of medication.

Diagnosis of Psychosis
- Psychosis needs to be differentiated from delirium and consists of hallucinations and/or delusions (known as positive symptoms of schizophrenia).
  - Patients experiencing psychosis may be difficult to engage. If the symptoms are due to schizophrenia, the patient will have disorganized thoughts, making communication difficult, and depression symptoms (negative symptoms of schizophrenia).

Schizophrenia
- Schizophrenia is one of the most debilitating psychiatric illnesses.
- Symptoms are conceptualized as either *positive* or *negative* symptoms.
  - Positive symptoms are characterized by delusions, hallucinations (either auditory and/or visual), speech that is disorganized and/or nonsensical, and disorganized behavior.
  - Negative symptoms refer to poverty of speech, lack of motivation, lack of emotional expression and feelings of pleasure, and impairments in cognitive functioning.

Other Disorders With Psychotic Features
- Major depression with psychotic features—psychosis present during mood disorder. Symptoms must be present for 2 weeks.
- Mania with psychosis—psychosis present during a manic episode of bipolar disorder.
- Brief psychotic disorder—symptoms present for at least 2 weeks, but with complete remission in 1 to 3 months. Often preceded by significant psychosocial stressors.

Differential Diagnosis
- Bipolar I disorder
- Depression with psychotic features
- Psychotic disorder vs schizophrenia
- Schizoaffective disorder
- Delirium
- Hypoglycemia
- Sepsis
- Medication interactions or withdrawal
- Substance use
- Electrolyte imbalances
- Autoimmune disorders (multiple sclerosis, systemic lupus erythematosus)
- Endocrine disorders (Cushing's disease, diabetes mellitus, thyroid disease)
- Neurologic disorders (dementia, encephalitis, epilepsy, Parkinson's disease)
- Nutritional conditions (Vitamin B deficiency)
- Oncologic conditions (small lung cancer, ovarian teratoma)

Clinical Management
Nonpharmacologic Treatment
- Strategies to cope with and distract from hearing voices, such as headsets, watching TV, listening to music
- Relaxation techniques
- Exercise
- Maintain a structured routine.
- Psychoeducation that voices and delusions cannot be reasoned with
- Remove distractions when trying to concentrate.
- Family psychoeducation to offer empathy, avoid criticism, and focus on feelings, not thought content

Pharmacological Treatment
Antipsychotic medications are the treatment of choice for schizophrenia.

First-Generation Antipsychotics
- Also known as "typical antipsychotics," dopamine antagonists block synaptic D2 receptors, which results in a decrease in positive symptoms of schizophrenia (psychosis) in the central nervous system.
- Medications include haloperidol, fluphenazine, and chlorpromazine.
- Side Effects
  - Produce extrapyramidal side effects. Some are used as antiemetics and antihistamines.
  - High risk of extrapyramidal symptoms (EPS), or movement-related symptoms, such as tardive dyskinesia, which may be permanent.
  - Affects up to 75 percent of patients who are prescribed first-generation psychotics.
  - In some cases, the adverse effects of tardive dyskinesia are irreversible.
- **EPS symptoms**
  - Constipation
  - Blurred vision

- Dry mouth
- Nasal congestion
- Mydriasis
- Photophobia
- Orthostatic hypotension
- Tachycardia
- Urinary retention
- Urinary hesitation
- Sedation
- Weight gain
- Agranulocytosis
- **Central nervous system (CNS) symptoms**
  - Akathisia (uncontrollable need to move within 2 months of treatment with beta blockers, benzodiazepines [BZDs], anticholinergic drugs)
  - Dystonias (oculogyric or torticollis with treatment of antihistamines or antiparkinsonian drugs)
  - Drug-induced parkinsonism (tremor, rigidity, bradykinesia)
  - Tardive dyskinesia (long-term use irreversible [anticholinergics contraindicated])
  - Neuroleptic malignant syndrome (fatal side effect, hyperthermia, tremor, rigidity with treatment including Parlodel or Dantrium)
  - Seizures (when treated with clozapine; an EEG needed for doses over 600 mg per day).
- High potency drugs, such as fluphenazine, haloperidol, pimozide, thiothixene, and trifluoperazine, have more EPS and CNS symptoms.
- Low potency causes more sedation and hypotension.
- ECG and labs (WBC, Hgb, Hct) before treatment; monitor with WBC, TSH, LFTs, and prolactin labs after treatment.
- Dopamine blockade will cause gynecomastia, galactorrhea, amenorrhea, and weight gain.
- Dopamine antagonists are contraindicated in severe hypotension or hypertension, narrow-angle glaucoma, adynamic ileus, Parkinson's disease, prostatic hyperplasia, seizure disorder, bone marrow depression, and prolactin-dependent carcinoma of the breast.
- Use of nutmeg is contraindicated with haloperidol. Kava kava causes dystonia. Evening primrose oil can cause seizures. Don quai and St. John's wort cause photosensitivity.
- Most common side effects are sedation, orthostatic hypotension, anticholinergic side effects, akathisia, parkinsonism, agranulocytosis, and photosensitivity.
- Concurrent use of anticholinergic drugs will decrease their effectiveness but relieve some side effects.
- Benztropine is an anticholinergic.
- Benadryl is an antihistamine.
- Amantadine is a dopamine agonist.

Second-Generation Antipsychotics (Atypical Antipsychotics)

Also known as "**atypical antipsychotics**," they are special because they block dopamine D2 receptors (D2) and serotonin 5-HT2 receptors (5HT2), causing some reduction in negative symptoms of schizophrenia in the cortex. They are associated with less tardive dyskinesia or EPS.

- Paliperidone and aripiprazole have less tardive dyskinesia (TD) and extrapyramidal symptoms (EPS), and are well tolerated.
- Other atypical antipsychotics include olanzapine, risperidone, ziprasidone, aripiprazole, quetiapine, paliperidone, and clozapine.
  - Adverse effects include weight gain, metabolic syndrome, and hypercholesterolemia.
  - Clozapine is only prescribed for 1 week at a time to enforce compliance with weekly blood monitoring for agranulocytosis.
  - Risperidone has less muscarinic (cholinergic) affinity, so it has fewer anticholinergic side effects. It does not cause agranulocytosis, neuroleptic malignant syndrome (NMS), or tardive dyskinesia but raises prolactin levels.
  - Olanzapine does not cause agranulocytosis; less EPS.
- Associated with fewer movement disorder symptoms than first-generation antipsychotics.
- Requires routine monitoring of weight, lipid profile, glucose, LFTs, and prolactin levels on initiation, at least annually, and more frequently as indicated.
- Clozapine requires ongoing blood monitoring for potential agranulocytosis, and in rare cases, it can cause myocarditis; therefore, it should be used as a last line of treatment and requires registration in the FDA REMS system and reporting of WBC counts to the pharmacist dispensing it.
- The Abnormal Involuntary Movement Scale (AIMS) should be administered to patients prescribed first- and second-generation antipsychotics to aid in the early detection of tardive dyskinesia as well as for ongoing maintenance (**Figure 21-2**).

AIMS Examination Procedure

SHOULD BE COMPLETED BEFORE ENTERING THE RATINGS ON THE AIMS FORM.

Either before or after completing the Examination Procedure, observe the patient unobtrusively at rest (eg, in waiting room).

The chair to be used in this examination should be a hard, firm one without arms.

1: Ask patient whether there is anything in his/her mouth (ie, gum, candy, etc) and if there is, to remove it.

2: Ask patient about the current condition of his/her teeth. Ask patient if he/she wears dentures. Do teeth or dentures bother patient now?

3: Ask patient whether he/she notices any movements in mouth, face, hands, or feet. If yes, ask to describe and to what extent they currently bother patient or interfere with his/her activities.

4: Have patient sit in chair with hands on knees, legs slightly apart, and feet flat on floor. (Look at entire body for movements while in this position).

5: Ask patient to sit with hands hanging unsupported. If male, between legs, if female, and wearing a dress, hanging over knees. (Observe hands and other body areas.)

6: Ask patient to open mouth. (Observe tongue at rest within mouth.) Do this twice.

7: Ask patient to protrude tongue. (Observe abnormalities of tongue movement.)

*8: Ask patient to tap thumb, with each finger, as rapidly as possible for 10-15 seconds: separately with right hand, then with left hand. (Observe facial and leg movements.)

9: Flex and extend patient's left and right arms, one at a time. (Note any rigidity and rate it.)

10: Ask patient to stand up. (Observe in profile. Observe all body areas again, hips included.)

*11: Ask patient to extend both arms outstretched in front with palms down. (Observe trunk, legs, and mouth.)

*12: Have patient walk a few paces, turn, and walk back to chair. (Observe hands and gait.) Do this twice.

Figure 21-2 AIMS Scale.

*Movements that are observed in other areas of the body when the patient performs the requested activity.

William Guy, Ph.D.: *ECDEU Assessment Manual for Psychopharmacology* - Revised (DHEW Publ No ADM 76-338), US Department of Health, Education, and Welfare, 1976.

Abnormal Involuntary Movement Scale (AIMS)

Patient's Name (Please print) _____ Patient's ID information _____

Examiner's Name _____

Current Medications and Total mg/Day

Medication #1 _____ Total mg/Day _____ Medication #2 _____ Total mg/Day _____

Instructions: Complete the examination procedure before entering these ratings.

	None, Normal	Minimal (may be extreme normal)	Mild	Moderate	Severe
Facial and Oral Movements					
1. Muscles of Facial Expression e.g., movements of forehead, eyebrows, periorbital area, cheeks; include frowning, blinking, smiling, grimacing	☐0	☐1	☐2	☐3	☐4
2. Lips and Perioral Area e.g., puckering, pouting, smacking	☐0	☐1	☐2	☐3	☐4
3. Jaw e.g., biting, clenching, chewing, mouth opening, lateral movement	☐0	☐1	☐2	☐3	☐4
4. Tongue Rate only increases in movement both in and out of mouth, NOT inability to sustain movement	☐0	☐1	☐2	☐3	☐4
Extremity Movements					
5. Upper (arms, wrists, hands, fingers) Include choreic movements (i.e., rapid, objectively purposeless, irregular, spontaneous); athetoid movements (i.e., slow, irregular, complex, serpentine). DO NOT include tremor (i.e., repetitive, regular, rhythmic).	☐0	☐1	☐2	☐3	☐4
6. Lower (legs, knees, ankles, toes) e.g., lateral knee movement, foot tapping, heel dropping, foot squirming, inversion and eversion of foot	☐0	☐1	☐2	☐3	☐4
Trunk Movements					
7. Neck, shoulders, hips e.g., rocking, twisting, squirming, pelvic gyrations	☐0	☐1	☐2	☐3	☐4

SCORING:
- Score the highest amplitude or frequency in a movement on the 0–4 scale, not the average;
- Score Activated Movements the same way; do not lower those numbers as was proposed at one time;
- A POSITIVE AIMS EXAMINATION IS A SCORE OF 2 IN TWO OR MORE MOVEMENTS or a SCORE OF 3 OR 4 IN A SINGLE MOVEMENT
- Do not sum the scores: e.g., a patient who has scores 1 in four movements DOES NOT have a positive AIMS score of 4.

Overall Severity

8. Severity of abnormal movements	☐0	☐1	☐2	☐3	☐4
9. Incapacitation due to abnormal movements	☐0	☐1	☐2	☐3	☐4

	No Awareness	Aware, No Distress	Aware, Mild Distress	Aware, Moderate Distress	Aware, Severe Distress
10. Patient's awareness of abnormal movements (rate only patient's report)	☐0	☐1	☐2	☐3	☐4

Dental Status

11. Current problems with teeth and/or dentures? ☐Yes ☐No
12. Does patient usually wear dentures? ☐Yes ☐No

Comments: _____

Examiner's Signature _____ Next Exam Date _____

Figure 21-2 (continued)

Neuroleptic Malignant Syndrome

NMS is a potentially life-threatening situation that arises within 2 weeks of initiating or modifying a neuroleptic medication (i.e., typical or atypical antipsychotic medication). It requires immediate evaluation and treatment. It includes:

- severe muscle rigidity,
- fever in an intensive care unit (ICU),
- autonomic instability, and
- changes in level of consciousness.

Treatment and Follow-Up

Neuroleptic malignant syndrome is a medical emergency and requires a quick diagnosis. The patient requires hospitalization in an ICU.

- The causative medication is immediately discontinued.
- Patient may require:
  - mechanical ventilation,
  - antiarrhythmic medications,
  - IV fluid and electrolyte monitoring,
  - antipyretics and other fever-reducing strategies, such as ice packs and cooling blankets,
  - antihypertensives, if needed, to lower blood pressure, and
  - muscle or skeletal relaxant medications.

Anxiety Disorders

Etiology

Anxiety disorders are collectively the most common mental health problem in the United States, with 31.1 percent of U.S. adults affected at some time in their lives (NIMH, n.d.d). While many people experience normal reactions to stress, people with anxiety disorders experience excessive worry that is difficult to control and contributes to a range of physical, psychological, and social impairments.

Screening

Given the prevalence of anxiety in the primary care population, screening may help identify patients at risk of these disorders. A commonly used screening tool is the GAD-7, or the abbreviated GAD-2, a seven- or two-question instrument, respectively, designed for use in primary care. While developed to recognize symptoms of generalized anxiety disorder (GAD), this tool has also been shown to be effective in detecting symptoms of social anxiety, panic, and posttraumatic stress disorders.

Assessment

Like all psychiatric disorders, medical causes for symptoms must be ruled out before making a psychiatric diagnosis of anxiety.

Labs and Diagnostic Tests

- Lab work includes CBC-dif, CMP, TSH, ACTH, cortisol, ferritin, B12 with MMA levels, glucose levels, and ECG.
- Ferritin deficiency can be a cause of restlessness and present like ADHD.
- Sometimes, if anxiety is present upon awakening, a polysomnography may be indicated to rule out sleep apnea.
- Causes of fight-or-flight symptoms, such as panic attacks, need to have full consideration for adrenal dysfunction or anything that would trigger the hypothalamic pituitary axis's negative feedback system.

Physical Symptoms

- Heart palpitations
- Shortness of breath
- Shakiness
- Trembling
- Chest pain
- Nausea
- Dizziness
- Choking sensation
- Dry mouth
- Numbness
- Decreased sexual desire
- Sleep disturbance

Psychological Symptoms

- Worried thoughts that are difficult to control
- Derealization (feeling of being detached from oneself)
- Restlessness
- Difficulty concentrating
- Irritability
- Distressing memories

Social Symptoms

- Avoidance of activities
- Changes in routines

- Fear of leaving home
- Distorted blame of self or others
- Poor performance in work or school settings

Type of Anxiety Disorders

There are many different types of anxiety disorders, and often they may occur together. The most common include:

- *Generalized Anxiety Disorder:* Excessive worry and anxiety more days than not for at least 6 months (**Figure 21-3**).
- *Social Anxiety Disorder:* Intense anxiety and distress around a feared situation (i.e., being in groups of people) that is unreasonable or excessive and continues for at least 6 months.
- *Specific Phobia:* An intense fear reaction to a specific object or situation (i.e., flying, heights, animals, blood, injections) that causes an immediate anxiety response, and the avoidance of which impairs a person's normal routine.
- *Panic Disorder:* Sudden and intense fear that typically peaks in less than 10 minutes from onset with a range of physical and psychological symptoms.
- *Agoraphobia:* Fear of being in a situation where leaving would be difficult or embarrassing, including places such as home, transportation, standing in line, or being in a crowd.
- *Somatic Symptom Disorder:* Excessive fear or worry about health that occurs for greater than 6 months and which is disproportionate to either a diagnosed medical disorder or medically unexplained symptoms.
- *Separation Anxiety Disorder:* Intense fear of separating from parents, caregivers, or home that may develop in childhood or adulthood and leads to severe anxiety and agitation even when anticipating a separation.
- *Selective Mutism:* A childhood disorder that begins before age 5 in which a child experiences a lack of speech that is not due to a lack of knowledge or comfort in at least one social situation.

GAD-7

Over the last 2 weeks, how often have you been bothered by the following problems? (Use "✔" to indicate your answer)	Not at all	Several days	More than half the days	Nearly every day
1. Feeling nervous, anxious or on edge	0	1	2	3
2. Not being able to stop or control worrying	0	1	2	3
3. Worrying too much about different things	0	1	2	3
4. Trouble relaxing	0	1	2	3
5. Being so restless that it is hard to sit still	0	1	2	3
6. Becoming easily annoyed or irritable	0	1	2	3
7. Feeling afraid as if something awful might happen	0	1	2	3

(For office coding: Total Score T____ = ____ + ____ + ____)

Figure 21-3 GAD-7 and GAD 2.

Reproduced from Pfizer. (n.d.). GAD-7. Retrieved from phqscreeners.com.

Differential Diagnosis

- Acute gastritis
- Addison's disease
- Adrenal crisis
- Atrial fibrillation/tachycardia
- Depression
- Delirium
- Graves' disease
- Hyperthyroidism
- Folate deficiency
- Hyperparathyroidism
- Insomnia
- Obstructive sleep apnea
- Personality disorders
- Premenstrual dysphoric disorder
- Syndrome of inappropriate antidiuretic hormone
- Tourette syndromes
- Uremic encephalopathy
- B12 deficiency
- Ferritin deficiency

Clinical Management

Nonpharmacologic

Consider symptom severity, level of functioning, psychosocial stressors, degree of support, patient motivation, and patient preferences.

- Therapeutic modalities may include CBT or exposure therapy.
- Patients often benefit from developing stress management and relaxation skills as well.

Pharmacologic

- SSRIs, SNRIs, and buspirone are considered first-line medication options.
- Panic attacks and short-term management can be treated with alpha agonists, such as clonidine and prazosin.
- Beta blockers, such as propranolol, and antihistamines, like hydroxyzine, are also used as needed.
- Benzodiazepines are considered a last line and should be used for emergencies because they are addictive, associated with memory impairment, delirium, and falls (Edinoff et al., 2021).

Buspirone

- Generally well tolerated
- Typically prescribed in 2 to 3 divided doses
- Does not cause dependence or withdrawal symptoms
- May take 2 to 4 weeks to achieve efficacy

Benzodiazepines

- May be short, intermediate, or long-acting
- Often provides immediate relief
- Are not indicated for chronic management, given high abuse and dependency potential
- Caution should be used in the older adult population due to the increased risk of cognitive impairment.

Posttraumatic Stress Disorder

Etiology

Posttraumatic stress disorder (PTSD) occurs in people who have experienced or witnessed a traumatic event. The experience is emotionally or physically harmful or life-threatening. Examples include serious accidents, natural disasters, combat, sexual assault, and bullying.

PTSD Facts

- Lifetime prevalence of 6.8 percent in the general population of adults in America (NIMH, n.d.c).
- PTSD occurs in all ages.
- Women are twice as likely as men to experience PTSD.
- Latinos, African Americans, and Native Americans are more likely to develop PTSD.

Diagnosis of PTSD

The disorder is characterized by three main symptom categories: intrusive thoughts, hyperarousal, and avoidance in response to real or perceived threat of death, injury, or sexual violence. Patients often present with flashbacks, nightmares, increased startle response, and avoidance of speaking about the trauma, as well as persons or places that remind them of the traumatic experience.

Screening for PTSD

Routine screening is not recommended.

The PC-PTSD is a commonly used screening tool in primary care (Prins et al., 2003). An answer "yes" to three or more questions warrants follow-up and referral.

> 1. Have had nightmares about it or thought about it when you did not want to?
>   YES/NO
> 2. Tried hard not to think about it or went out of your way to avoid situations that reminded you of it?
>   YES/NO
> 3. Were constantly on guard, watchful, or easily startled?
>   YES/NO
> 4. Felt numb or detached from others, activities, or your surroundings?
>   YES/NO
>
> Reproduced from U.S. Department of Veterans Affairs. (2015). PTSD: National Center for PTSD. Primary Care PTSD Screen (PC-PTSD). Retrieved from http://www.ptsd.va.gov/professional/assessment/screens/pc-ptsd.asp

Differential Diagnosis

- Acute stress disorder
- Dissociative disorder
- Depression
- Generalized anxiety disorder
- Panic disorder
- Phobias
- Substance abuse
- Postconcussion syndrome
- Psychosis
- Obsessive-compulsive disorder

Clinical Management

Nonpharmacologic Treatment

- Evidence-based therapies for PTSD, including cognitive trauma-focused therapies, such as cognitive processing therapy (CPT), prolonged exposure therapy, and eye movement desensitization and reprocessing therapy (EMDR) (U.S.D.V.A., n.d.b).
- People have varying and complex responses to trauma, and the main goal of trauma-informed therapy is to reduce distress related to the event and to help the person cope with reminders of the trauma.

Pharmacologic Treatment

- SSRIs are frequently used to alleviate symptoms of PTSD.
- Paroxetine and sertraline are both FDA-approved for treating the disorder.
- Fluoxetine and venlafaxine are commonly used.
- Prazosin (Minipress) and propranolol (Inderal) are often used to help alleviate nightmares and improve sleep.
- Anxiolytics, such as benzodiazepines, may be used in appropriate patients for short-term symptom improvement only.

Pediatrics: Posttraumatic Stress Disorder in Children

PTSD often presents differently in children than in adults. The following symptoms are more common in children 6 years of age and older:

- Intrusive thoughts—distressing nightmares (content not required), flashbacks, physiological reactions
- Persistent avoidance of stimuli
- Negative alterations in cognitions—negative emotional states, loss of interest, withdrawn behavior
- Persistent reduction in expression and positive emotions
- Alterations in arousal and reactivity
- Irritable, hypervigilant, exaggerated startle response, sleep disturbance

Treatment and Follow-Up

- Use a care team to provide treatment and support for the child and the family.
- The child benefits from talk therapy and social support.
- TF-CBT (Trauma-focused CBT).
- Medications may be prescribed if there are PTSD sleep-related issues that CBT does not resolve.
- Family members can help the child by validating their feelings, providing a trusting and supportive environment, and advocating for them with teachers, coaches, other family members, and friends.
- Respect their need for privacy (especially with older children and teens).

Substance Abuse

Etiology

Addiction is frequently encountered within primary care. Abuse of illicit and prescription drugs is dangerous and rarely reported by patients without prompting. The following are several classes of commonly abused substances:

- *Alcohol*—Alcohol use is common, and defining alcohol use or misuse is often difficult. Guidelines have been developed to assist with definitions.
- *Low-risk drinking*—Defined for women as no more than three drinks per day and less than seven per week; for men, defined as no more than four drinks per day and less than 14 per week.

- *At-risk drinking*—Alcohol intake above the recommended guidelines.
- *Harmful drinking*—Alcohol use that creates physical, social, and relational problems.

Screening

The U.S. Preventive Services Task Force recommends routine screening.

The following screening tool is common for screening for alcohol use or misuse within the primary care setting:

CAGE Questionnaire

> Have you ever felt you should **Cut** down on your drinking?
>
> Have people **Annoyed** you by criticizing your drinking?
>
> Have you ever felt bad or **Guilty** about your drinking?
>
> Have you ever had a drink first thing in the morning to steady your nerves or to get rid of a hangover (**Eye opener**)?
>
> Reproduced from Dhalla, S., & Kopec, J. A. (2007). The CAGE questionnaire for alcohol misuse: A review of reliability and validity studies. *Clinical and Investigative Medicine, 30*(1), 33-41.

Opioid Use Disorder

- *Opioids*—Heroin, morphine, and opioid analgesics act on mu, kappa, and gamma. This produces euphoria and analgesia. Commonly abused prescription drugs include oxycodone, morphine, and other medications within this class.
- *Cannabinoids*—Marijuana acts on the cannabinoid receptors (CB1 and CB2) and inhibit adenylate cyclase. Dopamine and opioid mechanisms likely play a role in the reward pathways of cannabinoid use.
- *Psychostimulants*—Drugs such as cocaine and amphetamine act on dopamine, serotonin, and noradrenaline receptors, blocking reuptake. Amphetamines and methylphenidate are commonly abused prescription medications within this class.
- *Sedatives or Anxiolytics*—Benzodiazepines and barbiturates act on GABA receptors and are CNS depressants. These drugs are frequently abused, given their highly addictive properties; can impair memory and cognition; and cause autonomic depression. Muscle relaxers are also in this category of potentially abused prescription drugs.
- *Hallucinogens*—Drugs such as PCP, LSD (lysergic acid diethylamide), ecstasy, and psilocybin (magic mushrooms, shrooms, etc.) often cause dissociation and altered perceptions.
- *Tobacco and Nicotine*—Cigarettes, chewing tobacco, and vapes are examples and are associated with addiction and carcinogenic exposure.

Screening for substance use is essential during primary care visits. The following acronym is useful for assessing and screening for potential abuse of drugs and/or alcohol.

- C—Have you ever ridden in a CAR driven by someone (including yourself) who was "high" or had been using alcohol or drugs?
- R—Do you ever use alcohol or drugs to RELAX, feel better about yourself, or fit in?
- A—Do you ever use alcohol/drugs while you are by yourself, ALONE?
- F—Do you ever FORGET things you did while using alcohol or drugs?
- F—Do your family or FRIENDS ever tell you that you should cut down on your drinking or drug use?
- T—Have you gotten into TROUBLE while you were using alcohol or drugs?

Knight, J. R., Sherritt, L., Shrier, L. A., Harris, S. K., & Chang, G. (2002). Validity of the CRAFFT substance abuse screening test among adolescent clinic patients. Archives of pediatrics & adolescent medicine, 156(6), 607–614. © John R. Knight, MD, Boston Children's Hospital, 2022. Reproduced with permission from the Center for Adolescent Behavioral Health Research (CABHRe), Boston Children's Hospital. crafft@childrens.harvard.edu http://www.crafft.org. For more information and versions in other languages, see http://www.crafft.org.

Diagnosis

- Substance abuse is defined as consuming larger amounts and for longer periods than intended. Persistent desire to cut down or regulate use.
- Unsuccessful attempts at cutting down in the past
- Spending a great deal of time obtaining, using, or recovering from the effects of substance use
- Persons diagnosed with alcohol use disorder may be deficient in thiamine and magnesium. Lab testing should include thiamine and magnesium levels.
- Detoxification is usually treated with Librium or Valium.

Clinical Management

Lab testing includes CBC, gamma-glutamyl transferase (GGT), AST, ALT levels, and urine drug screen.

Nonpharmacologic

- Referral to 12-step programs (lived experience programs)
- Harm reduction

- CBT, motivational interviewing, contingency management, and mindfulness
- Music-based therapy interventions may help reduce cravings (Megranahan et al., 2023).

Pharmacologic

Pharmacologic treatment falls under the category of harm reduction techniques and is more effective than nonpharmacologic modalities (Megranahan et al., 2023).

Opioid Substitution Therapy

- Buprenorphine with naltrexone (Suboxone) and methadone maintenance are both treatments offered to patients struggling with opioid addiction by blocking the mu (μ) receptors in the brain.
- The medication works by blocking the euphoric effects of alcohol and opioids, relieves physiologic cravings, and normalizes body functions without the negative and euphoric effects.
- There is no maximum recommended duration of maintenance treatment, and it may be indefinite.
- The goal of treatment is complete recovery from opioid dependence.
- There are different risks, benefits, and considerations for each medication.
- Naloxone prescriptions are essential in the case of overdose.
- Treatment options should be discussed with patients, including access, insurance considerations, risk of diversion, feasibility of treatment, and the patient's treatment goals.
- Monitoring for recurrence prevention is essential. Motivational interviewing techniques are effective, including empathy, rolling with resistance, developing discrepancy, and engaging with self-efficacy.

Alcohol Misuse Therapy

- Disulfiram, naltrexone, and acamprosate are used to reduce the cravings for alcohol.
- Alcohol withdrawal syndromes occur within 4 to 48 hours after the last drink and present with tremors, tachycardia, hallucinations, confusion, disorientation, and seizures.

Evaluation and Follow-Up

- Patients receiving medication-assisted treatment should be in psychotherapy or counseling for substance misuse.
- Toxicology urine screens should be done on follow-up visits for opioid use disorder treatment.

Suicide Risk and Prevention

Etiology

Suicide is death caused by injuring oneself with the intent to die. Suicide risk is a multifaceted problem with biologic, genetic, psychological, social, and environmental interactions. Major risk factors are male gender, psychopathology, prior suicide attempt, and means to commit suicide. Protective factors include effective problem-solving, reasons for living, a strong sense of cultural identity, support and connection, religious and moral objection to suicide, and access to high-quality health care.

Suicide Facts

- There is 1 death every 11 minutes due to suicide.
- 12.3 million people have seriously thought about suicide.
- 1.7 million attempted suicide.
- There have been 48,183 deaths by suicide.
- Assessment for suicide is imperative when a provider feels that a patient is at risk. Patients who are depressed should be asked explicitly about suicide. Using the acronym "SAL" assists providers in conducting a risk assessment:
  - **S**pecificity—Is there a suicide plan? How detailed is this plan (time, place, means, intention to write a suicide letter, saying goodbye to family and friends)?
  - **A**vailability—If there is a plan, are the means readily available (access to weapon, medication, etc.)?
  - **L**ethality—Is the plan intended to be lethal? What degree is the lethality (firearm, medication, jumping from a high building)?

Risk Factors

- Race and ethnicity—White males are at the greatest risk; minorities and immigrants are also at risk.
- Age—men over 65, the greatest risk for suicide
- Psychiatric diagnoses
- History of psychiatric hospitalizations
- Previous suicide attempt
- Family history of suicide
- Substance use disorders
- Chronic pain or illness
- Loss or bereavement
- Children and teens on antidepressant treatment may be at risk for suicide, and there is a black box warning on all antidepressants (Li et al., 2022).

Warning Signs
- Impulsive behaviors
- Acute anxiety
- Social isolation
- Changes in sleep patterns
- Lack of future-oriented thinking
- Suicidal planning or gesturing
- Anger, rage

Patient Education and Safety Measures
- Make an emergency referral when the patient is at risk to themselves.
- Create a contract between the provider and the patient that commits to not harming oneself and seeking immediate attention if suicidal thoughts/urges increase.
- Bar access to firearms, sharp objects, and medication (prescribed and over the counter) if the patient is at imminent risk.
- Limit prescription to a 7-day supply if there is a potential danger of overdose.
- Provide emergency contact numbers in case suicidal symptoms increase.
- Avoid 90-day dispenses and automatic refills.

Evaluation and Follow-Up
- Follow up within 24 hours of the appointment.
- Ensure patients and family have access to text or call 988, the national suicide hotline.

Neurodevelopmental Disorders

Etiology
The neurodevelopmental disorders begin in early childhood and may have a wide-ranging impact on brain function. Disorders in this group include intellectual disability, communication disorders, autism spectrum condition, ADHD, specific learning disorder, and motor disorders. There is much comorbidity among these disorders, with a focus on targeted symptom management.

Tourette Syndrome
Tourette syndrome is a persistent tic disorder characterized by tics or unwanted sounds. A tic is a sudden, rapid, and nonrhythmic repetitive motor movement or vocalization.

Tourette Syndrome Facts
- Affects about 1.4 million people.
- Affects 1 in 50 children aged 5 to 14 years.
- Boys are affected more than girls.
- Rates are similar across racial and ethnic groups.

Diagnosis of Tourette Syndrome
For a diagnosis of Tourette syndrome, multiple motor tics and one or more vocal tics must be present at some point (though not necessarily at the same time) *for more than 1 year*. Tics often wax and wane but have persisted in the patient for more than 1 year since onset.

Screening
There are no recommendations for routine screening of Tourette syndrome.

Differential Diagnosis
- Transient tic disorder
- Anxiety
- ADHD
- Autism spectrum disorder
- Cocaine toxicity
- Huntington's disease dementia
- Obsessive-compulsive disorder
- Wilson's disease
- Stimulants

Clinical Management

Nonpharmacologic
Habit reversal therapy is usually the first-line treatment for those who experience an urge or sensation before tics.

Pharmacologic
Typical and atypical antipsychotics can be used to alleviate symptoms. Haloperidol, pimozide, and aripiprazole are FDA approved for tics. Alpha-adrenergic agonists, like guanfacine and clonidine, are also used, although less effective than antipsychotics, but have a safer side-effect profile.

Evaluation and Follow-Up
- Children may need the support of individualized education plans at school.
- Follow-up visit frequency may depend on medication monitoring needs, with antipsychotics requiring closer follow-up:
  - Abdominal girth, BMI.
  - Laboratory monitoring for lipids and blood glucose levels.
  - Assessment for abnormal movements

Autistic Spectrum Condition

According to the CDC, autism spectrum disorder (ASD) affects 1 in 36 children, with a higher risk in males as well as siblings, especially twins (CDC, n.d.c).

Autism Facts

- There is no difference across racial or ethnic groups.
- ASD is 4 times more common in boys than girls.

Diagnosis of Autism

Children must meet the DSM-5 criteria as follows:

- *Social communication:* Deficits in reciprocity, non-verbal communication, and developing and understanding relationships
- *Restrictive/repetitive interests:* Stereotyped or repetitive movements, use of objects, or speech; insistence on sameness; inflexible routines; ritualized patterns or behavior; fixated interests; hyper or hyperreactivity to sensory input

Clinical Presentation/Assessment Findings

Screening

- The CDC recommends screening specifically for ASD at ages 18 and 24 months, with additional screening if behavioral symptoms are present or if there is high risk (i.e., prematurity, sibling with ASD).
- The recommended screening tool for children 16 to 30 months old is the Modified Checklist for Autism Spectrum Disorder in Toddlers (M-CHAT). As with all rating scales, this tool is not diagnostic (**Figure 21-4**). While many children may score as high risk, many will not meet diagnostic criteria following a comprehensive evaluation.

Assessment

- ASD diagnosis requires a multidisciplinary assessment, including referrals to genetics, neurology, audiology, developmental pediatrics or child psychiatry, and speech therapy. Many urban areas have specialized teams that help assess for ASD.
- Physical exam and differential diagnosis for ASD should include evaluations for dysmorphology, seizures, family history, infections (encephalopathy or meningitis), endocrine (hypothyroidism), metabolic (homocystinuria), traumatic (head injury), toxic (fetal alcohol syndrome), and genetic (chromosomal abnormality). Genetic screening should include a G-banded karyotype, Fragile X, and chromosomal microarray.

Differential Diagnosis

- Anxiety
- Obsessive-compulsive disorder
- Rett syndrome
- Prader-Willi syndrome
- Fragile X syndrome
- Lead toxicity
- Down syndrome
- Dissociative identity disorder
- Cri-du-chat syndrome

Clinical Management

Nonpharmacologic

- Comprehensive and early interventions that address core deficits, including social communication, play skills, and maladaptive behavior
  - Applied Behavioral Analysis
  - The Early Start Denver Model
  - Social skills programs
  - Augmentative and alternative communication
  - Behavior momentum intervention
  - Direct instruction
  - Music-medicated intervention
  - Sensory integration
- Many of the interventions require occupational therapy.
- Speech therapy for social pragmatics

Pharmacologic

There is no pharmacologic treatment for ASD itself. Medications are selected on a case-by-case basis to improve target symptoms. Target symptoms may include hyperactivity and inattention, maladaptive behaviors, or sleep. Medications for these symptoms are mostly prescribed off-label. Only risperidone and aripiprazole are FDA approved for treating irritability in ASD, including tantrums and self-injurious behavior.

Evaluation and Follow-Up

- Children will benefit from individualized education plans at school.
- Interdisciplinary referrals are needed for therapies.
- Follow-up visit frequency may depend on medication monitoring needs, with antipsychotics requiring closer follow-up:
  - Abdominal girth, BMI

M-CHAT-R™

Please answer these questions about your child. Keep in mind how your child usually behaves. If you have seen your child do the behavior a few times, but he or she does not usually do it, then please answer **no**. Please circle **yes** or **no** for every question.

1. If you point at something across the room, does your child look at it? Yes No
   (**FOR EXAMPLE**, if you point at a toy or an animal, does your child look at the toy or animal?)
2. Have you ever wondered if your child might be deaf? Yes No
3. Does your child play pretend or make-believe? (**FOR EXAMPLE**, pretend to drink from an empty cup, pretend to talk on a phone, or pretend to feed a doll or stuffed animal?) Yes No
4. Does your child like climbing on things? (**FOR EXAMPLE**, furniture, playground equipment, or stairs) Yes No
5. Does your child make unusual finger movements near his or her eyes? (**FOR EXAMPLE**, does your child wiggle his or her fingers close to his or her eyes?) Yes No
6. Does your child point with one finger to ask for something or to get help? (**FOR EXAMPLE**, pointing to a snack or toy that is out of reach) Yes No
7. Does your child point with one finger to show you something interesting? (**FOR EXAMPLE**, pointing to an airplane in the sky or a big truck in the road) Yes No
8. Is your child interested in other children? (**FOR EXAMPLE**, does your child watch other children, smile at them, or go to them?) Yes No
9. Does your child show you things by bringing them to you or holding them up for you to see — not to get help, but just to share? (**FOR EXAMPLE**, showing you a flower, a stuffed animal, or a toy truck) Yes No
10. Does your child respond when you call his or her name? (**FOR EXAMPLE**, does he or she look up, talk or babble, or stop what he or she is doing when you call his or her name?) Yes No
11. When you smile at your child, does he or she smile back at you? Yes No
12. Does your child get upset by everyday noises? (**FOR EXAMPLE**, does your child scream or cry to noise such as a vacuum cleaner or loud music?) Yes No
13. Does your child walk? Yes No
14. Does your child look you in the eye when you are talking to him or her, playing with him or her, or dressing him or her? Yes No
15. Does your child try to copy what you do? (**FOR EXAMPLE**, wave bye-bye, clap, or make a funny noise when you do) Yes No
16. If you turn your head to look at something, does your child look around to see what you are looking at? Yes No
17. Does your child try to get you to watch him or her? (**FOR EXAMPLE**, does your child look at you for praise, or say "look" or "watch me"?) Yes No
18. Does your child understand when you tell him or her to do something? (**FOR EXAMPLE**, if you don't point, can your child understand "put the book on the chair" or "bring me the blanket"?) Yes No
19. If something new happens, does your child look at your face to see how you feel about it? (**FOR EXAMPLE**, if he or she hears a strange or funny noise, or sees a new toy, will he or she look at your face?) Yes No
20. Does your child like movement activities? (**FOR EXAMPLE**, being swung or bounced on your knee) Yes No

Terminology update, March 2025

Figure 21-4 M-CHAT.

© 2009 Diana Robins, Deborah Fein, & Marianne Barton. See www.mchatscreen.com for permissions of use.

- Laboratory monitoring for lipids and blood glucose levels
- Assessment for abnormal movements

Domestic Violence and Intimate Partner Violence

Etiology

Intimate partner violence (IPV) crosses all lines of ethnicity, age, and class. The Centers for Disease Control and Prevention defines IPV as physical violence, sexual violence, stalking, and psychological aggression (including coercive acts) by a current or former intimate partner. Screening for IPV is paramount within the trusting alliance of the NP–patient relationship to avoid potential death, injury, and long-term physical and emotional health consequences (**Box 21-1**).

Personality Disorders

Etiology

Personality disorders are characterized by maladaptive, inflexible relational patterns that impair a person's global functioning. Genetic, social, environmental, and psychological domains typically influence personality disorders. Personality disorders are commonly encountered in primary care. Symptoms may elicit strong feelings in the primary care provider and may make it challenging to diagnose and treat medical and other psychiatric illnesses. **Table 21-1** provides descriptions of personality disorders.

Diagnosis

- *Antisocial*—Patterns of exploiting others without regard to the boundaries, needs, or feelings of others. Often manipulative, with tendencies toward violence and aggressive behaviors.
- *Avoidant*—Patterns of intense social anxiety and concern about how others perceive them. Fear of rejection and social anxiety impair typical social relationships.
- *Borderline*—Marked by feelings of emptiness and fears of separation. Often impulsive and reckless. Characterized by "splitting," or fluctuating between idealistic adoration of others and intense anger and rage.
- *Dependent*—Self-sacrificing to atypical degree, often submissive, afraid to be alone.
- *Histrionic*—Patterns of overly flirtatious, seductive behaviors meant to draw attention. Often experiences suicidality.
- *Narcissistic Personality Disorder*—Patterns of behavior marked by grandiosity, feeling superior to others. As a result, often exploitative and extremely sensitive to criticism.
- *Obsessive-Compulsive*—Patterns of rigid, inflexible need for correctness and perfectionism. As a result, can be critical of themselves and others.
- *Paranoid*—Mistrusting and suspicious of others. As a result, can become violent and aggressive to others.

Box 21-1 HITS Tool for Intimate Partner Violence Screening

HITS Tool for Intimate Partner Violence Screening: Please read each of the following activities and fill in the circle that best indicates the frequency with which your partner acts in the way depicted.

How often does your partner?

	Never	Rarely	Sometimes	Fairly often	Frequently
1. Physically hurt you?	O	O	O	O	O
2. Insult or talk down to you?	O	O	O	O	O
3. Threaten you with harm?	O	O	O	O	O
4. Scream or curse at you?	O	O	O	O	O
	1	2	3	4	5

Each item is scored from 1-5. Thus, scores for this inventory range from 4-20. A score of greater than 10 is considered positive.

Reproduced from Clinical Research and Methods (Fam Med 1998;30(7):508-12.) HITS is copyrighted in 2003 by Kevin Sherin MD, MPH. For permission to use HITS, email kevin_sherin@doh.state.fl.us.
*HITS is used globally in multiple languages, 2006.

Table 21-1 Descriptions of Personality Disorders

Cluster A—odd or eccentric	Cluster B—dramatic, emotional, or erratic	Cluster C—anxious or fearful
Paranoid - Pervasive pattern of mistrust and suspiciousness - Begins in early adulthood - Presents in a variety of contexts Schizoid - Detachment from social relationships - Restricted range of emotional expressions Schizotypal - Social and interpersonal deficits - Cognitive or perceptual distortions and eccentricities	Antisocial - Disregard for rights of others - Violation of rights of others - Lack of remorse for wrongdoing - Lack of empathy Borderline - Instability of interpersonal relationships, self-image, and affect - Marked impulsivity Histrionic - Excessive emotionality - Attention-seeking behavior Narcissistic - Grandiosity - Need for admiration	Avoidant - Social inhibition - Feelings of inadequacy - Hypersensitivity to criticism Dependent - Excessive need to be taken care of - Submissive behavior - Fear of separation Obsessive-compulsive - Preoccupation with orderliness and perfectionism - Mental and interpersonal control

Data from Widiger, T. A., Hines, A., & Crego, C. (2023). Evidence-Based Assessment of Personality Disorder. Assessment, 31(1), 191-198. https://doi.org/10.1177/1073191123117646

- *Schizoid*—Avoidant and asocial. Tends to keep to self and is extremely reclusive.
- *Schizotypal*—Often possesses odd beliefs, superstitions, and ideas of reference. Struggles socially, with perceptual disorders common.

Clinical Management

There are no lab or diagnostic tests, and a psychiatrist or psychiatric NP typically makes the diagnosis.

Nonpharmacologic
- The most widely used psychotherapy for borderline personality disorder is evidence-based dialectical behavior therapy.
- Schema-focused therapy has the most evidence for borderline personality disorder (Zanarini, 2009).
- Stress management, mindfulness, and yoga are effective treatments.

Pharmacologic
- There are no specific medications for personality disorders.
- Treatments include those for their comorbidities.

Evaluation and Follow-Up

Frequency and intervals depend on medication safety profiles and the need for monitoring.

BRIEF ADULT CASE STUDY

A 66-year-old divorced and retired White male states, "I just can't shake this feeling like I would be better off if I just didn't wake up ever again. The only thing that keeps me going is babysitting my grandson on Thursdays." When asked if he had lost interest in things he previously enjoyed, he replied, "Well, maybe, my appetite is gone. I used to enjoy a six-pack to unwind on Friday nights, but I don't even look forward to that anymore." His medications include sertraline 50 mg daily. His TSH level is 68, but his other labs are normal.

Considerations for the Nurse Practitioner
- White older males are the most likely to end their lives.
- His loss of appetite may be due to an exacerbation of depression.
- The nurse practitioner should ask him directly if he has any suicidal plans and about his means to carry out a plan.
- The nurse practitioner should focus on strengthening his protective factors, such as helping him recognize that he is an asset to his family.

- The nurse practitioner should check his actual medication adherence and ask about side effects.
- He has hypothyroidism and should be started on levothyroxine before intensifying his antidepressant.
- He should be further assessed for alcoholism and/or binge drinking patterns.

BRIEF PEDIATRIC CASE STUDY

A parent brings their 4-year-old to the clinic with a chief complaint of eye blinking. She states that her child has been getting into trouble in his preschool class for talking too much. She is concerned about these changes in his behavior. There have been no changes to his sleep pattern or dietary habits. He is generally well-behaved at home and not very talkative. His height and weight follow his normal curve, and he is afebrile with normal vital signs. His mother states the teacher told her, "He must have ADHD and should go on stimulants." He has a family history of ASD and Tourette syndrome.

Considerations for the Nurse Practitioner
- ADHD diagnoses require that the symptoms present across settings.
- The Vanderbilt screening could be provided, but a diagnosis cannot be confirmed because he does not have the behaviors at home.
- The eye-blinking may be a tic, which could be the result of stress, anxiety, or Tourette syndrome.
- Because he is talkative, he is not likely to need to be screened for autism.
- His mother should be encouraged to meet with his teacher to explore stressors in the child's school environment.

Review Questions

1. A family nurse practitioner (FNP) is seeing a 33-year-old patient for a follow-up visit for her depression. The patient began sertraline (Zoloft) 50 mg 4 weeks ago and reports a partial response. The NP does which of the following?
   A. Increases the dosage
   B. Advises switching to a different medication
   C. Considers augmenting with another agent
   D. Refers to a psychiatric provider

2. A 55-year-old male patient returns for follow-up after starting an antidepressant after one week. He reports occasional headaches and worries that it is not working. The family NP advises all *but* which of the following?
   A. "Side effects are common but often go away in a couple of weeks."
   B. "Successful treatment often involves a dose adjustment."
   C. "Patients typically show improvement in the first week, so it is time to consider a switch."
   D. "Do not stop taking the medication without calling me."

3. A 61-year-old male patient is following up 6 months after discharge from the hospital after having a heart attack. The FNP would like to begin an SSRI for his symptoms of depression. He is also taking clopidogrel (Plavix). The NP proceeds cautiously, recognizing which of the following risks?
   A. Sleep disturbance
   B. Serotonin syndrome
   C. Increased risk of bleeding
   D. Akathisia

4. A patient who is being treated with lithium 600 mg twice daily has a trough lithium level of 0.9 mEq/L. The patient is currently euthymic. The NP does which of the following?
   A. Decreases the medication to prevent toxicity
   B. Discontinues the medication to prevent toxicity
   C. Maintains the current dosage because the plasma level is within range
   D. Maintains the current dosage because the benefit outweighs the risk

5. The FNP orders all but the following lab work for an annual follow-up visit of her patient on lithium treatment.
   A. Thyroid function tests
   B. Urine creatinine
   C. Urine specific gravity
   D. Lipid panel

6. A 19-year-old male college student expresses concerns about being unable to talk to others, avoidance of joining activities he likes, fear of speaking in class, and avoiding approaching professors. His grades are poor due to concentration and lack of participation. His diagnosis is which of the following?
   A. Generalized anxiety disorder (GAD)
   B. Social anxiety disorder
   C. Attention-deficit/hyperactivity disorder (ADHD)
   D. Antisocial personality disorder

7. A 42-year-old female presents for follow-up after two emergency room visits for shortness of breath, heart palpitations, sweating, and fear of dying. A comprehensive workup shows no cause of medical illness. A urine drug screen before the office visit is positive for marijuana. The patient states, "Ativan really helped in the emergency room. Will you continue it?" What does the FNP advise?
   A. "Ativan is a safe and effective treatment for your panic attacks."
   B. "Serotonin reuptake inhibitors (SSRIs) are a better option for the long-term management of your panic disorder."
   C. "Psychotherapy can help you cope with feelings of panic."
   D. "Marijuana may be causing your anxiety or making it worse. Let's talk more about your use."

8. Older adults are at increased risk of impaired cognition and falls due to which of the following medications?
   A. Fluoxetine
   B. Duloxetine
   C. Lorazepam
   D. Buspirone

9. During a well-child visit, the mother of a 17-month-old shares concerns that her daughter is not yet pointing to objects to ask for what she wants and is very difficult to comfort. The FNP takes which of the following as the next step?
   A. Assures the mother that this is typical for a child of her age
   B. Administers the M-CHAT
   C. Administers the ASQ
   D. Schedules a visit in 6 months to see if the child has improved communication

10. A 42-year-old nonverbal male with autism spectrum disorder (ASD) who lives in adult foster care presents with symptoms of increased aggression following recent changes in staffing at the home. Despite modifications to his behavior plan, for the past 2 months, he has been hitting other residents and staff members. He is at risk of losing his placement. The FNP initiates which of the following?
    A. Risperdal 0.5 mg
    B. Prozac 40 mg
    C. Clonazepam 1 mg
    D. Haldol 5 mg

11. A 7-year-old female comes in to see the FNP because she is having problems in school. Her father is concerned that she has attention-deficit/hyperactivity disorder (ADHD) because she has trouble concentrating and sitting still in class. The FNP does what as an initial step?
    A. Observes and documents how the child interacts in the exam room
    B. Sends a validated rating scale to the teacher to obtain collateral information
    C. Prescribes a stimulant medication
    D. Refers the child to a psychiatrist for additional evaluation

12. A 20-year-old college student is home for the summer and schedules an appointment to see his FNP because he is concerned about ADHD. He was previously an A student in high school, but he has noticed that lately he is unmotivated, has trouble concentrating, and has experienced a decline in grades. The FNP:
    A. Suspects depression and requests the student complete a PHQ-9.
    B. Suspects depression and prescribes an antidepressant.
    C. Suspects malingering and calls his mother.
    D. Suspects malingering and orders a random urine drug screen.

13. The FNP is interviewing a 10-year-old female with a recent history of physical abuse. Which of the following symptoms is seen primarily in adults with PTSD but not in children?
    A. Sense of foreshortened future
    B. Unwillingness to speak about the traumatic event
    C. Nightmares
    D. Increased startle response

14. The parents of a 14-year-old with a history of Tourette syndrome are asking about their child's prognosis. Which is the most appropriate response?
    A. "This is a chronic disorder you will likely experience throughout your lifetime."
    B. "Tics typically wax and wane, so you are likely to experience tics throughout your lifetime during stressful periods."
    C. "Most commonly, tics begin to decrease in adolescence. Most people are symptom-free in adulthood, although others will experience tics throughout their lifetime."
    D. "Tics will improve considerably with safe and effective medication."

15. Which of the following patients most urgently requires a follow-up suicide risk screening?
    A. A 30-year-old female who is grieving the loss of her father. She is diagnosed with major depressive disorder.
    B. A 30-year-old male who has a history of multiple psychiatric hospitalizations and who reports he has not attended work for 2 weeks and has avoided friends and family.
    C. A 54-year-old woman who is going through a divorce and is involved in an intense custody battle. She is experiencing intense rage at her children's father.
    D. A 20-year-old male with a history of substance abuse who reports sleep disturbances after beginning sobriety 30 days ago.

16. The NP who is employed at the VA hospital is seeing a 24-year-old male returning from overseas who reports intense nightmares. He is afraid to sleep at night and feels he is functioning poorly both at home and at work. Which of the following is the most appropriate response by the NP?
    A. "I would like to recommend sertraline for your symptoms. Sleep should improve as your symptoms improve."
    B. "I recommend Ativan for sleep since it is a fast-acting medication."
    C. "I would like to refer you to a therapist to help you with your symptoms. In the meantime, I would like to start prazosin to improve sleep and decrease nightmares."
    D. "Cognitive behavioral therapy (CBT) is the best treatment for your symptoms. I would like to refer you to a therapist."

17. Which of the following patients presenting with psychosis would warrant further screening for schizophrenia?
    A. A 19-year-old male presenting with grossly disorganized speech, flat affect, and who appears suddenly suspicious of family and friends.
    B. A 20-year-old male with a history of severe mood disturbances, presenting with rapid speech and grandiosity, telling the office personnel that he has been appointed to solve the country's immigration problem.
    C. A 44-year-old female who is suspicious that her coworkers are trying to sabotage her employment after discovering a handwritten note in her employer's office.
    D. A 35-year-old male with treatment-resistant depression who has begun to experience auditory hallucinations.

18. Which information is accurate regarding screening for intimate partner violence (IPV)?
    A. Typically, IPV occurs in heterosexual relationships.
    B. Low socioeconomic status is stressful, so providers should monitor for IPV more carefully when working with low-income families.
    C. IPV occurs in all ages and ethnicities, regardless of socioeconomic status.
    D. IPV is particularly problematic in same-sex relationships.

19. The NP is seeing a 23-year-old female with borderline personality disorder who reports that she wishes she were dead because her partner just ended a short but intense relationship with her. What is the most appropriate response?
    A. Perform a careful risk assessment even if it appears that she is trying to gain attention and has no plan or intention to harm herself.
    B. Recognize that suicidal ideation and impulsivity are very common in patients diagnosed with borderline personality disorder. Validate her feelings and screen her carefully for intention, plan, and other self-injurious behavior.
    C. Acknowledge her feelings but give little attention to her "acting out" and suicidal threats.
    D. Inform her family of her threats so she can be monitored at home. Give emergency numbers in case suicidality increases.

20. A 30-year-old female reports enjoying a "couple of drinks" when she goes out with friends. This occurs 3 or 4 times a week. She states that she has missed work a few times due to hangovers, and her partner ended their relationship because she didn't like her "partying so much." What is the most appropriate action by the NP?
    A. Explain to her that this behavior is considered at-risk drinking because she is above the recommended limit for alcohol intake for females.
    B. Realize that she has to recognize harmful drinking on her own.
    C. Ask her if she believes the drinking is getting in the way of her job and relationships. Explain to her what harmful drinking means. Perform the CRAFFT and CAGE questionnaire. Screen for other potential substance use.
    D. Refer her for substance misuse treatment.

21. A 13-year-old female presents to the NP's office and reports she has been "hearing voices." The NP screens for psychosis. Which of the following descriptions of the "voice" concerns the treating NP?
    A. "It's like a voice telling me that I am ugly and stupid."
    B. "I hear it a lot. It sounds like a whisper, but then it tells me I should hurt people."
    C. "I only hear the voice when I'm really sad, but it sounds like my mom's voice trying to cheer me up."
    D. "It's the "inner voice" that helps me do the right thing."

22. The NP is seeing a 14-year-old male with a recent onset of both motor and vocal tics who is requesting a medication to "make the tics go away." What is the most appropriate response?
    A. "I can see that the tics are really bothering you. The best thing we can do is start a form of therapy known as 'habit reversal therapy (HRT).' If that doesn't work, then we can try a medication."
    B. "I can see that the tics are really bothering you. Let's try a therapy known as habit reversal therapy and a medication called risperidone, which will help decrease the tics."
    C. "I know the tics are bothering you, but there is a good chance they will go away on their own and we won't need medication."
    D. "Tics are not really a big problem. You can learn how to control it."

23. The NP initiates Lamictal for a patient. Which of the following is critical information that should be shared with the patient?
    A. "We have to monitor routine blood levels for this medication."
    B. "This medication has to be titrated slowly because it can cause agranulocytosis."
    C. "This medication has to be titrated slowly, and you should monitor for signs of a rash."
    D. "This medication can cause infertility."

24. Which of the following classes of medications would the NP avoid if a patient makes the following statement: "I'll take the pills as long as it doesn't interfere with my life too much. I'm not great at following rules."
    A. Selective norepinephrine reuptake inhibitor (SNRI)
    B. SSRI
    C. Second-generation antipsychotics
    D. MAOI

25. Which of the following laboratory tests is NOT required when a patient is receiving therapy with an atypical antipsychotic?
    A. Prolactin
    B. Oral glucose tolerance test
    C. Hepatic panel
    D. Weight

Answers and Rationales

1. Answer A is correct. The next step would be to increase the dosage until a full response is achieved.

    Answer B is incorrect. The patient and clinician must discuss that SSRI therapy may take 2 to 4 weeks before obtaining an effective response.

    Answer C is incorrect. If the patient does not effectively respond to the dosage increase, another agent may be added after 4 to 8 weeks of initial therapy.

    Answer D is incorrect. A psychiatric provider may be beneficial for this patient; however, at this point, the patient does verbalize a partial response to the SSRI therapy, and therefore, it should be continued.

2. Answer C is correct. It generally takes at least 2 weeks to show a response, though for many patients it takes at least 4 to 6 weeks of therapy with an SSRI or an SNRI.

    Answers A, B, and D are all incorrect. These statements are all true regarding the initiation of antidepressant therapy. There may be side effects, a dosage adjustment may be needed, and abruptly stopping the medication may cause discontinuation syndrome (flu-like symptoms including nausea, vomiting, and fatigue).

3. Answer C is correct. Patients taking an SSRI along with an antiplatelet agent are at increased risk of bleeding. While they are not absolute contraindications to be taken together, the NP should weigh the risks of bleeding and untreated depression, monitor INR, and ask the patient to report signs of bleeding promptly.

    Answer A is incorrect. Sleep disturbances are common for patients who have depression or an anxiety disorder. It is often helped by SSRI therapy. Adding Plavix to the SSRI therapy would not cause an increase in sleep disturbance.

Answer B is incorrect. Serotonin syndrome occurs when there is an increased amount of circulating serotonin. This can be the result of adding an SSRI or when weaning from one SSRI to switch to another. Adding Plavix will not cause an increase in serotonin.

Answer D is incorrect. Akathisia is a feeling of nervousness, restlessness, and involuntary movements often manifesting in the legs. It differs from restless leg syndrome in that it occurs during waking hours. First-generation antipsychotic medications primarily cause it and are not attributed to the combination of SSRI therapy with Plavix.

4. Answer C is correct. The recommended therapeutic range of lithium is between 0.5 and 1.2 mEq/L. No dosage adjustment is necessary.

Answer A is incorrect. The patient's lithium level is in a therapeutic range, and therefore, decreasing the dosage would be inappropriate.

Answer B is incorrect. Discontinuing the medication is inappropriate. The patient is euthymic.

Answer D is incorrect. The patient should continue the current dosage because the benefits outweigh the risks associated with lithium therapy. The question stem does not indicate that the patient is experiencing any negative side effects of lithium therapy.

5. Answer D is correct. A lipid panel is not indicated for lithium initiation or maintenance. However, lithium is associated with weight gain, and it is prudent to screen for dyslipidemia in patients who are overweight or obese.

Answer A is incorrect. Lithium increases the secretion of intrathyroidal iodine, inhibiting the release of T3 and T4 and increasing the risk for hypothyroidism. A thyroid function panel should be checked upon initiation, at least annually, and if symptomatic.

Answers B and C are incorrect. Lithium alters sodium transport across cell membranes and increases acute and chronic kidney disease risk. Urine creatinine and urine specific gravity should be checked on initiation, at least annually, and if symptomatic.

6. Answer B is correct. Social anxiety disorder is characterized by intense anxiety and distress around the fear situation; recognition that the fear is unreasonable or excessive; and social, academic, or occupational impairment related to avoidance of activities associated with the fear.

Answer A is incorrect. GAD and social anxiety have a lot of overlap in their symptomology. However, GAD occurs even when the patient is alone and not exposed to social interactions.

Answer C is incorrect. ADHD manifests as not being able to sit still, acting without thinking, interrupting conversations, and excessive talking. Although any thought disorder can overlap, the manifestation of ADHD is not consistent with the withdrawal aspect of social anxiety disorder.

Answer D is incorrect. Antisocial personality disorder is a condition where the person may be manipulative, deceitful, or harmful to others and feels no remorse for their actions.

7. Answer D is correct. Substances such as marijuana may cause symptoms of anxiety and panic. A timeline of psychiatric symptoms and substance use is needed to differentiate psychiatric disorders from a physical cause.

Answer A is incorrect. Benzodiazepines may be used for panic attacks, but they are only used for a short time due to the risks of physical and mental dependence. In this case, it is best first to remove a potentially causative factor for the panic, such as the use of marijuana.

Answer B is incorrect. SSRIs and SNRIs are preferred treatments for panic disorder and may be beneficial for this patient after the potentially causative factor (marijuana) has been removed.

Answer C is incorrect. Psychotherapy, and particularly CBT, is an effective treatment for panic disorder. It should be recommended for this patient if the panic attacks continue despite the discontinuation of marijuana.

8. Answer C is correct. Elder adults are at increased risk of adverse effects, including cognitive impairment, from benzodiazepines.

Answer A is incorrect. Fluoxetine (Prozac) is an SSRI, and although all SSRIs may have many side effects, it is not known to increase the risk of falls or impair cognition in older adults.

Answer B is incorrect. Duloxetine (Cymbalta) is an SNRI. It is an effective treatment for depression, fibromyalgia, and painful diabetic peripheral neuropathy. It is not associated with impaired cognition or increased risk of falls in older adults.

Answer D is incorrect. Buspirone (Buspar) is an anxiolytic used to treat anxiety disorders such as

GAD. Side effects may include movement disorders, nausea, headaches, and difficulty concentrating. It is not associated with impaired cognition or increased risk for falls in older adults.

9. **Answer B is correct.** Early signs of autism spectrum disorder may include deficits in social and communication skills, including not being comforted by others and not pointing or responding to pointing. The M-CHAT may be utilized for toddlers aged 16 to 30 months. While the FNP may call the child back in 6 months, early intervention is of primary importance, and a referral is indicated if a child scores high on developmental screening.

   Answer A is incorrect. These are not typical behaviors for a 17-month-old child.

   Answer C is incorrect. The ASQ assessment is a parent-centered developmental screening tool for assessing delays and acknowledging milestones in children aged 1 month to 5 ½ years. The FNP is concerned that this child exhibits symptoms of autism spectrum disorder, and therefore, the M-CHAT is the effective screening tool to be used for this child.

   Answer D is incorrect. Early intervention and referral are essential for a child with a high M-CHAT score. Therefore, waiting six months is inappropriate for this 17-month-old child.

10. **Answer A is correct.** Risperdal is FDA-approved for the treatment of irritability, including aggression, self-injurious behavior, and temper tantrums, in both adults and children with autism spectrum disorder.

    Answer B is incorrect. SSRIs are used to treat depression and/or anxiety disorders. They are not FDA approved for the treatment of increased aggression.

    Answer C is incorrect. Clonazepam is indicated for short-term management of epilepsy, anxiety, obsessive-compulsive disorder, and panic disorder. It is not appropriate therapy for long-term use and is not approved for the treatment of irritability or aggression.

    Answer D is incorrect. Conventional antipsychotics like haloperidol are used less frequently after the efficacy of the second-generation antipsychotic, such as risperidone, was established and approved by the FDA for the treatment of aggression toward self and others in individuals with autism.

11. **Answer A is correct.** The initial step in diagnosing ADHD is a physical exam that notes behavioral observations. However, symptoms may not be present in a brief office visit.

    Answer B is incorrect as an *initial* step. Further steps include a caregiver interview and obtaining caregiver and teacher rating scales, such as the Conners or Vanderbilt Rating Scales.

    Answer C is incorrect. A stimulant medication, such as Adderall or Ritalin, may be an effective treatment if the child does have ADHD. However, this is not the initial step since the child first must have an accurate diagnosis.

    Answer D is incorrect. The initial step is to evaluate the child's behavior. A psychiatric referral is not necessary.

12. **Answer A is correct.** While a person with ADHD may have difficulty initiating work and completing tasks, a person with depression is more likely to experience decreased motivation and related functional impairment.

    Answer B is incorrect. The FNP may suspect depression, but first needs to do an extensive history and physical examination (PE) to assess the etiology of this patient's lack of motivation and decline in function. Prescribing an antidepressant medication before a diagnosis of depression is inappropriate.

    Answer C is incorrect. The patient is seeking help for a decline in his function that has manifested as a decline in grades. This is not typical of malingering behavior. Calling the patient's mother when the patient is 20 years old is inappropriate and illegal unless the patient requests it and has written HIPAA consent to do so.

    Answer D is incorrect. There is no evidence that the patient is malingering since most malingering behavior is done to seek external benefits, such as avoiding work. There is no evidence that this patient has used any drugs, so ordering a random drug screen would only serve to alienate this patient from the FNP.

13. **Answer A is correct.** Children often do not present with a sense of foreshortened future. The developmental context of the child's perspective is important to consider.

    Answers B, C, and D are typical symptoms seen in children presenting with PTSD.

14. **Answer C is correct.** Tics typically begin to decrease in adolescence. It is important to inform

both children and parents of the prognosis and that there is a chance the child will not experience tics in adulthood.

Answer A is incorrect. Tics may disappear as the child ages into adulthood.

Answer B is incorrect. Although it is true that tics typically wax and wane, this is more common in young children, and there are usually fewer episodes of tics as the child ages into adulthood.

Answer D is incorrect. No medications have been approved for the treatment of the tics seen in Tourette syndrome, and no medications are without side effects. Psycho-behavioral therapy is often the most effective treatment.

15. Answer B is correct. Both social isolation and past psychiatric hospitalization are warning signs of suicide risk.

    Answer A is incorrect. This patient requires additional assessment in the context of safety and suicide risk, but is not as worrisome as the patient identified in answer B.

    Answer C is incorrect. This patient can be assessed for a suicide risk and depression screening but would likely benefit from psycho-behavioral therapy to deal with anger management.

    Answer D is incorrect. This patient should be assessed for depression and suicide risk; however, the patient is currently sober and, therefore, needs support and ongoing therapy to maintain sobriety. This person is at risk for the recurrence of substance misuse.

16. Answer C is correct. Initiating prazosin is the best choice given the patient's report of debilitating nightmares.

    Answer A is incorrect. Sertraline is prescribed for PTSD, but a thorough assessment of PTSD symptoms is warranted before sertraline is initiated.

    Answer B is incorrect. Ativan is highly addictive and not the best choice for this clinical situation.

    Answer D is incorrect. Referring to a therapist is important, given that the patient will need ongoing follow-up care; however, the patient needs immediate therapy to promote sleep.

17. Answer A is correct. This patient is presenting with both positive and negative symptoms typical of schizophrenia.

    Answer B is incorrect. This answer more accurately reflects a patient experiencing a manic episode of bipolar illness.

    Answer C is incorrect. This requires further investigation but does not necessarily reflect paranoid ideation.

    Answer D is incorrect. This requires further follow-up because psychosis can be a symptom of severe depression. The patient is more likely to experience depression with psychotic features.

18. Answer C is correct. IPV is present in all ages, sexual orientations, and ethnicities.

    Answers A, B, and D are incorrect since IPV is present in all ages and sexual orientations and is not more prevalent in low-income families.

19. Answer B is correct. This is the most appropriate therapeutic response. It is important to validate the patient's feelings while screening for suicidality.

    Answers A and C are incorrect and assume that the patient is not at risk, which is a potentially false assumption.

    Answer D is important, but only after responding therapeutically to the patient and assessing for risk.

20. Answer C is correct. Assessing where the patient is regarding at-risk substance misuse behavior is important. The first step should be an honest, nonthreatening conversation, and then an assessment to determine the risk of substance misuse.

    Answer A is incorrect. The best approach to helping this client is to build a therapeutic alliance and perform a complete assessment.

    Answer B is incorrect. The patient has opened a dialogue regarding the effects of her drinking; ignoring this would be inappropriate and potentially harmful.

    Answer D is incorrect. A referral to a substance use specialist will be helpful going forward; however, a thorough assessment of her misuse is essential prior to initiating the referral.

21. Answer B is correct. Auditory hallucinations that are commanding in nature and involve voices instructing the person to harm themselves or others are most concerning and require further assessment and management.

    Answer A is incorrect. Although it is concerning and warrants further assessment, it is not as concerning as command hallucinations with dangerous content that instruct patients to hurt themselves or others.

Answer C is incorrect and not indicative of an auditory hallucination.

Answer D is incorrect and is not an auditory hallucination by definition.

22. Answer A is correct. HRT is first-line therapy. If this fails to result in adequate progress, medication can be considered.

    Answer B is incorrect. Concomitant therapy may be appropriate only after HRT has failed to produce an adequate response.

    Answer C is incorrect. The patient verbalizes that he finds the tics distressing and is seeking help. Telling the patient that the tics will go away on their own in time is not helpful and may not be true.

    Answer D is incorrect. This response invalidates the patient's feelings and is, therefore, not appropriate.

23. Answer C is correct. Lamotrigine (Lamictal) has been known to cause Stevens-Johnson syndrome, a serious and potentially fatal rash.

    Answer A is incorrect. Lamotrigine does not require ongoing blood testing beyond the initial baseline testing that should be done for all mood stabilizing drugs.

    Answer B is incorrect. Lamotrigine does not cause agranulocytosis, and no laboratory monitoring is required.

    Answer D is incorrect. Lamotrigine does not cause infertility.

24. Answer D is correct. MAOIs require that patients avoid foods high in tyramine. These include some cheeses, meats, and soy-based products. Failure to follow these guidelines can result in a hypertensive crisis.

    Answer A is incorrect. SNRI therapy does not require that the patient make changes in diet.

    Answer B is incorrect. SSRI therapy does not require dietary changes. However, the patient needs to be counseled that abrupt withdrawal from an SSRI can lead to discontinuation syndrome, and the NP would need to be consulted if the patient is considering discontinuing the medication.

    Answer C is incorrect. Second-generation antipsychotics are also known as atypical antipsychotics. Second-generation antipsychotics treat both the positive and negative symptoms of schizophrenia. Second-generation antipsychotic medications have a decreased risk of extrapyramidal side effects when compared with first-generation antipsychotics.

25. Answer B is correct. Although a patient should have their glucose monitored while on a second-generation antipsychotic medication, an oral glucose tolerance test is not necessary. Fasting blood glucose and an HgbA1C value would be adequate for monitoring the patient.

    Answers A, C, and D should all be monitored while the patient is taking a second-generation antipsychotic. Weight gain is common. LFTs and prolactin levels should be monitored when clinically appropriate.

Resources

American College of Obstetricians and Gynecologists. (n.d.). *Postpartum depression.* https://www.acog.org/womens-health/faqs/postpartum-depression.

American Psychiatric Association. (2013). *Diagnostic and Statistical Manual of Mental Disorders* (5th ed.). American Psychiatric Association.

American Society of Addiction Medicine (2020). *The ASAM National Practice Guideline for the Treatment of Opioid Use Disorder.* American Society of Addiction Medicine.

Boland, Robert, et al. (2022) *Kaplan & Sadock's Synopsis of Psychiatry* (12th ed.). Lippincott Williams & Wilkins, a Wolters Kluwer business, https://psychiatry.lwwhealthlibrary.com/book.aspx?bookid=3071&sectionid=0

Carbonell, A., Navarro-Perez, J. J., & Mestre, M-V. (2020). Challenges and barriers in mental healthcare systems and their impact on the family: A systematic integrative review. *Health & Social Care in the Community, 28*(5), 1366–1379.

Carlat, D. J. (1998). The psychiatric review of symptoms: A screening tool for family physicians. *American Family Physician, 58*(7), 1617–1624.

Carlat, D. J. (2023). *The psychiatric interview* (5th ed.). Wolters Kluwer Health.

Center for Adolescent Substance Use Research. (2025). *CRAFFT: Substance use screening tool for adolescents.* Retrieved May 6, 2025, from https://crafft.org/

Centers for Disease Control and Prevention. (2022). "Infographic: Identifying Maternal Depression." *CDC Archive*, May 2, 2022. https://archive.cdc.gov/www_cdc_gov/reproductivehealth/vital-signs/identifying-maternal-depression/index.html

Centers for Disease Control and Prevention. (2024, November 19). *Data and statistics on ADHD.* CDC. https://www.cdc.gov/adhd/data/index.html

Centers for Disease Control and Prevention (CDC). (n.d.c). *Autism spectrum disorder (ASD). Data and statistics.* https://www.cdc.gov/autism/data-research/?CDC_AAref_Val=https://www.cdc.gov/ncbddd/autism/data.html

Centers for Disease Control and Prevention (CDC). (n.d.d). *Suicide prevention. risk and protective factors.* https://www.cdc.gov/suicide/risk-factors/?CDC_AAref_Val=https://www.cdc.gov/suicide/factors/index.html

Centers for Disease Control and Prevention (CDC). (n.d.e). *Facts about suicide.* https://www.cdc.gov/suicide/facts/index.html

Centers for Disease Control and Prevention (CDC) (n.d.f). *Tourette syndrome. Data and statistics.* https://www.cdc.gov/tourette-syndrome/data/?CDC_AAref_Val=https://www.cdc.gov/ncbddd/tourette/data.html

Conners, C. K. (2001). Development of the CRS-R. In C. K. Conners (Ed.). *Conners' Rating Scales-Revised* (pp. 83–98). Multi-Health Systems.

Costantini, L., Pasquarella, C., Odone, A., Colucci, M. E … & Amerio, A. (2021). Screening for depression in primary care with Patient Health Questionnaire-9 (PHQ-9): A systematic review. *Journal of Affective Disorders, 279,* 473–483.

Cox, J. L., Holden, J. M., & Sagovsky, R. (1987). Detection of postnatal depression: Development of the 10-item Edinburgh Postnatal Depression Scale. *British Journal of Psychiatry, 150,* 782–786.

Das, S. K., Sampath, A., Zaman, S. U., Pati, A. K., & Atal, S. (2023). Genetic predisposition for the development of lamotrigine-induced Stevens-Johnson syndrome/toxic epidermal necrolysis: A systematic review and meta-analysis. *Future Medicine, 20*(2). https://www.doi.org/10.2217/pme-2022-0126

Dhalla, S., & Kopec, J. A. (2007). The CAGE questionnaire for alcohol misuse: A review of reliability and validity studies. *Clinical and Investigative Medicine, 30*(1), 33–41.

Dome, P., Rihmer, Z., & Gonda, X. (2019). Suicide risk in bipolar disorder: a brief review. *Medicina, 55*(8), 403.

Edinoff, A. N., Nix, C. A., Hollier, J., Sagrera, C. E., Delacroix, B. M., et al. (2021). Benzodiazepines: Uses, dangers, and clinical considerations. *Neurology International, 13*(4), 594–607.

Hirota, T., & King, B. H. (2023). Autism spectrum disorder. A review. *Journal of American Medical Association, 329*(1), 157–168.

Hirschfeld, R. M., Calabrese, J. R., Weissman, M. M., Reed, M., Davies, M. A., Frye, M. A., Keck, P. E., Jr, Lewis, L., McElroy, S. L., McNulty, J. P., & Wagner, K. D. (2003). Screening for bipolar disorder in the community. *The Journal of Clinical Psychiatry, 64*(1), 53–59. https://doi.org/10.4088/jcp.v64n0111

Hirschfeld, R. M., Holzer, C., Calabrese, J. R., Weissman, M., Reed, M., … & Hazard, E. (2003). Validity of the mood disorder questionnaire: A general population study. *American Journal of Psychiatry, 160*(1), 178–180.

Howard, L. M., & Khalifeh, H. (2020). Perinatal mental health: A review of progress and challenges. *World Psychiatry, 19*(3), 313–327.

Kabir, K., Sheeder, J., & Kelly, L. S. (2008, September). Identifying postpartum depression: Are 3 questions as good as 10? *Pediatrics, 122*(3):e696–702. doi:10.1542/peds.2007-1759. PMID: 18762505.

Li, K., Zhou, G., Xiao, Y., Gu, J., Chen, Q., et al. (2022). Risks of suicidal behavior and antidepressant exposure among children and adolescents: A meta-analysis of observational studies. *Frontiers Psychiatry, 26*(13). https://www.doi.org/10.3389/fpsyt.2022.880496

Lowe, B., Decker, O., Muller, S., Brahler, E., Schellberg, D., Herzog, W., & Herzberg, P. Y. (2008). Validation and standardization of the generalized anxiety disorder screener (GAD-7) in the general population. *Medical Care, 46*(3), 266–274.

Missler, M. A., van Straten, A., Denissen, J. J. A., Donker, T. & Beijers, R. (2020). Effectiveness of a psycho-educational intervention for expecting parents to prevent postpartum parenting stress, depression and anxiety: A randomized controlled trial. *BMC Pregnancy and Childbirth, 20,* Article No. 658. https://doi.org/10.1186/s12884-020-03341-9

Megranahan, K., Megranahan, D., & Cooper, A. (2023). Non-pharmacological interventions for problematic substance use: A rapid overview of Cochrane Systematic Reviews. *International Journal of Mental Health Addiction.* https://doi.org/10.1007/s11469-023-01090-2

Miller, J. N., & Black, D. W. (2020). Bipolar disorder and suicide: A review. *Current Psychiatry Reports, 22,* 1–10.

National Institute of Mental Health (NIMH) (n.d.a). *Major depression.* https://www.nimh.nih.gov/health/statistics/major-depression.

National Institute of Mental Health (NIMH) (n.d.b). *Bipolar disorder.* https://www.nimh.nih.gov/health/statistics/bipolar-disorder

National Institute of Mental Health (NIMH) (n.d.c). *Post-traumatic stress disorder.* https://www.nimh.nih.gov/health/statistics/post-traumatic-stress-disorder-ptsd

National Institute of Mental Health (NIMH). (n.d.d). *Any anxiety disorder.* https://www.nimh.nih.gov/health/statistics/any-anxiety-disorder

National Institute of Mental Health (NIMH) (n.d.e). *Attention-deficit/hyperactivity disorder (ADHD).* https://www.nimh.nih.gov/health/statistics/attention-deficit-hyperactivity-disorder-adhd#:~:text=The%20overall%20prevalence%20of%20current%20adult%20ADHD%20is,aged%2018%20to%2044%20years%20was%208.1%25.%206

National Institute of Mental Health (NIMH) (n.d.f). *Disruptive mood dysregulation disorder.* https://www.nimh.nih.gov/health/topics/disruptive-mood-dysregulation-disorder-dmdd

Nemeroff, C. (2020). The state of our understanding of the pathophysiology and optimal treatment of depression: Glass half full or half empty? *American Journal of Psychiatry, 177*(8), 671–685.

Nestsiarovich, A., Gaudiot, C. E. S., Baldessarini, R. J., Vieta, E., & Zhu, Y. (2022). Preventing new episodes of bipolar disorder in adults: Systematic review and meta-analysis of randomized controlled trials. *European Neuropsychopharmacology, 54,* 75–89.

O'Connor, E. A., Perdue, L. A., Coppola, E. L., Henninger, M. L., Thomas, R.G., et al. (2023). Depression and suicide risk screening. Updated evidence report and systematic review for the U.S. Preventive Services Task Force. *Journal American Medical Association, 329*(23), 2068–2085.

Palagini, L., Manni, R., Aguglia, E., Amore, M., Brugnoli, R., Bioulac, S., Bourgin, P., Micoulaud Franchi, J. A., Girardi, P., Grassi, L., Lopez, R., Mencacci, C., Plazzi, G., Maruani, J., Minervino, A., Philip, P., Royant Parola, S., Poirot, I., Nobili, L., Biggio, G., … Geoffroy, P. A. (2021). International Expert Opinions and Recommendations on the Use of Melatonin in the Treatment of Insomnia and Circadian Sleep Disturbances in Adult Neuropsychiatric Disorders. *Frontiers in Psychiatry, 12,* 688890. https://doi.org/10.3389/fpsyt.2021.688890

Prins, A., Ouimette, P., Kimerling, R., Cameron, R. P., Hugelshofer, D. S., Shaw-Hegwer, J., … & Sheikh, J. I. (2003). The primary care PTSD screen (PC-PTSD): Development and operating characteristics (PDF). *Primary Care Psychiatry, 9,* 9–14. https://www.ptsd.va.gov/professional/articles/article-pdf/id26676.pdf

Prins, A., Ouimette, P., Kimerling, R., Cameron, R. P., Hugelshofer, D. S., Shaw-Hegwer, J., … & Sheikh, J. I. (2004). The primary care PTSD screen (PC-PTSD): Corrigendum (PDF). *Primary Care Psychiatry, 9,* 151.

Spitzer, R. L., Williams, J. B. W., & Kroenke, K. (1999). *Patient Health Questionnaire (PHQ-9)*. Pfizer Inc. https://www.med.upenn.edu/cbti/assets/user-content/documents/phq-9.pdf.

Stahl, S. M. (2021). *Stahl's essential psychopharmacology: Neuroscientific basis and practical applications* (5th ed.). Cambridge University Press.

Steinbrenner, J. R., Hume, K., Odom, S. L., Morin, K. L., Nowell, S. W., Tomaszewski, B., Szendrey, S., McIntyre, N. S., Yücesoy-Özkan, S., & Savage, M. N. (2020). *Evidence-based practices for children, youth, and young adults with autism*. The University of North Carolina at Chapel Hill, Frank Porter Graham Child Development Institute, National Clearinghouse on Autism Evidence and Practice Review Team. Retrieved May 6, 2025, from https://files.eric.ed.gov/fulltext/ED609029.pdf

Swartz, H. A., & Swanson, J. (2014). Psychotherapy for bipolar disorder in adults: A review of the evidence. *Focus (American Psychiatric Publishing), 12*(3), 251–266.

U.S. Department of Veterans Affairs (USDVA) (n.d.a). PTSD: National center for PTSD. *Clinician's guide to medications for PTSD*. https://www.ptsd.va.gov/professional/treat/txessentials/clinician_guide_meds.asp

U.S. Department of Veterans Affairs (USDVA) (n.d.b). PTSD: National center for PTSD. *Overview of psychotherapy for PTSD*. https://www.ptsd.va.gov/professional/treat/txessentials/overview_therapy.asp

Volkmar, F., Siegel, M., Woodbury-Smith, M., King, B., McCracken, J., & State, M. (2014). Practice parameter for the assessment and treatment of children and adolescents with autism spectrum disorder. *Journal of the American Academy of Child and Adolescent Psychiatry, 53*(2), 237–257.

Walter, H. J., Bukstein, O. G., Albright, A. R., Keable, H., Ramtekkar, U., ... & Rockhill, C. (2020). Clinical practice guidelines for the assessment and treatment of children and adolescents with anxiety disorders. *Journal of the American Academy of Child & Adolescent Psychiatry, 59*(10), 1107–1124.

Wolraich, M. L., Lambert, W., Doffing, M. A., Bickman, L., Simmons, T., & Worley, K. (2003). *Vanderbilt ADHD Diagnostic Parent Rating Scale (VADPRS)* [Database record]. APA PsycTests. https://doi.org/10.1037/t67076-000

Zanarini, M. C. (2009). Psychotherapy of borderline personality disorder. *Acta psychiatrica Scandinavica, 120*(5). https://www.doi.org/10.1111/j.1600-0447.2009.01448.x

PART V

Practice Exams

Congratulations on completing Parts I through IV of the *Family Nurse Practitioner Certification Review Guide, Second Edition*! You are reaching a critical moment in your career: board certification.

To help you prepare for the board certification exam, Navigate TestPrep is an online testing engine designed to help you practice and assess your knowledge at your own pace (**Figure V-1**). Every new print copy includes access to Navigate TestPrep. If your textbook does not contain access to purchase a code, please contact Jones & Bartlett Learning's Customer Service Department at customerservice@jblearning.com or 1-800-832-0034.

Navigate TestPrep provides questions designed specifically for family nurse practitioner certification exams, providing the best, most realistic test prep experience. It aligns with the blueprints for the American Nurses Credentialing Center Examination (ANCC) and American Academy of Nurse Practitioner Certification Board (AANPCB) family nurse practitioner certification examinations.

With more than 780 questions, this Navigate TestPrep offers the right resources to pass your board certification exam and prepare for your career.

Navigate TestPrep

The *Navigate TestPrep for Family Nurse Practitioner Certification Review Guide, Second Edition*, includes practice tests, predictor exams, and complete assessment tests, as described below.

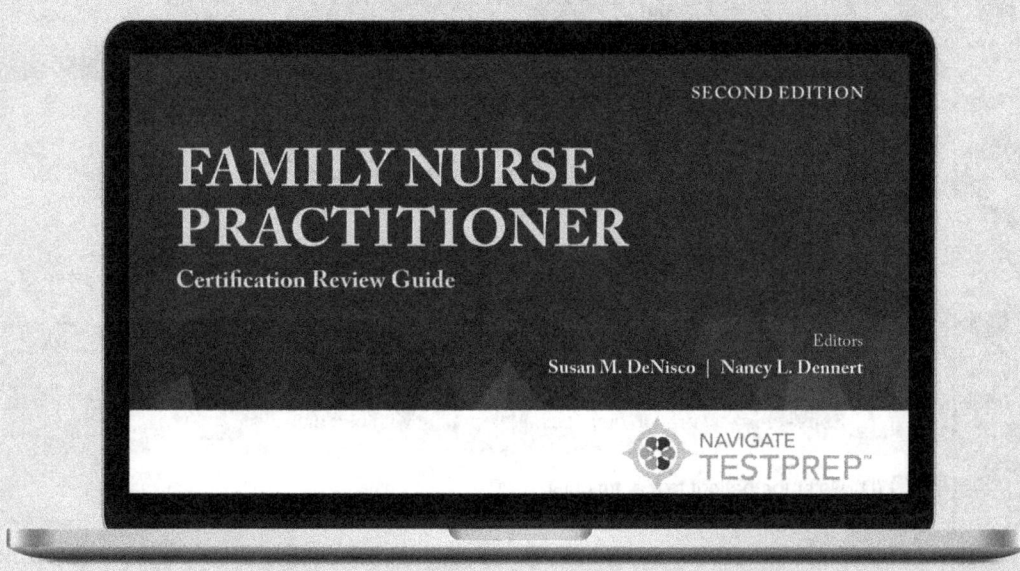

Figure V-1 Navigate TestPrep.

Practice Tests

The **Chapter Review Questions** from the printed text are provided as practice tests in the online environment.

- Select a specific topic or create a randomized practice test (**Figure V-2**).
- Choose tutorial mode or test mode.

Various features include a timer, calculator, confidence meter, notes area, the ability to flag questions you wish to revisit, and the ability to choose exactly how many questions you want to include in your practice test.

Practice tests provide immediate feedback, helping you identify where to focus your study (**Figure V-3**).

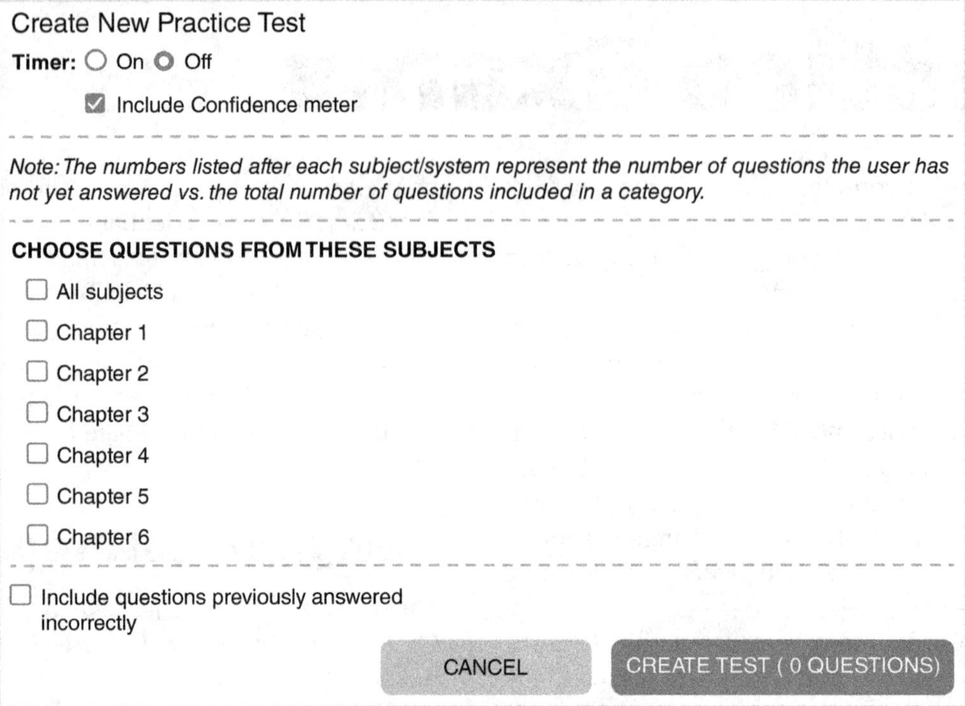

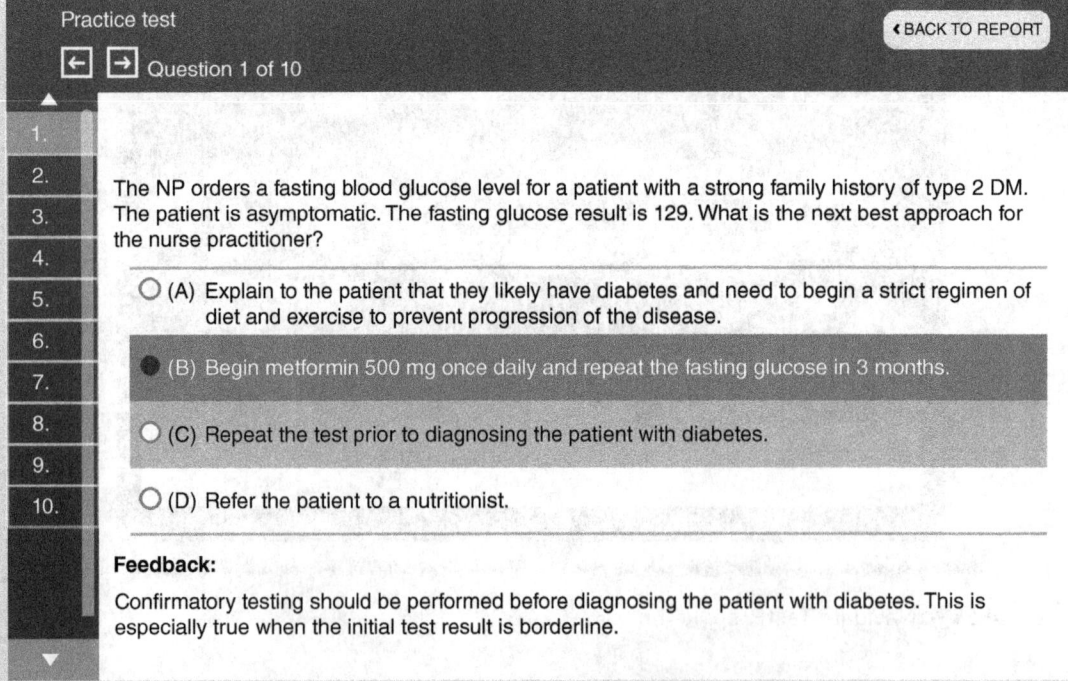

Figure V-2 Sample of creating a practice test in Navigate TestPrep.

Figure V-3 Sample of question feedback in Navigate TestPrep.

AANPCB and ANCC Predictor Exams

Navigate TestPrep for Family Nurse Practitioner Certification Review Guide, Second Edition, offers two predictor exams engineered like the ANCC and AANPCB family nurse practitioner certification exams.

To set the stage for your greatest success, this Navigate TestPrep is predictive of the ANCC and AANPCB certification exams, with questions covering all domains in the same percentage as the actual certification exams. Domains covered in the TestPrep include:

- Assessment (both ANCC and AANPCB)
- Diagnosis (both ANCC and AANPCB)
- Clinical management: Planning and Implementation (both ANCC and AANPCB)
- Evaluation and procedures (AANPCB)
- Professional role (ANCC)

Complete Assessment Tests

The Navigate TestPrep includes a complete assessment test in an online test-taking environment similar to the board exams, so you know what to expect on test day.

To generate the complete assessment test, a random assortment of questions is pulled from all Practice Tests (including the predictor exams).

Feedback is delivered after completing the exam to more closely mimic an actual exam (**Figure V-4**). Practice as many times as you like.

Best of luck!

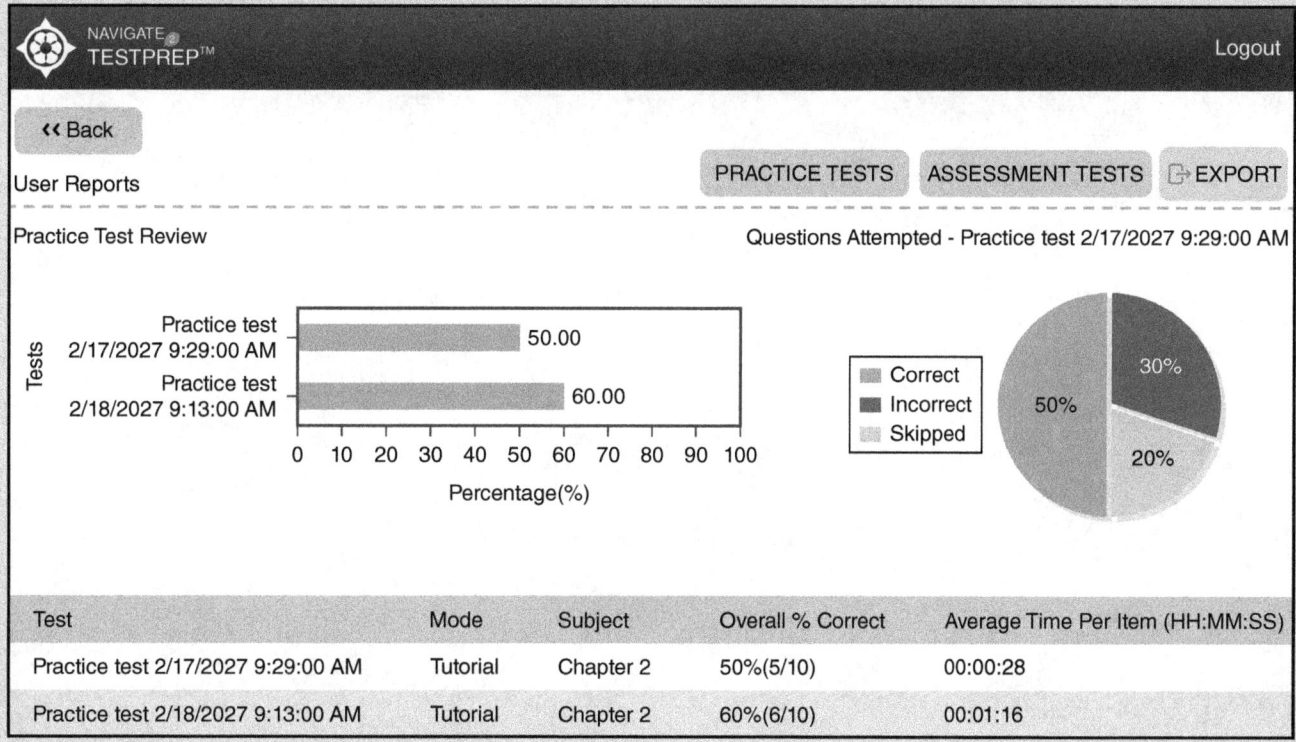

Figure V-4 Sample user report from Navigate TestPrep.

Index

Note: Page numbers followed by b, f, or t indicate material in boxes, figures, or tables, respectively.

A

abdominal aortic aneurysm (AAA), 41
   cauda equina syndrome, 203
   clinical lumbar instability, 203
   spinal stenosis, 202
   spondylolisthesis, 202
abdominal pain, 165
Abnormal Involuntary Movement Scale (AIMS), 437, 438–439f
abnormal uterine bleeding
   clinical management, 339
   clinical presentation, 339
   etiology, 339
   evaluation and follow-up, 339
absorption, overview, 353–354
abuse, child. See child abuse
AC joint injury/dislocation, 197
acarbose (Precose), 239
Accreditation Commission for Education in Nursing (ACEN), 18
achilles tendinopathy, 192
acid-fast bacilli (AFB), 131
ACL. See anterior cruciate ligament (ACL)
acne vulgaris, 309–310
actinic keratosis, 308
activated partial thromboplastin time (aPTT), 339
Actos (pioglitazone)
   for diabetes mellitus, 239
acute abdomen, in older adults, 416
acute bronchitis, 133–134
   in pediatrics, 390
acute cervical disc herniation/radiculopathy, 205
acute kidney injury (AKI)
   evaluation of, 277
   follow-up, 278
   prevention of, 278
   signs/symptoms of, 277
   treatment for, 277–278

acute otitis media (AOM)
   complications of, 90
   defined, 88
   diagnostic studies, 90
   differential diagnosis, 89
   etiology of, 88
   expected course, 86
   historical data, 89
   incidence of, 88
   indications for referral, 86
   management of, 90
   patient education, 92
   physical assessment, 89
   risk factors of, 88–89
acute pharyngitis
   clinical Pearls, 98
   defined, 98
   etiology of, 98
   incidence of, 98
   risk factors of, 98
acute rhinosinusitis (ARS)
   classification of, 93
   complications of, 93, 94
   defined, 93
   diagnostic studies, 72
   differential diagnosis of, 94
   etiology of, 93
   follow-up, 94
   historical of, 94
   indications for referral, 94
   management of, 94
   patient education, 95
   physical assessment, 94
acute stomatitis
   etiology of, 96
   incidence of, 96
   indications for referral, 98
   management of, 97
acyanotic defects, 385–386
Acyclovir (Zovirax), 69, 291
Addison's disease, 244–245
adhesive capsulitis/frozen shoulder, 197

adolescent
   physical growth and development, 382
   respiratory rate, 383t
   social and emotional development, 382–383
adrenal disorders, 244–245
adults
   diabetes mellitus in, 235–236
   referral, red flags for, 218
advance care planning, of older adults, 416
Advanced Practice Registered Nurse (APRN), 18
advanced practice state licensure, 19–20
adverse drug events (ADEs), 409
adverse drug reaction (ADR), 58
Advisory Committee on Immunization Practices (ACIP), 37, 126
Affordable Care Act (ACA), 21, 406
Agency for Healthcare Research and Quality (AHRQ), 57
agoraphobia, 441
alanine aminotransferase (ALT), 166
alcohol, use of, 443
alkaline phosphatase, 166
allergic conjunctivitis, 101
allergic rhinitis
   defined, 95
   diagnostic studies, 96
   differential diagnosis of, 96
   follow-up, 98
   incidence of, 95
   indications for referral, 98
   management of, 96
   physical assessment, 95
   risk factors of, 95
allied health provider, 23
allopurinol, for uric acid stones, 276
alopecia areata, 314
alpha-fetoprotein (AFP), 345
alpha-glucosidase inhibitors, for diabetes mellitus, 239

alpha thalassemia, 257
Alzheimer's disease (AD), 222–223
   depression in, 412
   moderate AD, 223
   treatment for, 223
amenorrhea
   clinical management, 338–339
   etiology, 338
   evaluation and follow-up, 339
American Academy of Nurse Practitioner Certification Board (AANPCB), 3
American Academy of Pediatrics (AAP), 381
American Association of Colleges of Nursing (AACN), 17, 18, 22
American Association of Nurse Practitioners (AANP), 22–23
American Cancer Society (ACS), 37, 368
American College of Cardiology (ACC), 414
American College of Obstetrics and Gynecology (ACOG), 37
American Diabetes Association and American Geriatrics Society, 414
American Heart Association (AHA), 414
American National Standards Institute, 86
American Nurses Credentialing Center Examination (ANCC), 3, 4
amoxicillin, for urinary tract infections, 274
ampicillin, for meningitis, 221–222
anal fissures, 179–180
anatomy
   breasts, 325
   cervix, 325
   ovaries, 326
   uterus, 325
anemia, 255, 256t
   aplastic, 257, 263, 264
   of chronic disease, 259–260
   Cooley's. *See* thalassemia major
   G6PD deficiency, 260–261
   hemolytic, 260
   iron deficiency, treatment of, 257
   macrocytic, 258
   microcytic, 257
   normocytic, 259–261
   sickle cell, 261
   vitamin B12 deficiency, 258
anemia of chronic disease (ACD), 259–260
angioedema, 81

angiotensin converting enzyme (ACE) inhibitor, 7, 63
   for blood pressure, 236
   for GFR, 277
angiotensin receptor blocker (ARB), 63
   for blood pressure, 237
   for GFR, 277
angle closure glaucoma, 103
ankle sprain lateral/medial, 193
ankylosing spondylitis, 201
anticoagulants, 65, 66t
   for epistaxis, 92
   for stroke, 220
anticonvulsants
   for disruptive mood dysregulation disorder, 433
   for prophylaxis, 225
antidepressants
   for breast-feeding women, 431
   for prophylaxis, 225
antimalarials
   and G6PD deficiency anemia, 261
antimicrobials, 66–67
   antibiotics, 67
   antifungals, 67–69
   antivirals
      influenza, 69
      oral, 69
      topical, 69
antipsychotics
   for disruptive mood dysregulation disorder, 433
   first-generation, 436–437
   second-generation, 437
antiretroviral therapy (ART), 297
antisocial personality disorder, 449
anxiety disorders
   assessment, 440
   management, 442
   screening, 440
aorta, coarctation of, 387
aortic regurgitation, 138
aortic stenosis (AS), 144, 386
aphthous stomatitis, 96
   complications of, 97
   defined, 96
   diagnostic studies, 97
   differential diagnosis of, 97
   follow-up, 98
   physical assessment, 97
   prevention/patient education, 96–98
   risk factors of, 97
apixaban, for stroke, 220
appendicitis, 170–171
APRN Compact Model, 19
APRN Joint Dialogue Group Report, 19
aspartate aminotransferase (AST), 166
Aspergillus, 91

aspirin, for stroke, 220
asthma, 117
   assessment of control, 124
   asthma-related death, risk factors for, 121t
   classifications of severity, 117
   clinical pearl, 124
   defined, 117
   diagnosing asthma, 121t
   diagnostic testing, 121
   measures of severity, 121
   in pediatrics, 388
   signs of severity, 119
   treatment, 122
   viral respiratory infection, 122
Asthma Control Questionnaire (ACQ), 124
Asthma Control Test (ACT), 124
at-risk drinking, 444
atopic dermatitis, 311
atrial fibrillation
   diagnostics of, 155
   etiology, 154
   prevention, 155
   treatment, 155
atrial-septal defect (ASD), 385–386
atrioventricular septal defect (AVSD), 386
atrophic rhinitis, 96
atrophic vaginitis
   clinical management, 335
   clinical presentation, 334–335
   etiology, 334
atrophy, 307
attention-deficit/hyperactivity disorder (ADHD), 434–435
   hyperactivity and impulsivity, 434
   inattention, 434
   nonpharmacologic treatment, 435
   pharmacologic treatment, 435
atypical presentation of acute illness, in older adults, 415
Atypical Squamous Cells of Undetermined Significance (ASCUS), 327
autistic spectrum disorder
   assessment, 447
   diagnosis of, 447
   screening, 447, 447f
Avandia (rosiglitazone), for diabetes mellitus, 239
avoidant personality disorder, 449
azithromycin, 288

Baby Friendly Hospital Initiative, 385
bacterial conjunctivitis, 101

bacterial pharyngitis, assessment of, 98–99
bacterial vaginosis
  clinical management, 337
  clinical presentation, 337
  etiology, 337
  evaluation and follow-up, 337
bactrim, for urinary tract infections, 274
Baloxavir (Xofluza), 69
bamboo spine, 201
Barlow maneuver, 385
Barrett's Esophagus, 168
basal cell, 308–309
basopenia, 263
basophilia, 263
beclomethasone, 177
Bell's palsy, 226
benign paroxysmal positional vertigo (BPPV), 82–84
  defined, 82
  diagnostic studies of, 83
  etiology of, 83
  expected course, 84
  historical data, 83
  incidence/prevalence of, 83
  indications for referral, 84
  management of, 83
  patient education, 84
  physical assessment of, 57
  risk factors, of, 83
benign prostatic hypertrophy, 3 66–367
benzathine penicillin G, 294
benzodiazepines, for anxiety disorders, 442
beta thalassemia, 257
biguanides, for diabetes mellitus, 238
bilateral heel pain, 192
bipolar disorder, 431–432
blood pressure
  assessment, for diabetes mellitus, 236–237
  of children, 383t
blood pressure (BP), 330
blood urea nitrogen (BUN), 367
blue bloaters, 125
body mass index (BMI), 383
borderline personality disorder, 449
boutonniere deformity, 198–199
Bowen's disease. See squamous cell carcinoma in situ
brain tumors, 219
breast, fibrocystic changes of
  clinical management, 333
  clinical presentation, 333
  etiology, 332–333
  evaluation and follow-up, 333

breast cancer
  clinical management, 333–334
  clinical presentation, 333
  etiology, 333
  evaluation and follow-up, 334
breastfeeding, 354–355, 385
brief psychotic disorder, 436
bright Futures, 381
bronchiolitis, in pediatrics, 389
Brudzinski's sign, 221
bulla, 307
bullous impetigo, 392
bullous myringitis, 89
bupropion (Wellbutrin), for attention-deficit/hyperactivity disorder, 435
buspirone, for anxiety disorders, 442
Byetta (exenatide), for diabetes mellitus, 238

C

CAGE questionnaire, 444–445
cancer antigen (CA) 125, 6
Candida, 97
*Candida albi*cans, 91, 96
*Candida glab*rata, 96
*Candida tropic*alis, 96
caput succedaneum, physical examination of, 385
carbamazepine (Tegretol)
  for disruptive mood dysregulation disorder, 433
  for trigeminal neuralgia, 226
carcinoembryonic antigen (CEA), 6
cardiovascular disease (CVD), 40–41
cardiovascular disorders, primary care, 143–157
carpal tunnel syndrome, 198
cataracts, 103
cauda equina syndrome, 203
cefoxitin, 288
ceftriaxone, 288
cellulitis, 310
Centers for Disease Control (CDC), 37, 61
Centers for Medicare and Medicaid Services (CMS), 20, 406, 407
centor criteria, 99
cephalohematoma, physical examination of, 384
cephalosporin
  first-generation for urinary tract infections, 274
  third-generation for meningitis, 221–222
cerebrovascular accident (CVA), 343, 329

Certification, 3
  body system, primary care diagnoses on, 4
  retaking, of, 7
certified nurse midwives (CNMs), 19
certified nurse practitioners (CNPs), 19
certified registered nurse anesthetists (CRNAs), 19
cervical spine
  acute cervical disc herniation/radiculopathy, 205
  spinal stenosis, 205–206
  torticollis, 205
chalazion, 104–105
Charcot neuropathic osteoarthropathy, 192–193
chest pain
  in children, 387
  evaluation of, 152–154
chest radiography, 127
child abuse
  differential diagnoses, 394
  emotional, 393
  physical, 393
  role of FNP, 393–394
  sexual, 393
children, diabetes mellitus in, 236
Chlamydia trachomatis, 98, 287, 288
chlamydial infections
  etiology of, 287
  evaluation of, 288
  follow-up, 288
  present illness, history of, 287
  risk factors of, 288
cholecystitis, 166–167
cholescintigraphy (HIDA scan), 166–167
cholesterol assessment, for diabetes mellitus, 237
cholesterol management
  assessment, 149–150
  follow-up, 150–152
  goals, 149
  initiation of statin therapy, 150t
  treatment, 150
cholinesterase inhibitor
  for Alzheimer's disease, 223
  for neurocognitive disorders, 411
chronic bronchitis, 125–126, 126t
chronic cough, 133, 133t
chronic disease, older adults and, 413–414
chronic kidney injury (CKI)
  evaluation of, 277
  follow-up, 278
  prevention of, 278
  stages of, 278t
  treatment for, 277–278

chronic obstructive pulmonary
    disease (COPD), 7, 64,
    124–125
  cause of, 124
  chest X-ray findings of, 131, 132t
  chronic bronchitis, 125–126, 126t
  classification of COPD severity,
    GOLD guidelines, 126t
  COPD Assessment Test, 126
  emphysema, 125
  follow-up and education, 126
  management and treatment of, 126
  pulmonary rehabilitation, 126
  severity, 125
  symptoms of, 117
ciprofloxacin, for meningitis, 222
clinical lumbar instability, 203
clinical nurse specialists (CNSs), 19
clonidine (Catapres), for
    attention-deficit/hyperactivity
    disorder, 435
clopidogrel, for stroke, 220
clostridium difficile, 177
  infection, 170
cluster headache, 225
coagulopathies, 65
coarctation of aorta, 387
cochlea, 81, 86
Code of Federal Regulations, Section
    1300.01(b28), 20
cognitive behavioral therapy
    (CBT), 356
  for disruptive mood dysregulation
    disorder, 442
  for major depressive disorder
    and persistent depressive
    disorder, 427
colon cancer
  clinical manifestations of, 172
  defined, 172
  differential diagnosis of, 172
  treatment and follow-up, 172–173
Commission on Collegiate Nursing
    Education (CCNE), 18
communication techniques, of older
    adults, 406
community acquired pneumonia
    (CAP), 7, 127–128, 128t
  chest radiography, 127
  diagnosing, 127–128
  physical examination findings, 128
  treatment for, mycoplasma
    pneumonia, 128
compartment syndrome, 193
complete blood count (CBC),
    339, 366
concussion, 206, 220–221
conductive hearing loss, 85

congenital heart defects (CHD), in
    pediatrics
  acyanotic defects, 385–386
  aortic stenosis, 386
  chest pain, 387
  coarctation of aorta, 387
  cyanotic defects, 386
  hypertension, 388
  hypertrophic obstructive
    cardiomyopathy, 387
  innocent murmurs, 387
  primary care for, 387
  pulmonic stenosis, 386–387
  tetralogy of fallot, 386
  tricuspid atresia, 386
conjunctivitis, 101–102
Conners Rating Scale, 434
Consensus Model, 19
constipation, 167
contraception, 355–356
  combined harmonal contraceptives
    advantages, of, 329
    barrier methods, 331–332
    contraindications, to, 329
    disadvantages, of, 329–330
    intrauterine device, 331
    overview, 328–329
    progesterone-only, 330–331
Cooley's anemia. See thalassemia major
COPD Assessment Test (CAT), 126
corneal abrasion, 104
corneal foreign body, 104
coronary artery disease, 153–154
corticosteroids, for temporal
    arteritis, 226
Corynebacterium, 98
costochondritis (rib dysfunction), 203
cough, 133
coxsackievirus, 392
cranial nerves, 217–218
Crohn's disease, 178
croup, 389
crust, 307
cryptorchidism, 369
Cullen's sign, 166
Cushing's syndrome (CS), 245
cyanotic defects, 386
cyclosporine, 177
cyclothymic disorder, 432
cysts, 307, 310
cytochrome P450 (CYP450), 56

D

dabigatran, for stroke, 220
DEA Drug Scheduling, 54t
death, leading causes of older adults, 403

deep vein thrombosis (DVT), 65
deepest vertical pocket (DVP), 349
degenerative joint disease (DJD), 200
degenerative lumbar disc disease, 201
dehydroepiandrosterone (DHEA), 341
delirium, 223, 410
dementia, 222
  frontotemporal, 223
  with Lewy body, 223
  vascular, 223
dependent personality disorder, 449
depigmentation, general patterns
    of, 314
depression, 412
dermatitis, 310–311
dermatophytosis, 313
diabetes, 414
  in pregnancy. See gestational
    diabetes (GDM)
diabetes mellitus
  ABC's of, 236–237
  in adults, 235–236
  in children, 236
  diagnosis of, 235
  facts, 235
  pharmacologic agents for, 239–241
  screening recommendations for,
    235–236
  types of, 236
diabetic ketoacidosis (DKA), 237
The Diagnostic and Statistical Manual
    of Mental Disorders, 5th edition
    (DSM-5), 410
diastolic BP (DBP), 329
digital rectal exam (DRE), 368
diphenhydramine, 392
diplopia, 81
dipyridamole, for stroke, 220
disease prevention, 37
disequilibrium, 82
disruptive mood dysregulation
    disorder, 432
distal radius fracture, 198
diverticulitis, 171–172
Docosanol (Abreva), 69
domestic violence, 449
  and intimate partner violence,
    449, 449b
donepezil (Aricept), 411
donepezil/memantine (Namzaric), 412
doxycycline, 288, 313
DPP-4 inhibitors (dipeptidyl
    peptidase)
  for diabetes mellitus, 238
Drug Enforcement Administration
    (DEA), 53
drug enforcement agency (DEA)
    licensure, 20

drug-to-drug interactions, 58–60, 59t
dry eyes, 102
dry skin. See xerosis
dual-energy x-ray absorptiometry (DEXA), 343
duodenal ulcer disease, 169
Dupuytren's contracture, 199–200
dysmenorrhea
   clinical management, 338
   clinical presentation, 338
   etiology, 338
dysthymia, 412

E

ear
   acute otitis media, 88–92
   benign paroxysmal positional vertigo (BPPV), 82–84
   ENT emergencies, 81
   hearing loss, 85–86
   otitis externa, 90–91
   otitis media with effusion, 88–92
   peripheral vertigo, 82, 84–85
   peripheral vestibular system, 81–82
   sensorineural hearing loss, 86–87
eczema. See atopic dermatitis
ejection fraction (EF), 64
elbow
   clinical presentation, 206
   lateral epicondylalgia/tennis elbow, 206–207
   treatment of, 207
electrocardiogram (EKG), 6
emotional abuse, of children, 393
emphysema, 125
end-of-life care, of older adults, 416
endocrine system, 235–245
   adrenal disorders, 244–245
   diabetes mellitus, 235–236
   hyperthyroidism, 242–243
   hypoglycemia, 239–240
   hypothyroidism, 241–242
   thyroid disorders, 240–241
endometriosis
   clinical management, 340
   clinical presentation, 340
   etiology, 339–340
   evaluation and follow-up, 340
eosinopenia, 263
eosinophilia, 263
eosinophils, 117, 262–263
epididymitis, 368
epigastric pain, 166
epiglottitis, 81

epistaxis
   complications of, 93
   defined, 92
   diagnostic studies, 93
   differential diagnosis of, 93
   etiology of, 92
   incidence of, 92
   indications for referral, 93
   management of, 93
   patient education for, 93
   physical assessment, 92
   risk factors of, 92
Epley maneuver, 83
epstein pearls, 385
erectile dysfunction (ED)
   erections, physiology of, 371
   medications, for, 371
   types, of, 371
Erikson's stages of development, for children, 383
erosion, 307
erythema infectiosum. See parvovirus (fifth disease)
Escherichia coli
   and hospital-acquired UTI, 273
essential (benign) tremor
   diagnosis of, 227
   treatment for, 227
estimated date of delivery (EDD), 346
eustachian tube dysfunction (ETD), 88
examination, 3–4
   AANP and ANCC, difference between, 4
   certification. See Certification
   failing, reasons for, 7
   general strategies, 7
   informed decision, 4
   preparation, of, 6–7
   questions
      anticipate, to, 6
      life span considerations for, 5–6
   study, plan of, 4
   taking, of, 6–7
excoriation, 307
expedited partner therapy (EPT), 288
extrapulmonary tuberculosis, 130
eye, 100–105, 101
   cataract, 103
   chalazion, 104–105
   common eye terminology, 100–101
   conjunctivitis, 101–102
   defined, 200
   dry eyes, 102
   eye exam, 100
   glaucoma, 103
   herpes simplex keratitis (type I herpes simplex), 105
   herpes zoster keratitis (shingles), 106

   iritis, 104
   macular degeneration, 103
   optic neuritis, 106
   presbyopia, 100
   retinopathy, 102–103
   terminology of, 100
   visual field defects, 106

F

famciclovir (Famvir), 69, 291
family nurse practitioners (FNPs), 3
   advanced practice state licensure, 19–20
   basics, 407–408
   drug enforcement agency (DEA) licensure, 20
   ethics, 23–24
   health policy, 21
   mid-level provider and physician extender, 22–23
   to minors, 24
   National Provider Identification (NPI), 20
   responsibility to patients/care priorities, 23
   role in child abuse, 393–394
   role of, 407
   scope of practice, 18–19
farxiga (dapagliflozin), for diabetes mellitus, 238
FDA has an Adverse Event Reporting System (FAERS), 60–61
fecal immunochemical test (FIT), 173
fetal heart tones (FHTs), 346
fine motor development, in pediatrics, 382
fissure, 307
follicle stimulating hormone (FSH), 339
folliculitis, 310
Food & Drug Administration (FDA), 53
Food-to-Drug Interactions, 58–60
foot and ankle
   achilles tendinopathy, 192
   ankle sprain lateral/medial, 193
   bilateral heel pain, 192
   Charcot neuropathic osteoarthropathy, 192–193
   compartment syndrome, 193
   Morton (interdigital) neuroma, 191
   Ottawa ankle rules, 193
   Ottawa foot rules, 194
   plantar fasciitis, 192
FRAX WHO fracture risk assessment tool, 415

frontotemporal dementia, 223
The Future of Nursing: Leading Change, Advancing Health, 21

G

GAD-2, 440, 441f
GAD-7, 440, 441f
galactorrhea
    clinical management, 334
    clinical presentation, 334
    etiology, 334
    evaluation and follow-up, 334
galantamine (Razadyne), 411
gamma glutamic transpeptidase (GGT), 173
ganglion cyst, 200
gas exchange, intrathoracic (inferior) airway, 117
gastric ulcer, 169
gastroenteritis, 170
gastroesophageal reflux disease (GERD), 168–169
gastrointestinal system, 165–181
    abdominal pain, 165
    anal fissures, 179–180
    appendicitis, 170–171
    cholecystitis, 166–167
    colon cancer, 172–173
    constipation, 167–168
    Crohn's disease, 178
    diverticulitis, 171–172
    gastroenteritis, 170
    gastroesophageal reflux disease, 168–169
    haemorrhoids, 178–180
    hepatitis, 173–174
    inflammatory bowel disease, 177–178
    irritable bowel syndrome, 175–177
    liver enzymes, 166
    nonalcoholic steatohepatitis, 174–175
    peptic ulcer disease, 169
    physical examination, 165
generalized anxiety disorder, 432, 440
generally recognized as safe (GRAS), 53
gentamicin, for meningitis, 222
genu varum, 385
geriatric care, goals of, 405
gestational diabetes mellitus (GDM), 236, 350
    clinical management, 350–351
    clinical presentation, 350
    etiology, 350
    evaluation and follow-up, 351

giant cell arteritis. *See* temporal arteritis
glaucoma, 103
Glimepiride, for diabetes mellitus, 239
Glipizide, for diabetes mellitus, 239
Global Deterioration Scale, 222t
global Initiative for Asthma (GINA), 388
Global Initiative for Chronic Obstructive Lung Disease (GOLD), 125
Glomerular filtration rate (GFR), 57
GLP-1 RAs (glucagon-like peptide receptor agonists), 238
glucose-6-phosphate dehydrogenase (G6PD) deficiency anemia, 260
glutamic oxaloacetic transaminase (SGOT), 173
glutamic pyruvic transaminase (SGPT), 173
Glyburide, for diabetes mellitus, 239
Glyset (miglitol), for diabetes mellitus, 239
gonococcal infection
    clinical pearls, 289
    etiology of, 289
    evaluation of, 289
    follow-up of, 289
    physical assessment, 289
    present illness, history of, 289
gonorrhea/chlamydia, 91
Gower's sign, 203
gross motor development, in pediatrics, 382
group A *Streptococcus* (GAS), 98
guaiac-based fecal occult blood test, 173
guanfacine (Tenex, Intuniv), 435
Guidelines for the COVID-19 vaccine, 134

H

H. Pylori testing, 169
habit reversal therapy, for neurodevelopmental disorders, 446
haloperidol, for Alzheimer's disease, 223
harmful drinking, 444
head, physical examination of, 384
headache. *See also* migraine
    cluster, 225
    primary, 224
    red flags for, 226
    secondary, 224
    tension-type, 225

Health Care and Education Reconciliation Act, 21
health history, of older adults
    eliciting, 406
    key elements essential to, 405, 406
Health Insurance Portability and Accountability Act of 1996 (HIPAA), 20
health maintenance, 406
    geriatric, 406
health policy, 21
    Affordable Care Act (ACA), 21
health problems
    in eye, 100–105
    general approach to, 81
    in mouth, 96–98
    in nose, 92–93
health promotion, 37
    case study, in
        primary prevention, 44
        secondary prevention, 44
        tertiary prevention, 44
    disease prevention case study, and
        current medications, 44
        pertinent past medical history, 42–43
        pertinent physical exam findings, 44
        present illness, history of, 42
        system, pertinent review of, 44
        treatment recommendations, 44
    immunizations schedules and exam tips, 42
    prevention, levels of
        primary, 38
        primordial, 38
        quaternary, 39
        secondary, 38
        tertiary, 38
    specific diseases, prevention applied to, 38
    United States preventative task force common screening recommendations, for
        abdominal aortic aneurysm (AAA), 41
        adolescents and adults, unhealthy alcohol use in, 41
        cardiovascular disease (CVD), 40–41
        community dwelling adults, in, 41
        depression and suicide risk, 41
        human Immunodeficiency Virus (HIV) Infection, 41
        ovarian cancer, for, 41
        prediabetes and type 2 diabetes, 41

Index

prevent fractures in women, to, 41
prostate cancer, for, 41
USPSTF recommendations, clinical preventative services to
disease targeted, for, 39
screening, criteria for, 39
screening test (*See* Screening test)
healthcare provider (HCP), 288
hearing loss, 85–86
heart
physical examination of, 384
rate, of children, 383*t*
heart failure (HF), 60, 64–65, 145–148
atrial fibrillation. *See* atrial fibrillation
chest pain, evaluation of, 152–154
recommended therapy, 147*f*
stages in development of, 147*f*
helicobacter pylori infection, 169
hematocrit (Hct), 255
hematology, 255–264
anemia. *See* anemia
eosinophils, 262–263
hemoglobin, 255
laboratory testing, 255
lymphocytes, 263
mean corpuscular Hgb concentration, 255
mean corpuscular volume, 255
neutrophils, 262
peripheral smear, 256, 256*t*
red blood cells, 255
red cell distribution width, 256
reticulocyte count, 256–257
thrombocytosis, 263–264
white blood cells, abnormalities of, 261, 262*t*
hemoglobin (Hgb), 255
hemoglobin A1C, 236
hemolytic anemia, normocytic, 260
hemorrhagic stroke, 219
hemorrhoids, 178–180
hepadnaviridae, 173
heparin induced thrombocytopenia (HIT), 264
hepatitis
clinical manifestations of, 173
hepatitis A, 173
hepatitis B, 173–174, 174*t*
hepatitis C, 174
history, 173
liver function tests (LFTs), 173
hepatitis B (Hep B), 345
hepatitis C virus (HCV), 330
hepatojugular reflux, 166
herpes simplex keratitis (type I herpes simplex), 105

herpes simplex virus (HSV-1 and HSV-2), 290–292, 365
clinical Pearls, 292
etiology of, 290
evaluation of, 292
follow-Up, 292
patient education, 292
pharmacologic, management, 291
present illness, history of, 290
herpes zoster, 313–314
herpes zoster keratitis (shingles), 106
HF. *See* heart failure (HF)
High-Grade Squamous Intraepithelial Lesions (HSILs), 328
Higher-Level Thinking, 6
hip
hip dislocation, 196
hip impingement, 196
intertrochanteric fracture, 196
Legg-Calve-Perthes disease, 195–196
histrionic personality disorder, 449
hives. *See* urticaria
homocysteine (Hcy), 258
hordeolum, 104
human chorionic gonadotropin (HCG), 327
human immunodeficiency virus (HIV), 295–298, 345, 366
etiology of, 295–296
evaluation of, 297–298
follow-up, 297–298
patient Education, 297
pharmacologic, 297
present illness, history of, 296
risk factors of, 296
human papilloma virus (HPV), 69, 292–293
clinical pearls, 293
etiology of, 292
evaluation of, 293
follow-up, 293
patient education, 293
physical assessment, 292
present illness, history of, 292
hydrocele, 385, 369–370
hyperactivity, 434
hyperglycemic hyperosmolar states (HHS), 237
laboratory findings for, 237–238
hyperlipidemia, 65–66, 67*t*
hyperopia, 100
hypersensitivity, 60*t*
hypertension (HTN), 62–64, 62*t*, 148, 414
follow-up, 149
overview, 140
pediatric, 388

in pregnancy. *See* gestational hypertension
treatment goals, 149
hyperthyroidism, 242–243
ablative therapy with RAI 131 for, 243
thyroidectomy for, 243
hypertrophic obstructive cardiomyopathy (HCOM), 387
hypoglycemia, 239–240
hypomania, 432
hypospadias, 385
hypothyroidism, 241–242

I

idiopathic thrombocytopenic purpura (ITP), 264
imipramine (Tofranil), 435
for attention-deficit/hyperactivity disorder, 435
immune-mediated diabetes. *See* type 1 diabetes
immunizations, 383
immunoglobulin E (IgE), 117
impetigo, 313, 392
implantable cardiac defibrillator (ICD), 64
inattention, 434
infant
physical growth and development, 381–382
social and emotional development, 382–383
inflammatory bowel disease, 177–178
influenza antivirals, 69
inguinal hernias, 371
diagnosis, 371
initial preventive physical examination (IPPE), 406
innocent heart murmurs, 387
insulin, for diabetes mellitus, 239
integumentary
acne vulgaris, 309–310
actinic keratosis, 308
alopecia areata, 314
atopic dermatitis, 311
basal cell, 308–309
cellulitis, 310
cysts, 310
depigmentation, general patterns of, 314
dermatitis, 310–311
dermatophytosis, 313
folliculitis, 310
herpes zoster, 313–314

integumentary (continued)
  impetigo, 313
  melanoma, 309
  pityriasis rosea, 312
  psoriasis, 311–312
  rosacea, 310
  seborrheic dermatitis, 311
  seborrheic keratoses, 308
  skin cancers, 308
  skin tags, 313
  squamous cell carcinoma in situ, 309
  terminology, 307–308
  urticaria, 314
  vitiligo, 314
  warts, 313
  xerosis, 310
interpersonal therapy (IPT), 427
interpretation of tuberculin skin testing, 131, 131t
intertrochanteric fracture, 196
intimate partner violence (IPV), 449–450, 449b
intrathoracic (inferior) airway, 117
Invokana (canagliflozin), for diabetes mellitus, 238
iritis, 104
iron deficiency anemia (IDA), 256t
irritable bowel syndrome (IBS)
  differential diagnosis of, 175
  follow-up, 178
  management of, 175–176
ischemic stroke, 219

J

Januvia (sitagliptin), for diabetes mellitus, 238
Jardiance (empagliflozin), for diabetes mellitus, 238
juvenile diabetes. See type 1 diabetes

K

keloid, 307
Kernig's sign, 221
knee, 194–195
  osteoarthritis OA, 195

L

labor. See also pregnancy; maternal
labrum tear, 196–197
labyrinth, 82
labyrinthitis, 84

lactational mastitis
  clinical management, 355
  clinical presentation, 355
  etiology, 355
Lamotrigine (Lamictal), for disruptive mood dysregulation disorder, 433
language development, in pediatrics, 382
latent TB infection (LTBI), 132
lateral epicondylalgia/tennis elbow, 206–207
LCL. See lateral collateral ligament (LCL)
left lower quadrant (LLQ), 166
Legg-Calve-Perthes disease, 196
leukocytosis, 261–262
leukopenia, 262
levonorgestrel (LNG), 331
Lewy body, dementia with, 223
licensure, accreditation, certification, and education (LACE), 18
lichen sclerosus
  clinical management, 335–336
  clinical presentation, 335
  etiology, 335
  evaluation and follow-up, 336
lichenification, 307
ligament strain, 198
lightheadedness, 82
limited license provider, 23
lithium, 433
liver enzymes, 166
liver function tests (LFTs), 173, 329
LLQ. See left lower quadrant (LLQ)
long-acting beta-agonists (LABAs), 126
low back pain (LBP), 201
low-dose computed tomography (LDCT), 42
Low-Grade Squamous Intraepithelial Lesions (LSILs), 328
low-risk drinking, 443
Lower-Level Thinking, 6
Ludwig's angina, 81
lumbar spine, 201
lung cancer, 119–120
  cigarette smoking and, 129
  clinical pearls, 129
  screening, 129–130, 130t
  signs and symptoms of, 129t
lungs, physical examination of, 384
lymphocytes, 263
lymphocytopenia, 263
lymphocytosis, 263

M

macrobid, for urinary tract infections, 274
macrocytic anemia, 258–259

macular degeneration, 103
macule, 307
major depression with psychotic features, 436
major depressive disorder (MDD), 41
  clinical pearls, 430
  evaluation for, 430
  follow up, 430
  indication for, 430
  nonpharmacologic, 427
  in older adults, 412
  patient education, 427–429, 428–429f
  pharmacologic, 427
male reproductive system, anatomy of, 365
malignant otitis externa, 81
mallet finger, 199
mania, 432
  with psychosis, 436
Marfan's syndrome, 391
mast cells, 117
mean corpuscular Hgb concentration (MCHC), 256
mean corpuscular volume (MCV), 255–256
measles, 392
medial tibial stress syndrome (MTSS), 195
Medicare
  Annual Wellness Visit, 407
  preventive visit, 406
meglitinides, for diabetes mellitus, 239
melanoma, 309
melatonin, for concussion, 221
memantine (Namenda), 411
  for Alzheimer's disease, 223
Ménière's disease, 84–85
meningitis, 221
  irritation, signs of, 221
meniscus tear, 194
menopause
  clinical management, 342–343
  clinical presentation, 342
  etiology, 342
  evaluation and follow-up, 343
menstrual cycle, phases, 326–327
mental health
  anxiety disorders, 440–442
  attention-deficit/hyperactivity disorder, 434–435
  autistic spectrum disorder, 447
  bipolar disorder, 431–432
  cyclothymic disorder, 432
  disruptive mood dysregulation disorder, 432
  domestic violence and intimate partner violence, 449

major depressive disorder and persistent depressive disorder, 425
medication nonadherence, 434
mood disorders, 425
neurodevelopmental disorders, 446
personality disorders, 449, 450t
post-traumatic stress disorder, 442–443
psychotic disorders, 435–436
substance abuse, 443–444
mesalamine, 177
metabolism, 409
methicillin-resistant Staphylococcus aureus (MRSA), 61
methimazole (MMI), for hyperthyroidism, 243
methylmalonic acid (MMA), 258
methylxanthines, 124t
microcytic anemia, 257–258
mid-level practitioner, 20
mid-level provider (MLP), 22–23
migraine, 224–225. *See also* headache
mini-Nutritional Assessment Short Form, 405
minor depression, 412
mitral regurgitation, 144–145
mitral valve prolapse (MVP), 145
Moniliasis, 96
monocytes, 263
monocytopenia, 263
monocytosis, 263
montelukast, 123
Mood Disorder Questionnaire (MDQ), 431
Morton (interdigital) neuroma, 191
mouth
  aphthous stomatitis, 96–98
  oral candidiasis, 96–98
multiple sclerosis, 226–227
murmurs, 143
Murphy's sign, 166
musculoskeletal injuries, 191
  abdominal aortic aneurysm (AAA), 202
  cervical spine, 205
  concussion, 206
  degenerative joint disease (DJD), 200
  elbow, 206–207
  foot and ankle, 191–194
  hip, 195–196
  knee, 194–195
  lumbar spine, 201
  pelvis and sacrum, 201
  rheumatoid arthritis RA, 206
  shoulder, 196–197
  thoracic spine, 203–205
  wrist and hand, 198–200
Mycobacterium tuberculosis (MTB), 130, 131
Mycoplasma pneumoniae (*M. pneumoniae*), 98, 128
myopia, 100

N

N-methyl-D-aspartate (NMDA) antagonist, for neurocognitive disorders, 411
narcissistic personality disorder, 449
nateglinide (Starlix), for diabetes mellitus, 239
National Asthma Education and Prevention Program (NAEPP), 122
National League for Nursing Accrediting Commission (NLNAC), 18
National Organization for Nurse Practitioner Faculties (NONPF), 17
  nurse practitioners policy competencies, 22
National Osteoporosis Foundation, 415
National Provider Identification (NPI), 20, 54
Neisseria gonorrhoeae, 287, 289
nephrolithiasis, 275–276
nephrotoxic drugs, 61t
nervous system, 217–226
  adults referral, red flags for, 218
  Alzheimer's disease, 220–221
  Bell's palsy, 226
  brain tumors, 219
  concussion, 220–221
  cranial nerves, 217–218
  delirium, 223–224
  dementia, 222
  essential (benign) tremor, 227
  headache, 224
  meningitis, 221
  migraine, 224
  multiple sclerosis, 226–227
  neurological assessment, 217
  Parkinson's disease, 227
  romberg test, 217–218
  stroke, 219–220
  temporal arteritis, 226
  transient ischemic attack, 219–220
  trigeminal neuralgia, 226
Nesina (alogliptin), for diabetes mellitus, 238
neurocognitive disorders, in older adults, 411
neurodevelopmental disorders, 446

neuroleptic malignant syndrome (NMS), 440
neutropenia, 262
neutrophils, 262
newborn, 383, 383t, 384t
nitrofurans, and G6PD deficiency anemia, 261
nodule, 307
non-alcoholic fatty liver disease (NAFLD), 174
non-melanoma skin cancer (NMSC), 308
non-steroidal antiinflammatory (NSAIDs), 53
  for nephrolithiasis, 276
  for urolithiasis, 276
nonalcoholic steatohepatitis (NASH), 174–175
nonbullous impetigo, 392
nongonococcal urethritis (NGU), 365
normocytic anemias, 259–261
nose
  acute rhinosinusitis, 93–95
  allergic rhinitis, 95–96
  atrophic rhinitis, 96
  epistaxis, 92–93
  vasomotor rhinitis, 96
  upper respiratory infections (URIs). *See* upper respiratory infections (URIs)
Nucleic acid amplification test (NAAT), 352
nurse practitioner (NP), 37, 53
nystagmus, 385

O

obsessive-compulsive personality disorder, 449
obstetric (OB) care
  pregnancy. *See* pregnancy
  prenatal care. *See* Prenatal care
obstructive lesions, in pediatrics, 386–387
obturator sign, 166
olanzapine, for Alzheimer's disease, 223
older adults
  acute abdomen, 416
  adverse drug events in, 409
  age-related changes, 404t
  assessment tools to reduce medication risks in, 410
  associated problems with medication use, 410
  atypical presentation of disease in, 415

older adults (continued)
  chronic disease and, 413–414
  commonly prescribed drug
    categories for, 409
  communication techniques, 406
  considerations for older patient, 403
  creating relationship, 406
  depression, 412
  diabetes, 414
  eliciting health history, 406
  end-of-life care/advance care
    planning, 416
  falls, 415
  family nurse practitioner, role of, 407
  FRAX WHO fracture risk assessment
    tool, 415
  geriatric care, goals of, 405, 406
  health maintenance, 406
  hypertension, 414
  income, 403
  leading causes of death, 403
  marital status, 403
  medicare annual wellness visit, 407
  medicare basics, 407–408
  medicare preventive visit, 406
  multiple chronic care needs, 403
  neurocognitive disorders, 411
  osteoarthritis, 414
  osteoporosis, 414
  pneumonia, 416
  population growth for oldest old, 403
  prescribing practices in, 408
  profile of, 403
  STOPP/START tool, 410
  urinary tract infections in, 415–416
older patient, considerations for, 403
oligohydramnios vs.
  polyhydramnios, 349
omalizumab (Xolair), 124
Onglyza (Saxagliptin), for diabetes
  mellitus, 238
open angle glaucoma, 103
ophthalmoscope, 100
opioids
  for nephrolithiasis, 276
  substitution therapy, 445
  for urolithiasis, 276
optic neuritis, 106
oral antibiotics, 68t
oral candidiasis, 96–98
oral contraceptive pills (OCPs), 339
oral glucose tolerance test
  (OGTT), 350
oral thrush, 96
Ortolani's test, 385
oseltamivir (Tamiflu), 69
Osgood Schlatter disease, 194
osteoarthritis (OA), 414

osteomyelitis, 200
osteoporosis, 414
  clinical management, 343–344
  clinical presentation, 343
  etiology, 343
  evaluation and follow-up, 344
otitis externa, 90–92
otitis media with effusion (OME)
  complications of, 90
  defined, 88
  diagnostic studies, 89–90
  differential diagnosis of, 89–90
  etiology of, 88
  expected course, 86
  historical data, 89
  incidence of, 88
  management of, 90
  patient education, 92
  physical assessment, 89
  risk factors of, 88–89
otoliths, 82
Ottawa ankle rules, 193
Ottawa foot rules, 194
Ottawa knee rules, 195
ovarian cancer
  clinical management, 342
  clinical presentation, 341–342
  etiology, 341
  evaluation and follow-up, 342
over-the-counter (OTC), 53, 367

P

panic disorder, 441
papanicolaou test (Pap test), 339
papule, 307
paranoid personality disorder, 449
Parkinson's disease, 227
partial thromboplastin time (PTT), 339
parvovirus (fifth disease), 391
patch, 307
patellar fracture, 194–195
patellar subluxation, 194–195
patent ductus arteriosus (PDA), 386
Patient Health Questionnaire,
  428–429, 428–429f
pediatric hypertension, 388
pediatrics. See also adolescent; infant;
    newborn; preschoolers;
    school-age children; toddler
  anticipatory guidance topics, 385
  breastfeeding, 385
  child abuse, 392–393
  congenital heart defects, 385–388
  growth and development,
    381–382, 384t
  infectious diseases, 391

respiratory conditions, 388–391
respiratory rate, 383t
sports physical/preparticipation
  physical evaluation, 391
Tanner stages, of development, 335t
pelvic inflammatory disease (PID), 288
pelvis and sacrum, ankylosing
  spondylitis, 201
penciclovir (Danavir), 69
penicillin (PCN), 61
peptic ulcer disease (PUD), 169
perianal fissures, 179
peripheral smear, 256
peripheral vascular disease (PVD),
  64, 156
peritonsillar abscess, 81
persistent depressive disorder
  nonpharmacologic, 427
  pharmacologic, 427
personality disorders, 449
pharmacodynamics, 56
  elderly considerations, 57
  pediatric considerations, 56
  pregnancy considerations, 56
pharmacokinetics, 55–56
pharmacologic agents, metformin, for
  diabetes mellitus, 238
pharmacology
  evidence, levels of, 57, 58t
    ADR reporting, 60–62
    drug-to-drug interactions, 58–60
    food-to-drug interactions, 58–60
  nurse practitioner (NP)
    pharmacodynamics (See
      Pharmacodynamics)
    pharmacokinetics, 55–56
    pharmacotherapeutics, 54–55
    prescribing, for, 53–54
  primary care, medications in
    anticoagulants, 65
    antihypertensive drugs, in,
      63t, 64t
    antimicrobials. See Antimicrobials
    heart failure, 64–65
    hyperlipidemia, 65–66
    hypertension, 62–64, 62t
pharmacotherapeutics, 54–55, 55t
pharmacotherapy, for postpartum
  depression, 431
pharyngitis
  acute. See acute pharyngitis
  antibiotic therapy for, 99
  bacterial. See bacterial pharyngitis
  complications of, 99
  defined, 98
  diagnostic studies, 99
  differential diagnosis of, 99
  etiology of, 98

Index

follow-up, 98
incidence of, 98
indications for referral, 98
management of, 99
patient education, 100
risk factors of, 98
viral. *See* viral pharyngitis
phobia, specific, 441
physical abuse, of children, 393
physician extender, 22–23
picornavirus, 173
pigmentation, 307
pink puffers, 125
pityriasis rosea, 312
plantar fasciitis, 192
plaque, 308
platelet abnormalities, 263
pleura, 130
pneumocystis pneumonia (PCP), 297
pneumonia, 126–127, 127t
   diagnostic tests, 127
   in older adults, 416
   in pediatrics, 390–391
   symptoms, 127
polycystic ovarian syndrome
   clinical management, 341
   clinical presentation, 341
   etiology, 341
   evaluation and follow-up, 341
polypharmacy, 408
population health
   disease registries. *See* disease registries
   Healthy People 2020. *See Healthy People 2020*
post-traumatic stress disorder (PTSD), 442–443
postexposure prophylaxis (PEP), 298
   healthcare workers, 298
postnasal drip, 133
postpartum depression (PDD), 430
potassium citrate, for calcium stones, 276
potassium hydroxide (KOH), 339
preeclampsia
   clinical management, 351–352
   clinical presentation, 351
   etiology, 351
prediabetes
   diagnosis of, 235
   screening recommendations for, 235–236
prednisone, for Bell's palsy, 226
preexposure prophylaxis, 298
pregnancy care
   clinical method, of
      Naegele's Rule, 346
      uterine sizing, 346

drugs and vaccines
   FDA classification system, of, 348
   teratogens, 348
   vaccines, 348
laboratory testing/expected changes, of
   first prenatal visit, 345
   subsequent prenatal visit, 345–346
obstetric history, 344
patient education, 348–349
physiologic changes, of
   cardiovascular, 347
   ears, nose, throat, 347
   endocrine, 347
   gastrointestinal, 347
   integumentary, 347
   musculoskeletal, 347–348
   renal, 347
   respiratory, 347
   vital signs, 346–347
   weight gain and BMI, 346
signs, of
   positive, 344
   presumptive, 344
   probable, 344
prenatal care
   goals, of, 345
   visit schedule, 345
presbycusis, 86
presbyopia, 100
preschoolers
   physical growth and development, 382
   respiratory rate, 383t
   social and emotional development, 382–383
presyncope, 82
primary reflexes, 385
primitive reflexes, 385
problem-solving treatment (PST), 427
propylthiouracil (PTU), for hyperthyroidism, 243
prostate cancer, 367–368
prostate cancer tumor marker (PCTM), 6
prostate-specific antigen (PSA), 6, 41, 367
prostatitis, 366
Proteus mirabilis, 91
prothrombin time (PT), 339
proton pump inhibitor (PPI), 168
Pseudomonas aeruginosa, 91
psoas sign, 166
psoriasis, 311–312
psychosis, 431

psychotherapy
   for major depressive disorder and persistent depressive disorder, 427
   for postpartum depression, 431
psychotic depression, 412
psychotic disorders, 436–437
   first-generation antipsychotics, 436–437
   pharmacological treatment, 436
   second-generation antipsychotics (atypical antipsychotics), 437
pulmonary embolism (PE), 65
pulmonary tuberculosis, 130
pulmonic stenosis, 386–387
pulsus paradoxus, 121
pustule, 308
pyogenic bone infection, 200

Q

quadruple therapy, 169
quetiapine, for Alzheimer's disease, 223
quinolone
   for urinary tract infections, 274

R

radiculopathy, 201–202
RAI 131, ablative therapy with, for hyperthyroidism, 243
Rapid Plasma Reagin/Venereal Disease Research Laboratory (RPR/VDRL), 345
Raynaud's phenomenon, 200–201
rectification, 7
recurrent aphthous ulcers (RAU). *See* aphthous stomatitis
red blood cells (RBCs), 255
red cell distribution width (RDW), 256
renal function assessment, for diabetes mellitus, 236–237
renal/genitourinary urinary system, 273–280
   acute kidney injury, 276–277
   chronic kidney injury, 277–278
   function of, 273
   laboratory findings of, 273
   nephrolithiasis/urolithiasis, 275–276
   normal findings of, 273
   urinary incontinence, 278–279
   urinary tract infections, 273–274
repaglinide (Prandin), for diabetes mellitus, 239
research process. *See* scientific method

respiratory conditions, in pediatrics, 388–391
  acute bronchitis, 390
  asthma, 388
  bronchiolitis, 389
  croup, 389
  pneumonia, 390–391
respiratory examination, 117
respiratory rate, of children, 383t
respiratory syncytial virus (RSV), 134, 389–390
  in pediatrics, 389–390
respiratory system
  anatomy of, 117
  assessment of, 117
  basic Anatomy of, 117
  COVID-19 infection, 134
  diseases of, 117–124
    acute bronchitis, 133–134
    asthma, 117
    chronic cough, 133
    chronic obstructive pulmonary disease, 124–125
    community-acquired pneumonia, 127, 128t
    cough, 133
    lung cancer, 129
    pneumonia, 126–127, 127t
    tuberculosis, 130–131
  functions of, 117
  gas exchange, 117
  medical history for, 117, 118–119t
  physical examination, 119, 120t, 121
  respiratory examination, 117
  respiratory syncytial virus, 134
reticulocyte count, 256–257
retinal detachment, 106
retinoblastoma, 385
retinopathy, 102
RH-incompatibility
  clinical management, 349–350
  clinical presentation, 349
  etiology, 349
  evaluation and follow-up, 350
rheumatoid arthritis (RA), 206
rhinitis
  allergic, 95–96
  atrophic, 96
  vasomotor, 96
rhinosinusitis, acute. See acute rhinosinusitis
rifampin, for meningitis, 222
right lower quadrant (RLQ), 166
right upper quadrant (RUQ), 351
Rinne test, 83, 85
rivaroxaban, for stroke, 220

rivastigmine (Exelon), 411
  for Alzheimer's disease, 223
rocker-bottom foot, 192
rosacea, 310
Rosving's sign, 171
rotator cuff (RTC) injury, 197
routine health maintenance and laboratory procedures
  cervical cytology ("Pap Test"), 327
  human papillomavirus
    Bethesda system, 327–328
    colposcopy, 328
    DNA test, 327
    mammogram, 327
Rovsing's sign, 166

S

scale, 308
scar, 308
schizoid personality disorder, 450
schizophrenia, 436
schizotypal personality disorder, 450
school-age children
  physical growth and development, 382
  respiratory rate, 383t
  social and emotional development, 382–383
scoliosis, 204–205
scratch test, 166
screening test
  sensitivity, 39
  specificity, 39
scrotum/testes, disorders of
  cryptorchidism, 369
  epididymitis, 368
  hydrocele, 369–370
  spermatocele, 370
  testicular cancer, 368–369
  testicular tension, 369
  varicocele, 369
seborrheic dermatitis, 311
seborrheic keratoses, 308
selective mutism, 441
selective norepinephrine reuptake inhibitors (SNRIs)
  for depression, 413
  for major depressive disorder and persistent depressive disorder, 427
selective serotonin reuptake inhibitors (SSRIs)
  for depression, 413
  for major depressive disorder and persistent depressive disorder, 427
  for post-traumatic stress disorder, 442

sensorineural hearing loss (SNHL), 86–87
separation anxiety disorder, 441
serologic test, 169
serotonin modulator (trazodone), 413
serotonin syndrome, 430
serum alanine aminotransferase (ALT), 173
serum aspartate aminotransferase (AST), 173
sexual abuse, of children, 393
sexually transmitted infection (STI), 287–298, 339
  chlamydial infections, 287
  gonococcal infection, 289
  herpes simplex virus (HSV-1 AND HSV-2), 290–292
  human immunodeficiency virus, 295–298
  human papillomavirus, 292–293
  preexposure prophylaxis, 298
    healthcare workers, 298
  syphilis, 293–295
  trichomoniasis, 289–290
SGLT-2 Inhibitors (sodium-glucose co-transporter 2 inhibitors), for diabetes mellitus, 238–239
shingles, 204. See also herpes zoster
short-acting b-agonist (SABA), 117, 124
shoulder
  AC joint injury/dislocation, 197
  adhesive capsulitis/frozen shoulder, 197
  labrum tear, 196
  rotator cuff injury, 197
sickle cell anemia, 261
Sjögren's syndrome, 102
skin
  cancers, 308
  lesions, 177
  physical examination of, 384
  tags, 313
Snellen test, 100
SNOOP mnemonic, 224
social and emotional development, in pediatrics, 382–383
social anxiety disorder, 441
somatic symptom disorder, 441
specific phobia, 441
spermatocele, 370
spinal stenosis, 205–206
spondylolisthesis, 202
sports physical, preparticipation physical evaluation, 391
squamous cell carcinoma in situ, 309
Staphylococcus aureus, 91
State Controlled Substances licensure, 20

Index

stool antigen test, 169
stool DNA test (sDNA), 173
STOPP/START tool, 410
Streptococcus pneumoniae, 127
Streptococcus pyogenes, 91
stress fracture ribs, 204
stroke, 219–220
    management of, 220
    sensitive test for, 219
    testing of, 220
    types of, 219
subacute bacterial endocarditis prophylaxis, 145
substance abuse. *See also* alcohol abuse
    CAGE questionnaire, 444
    opioid substitution therapy, 445
    suicide risk and prevention, 445
sudden cardiac death, 387
sudden death, 391
suicide, risk and prevention, 445
sulfonamides, and G6PD deficiency anemia, 261
sulfonylureas, for diabetes mellitus, 239
swan neck deformity, 198–199
syphilis
    clinical pearls, 295
    etiology of, 293
    evaluation of, 295
    follow-up, 295
    pharmacologic, 294
    present illness, history of, 293

T

tachycardia, 127
tachypnea, 127
tacrolimus, 177
talipes equinovarus, 385
telangiectasia, 308
temporal arteritis, 226
tension-type headache, 225
test-taking strategies, for nurse practitioner students, 9–13
    beginning of, 10–11
    best practices for, 11
    day after examination, 13
    day before examination, 13
    day of examination, 13
    know your test-taking, 11–13
testicular cancer, 368–369
testicular tension, 369
tetralogy of fallot (TOF), 386
thalassemia major, 257–258
thalassemias, 257–258
theophylline, 124
therapeutic effects, 56

thiazide, for calcium stones, 276
thiazolidinediones, for diabetes mellitus, 239
thoracic disc herniation, 203–204
thoracic spine, 203–205
throat, pharyngitis, 98–100
thrombocytosis, 263–264
thrombotic thrombocytopenia purpura (TTP), 264
thyroid disorders, 240–241
thyroid stimulating hormone (TSH), 339
thyroidectomy, for hyperthyroidism, 243
ticlopidine, for stroke, 220
toddler
    physical growth and development, 382
    respiratory rate, 383t
    social and emotional development, 383
torticollis, 205
Tourette's syndrome, 446
toxoplasma encephalitis, 297
Tradjenta (linagliptin), for diabetes mellitus, 238
transient ischemic attack (TIA), 219, 329, 343
transposition of great arteries (TGA), 386
trichomoniasis
    clinical pearls, 290
    etiology, 289
    evaluation of, 290
    follow up, 290
    physical assessment, 290
    present illness, history of, 290
tricuspid atresia, 386
tricyclic antidepressants, 413
tricyclics—desipramine (Norpramin), 435
trigeminal neuralgia, 226
trigger finger/stenosing tenosynovitis, 199
triple therapy, 169
tuberculosis (TB), 7
    diagnosing, 131
    latent infection, treatment of, 132, 132t
    latent TB infection (LTBI), 132, 132t
    latent *versus* active TB, 130, 130t
    risk factor for, 130–131
tumor, 308
tympanic membrane, 81, 85, 89
type 1 diabetes, 236
type 2 diabetes, 236
    pharmacologic agents for, 239–241

U

ulcer, 308
ulcerative colitis (UC), 177
uncomplicated chlamydia infection
    clinical management, 352–353
    etiology, 352
    evaluation and follow-up, 353
urea breath test, 169
urethritis, 365
urinary incontinence (UI), 278
urinary tract infections (UTI), 273–274
    clinical management, 352
    clinical presentation, 352
    etiology, 352
    evaluation and follow-up, 352
    in older adults, 415–416
urolithiasis, 275–276
urticaria, 314
U.S. Preventative Services Task Force (USPSTF), 57, 59t, 327
U.S. Preventive Task Force (USPTF), 406
uterine fibroids
    clinical management, 340
    clinical presentation, 340
    etiology, 340
    evaluation and follow-up, 340

V

valacyclovir (Valtrex), 69, 291
valproate (Depakote), for disruptive mood dysregulation disorder, 433
valvular disorders, 144–148
    aortic regurgitation, 145
    aortic stenosis, 144
    chest pain, evaluation of, 152–154
    cholesterol management. *See* cholesterol management
    coronary artery disease, 156
    grading and classification, 147f
    heart failure (HF), 145–148
    mitral regurgitation, 144–145
    mitral valve prolapse (MVP), 145
    patient symptoms, 147f
    peripheral vascular disease (PAD), 156
    subacute bacterial endocarditis prophylaxis, 145
    treatment, 147f
    varicose veins, 157
valvular heart disease, 143–145
vancomycin, for meningitis, 221–222
Vanderbilt tool, 434
varicella zoster virus (VZV), 204
varicocele, 369, 385
varicose veins, 157

vascular dementia, 223
vasomotor rhinitis, 96
venous disorders, 156–157
venous thromboembolic event (VTE), 343
ventricular-septal defect (VSD), 386
verruca vulgaris. *See* warts
vertigo, 82
vesicle, 308
vestibular neuritis, 84
Victoza liraglutide, for diabetes mellitus, 238
viral conjunctivitis, 101–102
viral pharyngitis
    assessment of, 98, 99
    clinical pearls, 99
    complications of, 99
    diagnosis of, 98, 99
    history data, 99

visual field defects, 106
vitamin B12 deficiency anemia, 258
vitiligo, 314
vulvovaginal candidiasis
    clinical management, 336–337
    clinical presentation, 336
    etiology, 336
    evaluation and follow-up, 337

W

warfarin, for stroke, 220
warts, 313
weber test, 83, 85
wheal, 308
white blood cells (WBCs), 365
    abnormalities of, 261, 262*t*

Wilm's tumor, 385
Wolf Parkinson's White Syndrome (WPW), 60
Women's Preventive Services Initiative (WPSI), 37
wrist and hand
    carpal tunnel syndrome, 198
    deformities, 198–199
    distal radius fracture, 198
    Dupuytren's contracture, 199–200
    ligament strain, 198
    trigger finger/stenosing tenosynovitis, 199

X

xerosis, 310